UCLA Forum in Medical Sciences

UNIVERSITY OF CALIFORNIA, LOS ANGELES

THE RETINA

MORPHOLOGY, FUNCTION AND CLINICAL CHARACTERISTICS

UCLA FORUM IN MEDICAL SCIENCES

NUMBER 8

THE RETINA

MORPHOLOGY, FUNCTION AND CLINICAL CHARACTERISTICS

Proceedings of a Conference held November, 1966, in connection with the opening of the Jules Stein Eye Institute, University of California, Los Angeles, and sponsored in part by a grant to Dr. B. R. Straatsma by the National Institute of Neurological Diseases and Blindness.

EDITORS

BRADLEY R. STRAATSMA, MICHAEL O. HALL, RAYMOND A. ALLEN and FREDERICK CRESCITELLI

UNIVERSITY OF CALIFORNIA PRESS

BERKELEY AND LOS ANGELES

1969

EDITORIAL NOTE

This volume contains material presented at the Inaugural Scientific Program of the Jules Stein Eye Institute. Convened in conjunction with the dedication of the Institute, this multidisciplinary symposium commences with studies of retinal structure, progresses to the dynamics of retinal function, and concludes with clinical appraisal of the retina. Successive papers range from the fundamental roots of biological information to the practical medical applications of this knowledge.

CITATION FORM

Straatsma, B. R., Hall, M. O., Allen, R. A., and Crescitelli, F. (Eds.), *The Retina: Morphology, Function and Clinical Characteristics*. UCLA Forum Med. Sci. No. 8, University of California Press, Los Angeles, 1969.

University of California Press
Berkeley and Los Angeles, California

University of California Press, Ltd.
London, England

Library of Congress Catalog Card Number: 75-626717
Printed in the United States of America

PARTICIPANTS IN THE CONFERENCE

BRADLEY R. STRAATSMA, *Chairman* and *Editor*
Jules Stein Eye Institute and Department of Ophthalmology,
UCLA School of Medicine
Los Angeles, California

MICHAEL O. HALL, *Co-Editor*
Jules Stein Eye Institute and Department of Ophthalmology,
UCLA School of Medicine
Los Angeles, California

RAYMOND A. ALLEN,* *Co-Editor*
Jules Stein Eye Institute and Department of Pathology,
UCLA School of Medicine
Los Angeles, California

FREDERICK CRESCITELLI, *Co-Editor*
Department of Zoology, University of California
Los Angeles, California

LEONARD APT
Jules Stein Eye Institute and Department of Ophthalmology,
UCLA School of Medicine
Los Angeles, California

NORMAN ASHTON
Department of Pathology, University of London
London, England

JOAQUÍN BARRAQUER
Clínica Barraquer
Barcelona, Spain

KENNETH T. BROWN
Department of Physiology
San Francisco Medical Center, University of California
San Francisco, California

* *Present address:* Mayo Clinic, Rochester, Minnesota.

Charles J. Campbell
Department of Ophthalmology
College of Physicians and Surgeons of Columbia University
New York, New York

Robert E. Christensen
Jules Stein Eye Institute and Department of Ophthalmology,
UCLA School of Medicine
Los Angeles, California

Adolph I. Cohen
Department of Ophthalmology
Washington University School of Medicine
St. Louis, Missouri

H. J. A. Dartnall
Medical Research Council Vision Research Unit
Institute of Ophthalmology
London, England

John E. Dowling
Wilmer Institute
Johns Hopkins University School of Medicine
Baltimore, Maryland

Peter Gouras
Ophthalmology Branch
National Institute of Neurological Diseases and Blindness
Bethesda, Maryland

David O. Harrington
Department of Ophthalmology
University of California School of Medicine
San Francisco, California

H. Keffer Hartline
The Rockefeller University
New York, New York

Joram Heller
Jules Stein Eye Institute and Department of Ophthalmology
UCLA School of Medicine
Los Angeles, California

Naganori Kirisawa
Department of Ophthalmology, Tohoku University
Sendai, Japan

ALLAN E. KREIGER
Jules Stein Eye Institute and Department of Ophthalmology
UCLA School of Medicine
Los Angeles, California

SHINJI KURIMOTO
Department of Ophthalmology, Tottori University
Yonago City, Japan

TOICHIRO KUWABARA
Howe Laboratory of Ophthalmology, Harvard Medical School
and Massachussetts Eye and Ear Infirmary
Boston, Massachussetts

MAURICE B. LANDERS
Jules Stein Eye Institute and Department of Ophthalmology,
UCLA School of Medicine
Los Angeles, California

ARTHUR LINKSZ
Department of Ophthalmology,
New York University Postgraduate Medical School
New York, New York

EDWARD F. MACNICHOL, JR.
The Thomas C. Jenkins Department of Biophysics
The Johns Hopkins University
Baltimore, Maryland

GERD MEYER-SCHWICKERATH
Department of Ophthalmology
Municipal Eye Clinic, Essen, University of Bonn
Bonn, West Germany

ISAAC C. MICHAELSON
Eye Department, Hadassah-Hebrew University Medical School
Jerusalem, Israel

WILFRIED F. H. M. MOMMAERTS
Department of Physiology, UCLA School of Medicine,
and Los Angeles County Heart Association Cardiovascular Research Laboratory
Los Angeles, California

FRANK H. MOYER*
Department of Biology, Washington University
St. Louis, Missouri

---

* *Present address:* Department of Biology, University of Missouri—St. Louis; St. Louis, Missouri.

Kenneth N. Ogle*
Section of Biophysics, Mayo Clinic and Mayo Foundation
and University of Minnesota
Rochester, Minnesota

Thomas H. Pettit
Jules Stein Eye Institute and Department of Ophthalmology,
UCLA School of Medicine
Los Angeles, California

Albert M. Potts
Eye Research Laboratories, University of Chicago
Chicago, Illinois

William A. H. Rushton
Department of Visual Physiology, University of Cambridge
Cambridge, England

Setsuko Shimizu
Department of Ophthalmology, Nagoya University
Nagoya, Japan

Fritiof S. Sjöstrand
Department of Zoology, University of California
Los Angeles, California

George Wald
Department of Biology, Harvard University
Cambridge, Massachusetts

Richard W. Young
Jules Stein Eye Institute and Department of Anatomy,
UCLA School of Medicine
Los Angeles, California

* Deceased.

JULES STEIN

Jules Stein, born April 26, 1896, graduated from the University of Chicago, Ph.B. (1915), and received the M.D. degree (1921) from Rush Medical College (now part of the University of Chicago). He later studied under Professor Ernest Fuchs in Vienna, where he was awarded the postgraduate diploma in ophthalmology by the Universität zu Wien. Dr. Stein then returned to Cook County Hospital as Chief Resident in Ophthalmology and became a Diplomate of the American Board of Ophthalmology.

Although he interrupted his medical career to embark on a career in business, he continued to maintain a strong interest in ophthalmology, and in 1960, cofounded and became Chairman of the Board of Research to Prevent Blindness, Inc.—a national voluntary health foundation devoted to stimulating research into the causes of blindness. This organization now awards unrestricted annual research grants and has aided the development of new ophthalmic research facilities at a number of universities.

In recognition of his distinguished contribution to the prevention of blindness, Dr. Stein has been awarded numerous honors, including the honorary degree of Doctor of Laws from the University of California (1968).

CONTENTS

MORPHOLOGY

FUNCTION

CLINICAL CHARACTERISTICS

DEVELOPMENT, STRUCTURE, AND FUNCTION OF THE RETINAL PIGMENTED EPITHELIUM

FRANK H. MOYER*†
Washington University
St. Louis, Missouri

The relationship of the pigment epithelium to the neural retina is evident in a variety of well-known observations and experiments by anatomists, cytologists, embryologists, physiologists, and clinicians. The bulk of the evidence derived from these investigations indicates that in the functioning vertebrate eye the pigment epithelium provides metabolic and functional support for the visual cells, but the molecular nature and the physiological details of the interactions are not yet clearly established. Fortunately, the convergence in modern research of the techniques of electron microscopy, cell fractionation, electrophysiology, and physical chemistry allow these questions to be examined with ever increasing precision and even, in some cases, to be answered, albeit tentatively and speculatively. An attempt will be made here to correlate recent research on the pigment epithelium and to use the data as the basis for further speculation about the nature of its interactions with the neural retina.

The origin of the pigment epithelium and the neural retina from a common source, the optic vesicle and their subsequent differentiation into morphologically and functionally discrete tissue layers epitomize a central topic of developmental biology, namely identification of the mechanisms by which divergent cell types arise and how they are stabilized in the differentiated state. These problems are of primary interest to developmental biology, and a brief treatment of the changes in the pigment epithelium during differentiation is included below. Because of space limitations, this discussion is limited to the interpretation of fine structure, and does not include the interesting problems of differentiation in tissue culture (10,59) and regeneration of the neural retina from the pigment epithelium (16).

---

* *Present affiliation:* University of Missouri—St. Louis; St. Louis, Missouri.

† I am grateful to Dr. Adolph Cohen and Dr. John Dowling for stimulating discussions and for donating some of the electron micrographs used in the paper. I also wish to thank Dr. Catherine Verhey for valuable criticism and assistance, Violet Moyer for drawing the diagrams, and Beverly Wright for typing the manuscript.

I wish to thank the *American Zoologist* for permission to use the electron micrographs of Figures 6 and 11. The original work from my laboratory discussed in this paper has been supported at various times by National Science Foundation grants GB 280, GB 1477, GB 4282, and GB 5512.

Structural and Functional Correlations in the Mature Pigment Epithelium

General Description

In its fully differentiated state the pigment epithelium is a columnar epithelium which lies in close contact with the visual cell layer vitread and, sclerad, with a basement lamella complex (Bruch's membrane), said to be derived from its own basement membrane and that of the choroid capillaries (11,47).

The plasma membrane of the epithelial cells is deeply infolded on the basal (sclerad) side and these infoldings are apparently continuous with elements of the endoplasmic reticulum (11,20,37,47,60). Mitochondria are heavily concentrated in this region of the cell (Figure 1). Laterally the plasma membrane forms a tight junction with the neighboring cells; the space between adjacent cells below the junctional area is variable. At the apical (vitread) side of the cell the plasma membrane spreads into long extensions which interdigitate with the outer segments of the rods and cones (Figures 2 and 3). In the lower vertebrates the pigment granules migrate into these extensions during light adaptation, and retreat

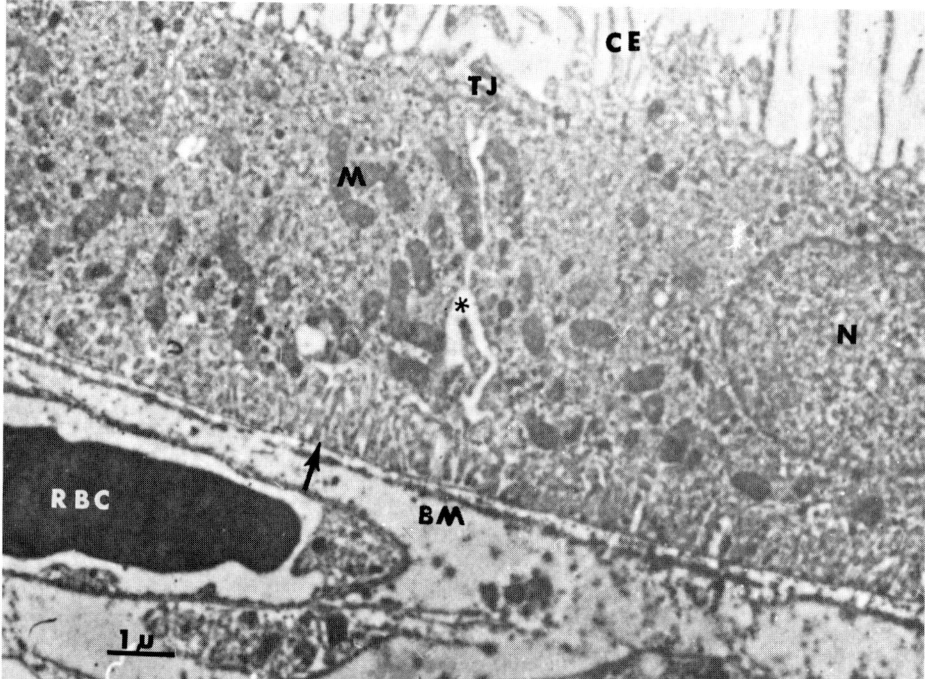

Figure 1. General features of the retinal pigment epithelium (albino mouse, 15 days post partum). Note the cytoplasmic extensions (*CE*) at the apical sides of the cells and the deep infoldings of the plasma membrane on the basal sides (arrow). The cells are connected by the tight junctions (*TJ*), below which the intercellular space is variable (*). An erythrocyte (*RBC*) is seen in the lumen of a capillary in the choroid at lower left. *BM:* Bruch's membrane; *M:* mitochondria; *N:* nucleus.

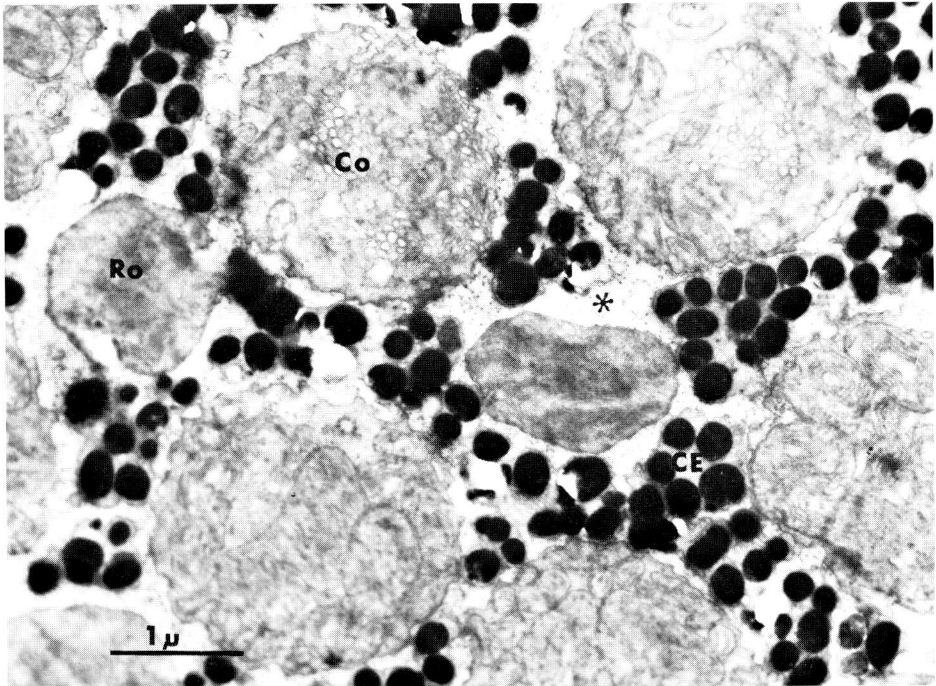

Figure 2. Section cut parallel to the plane of the pigment epithelium through the visual cell layer (adult gray squirrel), showing cross sections of the cytoplasmic extensions (*CE*) of the pigment epithelium cells where they interdigitate with the outer segments of the rods (*Ro*) and cones (*Co*). The level of this section is shown by the line *x-y* in Figure 3. Some of the mucopolysaccharide extracellular matrix that fills the gap between these cells is evident. (Electron micrograph by Dr. Adolph Cohen.)

from them during dark adaptation; this process has been described in detail by Walls (58).

The nuclei are located centrally or basically in the cells and ordinarily do not have well-developed nucleoli, marginal chromatin, or pores in the nuclear envelope; an interesting exception is discussed below. The endoplasmic reticulum is tubular and smooth-surfaced, and Golgi profiles are limited to small paranuclear areas.

Pigment granules, which are the characteristic inclusions of these cells, are predominantly melanin, although, at least in humans, lipofuscin appears with aging. Other inclusions are probably lysosomes and fragments of ingested visual cell outer segments. Most of these details are evident in Figures 1, 2, and 3.

Specializations of the Plasma Membrane

Pinocytosis. The fine structure of the plasma membrane shows two important features related to functional activity. The first of these is indicative of pinocytosis. Where it adjoins Bruch's membrane, the basal plasma membrane is deeply involuted (Figure 4A) and various stages in the formation of pinocytotic vesicles are often seen in this area (Figure 4B). Such vesicles are also found in the apical

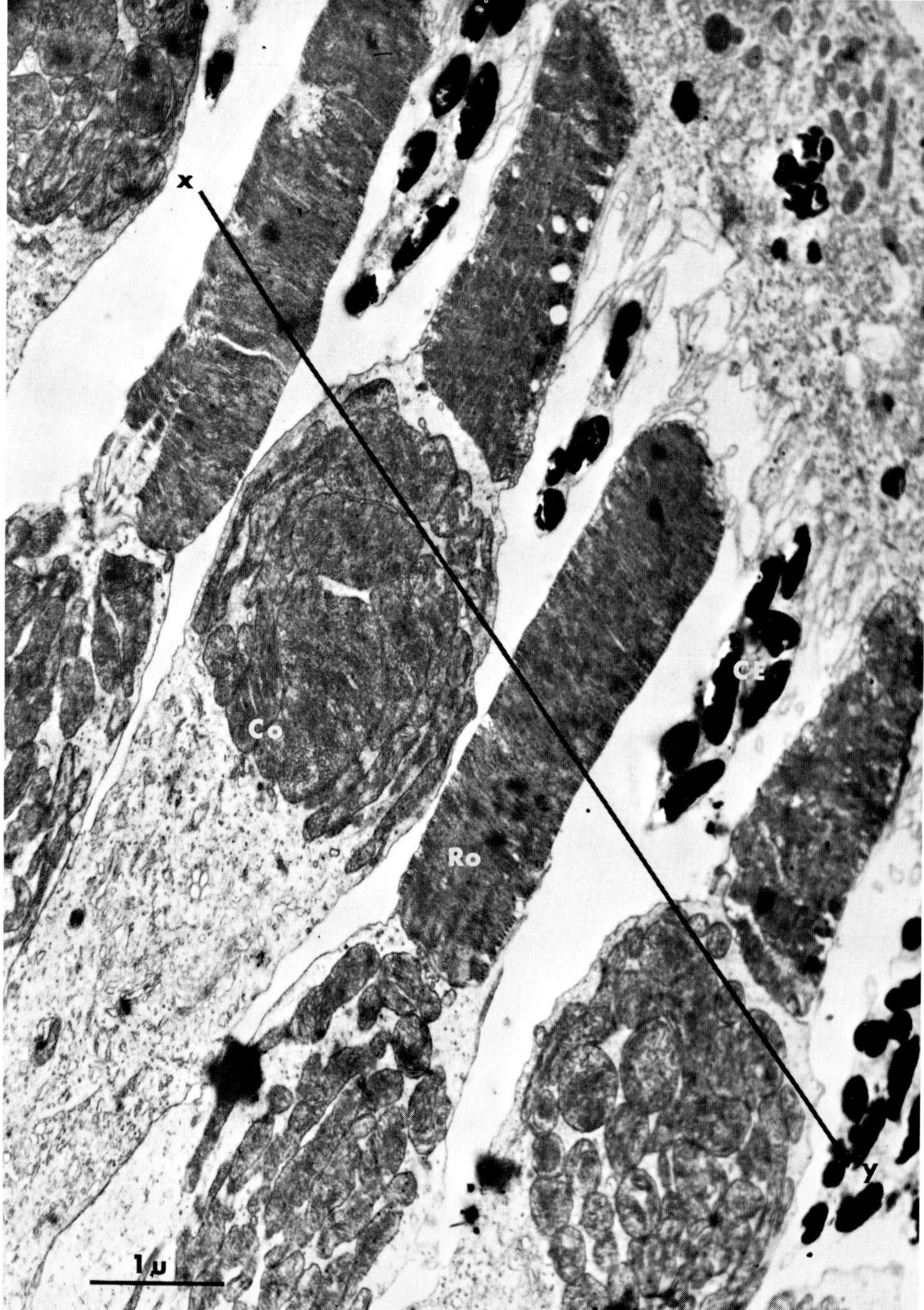

Figure 3. Cross section of the retina (adult gray squirrel), showing how the cytoplasmic extensions (*CE*) of the pigment epithelium interdigitate with the outer segments of the visual cells. The line *x-y* indicates the level of the tangential section shown in Figure 2. *Co:* Cones; *Ro:* rods. (Electron micrograph by Dr. A. Cohen.)

plasma membrane (Figure 4C). In the region where the vesicles are forming, the plasma membrane thickens, apparently because of the addition of electron-dense material. At the same time, regularly spaced "furry-looking spikes" appear on the cytoplasmic face of the membrane, which then seemingly invaginates into the cytoplasm and pinches off to form a vesicle with the dense thickening on the inside and the "spikes" pointing out into the cytoplasm (Figure 4B,C,D). These vesicles often may be deep in the Golgi region, located laterally or apically to the nucleus (see Figures 4D and 6). This observation apparently is a common one (for instance, figure 16 in 47), although no one seems to have called attention to it yet.

These vesicles are virtually identical to the pinocytotic vesicles implicated in yolk formation in insect oocytes (1,49,52). It has been suggested that the dense substance that thickens the membranes in these cases is a protein precursor of yolk, and that their characteristic appearance is indicative of the pinocytosis of protein (49). But the vesicles also are found in the brush border of proximal tubule epithelial cells in the mouse kidney (cf. Rhodin, 48, page 99, top left figure) and in chick fibroblasts grown in tissue culture (56). Thus, a more conservative view is that they simply indicate pinocytosis, and that their structure is not necessarily correlated to the chemical nature of the material being ingested. Their occurrence at both the apical and the basal membranes and in the central Golgi region certainly suggests that the cell is transporting materials from one side to the other. It is commonly assumed that the formation of the vesicle as described is characteristic of ingestion, but a similar morphology might indicate an egestion sequence, and the data at hand provide no assurance of the direction the ingested material is moving.

Electron micrographs of the capillary walls in the choroid reveal numerous fenestrations which strongly suggest the movement of material from the capillary into the extracellular area of Bruch's membrane. These fenestrations are bridged by diaphragms implying that the capillary endothelium plays a definite role in determining the nature and extent of this transfer of material (Figure 4A) (48: pp. 52–53). It is therefore tempting to conclude that material is being moved from the choroid capillary net through the pigment epithelium to the neural retina; certain evidence, however, suggests that material is being ingested at the apical end of the cell as well (see below). Hence it is probable that material ingested by pinocytosis is being moved simultaneously in both directions through these cells. The occurrence of vesicles in the Golgi region suggests that it is involved in the movement of these materials, perhaps in a manner analogous to its role in fat absorption in the intestinal epithelium (45). The possibility of pinocytotic transfer of material between choroid capillaries and neural retina receives strong morphological support from these observations, but they also raise the intriguing possibility of simultaneous flow in both directions. This possibility might be tested by electron microscope observations of the distribution of two morphologically distinct electron-dense markers (ferritin and thorotrast) applied to opposite sides of the isolated pigment epithelium-choroid complex at varying times prior to fixation.

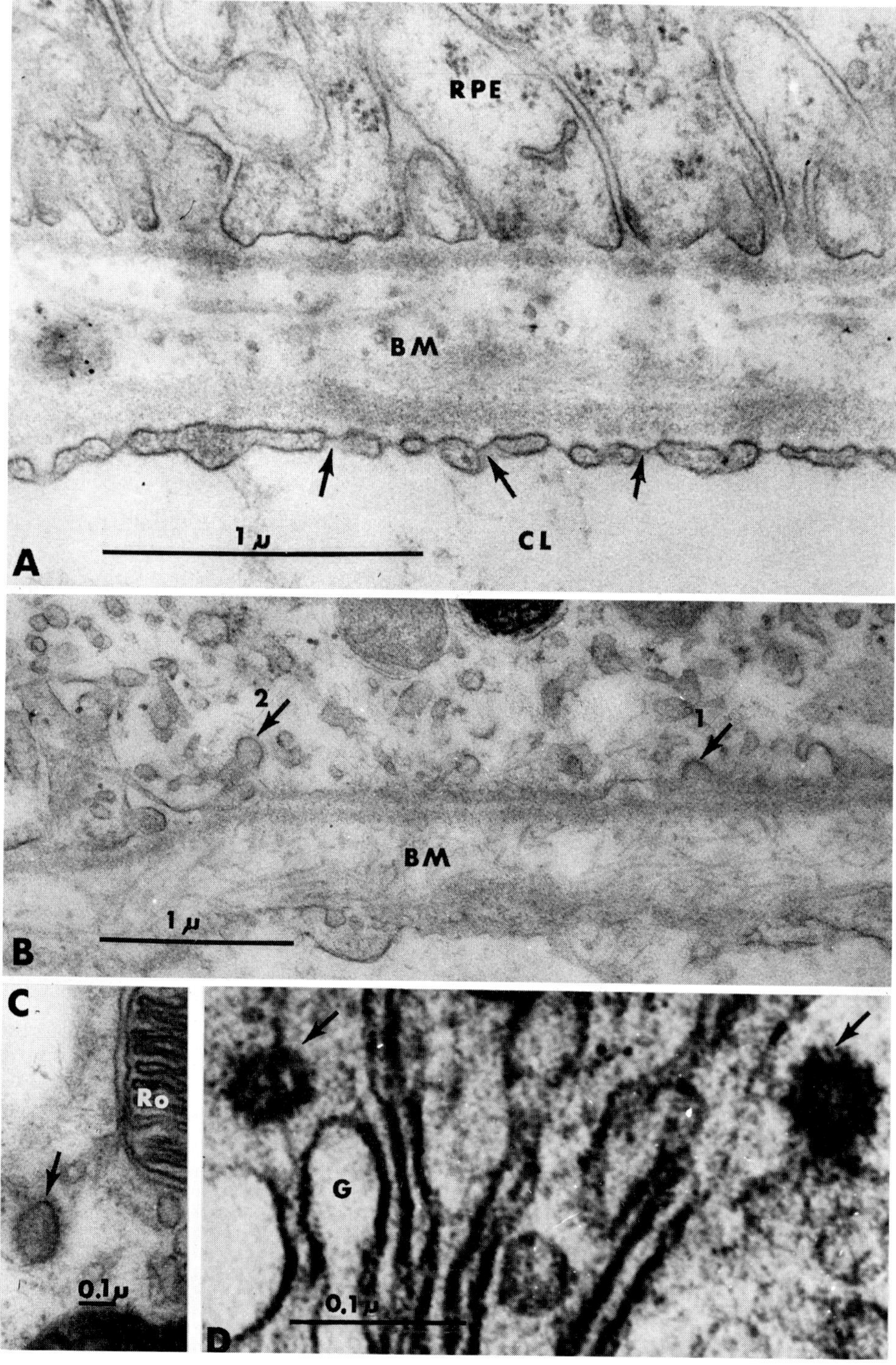

Figure 4 →

Tight Junctions. The second feature of interest in the structure of the plasma membrane of pigment epithelial cells is the complex of tight junctions and deeply infolded basal plasma membranes. When they are considered together with the basal distribution of mitochondria, the total impression is one of active transport. There are a number of observations which suggest that the pigment epithelium is the major source of the resting potential which can be measured across the intact eye (7,8,12,29,42).* Lasansky & de Fisch (29) actually measured ion flux across short-circuited, isolated, toad pigment epithelium-choroid complexes and found that the current of 40 μamp/cm^2 could be accounted for by the flux of chloride ions from the tissue complex into the medium on the sclerad side. They were unable to demonstrate a compensatory flow of cations in the opposite direction. On the basis of this demonstration of active transport of chloride ions they predicted a tight junction between adjacent pigment epithelial cells which would contain a so-called *zonula occludens.*

This tight junction was in fact located by Cohen (12), who found that the terminal bar was longer than is usual in epithelia and contained a well-defined *zonula occludens* (Figure 5). To test whether or not material could move between the cells at this point, Cohen (12a) exposed isolated frog retinas to lanthanum precipitates in suspension during and following fixation in gluteraldehyde, postfixed them in osmium tetroxide, and prepared them for electron microscopy. That the lanthanum precipitates could not penetrate the *zonula occludens* was evident in the electron micrographs because the dense lanthanum precipitate was localized in the intercellular spaces sclerad to the tight junctions. Thus it seems certain that the tight junctions of the neighboring epithelial cells are the physical basis for the resistance and capacitance of the retina: the so-called "R"-membrane of Brindley (7). It is also clear from the work on ion flux (29) that the pigment epithelium is engaged in active transport of ions, just as is suggested by its morphology. More will be said of this later.

The Endoplasmic Reticulum

General Features. In the mature pigment epithelium the endoplasmic reticulum is a densely tangled network of smooth-surfaced membranous tubules (see Figures 1, 5, and 6). It is contiguous with the deeply infolded plasma membrane

---

* See also Dr. Brown's paper, pp. 319–378.

Figure 4. *A:* Relationships of the basal plasma membrane of a pigment epithelium cell with Bruch's membrane (BM) and a choroid capillary (adult human eye); note the extensive infoldings of the plasma membrane of the pigment epithelium cell and the fenestrations in the capillary endothelium (arrows); CL: capillary lumen; RPE: retinal pigment epithelium. (Electron micrograph by Dr. A. Cohen.) *B:* Pigment epithelium-Bruch's membrane region of an immature retina (mouse, three days post partum); two stages in the formation of a characteristic pinocytotic vesicle are shown (arrows #1 and #2); compare the disordered arrangement of collagen in Bruch's membrane (BM) with the more ordered arrangement seen in *A. C:* Typical pinocytotic vesicle at the apex of a pigment epithelium cell (arrow) (adult gray squirrel); a portion of a rod (Ro) outer segment is visible. (Enlarged from an electron micrograph by Dr. A. Cohen.) *D:* Pinocytotic vesicles (arrows) in the Golgi region (G) of a pigment epithelium cell (adult frog). (Electron micrograph by Dr. John Dowling.)

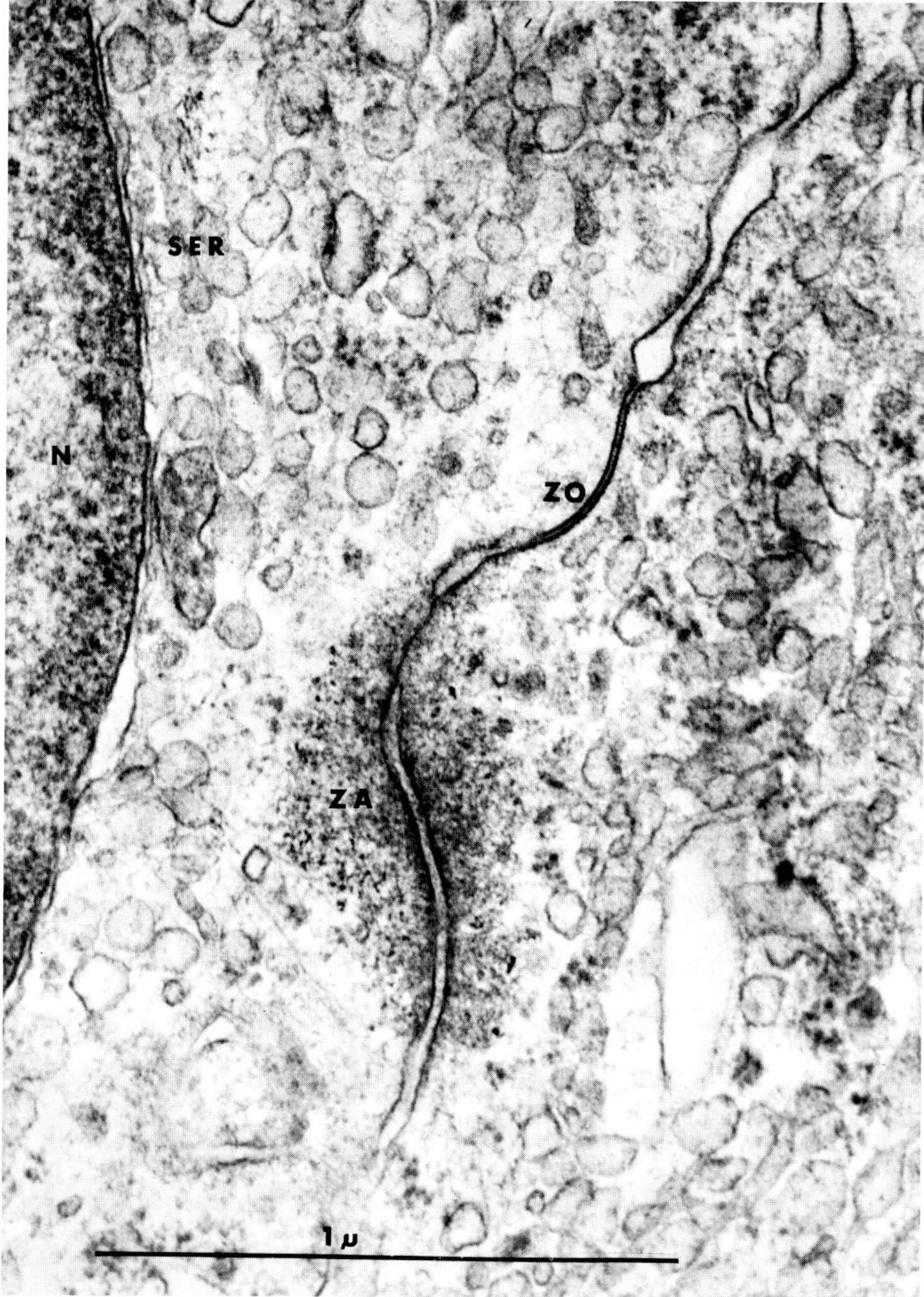

Figure 5. Details of the tight junction connecting cells of the pigment epithelium (adult human). Note the extensive *zonula occludens* (*ZO*). The typical vesicular profiles of the smooth-surfaced tubular endoplasmic reticulum (*SER*) characteristic of the adult pigment epithelium are well illustrated. *N:* Nucleus; *ZA:* zonula adherens. (Electron micrograph by Dr. A. Cohen.)

at the base of the cell and also at the apex (4,20,37,47,60). The Golgi region in these cells is limited to a small area apical or lateral to the nucleus. Often it is difficult to detect because of the extreme number of vesicular profiles of the endoplasmic reticulum present in the cells, but in serial sections a characteristic profile of stacked lamellae can usually be found (Figure 6). The general form and relationships of the reticulum suggest that it may function in the transport of materials between the retinal and choroidal sides of the cell. This suggestion is supported by the previously mentioned occurrence of pinocytotic vesicles in the Golgi region (Figures 4D and 6).

It is known that the Golgi region is the site of incorporation of hexoses destined to be used in mucopolysaccharide synthesis (40,41), and the extracellular material filling the spaces between the visual cells and the extensions of pigment epithelial cells is mucopolysaccharide (50). Young has shown* that some of this mucopolysaccharide is synthesized in visual cell inner segments, but it is possible that the specialized appearance of endoplasmic reticulum and Golgi in pigment epithelial cells may also reflect a synthetic contribution to this extracellular matrix by the pigment epithelium. The pronounced similarity in appearance of the reticulum in these cells with the smooth tubular reticulum of the glycogen areas of liver cells (17,18,23) supports this possibility. It could be tested by radioautography employing labeled hexoses and hexose amines.

Myeloid Bodies. These are a specialization of the endoplasmic reticulum occurring in lower vertebrates. Their fine structure in the frog has been well described (47): they consist of stacks of flattened vesicles which are continuous peripherally with the tubular endoplasmic reticulum (Figure, 6 inset) and have the three-dimensional configuration of a pair of cones joined at their bases (Figure 6); the membranes of the flattened vesicles are thicker than those of the surrounding endoplasmic reticulum (Figure 6, inset). Mostly on the basis of their structural resemblance to the visual cell outer segments, it has been suggested (47) that the myeloid bodies are photoreceptor elements and that they may contain rhodopsin. No direct evidence has been obtained on this point as yet but it is certainly a reasonable suggestion. Myeloid bodies probably do not occur in mammalian retinas. The occasional reports of their presence referred, in all cases examined by the author, to incorrectly identified fragments of visual cell outer segments or to the lysosome-like bodies described below (see 47 for a detailed discussion).

Annulate Lamellae. These are another specialization of the endoplasmic reticulum occasionally encountered in pigment epithelium cells (Figure 7). These structures closely resemble annulate lamellae seen in invertebrate oocytes and in cancer cells (see 36 for review and references). Annulate lamellae are usually found in cells actively synthesizing protein and may be associated with the synthesis of ribosomal and messenger RNA (57). The pigment epithelium cells in which they have been found contain fairly numerous ribosomes, as well as nuclei

* See pp. 177–210.

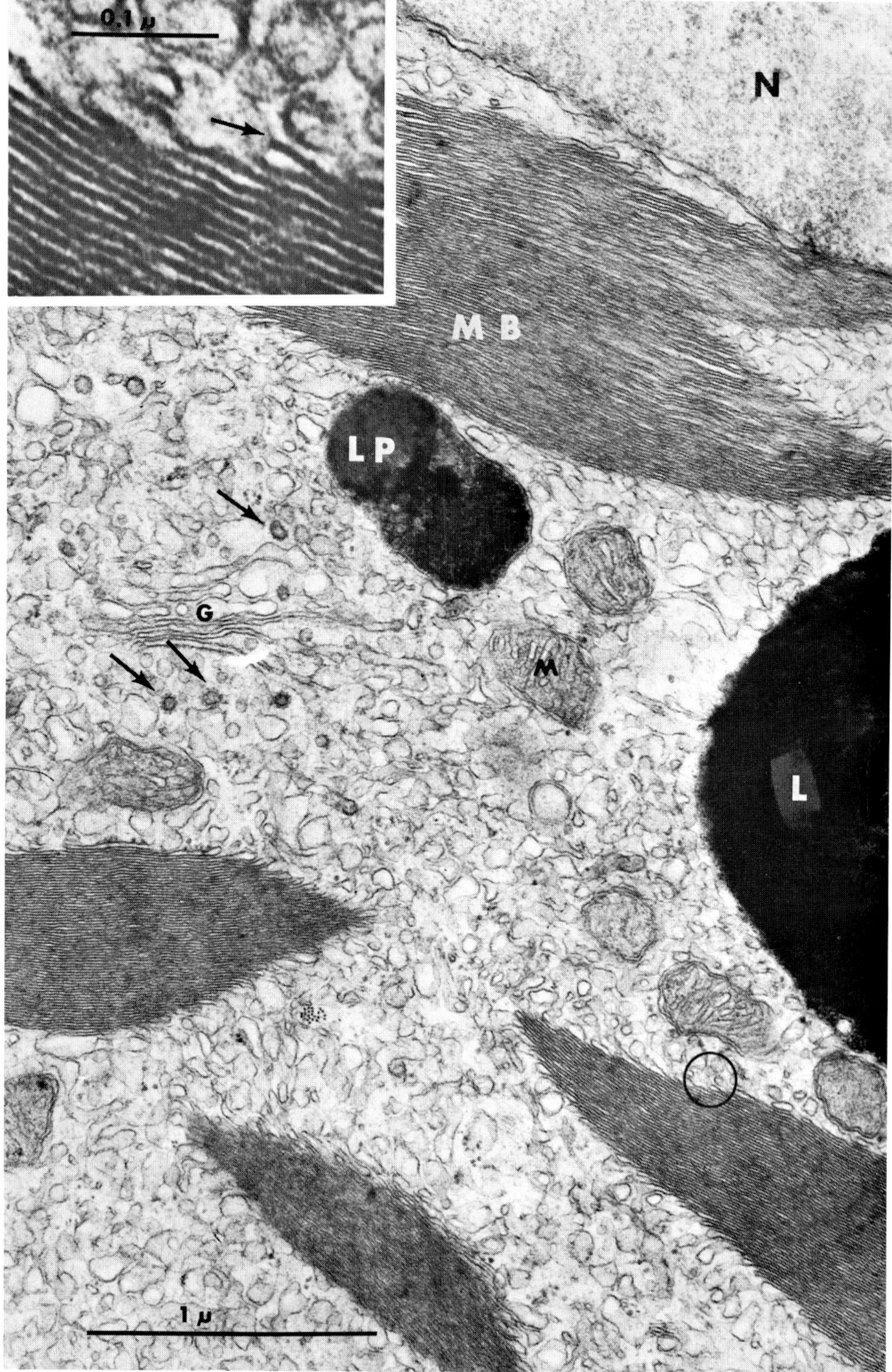

Figure 6 →

resembling the nuclei of cells active in protein synthesis in that they contain dense peripheral chromatin and prominent nucleoli. Annulate lamellae have been found in the retinas of humans from 12 to well over 60 years of age,* and in most cases could not be directly associated with retinal or other pathology. It is surprising to find cells of the pigment epithelium which appear to be synthesizing protein so long after the definitive stages in the differentiation of the eye. The physiological factors responsible for this unexpected morphology and its functional significance are problems of considerable interest. Hopefully, a similar situation will be found in some laboratory animal so that the problem may be approached by experimentation.

Specialized Inclusions of the Pigment Epithelium

LYSOSOMES. The pigment epithelium often contains inclusions which appear to be fragments of the outer segments of visual cells (Figure 8E). These fragments are presumably engulfed intact by the apical part of the cell, although the process has never been observed, which is rather surprising in view of the size of these inclusions. Also present in these pigment epithelial cells are various structures resembling lysosomes (19,43,44) (see Figure 8,A–D) or, more appropriately, perhaps, areas of focal cytoplasmic degradation (2,55). It seems reasonable to suggest that these inclusions represent a process in which the ingested fragments of outer segments of the visual cells are degraded and digested, with the final digestion products being removed to the choroid capillaries for redistribution. Such a process might be useful in regulating growth and renewal of visual cell outer segments. The inclusions are particularly evident in the pigment epithelial cells of dystrophic animals during the initial period of visual cell differentiation (21),† where they may be involved in ridding the retina of debris from the massive and abortive synthesis of rod outer segment material characteristic of this condition (30). Such an ingestion-digestion function of the pigment epithelium would help to explain its prominent changes in various pathological conditions.

Some support for these ideas comes from tracer experiments with radioisotopes. When radioactive amino acids are injected into rats, radioautography with the light microscope shows that in the retina they are first concentrated in the inner segments of the receptor cells. Within 24 hours they are displaced to the proximal part of the outer segment and then move distally, reaching the outer tip within a week after the injection; a few weeks later, the activity is no longer detectable

* A. I. Cohen, personal communication.
† Also, author's unpublished observations.

Figure 6. Part of a pigment epithelium cell (adult frog), showing the relationship of myeloid bodies (*MB*) to the endoplasmic reticulum. The region in the circle at lower right, magnified in the inset, possibly shows (arrow) an area of continuity between the membrane of the myeloid body and that of the endoplasmic reticulum; the inset also shows that the membranes of the myeloid body are thicker than those of the endoplasmic reticulum. Typical pinocytotic vesicles are indicated (arrows) in the Golgi region (*G*) of the cell. *L:* Lipid inclusion; *LP:* lysosome-like particle; *M:* mitochondrion; *N:* nucleus. (Electron micrograph by Dr. J. Dowling.) (From Moyer, 39.)

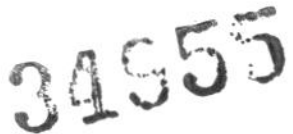

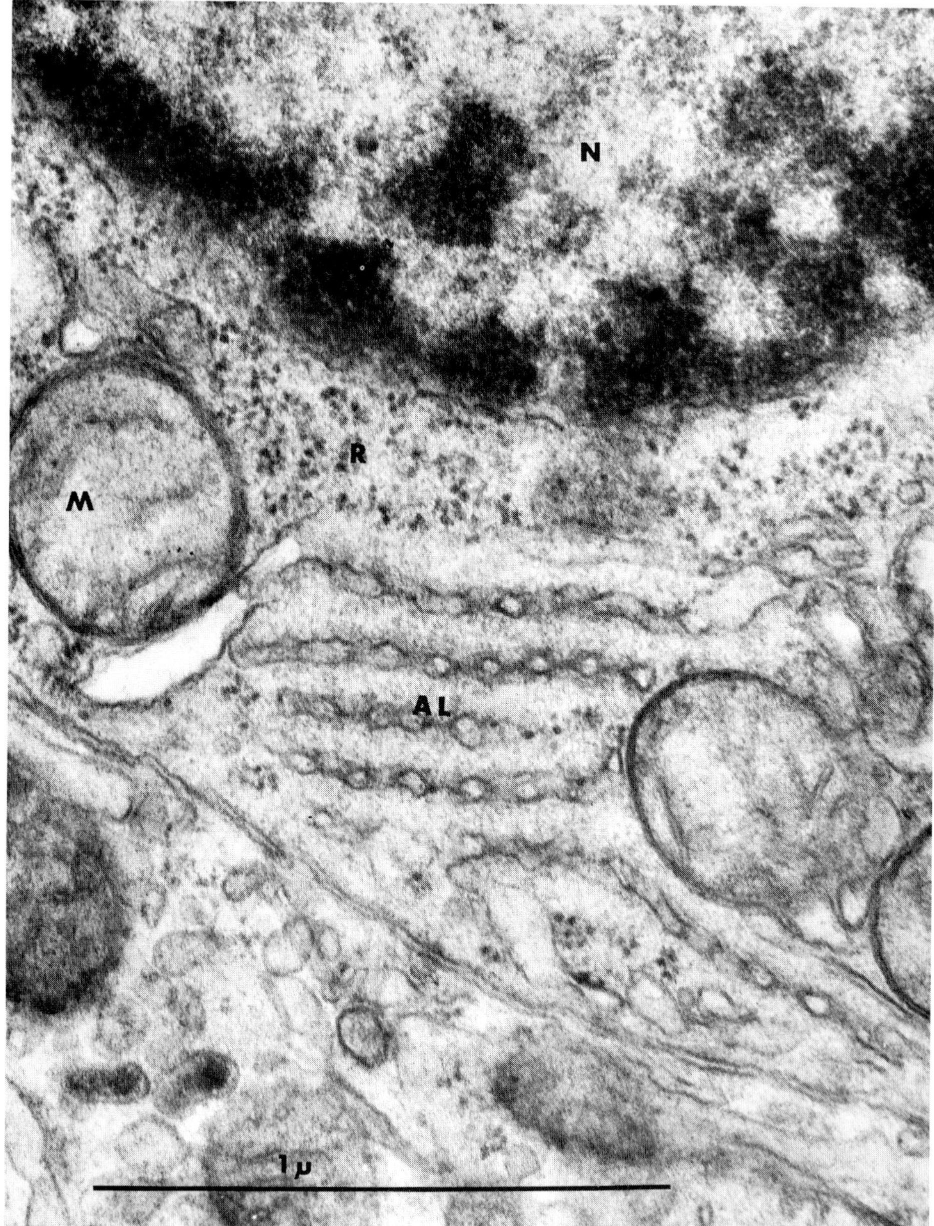

Figure 7. Annulate lamellae (*AL*) in a pigment epithelium cell (12-year-old human). The marginal chromatin in the nucleus (*N*) and the dense accretion of ribosomes (*R*) suggest protein synthesis. *M:* Mitochondrion. (Electron micrograph by Dr. A. Cohen.)

(22,62).* If the process of ingestion and digestion suggested above is correct, electron microscope radioautography should reveal activity over the inclusions approximately one week after the isotope injection, and this activity should disappear gradually in the following weeks.

---

*See also Dr. Young's paper, pp. 177–210.

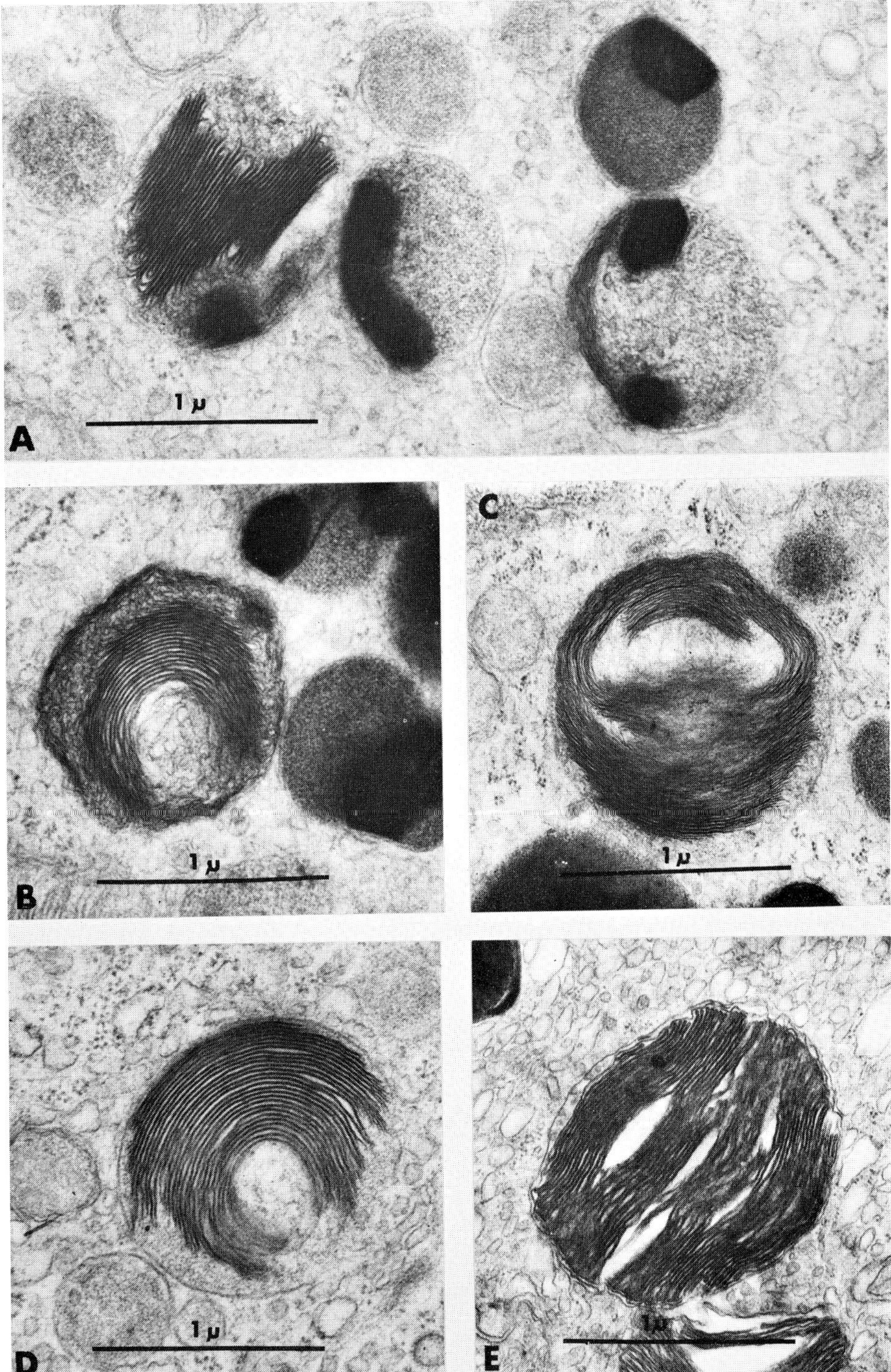

Figure 8. *A–D:* Lysosome-like inclusions in the pigment epithelium; adult rat. *E:* Fragment of rod outer segment ingested by the pigment epithelium; adult human. The ingestion-digestion sequence described in the text may be represented by the progressive changes from *E* to *A*. (Electron micrographs by Dr. J. Dowling.)

Pigment Granules. The term "pigment epithelium" is derived from the characteristic inclusions of these cells, the pigment granules. In most vertebrates these are melanin pigments rather than fuscins or lipofuscins (37,38,39). This conclusion is based on the fact that melanin is formed enzymatically by the oxidation of tyrosine through dihydroxyphenylalanine to indole-5,6-quinone and related compounds, and subsequent polymerization of these compounds to form the pigment (see 54 for an excellent discussion of melanin structure). Since the pigment epithelium contains tyrosinase (14), and since retinal pigment granules incorporate radioactive tyrosine (26) and are structurally similar to the granules of neural-crest derived melanocytes, which are known to produce melanin, it seems clear that they belong to the melanin group of pigments. Most persuasive in this connection is the fact that genes which alter the structure and enzymatic properties of the melanin granules in neural-crest derived melanocytes affect the pigment granules of the retina in the same way (39).

The human retina, in addition to melanin, contains lipofuscin. The distinction between melanins and lipofuscins has been made on the basis of staining reactions that are hard to interpret and difficult to reproduce; more important is the fact that the chemical basis for these reactions is not entirely clear (46,53).

An analysis of the fine structure of lipofuscin granules (25) has helped to clear up the confusion about staining characteristics of lipofuscin and melanin. Lipofuscin granules are less electron-dense than melanin granules, and are homogeneous in appearance; they are localized in the basal half of the cells, while melanin granules are generally found in the apical half. In sections treated with 0.25 per cent aqueous potassium permanganate, melanin was removed from the protein matrices of melanin granules but the lipofuscin granules remained unaffected. The appearance of lipofuscin in the retina is definitely correlated with age, as it is elsewhere in the nervous system.

Feeney, Grieshaber & Hogan (25) suggest that lipofuscin granules may be derived from the lysosome-like inclusions previously described, a view similar to Novikoff's (43). To support this idea, Feeney et al. offer their preliminary finding that some lipofuscin granules show acid phosphatase activity at the fine structural level of analysis. This observation would be more convincing were it supported by a clear demonstration of morphological types intermediate between the lysosome-like inclusions and lipofuscin granules. They also found a number of interesting "compound granules" which have the characteristics of both melanin and lipofuscin granules (25). In most of these compound granules the melanin forms the medulla and the lipofuscin the cortex. It seems quite likely, as they suggest, that the lipofuscin is somehow related to the breakdown of melanin pigment, and their data tend to support this idea because the amount of melanin per cell appears to decrease with age, while lipofuscin increases. The fact that both pigments frequently occur in the same granule clarifies substantially the confusion in the literature regarding the staining reactions of these pigments at the light microscope level. The problem is of interest to cell biologists and pathologists alike, but progress is considerably hampered by dependence on human autopsy and biopsy specimens.

The ontogeny of melanin granules and the genetic variations in their various attributes are of interest to developmental biologists, as they reveal various steps in the assembly of an organelle during cytodifferentiation. This process has been studied most thoroughly in mice and rats, because inbred strains carrying genes affecting pigmentation are readily available (20,21,37,38,39,51); data on granule ontogeny in human retinas are also available (25,31). After some initial confusion it is now generally agreed that melanin granules are formed by the aggregation of protein and lipoprotein subunits into fibers or fibrous sheets. Consequent to this aggregation, enzymatic activity appears and melanin begins to be deposited on the matrix. As it is deposited, the melanin blocks the active sites on the matrix by copolymerizing with the matrix protein. Melanin continues to be deposited until all the active sites are blocked and the underlying structure of the matrix is obscured (Figures 9 and 10). Evidence for this hypothesis is presented elsewhere in detail (39).

Various genes alter the size, shape, and distribution of melanin granules in the cells of the retina. In mice, the B locus (black or brown pigment), the C locus (albinism) and the P locus (pink-eyed dilution) probably act by altering the structure of protein chains included in the matrix of the granule (Figure 11). The D locus (maltese dilution) causes localized clumping of melanin in the basal rather than in the apical halves of retinal pigment cells. The mechanisms which produce clumping effects remain enigmatic.

One can scarcely doubt that similar genes act also in humans. Investigations of this problem, however, are severely curtailed by dependence on autopsy and biopsy specimens and by the complete absence of quantitative data on inheritance of phenotype. Data from the only investigation in which structure and distribution of melanin granules in the human retina was correlated with phenotype indicate that eye color is a consequence of the number and size of the pigment granules in the iris stroma, rather than of variations in the granules of the retinal pigmented epithelium (25). This is not surprising, in view of Mann's statement (35) correlating eye color with the differentiation of iris stromal melanocytes.

Hogan and coworkers (25) noted variations between individual specimens that probably have a genetic basis. In one case they state that the specimen ". . . consistently showed about one-quarter of the iris granules to have a loose granular internal substructure." This sounds intriguingly like a heterozygote between the dominant black and the recessive brown at the B locus in mice. Another specimen contained clumps of immature granules in every cell and therefore may have carried some sort of clumping gene such as *leaden* or *dilute* in the mouse. Finally, they observed that the pigment granules of the skin and hair follicles of a red-haired subject differed from those in the pigment epithelium of his blue eyes in a manner exactly analogous to the differences observed between hair follicle pigment and retinal pigment in mice carrying the gene A^y (at the *agouti* locus). This gene causes the synthesis of phaeomelanin rather than eumelanin in the hair follicle pigment cells. Thus the suggestion that red hair pigment in humans is phaeomelanin (3,5) receives strong support from this observation. Apparently humans have a genetic locus homologous to the *agouti* locus in other mammals. (The mouse genes referred to here are discussed in detail in 39.)

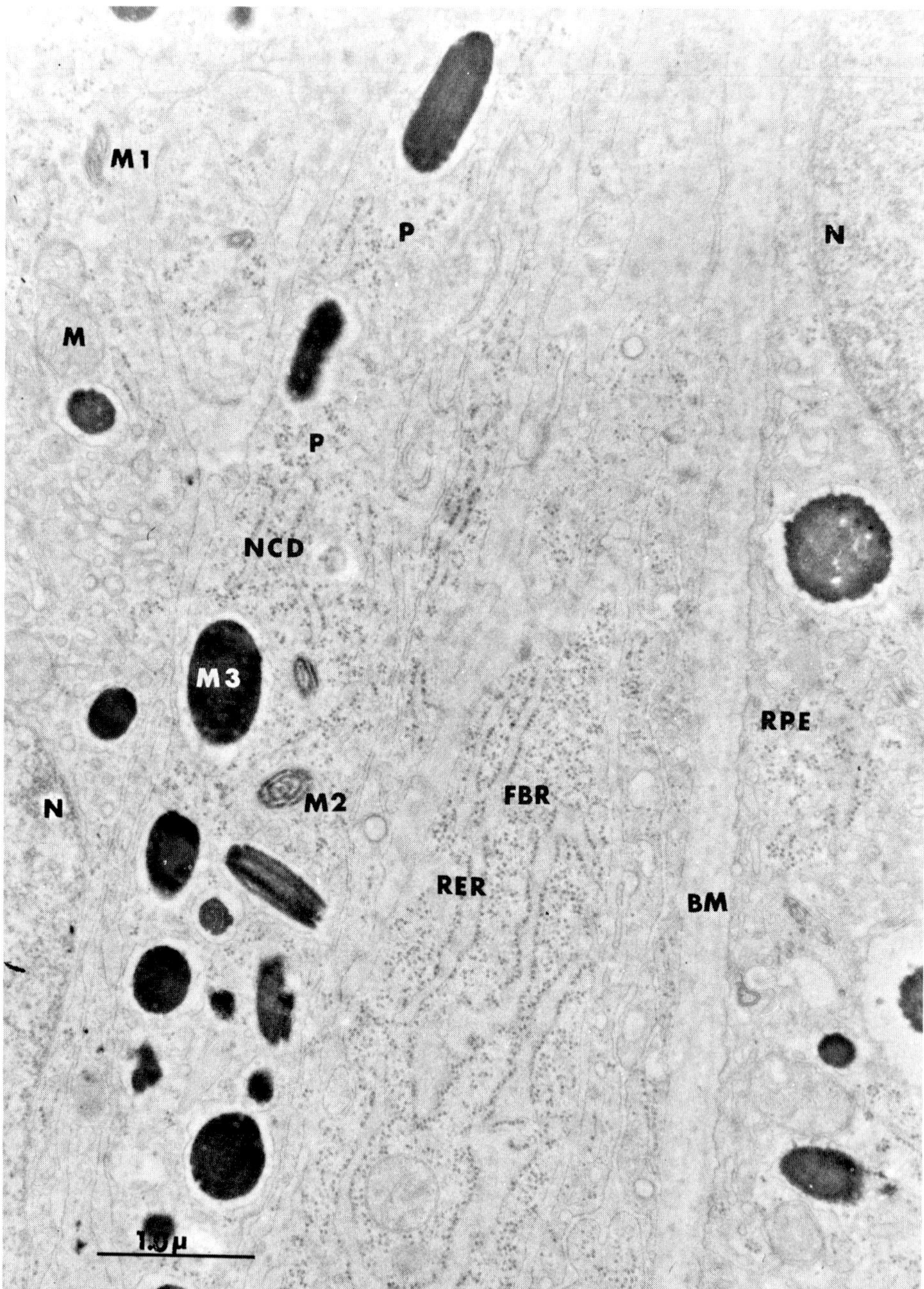

Figure 9. The pigment epithelium-Bruch's membrane-choroid complex of a late mouse fetus. Note the stages (*M1, M2, M3*) in development of the melanin granules in the choroidal pigment cells; note also the absence of an organized capillary bed at this early stage. The rough-surfaced endoplasmic reticulum (*RER*) is well developed in fibroblasts (*FBR*) in the choroid, which suggests that these may be involved in the synthesis of collagen for Bruch's membrane (*BM*). *M:* Mitochondria; *M1:* early melanin granule; *M2:* intermediate melanin granule; *M3:* mature melanin granule; *N:* nucleus; *NCD:* neural crest-derived melanocyte; *P:* neural crest-derived melanocyte; *RPE:* retinal pigmented epithelium. (From Moyer, 39.)

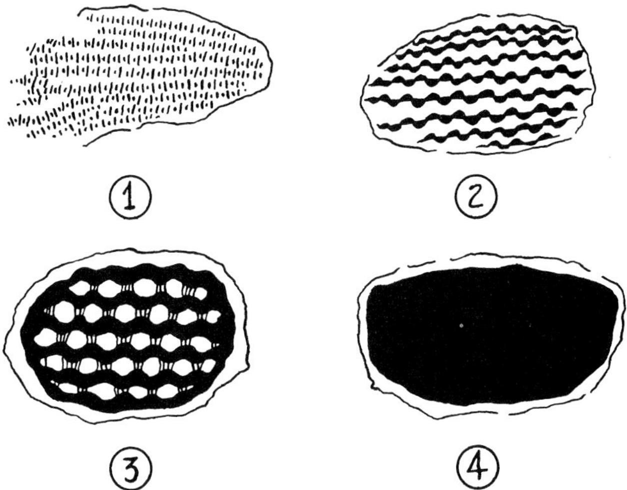

Figure 10. Schematic diagram of the stages in melanin granule synthesis. Stages 2, 3, and 4 are referred to in Figure 9 as M1, M2, and M3 respectively. Stage 1 occurs with low frequency in the retina but is common in melanomas and not infrequent in hair follicle melanocytes.

Function of Melanin Pigment

The function of melanin pigment in the retina is a matter of considerable speculation. It has been shown that the free radical content of melanin changes on illumination (13), which suggests that it may have photoactivity. In the lower vertebrates melanin migrates into the cytoplasmic extensions between the visual cell outer segments during light adaptation, and returns to a basal distribution during dark adaptation. It is generally agreed that such a distribution could increase visual acuity in high-intensity illumination by preventing reflection, and heighten sensitivity in low-intensity illumination by permitting reflection (see 58 for discussion and references).

Photochemical Response

The isolated pigment epithelium-choroid complex of the toad responds to flash illumination with a three-phase change in electrical potential. At physiological temperatures the very fast initial phase is masked by the second phase, but at 2.5° C all three are clearly visible (Figure 12). This response of the pigment epithelium differs from the early receptor potential of visual cells in its resistance to light adaptation, thus it is probably not due to rhodopsin. Since a similar response may be obtained from the eyes of pigmented rats but not from those of albino rats, melanin is a likely candidate for the photopigment (9).

This interesting finding takes on added significance in view of the fact that illumination of melanin granules isolated from beef eyes increases the free radical content of the melanin as measured by electron spin resonance (13). The time-course of this reaction is illustrated in Figure 13, and although it differs by several

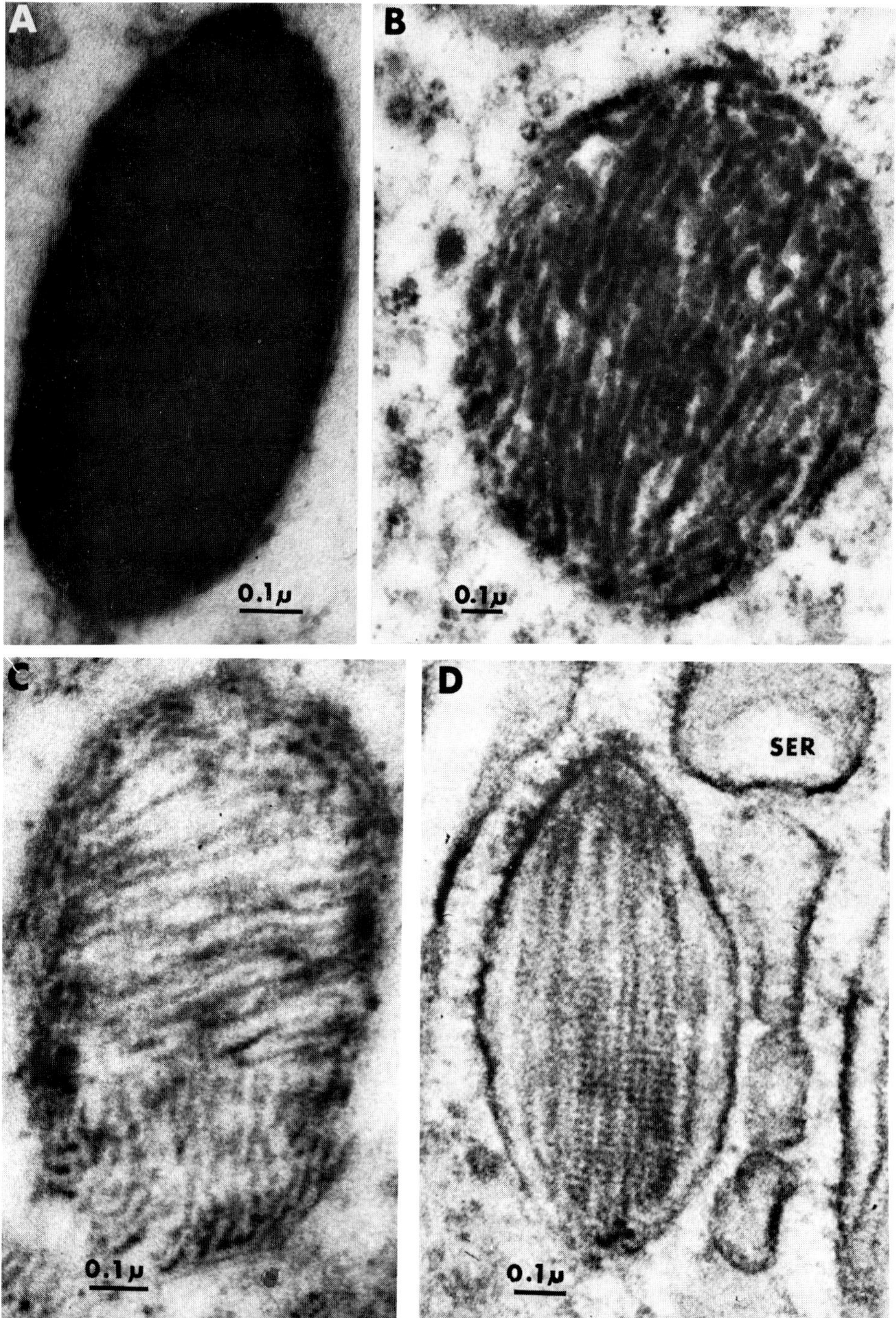

Figure 11 →

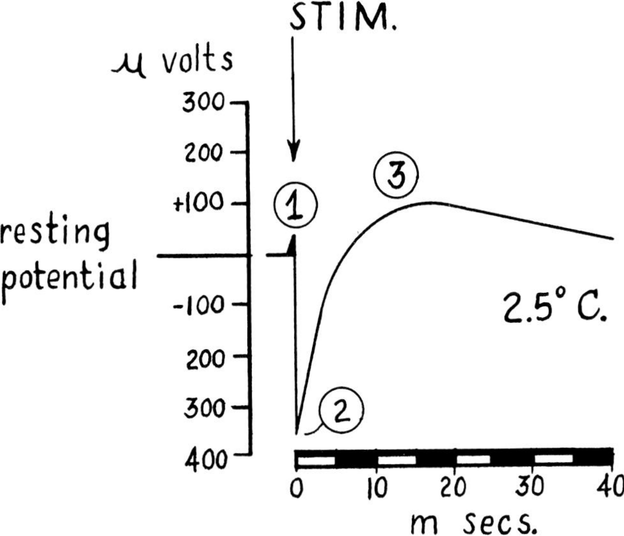

Figure 12. The "early non-retinal potential" of Brown & Gage. This change in potential is evoked from the isolated pigment epithelium-choroid complex of the toad by flash illumination. The three phases are indicated by number (see text). (Adapted from Brown & Gage, 9.)

orders of magnitude from the changes in electrical potential described above, the two phenomena may nevertheless be related.

If, on illumination, a number of monomeric units in the melanin went from the quinone configuration to the semiquinone free radical configuration, hydrogen ions would be taken up. The magnitude of this effect might very quickly be sufficient in a single cell to cause a drop in intracellular potential, which in turn might change the characteristics of the cell membranes and allow an influx of cations more than adequate to compensate for the initial potential drop. The overcompensation could then be corrected by a cation pump. These three processes would cause a progressive swing from the resting potential within the cell to negative, positive, and negative, respectively. The consequence of these changes, would be an extracellular swing to positive, negative, and positive, corresponding to the three phases found in the electrophysiological response (see Figure 12). These ideas are presented schematically in Figure 14.

Figure 11. Melanin granules showing correlation with genetic data. *A:* Mature black melanin granule in mouse retina; the dense homogenous appearance of the melanin is correlated with homozygosis for the full color allele B (black) at the B locus. *B:* Nearly mature brown melanin granule in mouse retina; the loose flocculent appearance of the melanin is correlated with homozygosis for the recessive allele b (brown) at the B locus. *C:* Intermediate melanin granule from the retina of a mouse homozygous for the recessive allele p (pink-eyed dilution) at the P locus; note that the fibers are not parallel as in *B* and *D*, but rather run in various directions. *D:* Mature melanin granule from the retina of a mouse homozygous for the recessive allele c (albinism) at the C locus; melanin is not synthesized in this mouse because of defective tyrosinase; the periodicity in the unpigmented protein matrix is clearly visible. SER: Smooth-surfaced endoplasmic reticulum. (From Moyer, 39.)

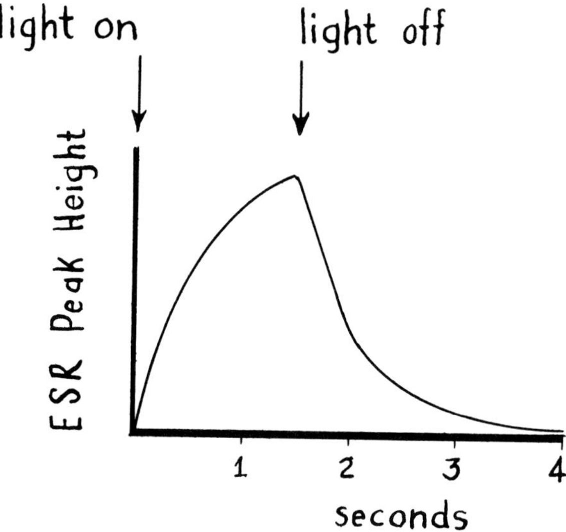

Figure 13. Time-course of increase and decay of free radicals resulting from pulse illumination of melanin granules isolated from bovine eyes (see text). (Adapted from the data of Cope, Sever & Polis, 13.)

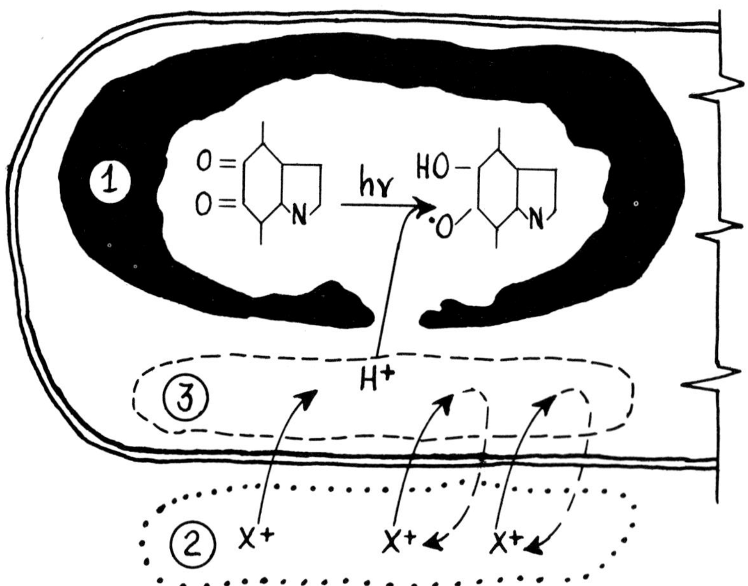

Figure 14. Schematic diagram illustrating the hypothesis presented (see text) to relate the change in free radical content of melanin following illumination (Figure 13) to the early non-retinal potential (Figure 12).

The large discrepancy in the time-courses of the two phenomena could be due to the dependence of the potential change on some integrity of structure that is disrupted when the melanin granules are isolated from the cell for electron spin resonance measurements. Melanin granules *in situ* are usually closely related to the membranes of the tubular endoplasmic reticulum (47), but in the course of isolation these membranes are invariably lost.* There may be some sort of electron transport relationship between the melanin, the granule matrix, and the surrounding membrane system that accounts for the extremely rapid electrical response. Of course, the number of free radicals necessary to initiate the reaction could be very small in comparison to the total number that can be generated.

Although this electrical response of the pigment epithelium is extremely resistant to light adaptation, the second and third phases decrease slightly in amplitude in a sequence of flashes of maximum intensity at 15-second intervals (9). If the ideas expressed above are correct, this change in amplitude could be increased by spacing the flashes only one or two seconds apart, so that there would be no time for the majority of free radicals formed to decay between flashes. A further test could be the simultaneous measurement and recording of changes in electron spin resonance and evoked potential from flash-illuminated, isolated retinas. Finally, the scheme presented in Figure 14 predicts that the characteristics of the evoked potential will show a definite pH dependence.†

Whatever its origin, the early potential from the pigment epithelium may account for the fact that rats and mice homozygous for retinal dystrophy genes, and consequently virtually without receptors, still show a marked pupillary reflex on strong direct illumination (28). A variety of epithelia in which the cells are connected by tight junctions have been shown to conduct electrical impulses from cell to cell. In these cases, the signals to the individual cells are added by the epithelium as a whole (34). The tight junctions connecting the cells of the pigment epithelium are continuous from the fundus to the iris and, at least in mice, there are tight junctions between these cells and iris muscle cells, both dilator and sphincter (12).‡ The early electrical response therefore may be transmitted directly to the iris muscle cells in a way that, directly or indirectly, induces contraction of the pupillary sphincter. The advantages of such a system as protection against sudden strong changes in illumination are obvious. This possibility should be relatively easy to test by means of properly placed electrodes in dystrophic mice and rats.

Photomechanical Response

The mechanism by which pigment granules move remains a mystery. Porter & Yamada (47) found that the pigment granules in frog retinas were bounded by membranes which occasionally appeared to be contiguous with the smooth tubular system of endoplasmic reticulum. Since myeloid bodies obviously were specializations of this reticulum, and since they resembled receptor cell outer segments in their stacked lamellar appearance, these authors tentatively suggested that the myeloid bodies were photoreceptors which mediated pigment migration through the agency of the tubular endoplasmic reticulum. Such a

* Author's unpublished observations.

† *Dr. Moyer's note after the Conference:* Since this manuscript was submitted, Stratton & Pathak (52a) have confirmed reversible photoenhancement of the ESR signal from melanin with visible light, and Crawford, Gage & Brown (16a) have demonstrated pH dependence of the pigment epithelium electrical response.

‡ Also, A. I. Cohen, personal communication, 1965.

process would require the presence of a light-sensitive pigment in the myeloid bodies but, although this is suggested by the observations of early investigators such as Kühne and Angelucci (cf. Porter & Yamada, 47), there is still no direct evidence available. Attempts to demonstrate rhodopsin in myeloid bodies by means of microspectrophotometry are undoubtedly plagued by the difficulty in distinguishing these organelles from ingested pieces of visual cell outer segments at the light microscope level. Perhaps an electron microscope study using labeled anti-rhodopsin antibodies could adequately test this possibility. Even if the myeloid bodies contain rhodopsin or a similar pigment it is difficult to see how they might mediate pigment migration. Porter & Yamada found no significant difference in the form or extent of the endoplasmic reticulum in the apical extensions of pigment epithelial cells when comparing tissues from light- and dark-adapted animals. Thus, it appears that pigment granule movement is independent of membrane distribution.

It seems that at least one other possibility should be considered. The work of Lasansky & de Fisch (29) showed sufficient efflux of chloride ions from the basal side of the pigment epithelium-Bruch's membrane complex to account for the current measured when the isolated epithelium is short-circuited. An equivalent movement of cations in the opposite direction probably takes place, but the responsible ionic species could not be identified in these experiments. However, it was noted that bicarbonate disappeared from the buffer on the apical (vitread) side of the isolated pigment epithelium and did not appear on the opposite side. This strongly suggests that hydrogen ions are released at the apex of the cells. The investigators found no change in pH in the absence of buffer, so they discounted this possibility, but the bicarbonate ion itself would be an effective buffer in this case, and a more sensitive test criterion would be whether or not carbon dioxide was given off at the apical side of the epithelium.

If the cation involved is the hydrogen ion, then a small pH gradient could exist, the apices of the cells being slightly more acid than their basal regions. *In situ* melanin granules are related closely to membranes (47), and such complexes would be expected to carry an electrical charge due to the ionization of polar groups. If this charge changes as a result of the illumination of melanin as discussed above, the migration of pigment might simply be a gross electrophoretic phenomenon involving a slight alteration in the "isoelectric point" of the granules, thus causing a change in their position relative to the pH gradient. Such a scheme requires that the pH gradient (i.e., the ion flux) be unchanged by light or dark adaptation; in the experiments mentioned above, changes in illumination did not affect the current due to the ion flux.

The Development of the Pigmented Epithelium

General Considerations

A variety of biochemical and morphological criteria indicate that there are three periods of transition in the development of the retina. The general morphological features of these periods in the development of the chick eye have been characterized as follows: *a.* Rapid cellular proliferation in the neural retina, appearance of axonal processes of prospective ganglion cells, the first appearance of Müller's fibers, a sharp decrease in mitotic activity of the pigment epithelium, and its transition from "low columnar" to "cuboidal" epithelium; *b*. the cells of the neural retina become layered, the inner plexiform layer forms, the ganglion cell layer is reduced to one-cell thickness, the size of pigment epithelial cells increases without change in thickness; *c*. differentiation of the rods and cones begins, development of inter-visual cell extensions from cells of pigment epithelium takes place (14). These transition periods are marked by distinct shifts in various enzymatic activities; for instance, choline esterase first appears in the retina during the second stage (27,32), and there is a rise in alkaline phosphatase activity in the third stage (14,33). The most striking chemical indication of these transition periods is the marked fluctuation of adenosine triphosphatase activity in the developing chick retina, where there are three peaks of activity, one of which is approximately correlated with each transition. The ATPase activity of the neural retina may be distinguished from that of the pigment epithelium on the basis of requirements for dibasic cations, and the fluctuations in the activity of the pigment epithelium are markedly greater than those in the neural retina (14).

Because of the obvious difficulties in working with fetuses, information on enzymatic and structural changes in mammals is largely confined to postnatal development, and thus is not nearly as complete as that available for birds. However, marked changes in enzymatic activity in the days following birth have been recorded; for example, as the visual cells begin to differentiate, malate dehydrogenase activity increases, and the activity of the NADP-linked dehydrogenases of the pentose shunt decreases. Moreover, there is a change in the pattern of lactate dehydrogenase isozymes, with the activity of LDH-5 decreasing (6).

Fine Structural Changes During Development

Inasmuch as changes in fine structure often appear to reflect changes in cellular metabolism, it would be desirable to make detailed electron microscope observations of the early differentiation of the retina. As yet, apparently no such study has been completed, although later stages in development have been described (61). Some limited observations on the pigment epithelium are available, however, from studies on the ontogeny of melanin granules (37,38).* In the mouse, at about 15 to 17 days *in utero* the cells of the pigment epithelium are columnar in form and contain large numbers of ribosomes and polysomes, some of which are contained on elements of rough-surfaced endoplasmic reticulum, while others appear to be free in the cytoplasm. The synthesis of melanin granule matrices has already begun, and in pigmented strains melanin is already being deposited on them. No Golgi region is apparent in the specimens I have examined. The overall appearance of the cells suggests fairly active protein synthesis, although no inclusions other than the melanin granule matrices can be correlated with the accumulating products of this synthetic activity. No desmosomes

* Also, author's unpublished observations.

or terminal bars in cells were observed at this stage, but there were frequent interdigitations of cytoplasmic extensions from the apical region of neighboring cells. Mitochondria tended to be elongated and oriented roughly parallel to the long axis of the cell. Stages in mitosis were occasionally encountered, thus this was probably the morphology of the first stage. These features may be seen in Figure 15.

In late fetal life there is a marked and rapid change in morphology in the pigment epithelium. The precise timing is uncertain because of apparent genotypic variations, but the change occurs at about 17 to 18 days *in utero* in the C57 B1/6 strain of mice. Most striking is the change in overall shape of the cells to a low "cuboidal" type of epithelium and the simultaneous appearance of smooth-surfaced vesicles and occasional elements of tubular endoplasmic reticulum. A number of ribosomes are still attached to the membranes, but the space between groups of them is greater than before. In this respect the change is similar to that occurring in developing liver cells when the membranes of the endoplasmic reticulum are being synthesized (17,18). While in previous publications (37,38,39) I had stated that these cells lacked Golgi areas, the use of improved techniques of fixation and embedding allowed me recently to find characteristic Golgi profiles

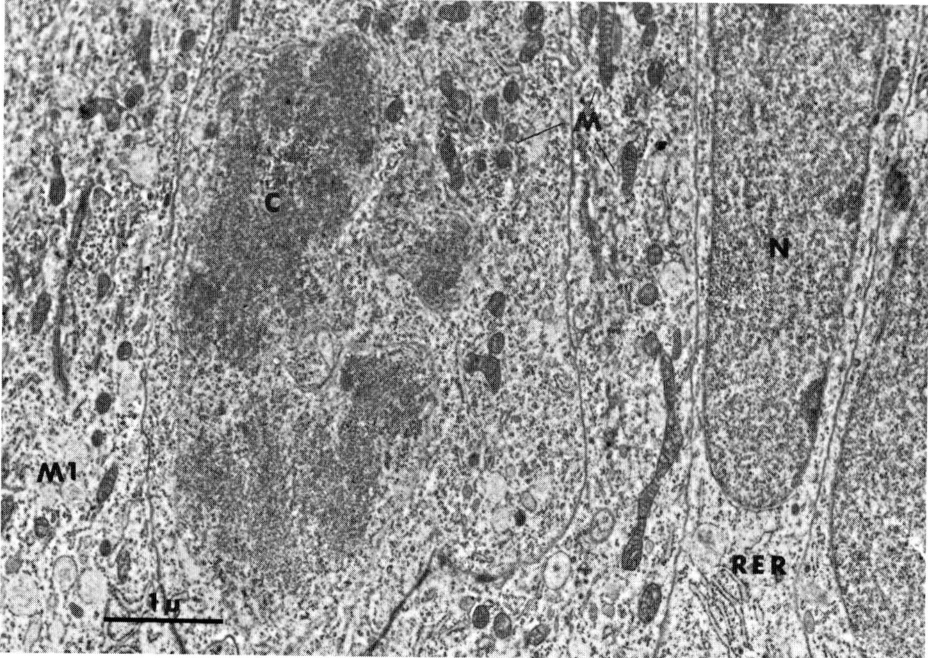

Figure 15. Pigment epithelium of an albino mouse 17 days *in utero*. Note the free ribosomes and the rough-surfaced endoplasmic reticulum (*RER*). Some early stages in the synthesis of the protein matrices of melanin granules may be seen; since this is an albino mouse, these granules will develop to the stage seen in Figure 11D but will not become pigmented. Note also the tall columnar morphology of the cells and the metaphase plate in the dividing cell in the left center of the field. *C:* Chromosome; *M:* mitochondria; *M1:* early melanin granule; *N:* nucleus.

in many of the cells, though they seem to be limited to small areas of cytoplasm near the nucleus. Many melanin granules in various stages of development are scattered through the cytoplasm at random, and in pigmented strains many of them have achieved their mature morphology (see below). The developing pigment granules are not related to the Golgi areas. Prolific folding of extensions of the plasma membrane are fairly common at the apices of the cells where they contact the developing neural retina. Junctional complexes form just basal to these areas. The nuclei do not have prominent nucleoli or marginal chromatin. A distinct basement membrane containing fibrils (presumably collagen) is present. At this stage, pinocytotic vesicles of characteristic morphology are evident for the first time (see Figure 4B). They are seen in the plasma membrane at the base of the cells. Mitochondria are randomly distributed throughout the cells. The general features of the pigment epithelium at this stage are evident in Figure 16.

The pigment epithelium retains these morphological features for 11 to 14 days. During this period the size of the cells increases, presumably in response to growth of the neural retina and pressure exerted by the developing vitreous body, a process described in detail for the chick by Coulombre et al. (15). Clearly, the volume of the individual cells must increase considerably during this period and, as their volume rises, the smooth tubular endoplasmic reticulum proliferates and

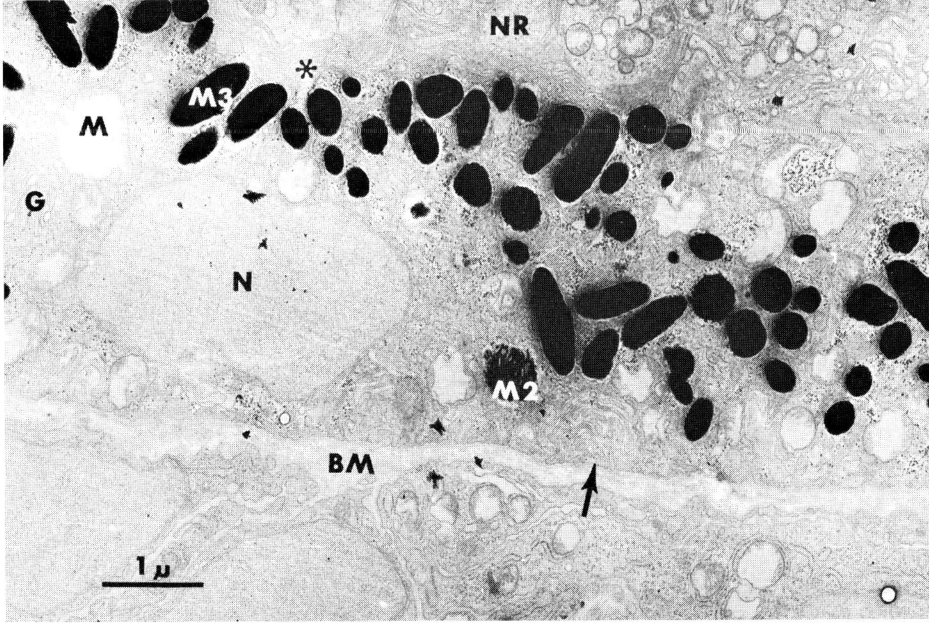

Figure 16. Pigment epithelium of a black mouse (C57 Bl/6) three days post partum. Note the extensive infolding of the basal plasma membrane (arrow) and the massive proliferation of plasma membrane at the apex of the cells (*). Note also that the melanin granules tend toward an apical localization. The swelling of the mitochondria (*M*) is probably an artifact caused by overexposure to glutaraldehyde fixative. *BM:* Bruch's membrane; *G:* Golgi region; *M2:* intermediate melanin granule; *M3:* mature melanin granule; *N:* nucleus; *NR:* neural retina.

the plasma membrane on the choroid side becomes extensively and deeply infolded. At the apex of the cell, where it contacts the developing visual cell layer, the massive complex of smooth membranes continues to develop. Presumably, this is the beginning of the process by which the pigment epithelial cells send out their long extensions between the visual cells. The Golgi region is localized close to the nuclear envelope and remains limited in extent. Pigment granules in the later stages of development are present and tend to be localized in the apical half of the cell. The early aggregative stages in pigment granule development are rarely encountered toward the end of this period.

Around eight to ten days *post partum* a very considerable increase in smooth tubular endoplasmic reticulum occurs, accompanied by very deep and extensive infolding of the plasma membrane facing the choroid. At the same time, the cytoplasmic extensions at the apex are forming. Mitochondria tend to become oriented along the plasma membrane basally and laterally, and the pigment granules begin to move into the apical cytoplasmic extensions. By 15 to 16 days *post partum* the pigment epithelium has achieved its mature morphology and interrelationship with the newly differentiated rods. These features are shown in Figure 1, which, being taken from an albino animal, does not show the melanin granules characteristic of pigmented strains.

It should be strongly emphasized that the sequence of differentiation described above has been deduced from limited observations of material selected solely to demonstrate stages in the development of pigment granules. It undoubtedly suffers from erratic sampling and from difficulties in comparing tissue taken from a variety of genotypes and processed by a variety of techniques. Nevertheless, it is provocative and suggests certain switches in the energy-utilizing processes of the pigment epithelium as it develops. The first period has a morphology quite characteristic of rapid protein synthesis with its attendant synthesis of ribosomes and messenger RNA. The second period shows all the characteristics of a switch to rapid membrane synthesis and an attendant synthesis of polysaccharides (17,18,40,41). I believe the appearance of the Golgi apparatus to be associated with the beginnings of this synthesis. The third stage has a morphology suggestive of further synthesis of polysaccharides, possibly those of the extracellular matrix between the epithelium and the visual cells; it is also the stage in which the characteristic morphology of transport is clearly established. Obviously these are only speculations and need to be tested by a well-organized study of the early differentiation of the eye in embryos and fetuses.

SUMMARY

The work reviewed in this paper suggests that the pigment epithelium functions in support of the neural retina by: *a.* engaging in the active transport of ions, particularly Cl^-; *b.* transporting large molecules by pinocytosis; *c.* participating in the phagocytosis and turnover of visual cell outer segment material; *d.* synthesizing at least part of the mucopolysaccharide matrix material that fills the extracellular spaces between the pigment cell extensions and the visual cells; *e.* varying visual sensitivity and acuity by the photomechanical response of melanin granules to meet varying conditions of illumination; and *f.* protecting the retina from damage resulting from sudden intense illumination by communicating its electrical response (for which melanin is probably the photopigment) directly to the iris muscles through a system of tight junctions. Furthermore, it suggests that the three phases in the differentiation of the pigment epithelium reflect a progressive shift in cellular metabolism from protein synthesis through membrane synthesis to extracellular matrix synthesis and transport. The ideas are highly speculative and require much further research.

Discussion

Wald: I can see the basis for a potential between a pigment granule and the cytoplasmic matrix in which it occurs, but how can this turn into the external circuit in which pigment epithelium potentials have been registered by Dr. Brown (8), among others?

Moyer: Good electron micrographs of frog pigment epithelium show that melanin granules are intimately associated with membranes (47). Furthermore, the plasma membrane at the basal and apical ends of the cells penetrates deeply into the cytoplasm of the cells, thus presumably making these regions more accessible to extracellular materials. Possibly the light-induced change in melanin triggers a depolarization of the membranes surrounding the granules which then spreads rapidly throughout the cell via the endoplasmic reticulum, and is communicated by it to the plasma membrane through the deep invaginations. If this depolarization caused a rapid change in the selective properties of the plasma membrane, the further events depicted in Figure 14 might then take place. This idea is similar in some respects to that proposed for skeletal muscle, where depolarization of the membrane in the region of the motor end plate is believed to spread along the t-system deep into the fibers, and to somehow trigger a change in the sarcoplasmic reticulum which allows calcium ions to diffuse into the myofibrils and trigger contraction (24).

REFERENCES

1. Anderson, E., Oocyte differentiation and vitellogenesis in the roach *Periplaneta americana*. *J. Cell Biol.*, 1964, **20**: 131–155.
2. Ashford, T. P., and Porter, K. R., Cytoplasmic components in hepatic cell lysosomes. *J. Cell Biol.*, 1962, **12**: 198–202.
3. Barnicot, N. A., and Birbeck, M. S. C., The electron microscopy of human melanocytes and melanin granules. In: *The Biology of Hair Growth* (W. Montagna and R. A. Ellis, Eds.). Academic Press, New York, 1958: 239–253.
4. Bernstein, M. H., Functional architecture of the retinal epithelium. In: *Structure of the Eye* (G. K. Smelser, Ed.). Academic Press, New York, 1961: 139–150.
5. Birbeck, M. S. C., and Barnicot, N. A., Electron microscope studies on pigment formation in human hair follicles. In: *Pigment Cell Biology* (M. Gordon, Ed.). Academic Press, New York, 1959: 549–561.
6. Bonavita, V., Molecular and kinetic properties of NAD-, and NADP-linked dehydrogenases in the developing retina. In: *Biochemistry of the Retina* (C. N. Graymore, Ed.). Academic Press, New York, 1965: 5–13.

7. Brindley, G. S., The passive electrical properties of the frog's retina, choroid and sclera for radial fields and currents. *J. Physiol.* (London), 1956: **134**: 339–352.
8. Brown, K. T., An early potential evoked by light from the pigment epithelium-choroid complex of the eye of the toad. *Nature* (London), 1965, **207**: 1249–1253.
9. Brown, K. T., and Gage, P. W., An earlier phase of the light-evoked electrical response from the pigment epithelium-choroid complex of the eye of the toad. *Nature* (London), 1966, **211**: 155–158.
10. Cahn, R. D., and Cahn, M. B., Heritability of cellular differentiation: clonal growth and expression of differentiation in retinal pigment cells *in vitro*. *Proc. Nat. Acad. Sci. USA*, 1966, **55**: 106–114.
11. Cohen, A. I., The fine structure of the extrafoveal receptors of the Rhesus monkey. *Exp. Eye Res.*, 1961, **1**: 128–136.
12. ———, A possible cytological basis for the 'R' membrane in the vertebrate eye. *Nature* (London), 1965, **205**: 1222–1223.
12a. ———, New evidence supporting the linkage to extracellular space of outer segment saccules of frog cones but not rods. *J. Cell Biol.*, 1968, **37**: 424–444.
13. Cope, F. W., Sever, R. J., and Polis, B. D., Reversible free radical generation in the melanin granules of the eye by visible light. *Arch. Biochem. Biophys.*, 1963, **100**: 171–177.
14. Coulombre, A. J., Correlations of structural and biochemical changes in the developing retina of the chick. *Am. J. Anat.*, 1955, **96**: 153–189.
15. Coulombre, A. J., Steinberg, S. N., and Coulombre, J. L., The role of intraocular pressure in the development of the chick eye. V. Pigmented epithelium. *Invest. Ophthal.*, 1963, **2**: 83–89.
16. Coulombre, J. L., and Coulombre, A. J., Regeneration of neural retina from the pigmented epithelium in the chick embryo. *Develop. Biol.*, 1965, **12**: 79–92.
16a. Crawford, J. M., Gage, P. W., and Brown, K. T., Rapid light-evoked potentials at extremes of pH from the frog's retina and pigment epithelium, and from a synthetic melanin. *Vision Res.*, 1967, **7**: 539–551.
17. Dallner, G., Siekevitz, P., and Palade, G. E., Biogenesis of endoplasmic reticulum membranes. I. Structural and chemical differentiation in developing rat hepatocyte. *J. Cell Biol.*, 1966, **30**: 73–96.
18. ———, Biogenesis of endoplasmic reticulum membranes. II. Synthesis of constitutive microsomal enzymes in developing rat hepatocyte. *Ibid.*: 97–118.
19. de Duve, C., Lysosomes, a new group of cytoplasmic particles. In: *Subcellular Particles* (T. Hayashi, Ed.). Ronald Press, New York, 1959: 128–159.
20. Dowling, J. E., and Gibbons, I. R., The fine structure of the pigment epithelium in the albino rat. *J. Cell Biol.*, 1962, **14**: 459–474.
21. Dowling, J. E., and Sidman, R. L., Inherited retinal dystrophy in the rat. *Ibid.*: 73–110.
22. Droz, B., Dynamic condition of proteins in the visual cells of rats and mice as shown by radioautography with labeled amino acids. *Anat. Rec.*, 1963, **145**: 157–168.
23. Fawcett, D. W., *An Atlas of Fine Structure; The Cell.* Saunders, Philadelphia, 1966.
24. Fawcett, D. W., and Revel, J. P., The sarcoplasmic reticulum of a fast-acting fish muscle. *J. Biophys. Biochem. Cytol.*, 1961, **10** (4/II): 89–109.
25. Feeney, L., Grieshaber, J. A., and Hogan, M. J., Studies on human ocular pigment. In: *The Structure of the Eye; II. Symposium* (J. W. Rohen, Ed.). Schattauer, Stuttgart, 1965: 535–548.

26. Fitzpatrick, T. B., and Kukita, A., Tyrosinase activity in vertebrate melanocytes. In: *Pigment Cell Biology* (M. Gordon, Ed.). Academic Press, New York, 1959: 489–524.
27. Francis, C. M., Cholinesterase in the retina. *J. Physiol.* (London), 1953, **120**: 435–439.
28. Karli, P., Stoeckel, M. E., and Porte, A., Dégénérescence des cellules visuelles photoréceptrices et persistance d'une sensibilité de la rétine a la stimulation photique. Observations au microscope électronique. *Zschr. Zellforsch.*, 1965, **65**: 238–252.
29. Lasansky, A., and de Fisch, F. W., Studies on the function of the pigment epithelium in relation to ionic movement between retina and choroid. In: *The Structure of the Eye; II. Symposium* (J. W. Rohen, Ed.). Schattauer, Stuttgart, 1965: 139–144.
30. Lasansky, A., and De Robertis, E., Submicroscopic analysis of the genetic distrophy of visual cells in C3H mice. *J. Biophys. Biochem. Cytol.*, 1960, **7**: 679–684.
31. Lerche, W., Electronenmikroskopische Untersuchungen zur Differenzierung des Pigmentepithels und der äusseren Körnerzellen (Sinneszellen) im menschlichen Auge. *Zschr. Zellforsch.*, 1963, **58**: 953–970.
32. Lindeman, V. F., The cholinesterase and acetylcholine content of the chick retina with especial reference to functional activity as indicated by the pupillary constrictor reflex. *Am. J. Physiol.*, 1947, **148**: 40–44.
33. ———, Alkaline and acid phosphatase activity of the embryonic chick retina. *Proc. Soc. Exp. Biol. Med.*, 1949, **71**: 435–437.
34. Lowenstein, W. R., Socolar, S. J., Higashino, S., Kanno, Y., and Davidson, N., Intercellular communication: renal, urinary bladder, sensory, and salivary gland cells. *Science*, 1965, **149**: 295–298.
35. Mann, I. C., *The Development of the Human Eye*. Cambridge Univ. Press, London, 1928.
36. Merkow, L., and Leighton, J., Increased numbers of annulate lamellae in myocardium of chick embryos incubated at abnormal temperatures. *J. Cell Biol.*, 1966, **28**: 127–137.
37. Moyer, F. H., Electron microscope observations on the origin, development, and genetic control of melanin granules in the mouse eye. In: *Structure of the Eye* (G. K. Smelser, Ed.). Academic Press, New York, 1961: 469–486.
38. ———, Genetic effects on melanosome fine structure and ontogeny in normal and malignant cells. *Ann. N. Y. Acad. Sci.*, 1963, **100**: 584–606.
39. ———, Genetic variations in the fine structure and ontogeny of mouse melanin granules. *Am. Zool.*, 1966, **6**: 43–66.
40. Neutra, M., and Leblond, C. P., Synthesis of the carbohydrate of mucus in the Golgi complex as shown by electron microscope radioautography of goblet cells from rats injected with glucose-H^3. *J. Cell Biol.*, 1966, **30**: 119–136.
41. ———, Radioautographic comparison of the uptake of galactose-H^3 and glucose-H^3 in the Golgi region of various cells secreting glycoproteins or mucopolysaccharides. *Ibid.*: 137–150.
42. Noell, W. K., Studies on visual cell viability and differentiation. *Ann. N. Y. Acad. Sci.*, 1958, **74**: 337–361.
43. Novikoff, A. B., Lysosomes and related particles. In: *The Cell, Vol. 2: Cells and Their Component Parts* (J. Brachet and A. E. Mirsky, Eds.). Academic Press, New York, 1961: 423–488.

44. NOVIKOFF, A. B., ESSNER, E., and QUINTANA, N., Golgi apparatus and lysosomes. *Fed. Proc.*, 1964, **23**: 1010–1022.

45. PALAY, S. L., and KARLIN, L. J., An electron microscope study of the intestinal villus. II. The pathway of fat absorption. *J. Biophys. Biochem. Cytol.*, 1959, **5**: 373–384.

46. PEARSE, A. G. E., *Histochemistry; Theoretical and Applied.* Churchill, London, 1960.

47. PORTER, K. R., and YAMADA, E., Studies on the endoplasmic reticulum. V. Its form and differentiation in the pigment epithelial cells of the frog retina. *J. Biophys. Biochem. Cytol.*, 1960, **8**: 181–205.

48. RHODIN, J. A. G., *An Atlas of Ultrastructure.* Saunders, Philadelphia, 1963.

49. ROTH, T. F., and PORTER, K. R., Yolk protein uptake in the oocyte of the mosquito *Aedes aegypti* L. *J. Cell Biol.*, 1964, **20**: 313–332.

50. SIDMAN, R. L., Histochemical studies on photoreceptor cells. *Ann. N. Y. Acad. Sci.*, 1958, **74**: 182–195.

51. SIDMAN, R. L., and PEARLSTEIN, R., Pink-eyed dilution (p) gene in rodents: increased pigmentation in tissue culture. *Develop. Biol.*, 1965, **12**: 93–116.

52. STAY, B., Protein uptake in the oocytes of the Cecropia moth. *J. Cell Biol.*, 1965, **26**: 49–62.

52a. STRATTON, K., and PATHAK, M. A., Photoenhancement of the electron spin resonance signal from melanins. *Arch. Biochem. Biophys.*, 1968, **123**: 477–483.

53. STREETEN, B. W., The sudanophilic granules of the human retinal pigment epithelium. *Arch. Ophthal.* (Chicago), 1961, **66**: 391–398.

54. SWAN, G. A., Chemical structure of melanins. *Ann. N. Y. Acad. Sci.*, 1963, **100**: 1005–1019.

55. SWIFT, H., and HRUBAN, Z., Focal degradation as a biological process. *Fed. Proc.*, 1964, **23**: 1026–1037.

56. TERRY, R. B., *Fine Structure of Chick Embryo Cells Differentiating in Vitro with Observations on Cultures Infected with Rous Sarcoma Virus.* Ph.D. Dissertation, Univ. of Illinois, Urbana, 1966.

57. VERHEY, C. A., and MOYER, F. H., Fine structure changes during sea urchin oogenesis. *J. Exp. Zool.*, 1967, **164**: 195–226.

58. WALLS, G. L., *The Vertebrate Eye and Its Adaptive Radiation.* Cranbrook Press, Bloomfield Hills, 1942.

59. WHITTAKER, J. R., Loss of melanotic phenotype *in vitro* by differentiated retinal pigment cells: demonstration of mechanisms involved. *Develop. Biol.*, 1967, **15**: 553–574.

60. YAMADA, E., The fine structure of the pigment epithelium in the turtle eye. In: *The Structure of the Eye* (G. K. Smelser, Ed.). Academic Press, New York, 1961: 73–84.

61. YAMADA, E., and ISHIKAWA, T., Some observations on the submicroscopic morphogenesis of the human retina. In: *The Structure of the Eye; II. Symposium* (J. W. Rohen, Ed.). Schattauer, Stuttgart, 1965: 5–16.

62. YOUNG, R. W., Renewal of photoreceptor outer segments. *Anat. Rec.*, 1965, **151**: 484.

RODS AND CONES AND THE PROBLEM OF VISUAL EXCITATION

ADOLPH I. COHEN *
Washington University School of Medicine
St. Louis, Missouri

Understanding the function of a visual receptor, or of any primary receptor, involves the problem of elucidating the mechanisms by which the detection of some change for which the cell is competent is reflected in its nervous activity. Earlier reviews of this subject have been made by Moody (78) and Wald, Brown & Gibbons (110); this review will focus on those morphological aspects of rods and cones which might relate to visual excitation, without going into the numerous studies of receptors not relating to that problem.

Receptor Form and Its Significance

In general, visual receptors are elongated cells which present themselves axially to the incident illumination. Presumably, the evolutionary significance of this arrangement is that it permits closer packing of the cells and hence the opportunity for a more detailed sampling of the visual field.

The visual receptors are the initial functional element in the series of nerve cells constituting the visual system; they occupy positions in the ependymal layer, differentiating from cells lining the cavity of the optic vesicles, which are side chambers off the primitive neural tube. The receptors differentiate longitudinally into two major divisions. One portion extends into the ventricular space lying between the retina and the pigment epithelium, being therefore surrounded by extensive extracellular space, in contrast to the remaining portion, which consists of the cell body and nucleus, axon, and synaptic enlargement, all embedded in the retina proper and contiguous with neurons and glial cells. The border between the ventricle and retina proper is demarcated by a line of terminal bars indicating the external limiting membrane. The ionic composition of the extracellular medium in the ventricle is unknown, but Fine & Zimmerman (51) have presented evidence for mucopolysaccharide in this fluid. The portion of the receptors extending into the ventricle is typically subdivided by a narrow neck, which is a ciliary derivative, into the two regions known as the outer and inner segments.

* This work was supported by grant NB-04816-04 of the National Institute of Neurological Diseases and Blindness, and was performed during the tenure of a Career Development Award (5-K3-NB-3170) from the National Institutes of Health.

The outer segment tips, especially those of rods, are generally found to be contiguous with the cells of the pigment epithelium or with long microvillous processes of these cells.

The diameters of the receptor portions extending into the ventricle are double or treble the wavelengths of light (diameter of human rod outer segment = 1.3 μ). The fact that they may be surrounded by a medium whose refractive index may differ from that of the cytoplasm suggested (14) that complex optical phenomena involving wave-guiding by receptors might occur in this region—a theory since confirmed (43). The effects of these phenomena on light channelling or scattering with regard to details of the receptor function are being explored.

In the mosaic of receptors there occur in some forms certain non-random pairings which may involve similar (twin) or dissimilar (double) elements (111). These paired receptors are so closely applied to one another that a discontinuity in the refractive index, which might obtain between receptors more widely separated by the extracellular medium, would not occur; i.e., light would move through these paired cells as if they were one. The apparent significance of this arrangement is that it seems to permit two cells to sample identical portions of the visual field, with the information being presumably handled differently by each of them. In some cases, as in the pigeon, one of the paired elements has a large colored oil droplet, so positioned as to filter the light entering the outer segment; a comparison of information from this pair might provide local data on hue and brightness.

In some species (e.g., mice, rats) the ciliary region is long, and a micron gap may exist between the inner and outer receptor segments, bridged only by the connecting cilium. In others (e.g., frog), however, the ciliary region is so short that the inner and outer segments abut one another closely, thus minimizing the possibility of a refractive break due to the extracellular medium. Particularly in the latter case, the inner segments may guide and concentrate light entering the outer segments.

A nomenclature developed over many years for the description of receptor form has proven highly useful because of the tendency of receptor form to correlate with the physiological aptitudes of the retinas. The description followed from the morphological generalization that receptor outer segments tended to be either rod-like (Figure 17a) or conical (Figure 17b), and from Schultze's (97) observation that retinas dominated by the presence of rod-like receptors tended to occur in nocturnal animals, whereas diurnal animals possessed considerable numbers of cones; moreover, animals whose activities were essentially confined to daylight hours possessed cone-dominated retinas. From this correlation rods and cones came to be called scotopic and photopic receptors respectively, and the knowledge that rhodopsin is possessed by rods of many forms brought about a further tendency to assume that a rod-like receptor would contain this pigment. Despite the great and continuing value of Schultze's generalization, there are enough ambiguities of form and exceptions to the above tendencies and correlations to require caution in inferring receptor chemistry, or receptor or retinal physiology, from receptor form.

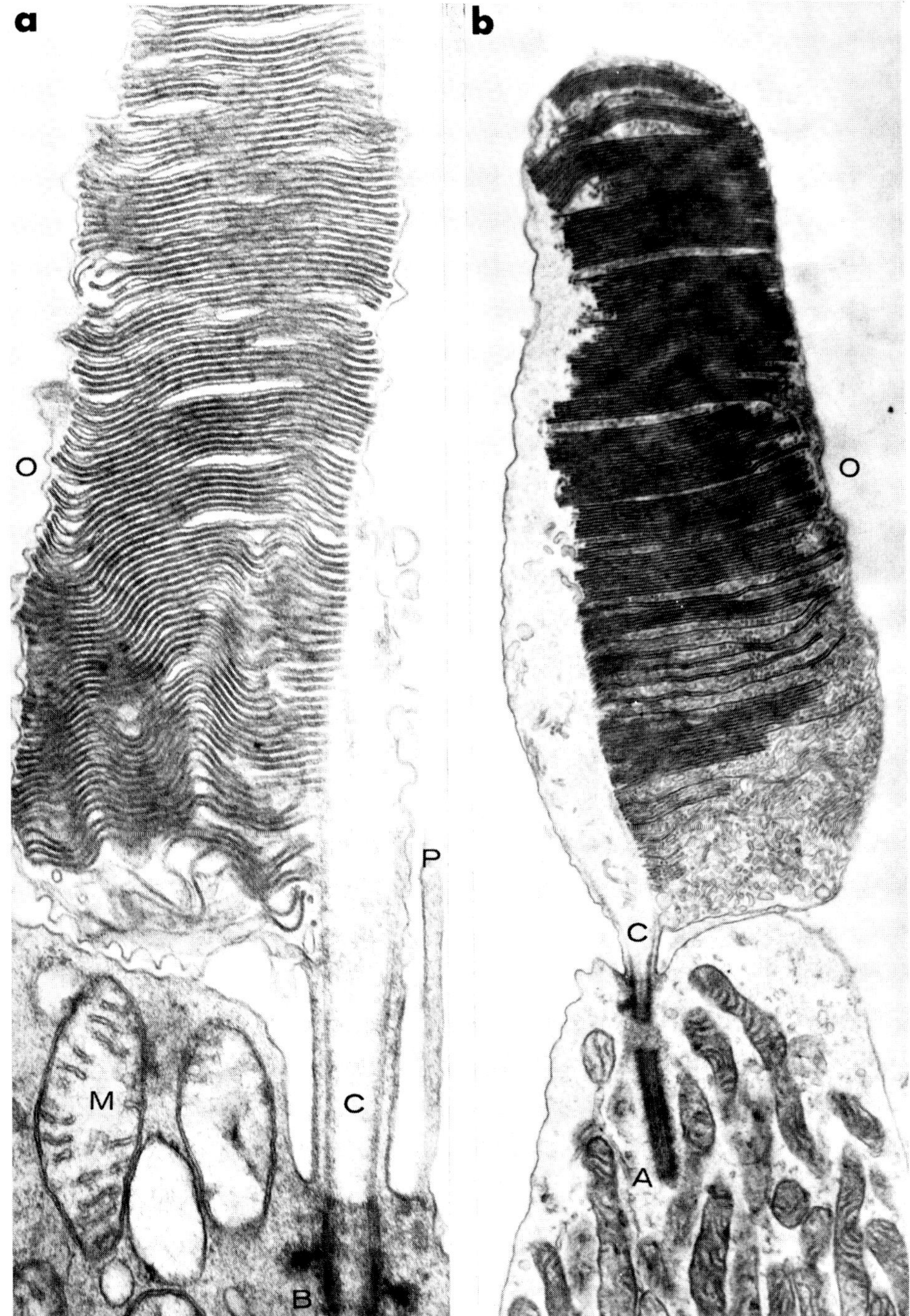

Figure 17. Electron micrographs of the human retina. *a:* A basal portion of the outer segment (O) of a rod joined to the inner segment by the cilium (C), a calycal process of the inner segment (P), the generative centriole or basal body (B), and a mitochondrion (M); × 44,400. *b:* An outer segment (O) of a peripheral cone joined by a cilium (C) to the inner segment; below the basal body are traces of rootlet fibrils and a large accessory centriole (A); × 15,800.

For example, receptors whose inner segments are of larger diameter than their outer segments tend to have an overall conical appearance in light microscopy; all the receptors of the American gray squirrel have this appearance, yet it is now known that chemical (29), physiological (54), psychological (2,98) and ultrastructural (22) evidence exists for a scotopic as well as a photopic system in this retina. Furthermore, the superior fixation procedures developed to meet the needs of electron microscopy have often suggested that the outer segments of some mammalian cones may not possess a strictly conical shape: the tips are truncated rather than pointed, and some seem to approach cylinders whose basal diameter increases only in the region of junction with the inner segments. The imperfect correlation of rod shapes with pigment is best exemplified by the well-known case of the red and green rods of frogs, whose similar fine morphology has recently been investigated by Nilsson (84).

Granit (55) has called attention to the tendency of cones to end in pedicles and rods in spherules as a means of distinguishing these classes. At times, this distinction is clearly useful, e.g., in primates the foveal receptors end in pedicles which relate them to cones despite their overall rod-like appearance, arising from the similar diameters of the outer and inner segments. On the other hand, the rods of pigeons (20) end in pedicles, as do some rod-like receptors in mice (26).

With reference to physiology, the terms scotopic and photopic receptors may be ambiguous, since they could refer to the response of a retinal system rather than to the physiology of isolated receptors. If recent claims of success in isolating receptor responses are confirmed (10,11,107), a classification by receptor action may become possible. With reference to photopigment content of individual receptors, this has to be established by light absorption characteristics and, while current evidence suggests that individual receptors do not contain more than one pigment, extremely few species and receptors have been studied in this respect.

The Location of Visual Pigment

It is now established beyond reasonable doubt that the receptor outer segments contain visual pigment, and extraction studies have amply demonstrated that the receptor outer segments are the source of most of the visual pigment. But is visual pigment confined to this location, or do small amounts occur elsewhere? The isolated irises of amphibia and certain fish, as first noted by Brown-Sequard (13), show pupillary activity in response to light, and Barr & Alpern (4) have demonstrated in the frog an action spectrum for this response consistent with the rhodopsin adsorption spectrum. In "rodless" mice, the presence of direct and consensual light responses and a degree of high-threshold vision with a rhodopsin action spectrum have led Karli, Stoeckel & Porte (62) to propose that the pigment epithelium may contain a rhodopsin whose bleaching initiates retinal activity; Karli (61) found that cutting the optic nerve abolished this residual vision.

Membrane aggregations termed myeloid bodies are found in the pigment epithelium cells of amphibia and birds (92,114). As these cells respond to light by redistributing melanin granules, it has been suggested that they may possess some visual pigment in their myeloid bodies; however, no action spectra are available for the melanin redistributions. On the other hand, as already noted, the pupillary action spectrum of the isolated frog iris gives a rhodopsin spectrum. The isolated toad iris also responds to light but, while like all irises it contains an extension of the pigment epithelium, no lamellar systems have been discerned (5). It thus seems possible that a small amount of rhodopsin may occur outside the rods and cones and even in the absence of obvious lamellar systems.

The bipolar cell has many morphological similarities to the conventional visual receptors, and in amphibia and birds at least some of these cells send processes, known as Landolt clubs, into the ventricle between receptors and the glial cells of Müller. In newts, the club process is, in fact, tipped with a cilium (60), which is of the 9 + 0 type. If the aforementioned observations of Karli (61) are correct, and light can somehow activate the retina in "rodless" mice, then bipolar neurons or other retinal neurons may contain some rhodopsin and might, under special circumstances, qualify as receptors.

The Structure of Outer Segments

Turning to the conventional visual receptors, it is now known that the pigment-containing outer segments have numerous bimembranous disks or flattened sacs (21). In saccule sections the membrane turns at the disk margins, forming a loop (Figure 18, a and b). While the dimensions of the loop may conform to a minimal turning radius related to the molecular architecture of the membrane, it is noteworthy that, even when the lumen of the saccules is distended, the edge structure appears to resist the expansion (33). Brown, Gibbons & Wald (12) also believe that their cross-sections of outer segments of frog rods indicate a specialized disk edge structure, but this appearance might well be artifactual: their photographs seem to show thick sections in which several disks are superimposed; as these saccules are not precisely registered or exactly parallel to the section plane, it would be easy to obtain an optical artifact giving the edge appearance they demonstrate. Robertson (93) initially noted a single membrane continuously pleating to form the saccules of the outer segments of frog rods, but later realized that this appearance was due to an optical artifact (94). The electron microscope reveals that, in the conical outer segments of infra-mammalian forms, these sacs represent infoldings of, or ingrowths from, the cell membranes (20,102) and the sac membrane and cell membrane are in continuity. This does not imply structural identity of these continuous membranes. In the few mammalian cones thus far examined, the basal (vitreal) sacs of the outer segments often show this continuity, but most distal saccules do not (19,22). It is not yet established, however, whether this simply represents a narrowing of the infolding zone which connects the saccule with the cell membrane, since a very narrow connecting neck could readily be missed in longitudinal sections. From the few vertebrate rods that have been studied, it has been impossible, except for the occasional very basal saccules, to discern persistent connections of the saccules and the cell membrane in either longitudinal or cross sections (23,84).

As a small connection of a saccule to the cell membrane may easily be missed in longitudinal section, cross-sections are preferable; the obtention of successful

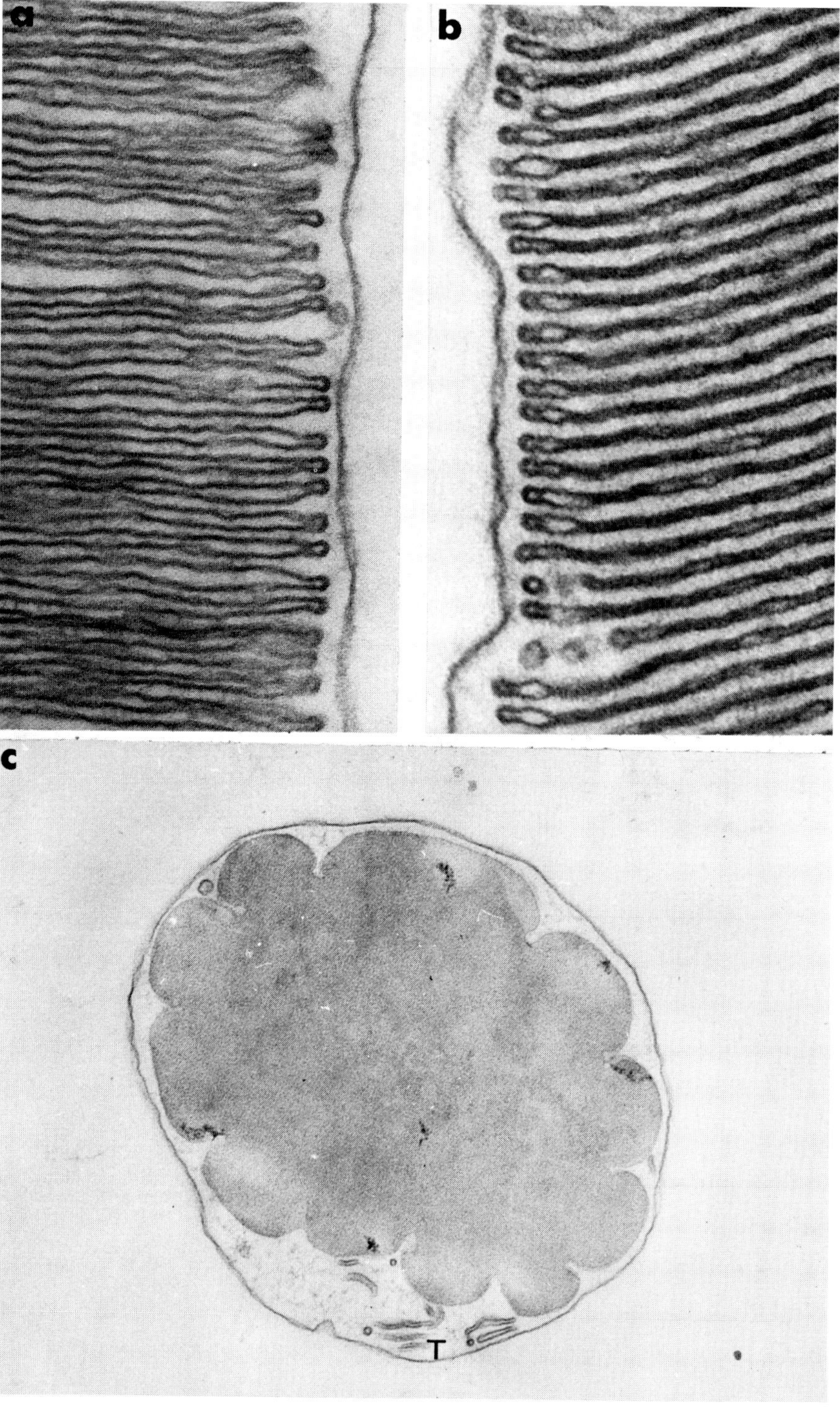

Figure 18 →

cross-sections is often frustrated, however, by a tendency of the saccules to dome or ripple, a problem that is more serious in the case of large rods such as those of amphibia or fish. J. P. Revel and M. J. Karnovsky* have developed a technique for creating dense and ultrafine depositions of lanthanum salts in the extracellular space of various tissues, a treatment that may be carried out either during or after fixation. I have recently applied it to frog retina, with interesting preliminary findings. Since electron micrographs show that all the saccules of frog cones are in continuity with the extracellular space (Figure 19a), one might expect a dark deposit in the potential lumen of the cone saccules—a prospect which has been confirmed by electron microscopy (Figures 19b,20). On the other hand, since only a few basal saccules of frog rods have been shown to be connected to the cell membrane (79), and assuming the electron microscopists have interpreted correctly their fixed material, only these few saccules should show lanthanum filling. This prediction seems generally to be valid, as can be seen in Figure 21. However, restricted regions of non-basal rod outer segments may also show filling with lanthanum (Figure 22), which is likely to be due to a local tear in the cell membrane, since this results in material in the intersaccule rather than the intra-saccule space. This infiltration seems to spread more readily between the fixed saccules than up and down the saccule column.

Several caveats must be introduced immediately. In my laboratory the lanthanum deposition technique was carried out during or following fixation in glutaraldehyde, and may therefore tell nothing about the possible patency of unfixed saccules.† Brindley & Gardner-Medwin (8) found the early receptor potential to survive formaldehyde fixation of frog retinas with but a slight shortening of its time-course, but Arden and coworkers (1) found that glutaraldehyde reduced the early receptor potential to a small, temperature-insensitive, and very fast positive response, closely resembling a photovoltaic response. The ability or failure to penetrate of certain sizes of lanthanum precipitates indicates nothing about the possible penetration capabilities of particles or ions of smaller size. The results with frog cones reveal nothing about cones of mammals, in which it has been difficult to demonstrate the connection of most of the distal saccules to the extracellular compartment.

The main difference between the saccules of rods and cones, which has persisted in the few rods studied in various vertebrates classes, is the presence of a scalloped outline of the rod sacs (see Figure 18c). Deep scalloping is seen in amphibia (91)

---

* Personal communication.

† *Added after the Conference:* I have recently found filling of the few cone saccules which survive exposure to lanthanum in the unfixed state, but no rod saccule filling.

Figure 18. *a:* Saccule edges of a human rod, fixed in buffered osmium tetroxide; note the obvious lumina of the saccules and the suggestion of rigidity of the saccule edges; × 122,900. *b:* Saccule edges of a human peripheral cone, fixed in buffered osmium; note that the lumina of the saccules tends to be less obvious than in rods, and again the suggestion of a rigid saccule edge; × 139,200. *c:* Cross section of the outer segment of a human rod, with one to two saccules superimposed in the section; note the scalloped saccule perimeter and the microtubular elements (T) derived from the cilium; × 57,600.

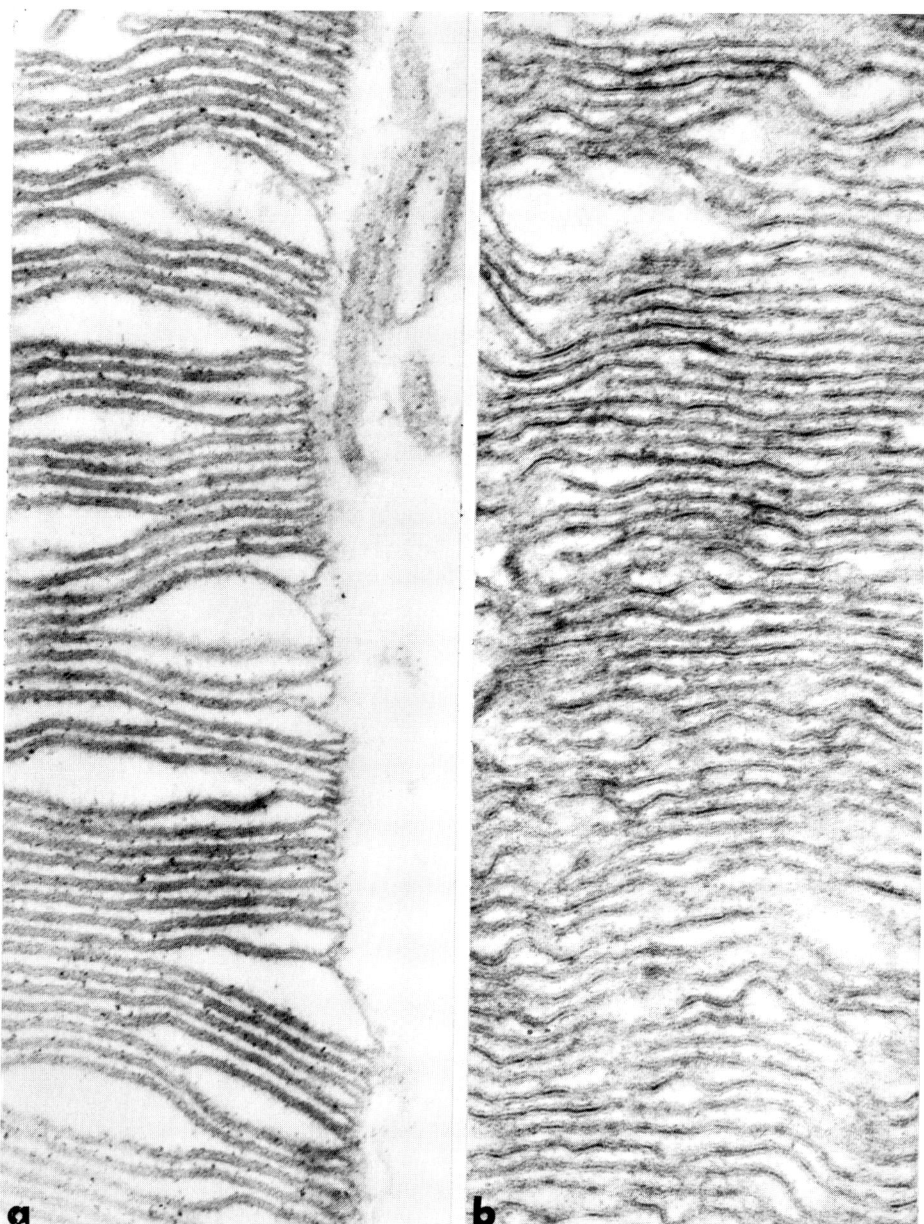

Figure 19. *a:* Edge of an outer segment of a frog cone from a retina not exposed to lanthanum; note that the cell membrane at the right appears to fold inwards to form the saccules; the fine black specks are artifacts, located both within and without the saccules; glutaraldehyde-osmium fixed; ×91,000. *b:* Portion of an outer segment of a frog cone from a retina exposed to lanthanum; note the dense interior of the saccules; glutaraldehyde-osmium fixed, ×99,400.

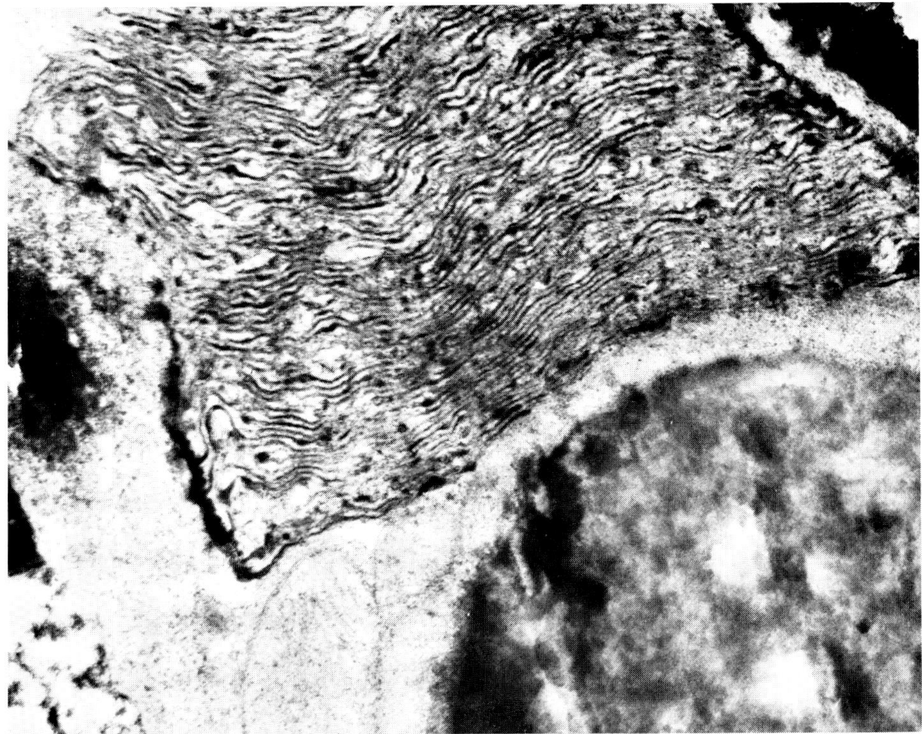

Figure 20. Outer segment of a frog cone from a retina exposed to lanthanum; note the heavy infiltration of the saccules with a black deposit. Glutaraldehyde-osmium fixed, × 40,100.

and fish,* a single notch in some rodents (18,37,99), and shallow scalloping in other species (19,20,23). Cone disks in cross-section (12,20) appear to have circular perimeters except at their points of attachment to cell membranes. In vertebrates, these saccules represent a great increase in the membranous area of the cell, while in invertebrate visual receptors there is an apparent analogy in the microvillous rhabdomes of the retinula cells. With certain fixatives, such as buffered osmium tetroxide, the flattened rod saccules show a greater lumen than do those of cones (Figure 18, a and b); this difference is less apparent, however, with potassium permanganate or with glutaraldehyde followed by osmium.

Since vertebrate rhodopsin, a carotenoid-protein, is an insoluble molecule requiring surface-active agents to bring it into colloidal suspension, and since rhodopsin constitutes a substantial portion of the outer segment's weight, it is reasonable to assume that rhodopsin is a structural protein found in membranes, and that the saccules are rich in it. However, this does not preclude the presence of rhodopsin in the cell membrane apparently forming the saccules nor, for that matter, the presence of rhodopsin in other parts of the receptor.

Studies with polarized light, though, indicate that most of the retinene has a non-random orientation, and this is consistent with the view that the bulk of this

* Author's unpublished observations.

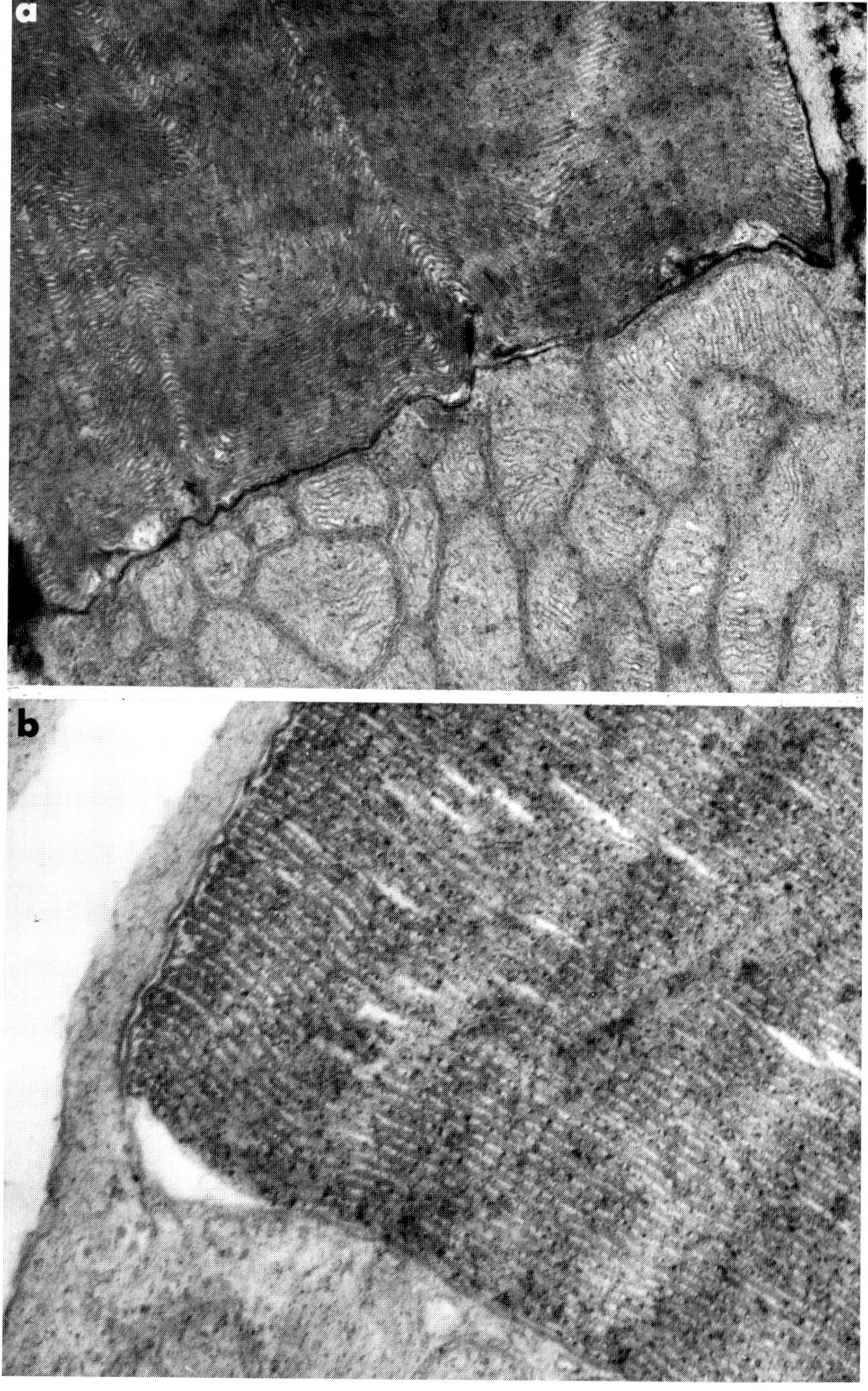

Figure 21 →

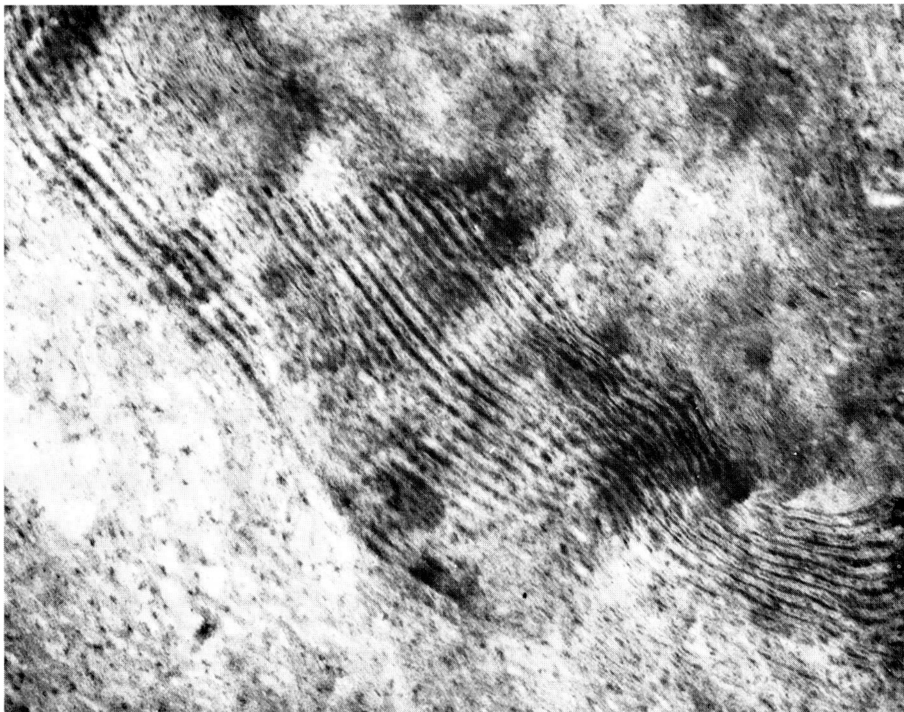

Figure 22. Anomalous portion of an outer segment of a frog rod from a retina exposed to lanthanum. A dense material has infiltrated the *intersaccule* space, presumably through a tear in the outer segment membrane, resulting in a negative staining effect. Glutaraldehyde-osmium fixed, × 92,000.

pigment is built into the disk membranes. The chromophores seem to lie in the planes of the lamellae (30,96,110) or at least parallel to them. Attempts to quantitate the number of rhodopsin chromophores which lie in or parallel to the planes of the saccules are handicapped by the following non-exclusive possibilities: the saccules may possess some curvature and not be strictly planar, the planes of groups of saccules within a single receptor may be slightly tilted with respect to the receptor axis, or the saccule planes within a group of receptors may not coincide because of slight differences in the individual receptor axes or in the saccule planes in individual receptors. Of course, the chromophore itself may not fit strictly within a plane due to its own three-dimensional configuration. Moreover, as an hour's treatment of dark-adapted outer segments with osmium tetroxide or potassium dichromate solutions does not change the segments'

Figure 21. *a:* The junction of the outer and inner segments of a frog rod from a retina exposed to lanthanum; a dense deposition can be seen between the outer and inner segments and on the outer segment surface; the saccules and mitochondrial area, however, show only a nonspecific precipitate similar to that seen in controls; glutaraldehyde-osmium fixed, × 41,400. *b:* The base of an outer segment of a frog rod from a retina not exposed to lanthanum; only nonspecific precipitation, both within and without the saccules, is evident; glutaraldehyde-osmium fixed, × 82,800.

apparent red color nor interfere with their subsequent ability to bleach, and since these substances readily attack vitamin A, it must follow that the carotenoid is well protected from these oxidants. It would be interesting to see whether the early receptor potential can survive these oxidants. In cross-sections of rods of the mudpuppy, *Necturus*, Brown, Gibbons & Wald (12) noted a system of deeply staining micelles in virtually crystalline array, which might contain porphyropsin. Nilsson (82) noted a globular fine structure for the receptor membrane, but this might be an optical artifact (94). Blasie and coworkers (6) have presented X-ray diffraction and electron microscopic evidence suggesting the presence of a 40 Å particle in the membrane of the frog rod.

Possible challenges to this view of outer segment architecture or to the simplest assumptions regarding pigment localization have been made by Lettvin (71) and by Brindley & Gardner-Medwin (8). As the early receptor potential appears in a very short time (ca. 50 μ/sec.), is relatively temperature-insensitive (87), has the action spectrum of rhodopsin, and is proportional to the pigment bleached (27), it appears likely that it originates in the formation of some dipole in the rhodopsin molecule or perhaps from a dipole perpendicular to and within the membrane. However, if the double membrane saccules in rods are free-floating entities cut off from extracellular space, and if pigment is symmetrically distributed within the membranes forming the saccules, any dipoles due to the action of light on the pigment in the upper membrane walls of the saccules would be cancelled by dipoles of opposite orientation forming in the lower membrane walls. But, as Lettvin (71) points out, if the potential lumen in every saccule had an actual connection to the extracellular space, the dipoles would be in a membrane border separating intra- and extracellular compartments, and an intracellular-extracellular charge asymmetry could arise. However, while electron microscopy is no less free from artifacts than electrophysiology or other complex techniques, the best evidence advanced shows no connections between the lumina of most rod saccules and the extracellular space.

In a recent study by Falk & Fatt (48) of potential changes due to hydrogen ion uptake following rhodopsin bleaching in outer segment suspensions of frog rods, they found that their results best fit a model where H^+ buffer diffused from an open end of a column, with diffusion through the walls being negligible. One might consider that the cell membrane over the outer segment also contains rhodopsin, and that this rhodopsin accounts entirely for the vertebrate early receptor potential (ERP) phenomenon, the saccule dipoles cancelling but the effect of the cell membrane dipoles persisting. It is doubtful, however, whether enough rhodopsin could be present in the cell membrane to account for the ERP. We must therefore consider rhodopsin or some portion of the rhodopsin molecule as not symmetrically oriented in both membranes of the saccules, which was the conclusion reached by Brindley & Gardner-Medwin (8); while this is possible, it is clearly surprising in view of the apparent formation of the saccules by the symmetrical process of invagination or ingrowth of cell membrane. It has been argued with respect to the later electrical responses of receptors that, if the rod saccules are separated from the cell membrane and contain all the rhodopsin, and if bleaching is linked to subsequent alterations in the cell membrane potential, a diffusion step must be involved. It is the appearance in microseconds and relative resistance to low temperatures of the first part of the biphasic ERP which makes diffusion of a significant number of ions most doubtful to some researchers of this phenomenon.*

Dr. Wald (109) has suggested that activation of an enzyme, or alteration of the transmembranal potential, or both, might be the mechanism of signal amplification in the rod. Although McConnell & Scarpelli (73) reported that rhodopsin might have light-influenced ATPase activity, two subsequent studies (7,52) have failed to confirm this. Hara (58) and Falk & Fatt (47) have reported conductivity increases in outer segments upon illumination. The latter authors found conductance changes independent of the medium with alternating currents above 5 kc/sec. and calculated a mobility of 10^{-4} cm^2/volt/sec.; this is in the range of some organic molecules but about one tenth the mobility of a hydrogen ion (42), and slower than movement in ordinary semiconductors (112). Rosenberg, Orlando & Orlando (95) have reported some evidence for photoconduction in partially dried outer segments of sheep rods. Some of these possibilities and the problems involved are considered by Hagins and Jennings (56,57).

A phenomenon similar to the second half of the biphasic ERP but highly resistant to light adaptation has reportedly occurred in isolated pigment epithelial-choroid complexes of toads (9). Since this epithelium contains myeloid bodies, the resistance to light adaptation argues against rhodopsin bleaching in this complex as a source of this potential. Lanthanum studies do not support the direct linkage of myeloid bodies to the extracellular compartment, although the tortuosity of the potential pathway could have defeated the experiment or the processing might have severed the connection.

In other studies pertinent to receptor cytoarchitecture Nover & Schultze (86) have reported protein synthesis in receptor inner segments, and Droz (40,41), also using radioautography, presented evidence for the migration of some of this labeled protein, described as possessing a "fast" turnover, first into the apical part of the inner segment and spreading, after a delay, from this point through the outer segment. Dr. Young (115,116) has confirmed and refined these data and reports a zone of labeled protein migrating up the outer segment, but no label in the pigment epithelium. Since ribosomes are not seen in the outer segment but are seen in the inner segment, it would not seem surprising that the inner segment might be the source of synthesis of some outer segment protein; Dr. Young's reports contain a suggestion that some of the migrant protein might be opsin and that formation of the saccules might be a continuous process with the formed saccules moving up the outer segment—indeed, he considers it possible that the entire outer segment is renewed in rats (116). Evidence bearing on the rate of turnover of opsin is lacking, however. The newly formed protein would enter the

* *Added after the Conference:* Goldstein (53) has recently obtained evidence that the early receptor potential of isolated frog retinas derives largely from cones. This would support the isolation of saccules of frog rods from the extracellular space as deduced from conventional electron microscopy and the failure of lanthanum precipitates to infiltrate these saccules.

outer segment through the cilium, which in photoreceptors has a core of low optical density and is devoid of central fibrils (23).

Occasionally, the cells of the pigment epithelium contain membranous entities superficially resembling the myeloid bodies of amphibia and birds. These have been reported in rats (38) and humans (50), and I have observed them in some mice. When critically examined in well-fixed preparations, they usually turn out to be within vacuoles and resemble fragments of receptor outer segments presumably phagocytized by the cells of the pigment epithelium. Does this represent a normal finding suggestive of continuous chewing up of receptor outer segment tips? Counter to this view is the failure of some human preparations in my laboratory to exhibit any of these membranous entities in most sections of the pigment epithelium. When they do occur, they may represent sequelae of occasional microdetachments, with outer segments tearing where they fit into "sockets" formed by pigment cell microvillae. These phenomena may not be so rare in other species. A stronger possibility is that the attrition of outer segment tips is not a continuous phenomenon but is influenced by diurnal rhythms or other physiological events, and that the phagocytized fragments are digested with some speed.

To summarize, if the saccules were in continuous formation (a view supported by the connection of the most basal saccules in both rods and cones to the cell membrane) and moving up the outer segments, they would either have to fuse with the apical cell membrane of the outer segment or break down in this area, or whole tips of outer segments would have to be continually breaking off with healing over the cell membrane.

While there is surprising evidence of the instability of the insoluble protein opsin in the absence of retinene (39), there is no quantitative evidence of the stability of rhodopsin in the dark. Is rhodopsin more unstable at the receptor tip? Most molecules of low solubility or structural proteins have a slow turnover. A constant attrition of the outer segment tips would, of course, not represent intrinsic instability of the rhodopsin molecule, although it would contribute to rhodopsin turnover in chemical studies. The undisputed presence of some bits and pieces of rod outer segments within some pigment epithelium cells also calls for caution in integrating chemical indications of the presence of rhodopsin in these cells in terms of the physiology of this epithelium. Noell and associates (85) have reported receptor deterioration in rats exposed to olonprged light, but it is not yet clear how the damage is accomplished, although rhodopsin bleaching seems to be the initiating step.

The Cilium and Inner Segment
Cell Fibrils, Microtubules and Reticulum

The connecting cilium is of considerable importance as the bridge linking the inner and outer segments. This is probably a weak point as regards breakage by mechanical trauma. Metabolic interchanges meant to circumvent the complications of twice crossing the cell membrane must perforce occur through this bridge and, if differences in transmembranal potentials exist with respect to the cell membrane of the outer segment and that in other parts of the receptor, steady currents would flow through this bridge. Any form of spreading perturbation of membrane potential, if such exists, would have to cross this bridge if it originates in the outer segment. Further speculations about other involvements of this region and the ciliary filaments are handicapped by our ignorance of ciliary physiology in general. As has been repeatedly pointed out, the cilium in the photoreceptor lacks the central fibril pair that is characteristic of motile cilia (31), and it has been noted (23) that the central core has a very empty appearance, with an interface evident where the core abuts on the remaining ciliary cytoplasm. Both the cilium and the motile cilia seem to originate from a centriole in ways apparently similar in all details, but how the ciliary filaments terminate in the outer segments has been little explored. In primates the nine pairs change rather quickly to nine singlets which terminate somewhere in the first third to half of the outer segment (23); in *Necturus* the filaments seem to extend half the height of the outer segments (12).

The inner segments of both rods and cones contain a pair of centrioles, one of which relates to the cilium linking the inner and outer segments. From these organelles arise cross-striated fibril systems of rootlets that course through the inner segments; their function is unknown. In extrafoveal human cones, the centrioles seem larger than in rods, but the rootlet systems seem less extensive than those of rods. In the mouse the rootlets in the inner segment are closely associated with long vacuoles (18). Mountford (81) has reported similar striated filaments associated with vacuoles, but in the axons and synaptic terminals of guinea pig photoreceptors. J. Olney* has also observed them in that location in nine-day-old mice.

In the apex of the inner segments there is the well-known collection of mitochondria known as the ellipsoid, which obviously plays a significant role in cell metabolism. Indeed, Enoch (44,45) has shown staining differences in the ellipsoid which depend on the activity or inactivity of a given photoreceptor. It may also be suspected that many of the reports in the classical literature on differences exhibited by rods and cones with conventional stains may be consequences of these receptor types exhibiting differential fixation quality based on differential metabolic activity prior to fixation. By the use of electron microscopy of rabbit retinas, Webster & Ames (113) found receptor changes consequent to experimental anoxia within three minutes; these were reversible up to 20 minutes.

Since there is a concentration of mitochondria within the apex of the inner segment, one is drawn to consider the interaction between mitochondrial activity and that of the outer segment. So far only Enoch (45) seems to have established such a relationship, and it seems reasonable to assume that in large part the products of mitochondrial activity feed into a metabolic pool and are not directly linked to a single visual signal. The mass of mitochondria seems related to the volume of the visual cell; extrafoveal cones with large inner segments, large axons, and large synaptic pedicles appear to have the greatest mass of mitochondria. I

---

* Personal communication.

have noted elsewhere (21) that energetic demands at the synaptic terminus may relate to this mitochondrial mass. Both Kühne (64) and Sjöstrand (100) have suggested that definitive nervous activity or impulses may originate in the inner segment, having been triggered by events in the outer segment. Carr, Ripps, Siegel & Weale (17), who have studied patients with two types of night blindness by reflection spectrophotometry and by electroretinography, demonstrate that it is possible to have apparently normal rhodopsin bleaching and regeneration and yet have other sources of failure in the signalling systems after the pigment. Tomita's recent work with fish (107) points to a hyperpolarization of the inner segments in response to light; he sees no sign of impulse activity of a conventional type. Similar absence of conventional impulses have been reported by Brown & Watanabe (10), who implanted electrodes in the foveal areas of monkey retinas.

Many cones of amphibians, reptiles and birds have a large oil droplet at the apex of the inner segment, which may give the appearance of blocking the passage of water soluble materials entering or leaving the outer segments. However, even the narrow channels between the edges of the droplets and the cell membrane add up to a greater area than the ciliary stalk.

The calycal processes are another feature of the apex of the inner segment, being a circlet of long microvillous projections of the inner segment which surround the base of the outer segment. Brown, Gibbons & Wald (12) have seen in *Necturus* about 27 of these processes (which they call dendrites) around the proximal halves of the outer segments; in rods they were closely applied to the outer segment surface and tended to occur one for each surface groove formed between saccule lobulations. In the human or macaque these processes number nine to twelve (19,23) but are not closely applied to the receptor surface. The fact that the calycal processes, like the ciliary filaments, do not extend the full length of the outer segment and are not tightly (meaning < 12.5 mμ) applied to the outer segment surface argues against their role in signal transmission.

Elsewhere in the inner segments of certain receptors in amphibia, reptiles and birds (111) are the complex accumulations of membranous systems and glycogen known as paraboloids but, not being universal constituents of visual receptors, it is doubtful that they play a direct role in visual excitation.

The ciliary filaments have the appearance of microtubules; though, apart from these, Kuwabara (65) has discerned many microtubules about 15 mμ in diameter in the inner segment, some of these running the length of the photoreceptor and ending just above the spherules and pedicles; Kuwabara reports that they are sparse near the receptor nuclei. In the morphological axon (Figure 23a) they are present in large numbers and seem non-randomly distributed. Endoplasmic reticulum is also evident throughout the length of the receptor, starting in the inner segment and going into the spherules or pedicles; at times this tortuous system appears to connect with the extracellular compartment. Thus, microtubular, endoplasmic reticulum, and filament-associated endoplasmic reticular systems are possible candidates for internal signalling pathways, if a system by which a signal may move through the cell is to be sought elsewhere than in the cell membrane.

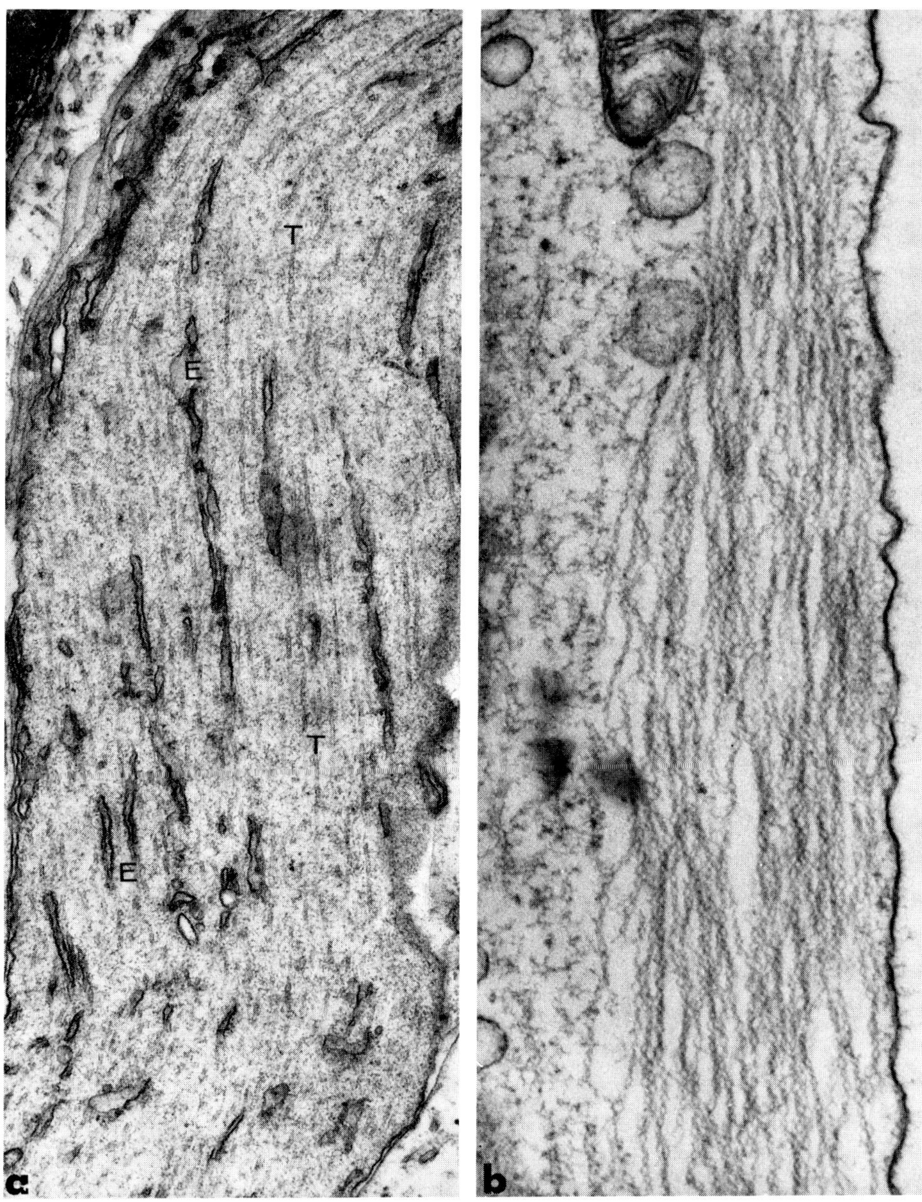

Figure 23. *a:* Portion of a morphological axon (Henle fiber) of a human cone; note the microtubular (T) and endoplasmic reticulum (E) systems coursing within the axon; × 58,000. *b:* Portion of an inner segment of a human rod with intertwined fibril pairs; these are also seen in other receptor regions and in most receptors of the retinas demonstrating them, and occasionally seem to be forming crystalline arrays, particularly in the spherules and pedicles; × 59,800.

The external limiting membrane—the line seen in thick sections and in low-resolution light microscopy—derives from the staining of the terminal bars between the receptors and glial cells of Müller; it forms a convenient boundary between the ventricle and retina proper. These terminal bars usually differ from the homologous system between the cells of the pigment epithelium in that a tight or occluded (10 mμ) zone is often not part of the bar; this junction is therefore probably less restrictive to the movement of ions and small molecules than that between the cells of the pigment epithelium (24,70). Below this level the receptors are contiguous with and separated by glial cells of Müller; the spaces between the receptors and glial cells are of the same order as those usually seen between elements of the central nervous system (about 20 mμ), and are probably adequate for carrying current in an unrestricted fashion. Thus, because of the absence of the tight junction as part of the terminal bar, external currents may flow between two receptor regions on opposite sides of the bar without significant restriction. An interesting variant of this situation occurs in toads, where Lasansky (69) notes that tight junctions may often occur between two Müller cells but not between receptors and Müller cells; I can confirm this as also true of the retina of the leopard frog (*R. pipiens*). This suggests that a second but weaker electrical barrier (R-membrane) may occur in the amphibian eye in addition to the one in the pigment epithelium-choroid complex (cf. Bysov & Hanitzsch, 15).

At the level of the terminal bars the receptors (except in the case of twin or double cones) are spaced in an ordered array and well isolated by the glial cells of Müller. Below this level, however, the precision of placement breaks down; illumination at these levels is presumably not channelled through individual receptors because of the absence of extensive extracellular gaps and consequent steps in refractive index, and therefore there would be no apparent value in maintaining precise order. The morphological axons (Figure 23a) of the rods and cones (Henle's fibers) connect the nuclear levels of the cells with their synaptic bases. In some forms (guinea pigs, mice) these axons can be extremely short, with the synaptic apparatus occurring near the cell nucleus. In other instances, as in the primate fovea, the axons may cover more than 125 μ from the cell nucleus to the synaptic termination. Indeed, a distance of some 200 μ may be spanned from the apex of the inner segment of a foveal cone of a macaque to its synaptic termination (90), which compares with, but certainly does not exceed the most extreme distances (about 300 μ) between the axon hillocks of Purkinje cells of the cerebellum and their dendritic tips (28); thus this distance alone does not preclude similar electrotonic signaling processes. However, not only did Brown & Watanabe (10) and Tomita (107) fail to detect spikes, but the former authors believe they can rule out electrotonic spread of current such as might be seen in physiological dendrites and cell somas (10). Thus the Henle fiber is a morphological axon only in the sense of its being a process connecting the cell soma and some centripetal terminus; their physiological character is quite unknown. The microtubular elements they contain are also seen after glutaraldehyde fixation in the dendrites of conventional neurons (66) and in certain glial processes.

The Receptor Terminals: Interreceptor Contacts and Synaptic Terminations

The synaptic bases of the photoreceptors generally lend themselves to the description "spherules" if they are small and rounded, or "pedicles" if they seem to have a flat base facing the processes of the second order neurons in the outer plexiform layer. In some retinas, like the pigeon's, only pedicle-like endings are seen despite the presence of rods (20). In others, like the human, rods end in spherules and cones in pedicles (76). In the mouse, where no Purkinje shift is seen (59) and no receptor corresponds to our usual notions of cone morphology, all appearing rod-like, numerous pedicles as well as spherules are seen (18,26). Likewise, the guinea pig has two classes of synaptic terminals (101).*

The terminals generally contain elements of the endoplasmic reticulum, small numbers of mitochondria, and numerous vesicles about 300–500 mμ in diameter. As similar vesicles have been encountered in nervous system processes in regions where synapsis is almost certainly occurring, they are now known as synaptic vesicles. It is suspected that they serve as carriers for neurohumors released on proper stimulation, but it is not clear whether vesicle breakdown is part of the release mechanism. In any event, Mountford (80) could find no statistical evidence for changes in vesicle size in receptors after various periods in the light or dark but, because of numerous factors affecting vesicle distribution which were not readily controlled, no attempt was made to see whether the vesicle concentration or amount had changed. De Robertis & Franchi (32) had previously reported size and distribution changes of vesicles in response to light.

In some human retinas, obtained from normal as well as abnormal eyes, interesting collections of strands of two intertwined fibers, one micron long, have been observed (Figure 23b), confined to the receptors and appearing to be embedded in a gel. Such collections have been observed most often in spherules and pedicles, but also near the cell nuclei and in inner segments. The individual fibers are 68 Å in diameter and in the photographic projections the two threads cross at intervals of about 200 Å. In two specimens these double strands seemed to be more tightly entwined and more regularly disposed, and were apparently undergoing incipient crystallization; crystalloids possibly resulting from these fibrils have also been observed. It is conceivable that they are viral, but double-stranded filaments are also known to occur in non-viral proteins. They do not resemble the filamentous organelles reported by Mountford (81) in the synaptic regions of the guinea pig's photoreceptors.

The most interesting questions about the receptor terminals deal with their synaptic connections. Before examining the possible synaptic relations of receptors

---

* *Added after the Conference:* A comment by Dowling (34) notes that two terminal classes are also seen in rats, and he speculates as to whether one class may be a rhodopsin-containing cone. Goldstein's recent finding (53) that cones, and not rods, seem largely responsible for the early potentials of isolated frog retinas, raises the question of whether rhodopsin cones are the main source of these potentials in rats. Such postulated cones would have to have saccules still connecting to the cell membrane.

with the neurites of bipolar and horizontal cells, an interesting relationship among receptors must be considered. Sjöstrand's (101) serial section analysis of the synaptic bases of guinea pig photoreceptors disclosed the fact that synaptic bases of the beta photoreceptors extend processes which terminate on alpha photoreceptor bases. Further work by Sjöstrand and Mountford (103) showed that short receptor processes may end on adjoining receptor terminals, while longer ones bypass several cells before terminating. The synaptic bases of pigeon photoreceptors likewise give rise to long processes which run horizontally (20). Processes from receptor terminals which contact terminals of other receptors have also been noted in the gray squirrel (22), mouse (26), human and macaque (25), and human (76); broadside contiguities of receptor bases have been seen in the frog (83).

These contacts exhibit an organized pattern. In the parafoveal area of the human, the synaptic bases of the foveal cones may be seen to be in contact with each other to form a network (Figure 24). As one moves peripherally and rod spherules appear, they tend to be contacted by processes from the cones which, however, continue to contact each other. In the peripheral human retina, it is quite easy to demonstrate by serial sectioning that at least some cone pedicles continue to contact each other and that, by processes and broadside contacts, they continue to contact nearby spherules. Some spherules receive several contacts and others none. Spherule-to-spherule contacts are very rare. In all cases, contacts consist of cell contiguities characterized by membrane densities on both sides (25). The intercellular gap is about 200 Å, i.e., not as tight as that in known electrotonic connections of nerve cells, despite the fact that the same fixative shows tight junctions elsewhere, as in the terminal bars of the pigment epithelium. However, by using other fixatives and osmolarities, the junctions can be made tight (25). Missotten (75) gives 100 Å as the distance between these contacts, but he has not studied this point critically. No synaptic vesicles are clustered at such points of contact—but neither are they clustered where the receptor is contiguous with the presumed neurites of bipolar and horizontal cells. In short, were the receptor a conventional nerve cell, one would immediately be inclined to regard these as desmosomes (maculae adhaerens) of significance for a knitting of the cells to resist mechanical force; there is still a very substantial probability that this is correct, and it is also Missotten's conclusion (75). However, the receptor makes no conventional synaptic contacts (25), and the contiguities in humans, while mostly lateral when two cones are involved, are made in many directions when rods and cones are linked. As a system for resisting lateral mechanical stress, the contacts would be redundant in terms of a similar function postulated for the terminal bars of the external limiting membrane, where not only receptors but glial cells are laterally knit. Only rare glial-to-receptor desmosomes have been seen (25). On the other hand, the extensiveness of the human contact system is not paralleled quantitatively in the macaque, though similar contacts are seen; this may be considered evidence against a signalling role for the system.

The high resolution of the central foveal area (89), as measured by interference pattern techniques which bypass the optics of the eye, argues for discreteness of

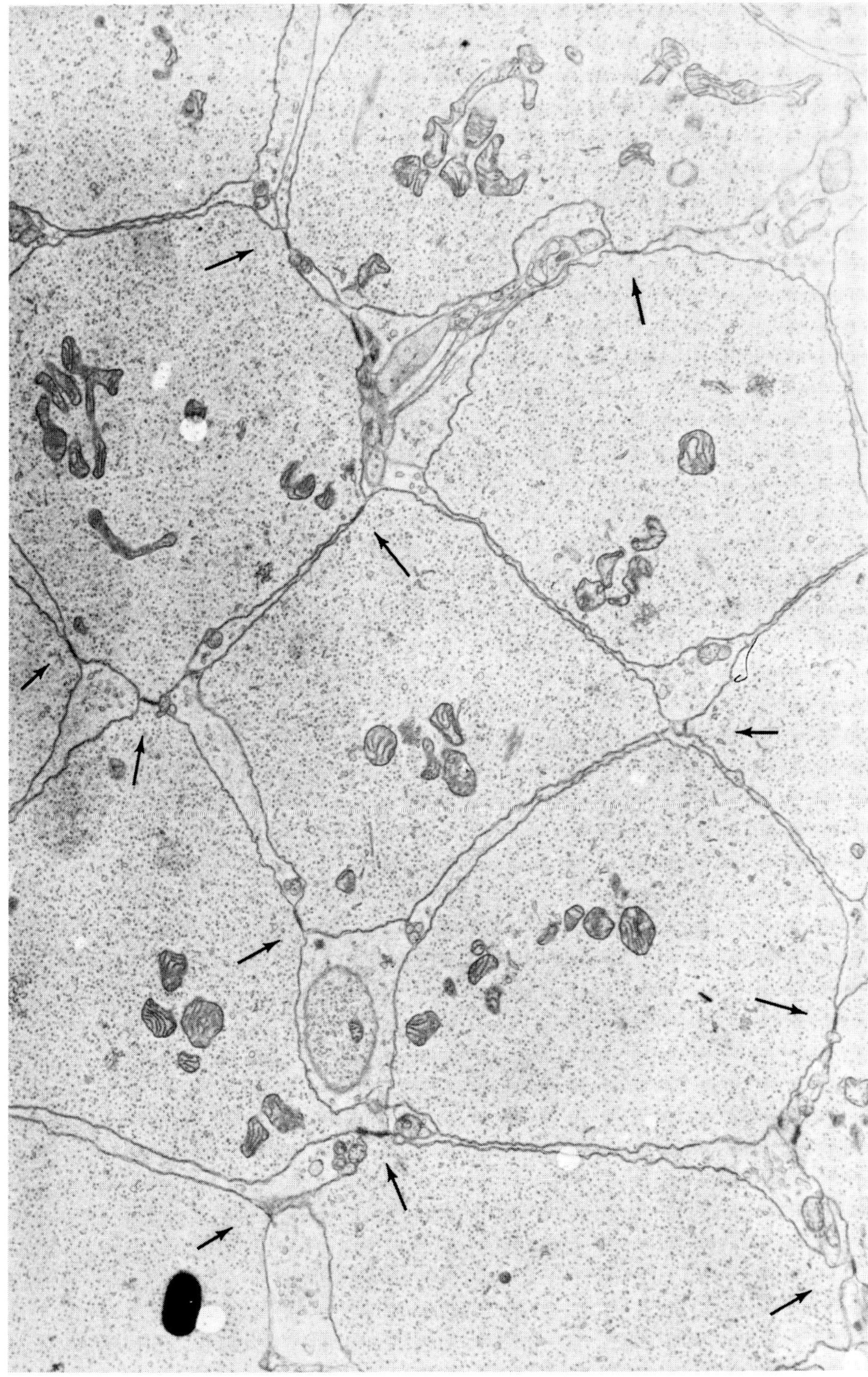

Figure 24. Section through the pedicles of human foveal cones in a parafoveal area. Note the numerous interreceptor contiguities demarked by membrane densities (arrows). Since these contacts are not confined to a single level of the pedicles, it must be appreciated that these specialized contacts constitute only a fraction of the contacts made; ×7800.

signals originating with individual foveal cones, as does their apparent content of but one of the varieties of cone pigments. The best resolution obtained approximates the distance between the centers of cones. It is not clear, however, whether this precludes all forms of interaction at receptor levels; indeed, interactions might facilitate line resolution. Little information is yet available on the electrical properties of desmosomes. Kuffler & Potter (63) studied a desmosome in the central nervous system of the leech which had a more complex structure than the desmosome at vertebrate interreceptor contacts; it joined glial and neural cells but current delivered to the glial cells did not modify the activity of the neurons to which they were joined.

Turning to the probable site of interaction between the photoreceptor and neurites of bipolar and horizontal cells, it should first be noted that neither of these second–order cells can be described as typical neurons, since no spikes have ever been reported to result from their activity. Indeed, the morphological similarities of bipolars to photoreceptors in terms of their synaptic terminals (26,35) and in the cilia-tipped Landolt clubs from some bipolars (60) predict a further resemblance in their electrical response. Dowling, Brown & Major (36) have reported the presence of synaptic vesicles, a neuronal character, in some outer plexiform synapses of horizontal cells of the cat and rabbit.

It is not clear how the photoreceptors influence the second-order cells. While the presence of vesicles suggests chemical transmission, there is no evidence for the nature of any neural humor of the receptor. The general paucity of cholinesterase staining in this area (46) would seem to suggest that acetylcholine may not be involved, but this has not been proven.

In examining the synaptic bases, the most striking observation is that the potential postsynaptic elements are for the most part deeply inserted into and enveloped by the receptor terminal, particularly in rods. This invites speculation on the importance of confining the site of interaction, which might mean that either the diffusion of a neurohumor is restricted or that there is low shunting of current. Indeed, while in most chemical synapses there is no apparent electrical coupling of pre- and postsynaptic elements (49), something of this type does occur in the chick ciliary ganglion (72), where the presynaptic element simulates a chalice or cup which tends to envelope a substantial portion of the postsynaptic element. However, there are many missing elements such as the resistances of the opposed membranes, which preclude a rational analysis of the synaptic area of receptors.

The deep insertion of neurites into the receptor bases was noted by De Robertis & Franchi (32) and Carasso (16), and later by Ladman (67), Sjöstrand (101), Lanzavecchia (68), and Cohen (18). In general, these early studies showed that in the receptor cytoplasm, opposite to the tip of the entering neurites, there was a lunate plate oriented perpendicularly to the receptor membrane (Figure 25), with the lunate concavity facing it. Ladman (67) named this object a synaptic lamella, which aptly corresponded to its three-dimensional structure, but other workers, impressed by the appearance of sections of this plate, have termed it a synaptic ribbon; both terms are still in use. It is typical of the lamella that an extension of its plane passes between the two neurites which end in apposition to it, although these can sometimes be two branches of the same process. Lanzavecchia (68) first noted that the lamella had a pentalaminate appearance in cross-section. The synaptic lamella seems to be surrounded by a clear area of 200 Å and this, in turn, by a halo of synaptic vesicles. Intervening between the lamella and the cell membrane to which it is perpendicularly oriented, there is a ribbon-like density which parallels the lamella concavity. It is of some interest that the synaptic lamella or very similar structures occur in many receptors, e.g., in hair cells of the guinea pig cochlear (104) and in lateral line receptors (3). They are also found in invertebrate eyes such as *Lycosa* (108) and in the neuropil of the lateral eye of the horseshoe crab.* Human spherules may have one to a few of these groupings of lamella and associated neurites, and separate processes of the same postsynaptic cells or branches of their neurites may participate at each junction. Pedicles have many such groupings. The complexity of the area is such that serial sectioning and other special techniques have been applied in attempts to identify the nature and disposition of the entering neurites. In addition to the pioneering study of Sjöstrand (101) on this problem, more recent investigations have been made by Missotten and his associates (74,77), Sjöstrand and Mountford (103), Stell (105,106),† and in our own laboratory.

Although in most cases neurites are believed to be involved in these arrangements, a Müller cell process has been traced into the receptor concavity in one instance (103). In spherules of guinea pigs, Sjöstrand (103) has reported a separation of the terminations of the entering processes into those ending below the lamella or ribbon (proximal processes) and those entering the spherule but not ending near the ribbon (distal processes). He recognizes subtypes with two proximal and two distal processes, others with one proximal and two distal processes, and still others with one process of each type. Where there is one proximal process, it passes beneath the lamella and faces it on both its lateral aspects; examples of this type of ending have been found in a pigeon terminal (20) and in human spherules. Although such processes may be proximal and distal with respect to the lamella, all entering processes are contiguous with the receptor membrane, as the cavitation they enter is not a simple cup but one in which evaginated fingerlike receptor processes weave among the entering elements. Sjöstrand (101) traced the distal entering neurites to bipolar cells. In an excellent study of human spherules and pedicles, Missotten (74,75) concluded that the most lateral and deeply inserted elements, proximal to the lamella, come from axon terminals of horizontal neurons, and the central and more distal elements from dendrites of bipolar cells. He felt that in cones some central elements may be horizontal cell dendrites; in spherules, he noted that the elements lateral to the synaptic lamella often had vesicles, whereas those in a similar position in cone pedicles seemed relatively free of them. The same is true in spherules and pedicles of the mouse (26) and in the alpha and beta receptors of the guinea pig (101). Missotten's belief that the lateral elements derive from horizontal cells is

* Unpublished observations.
† Also, personal communications from W. K. Stell.

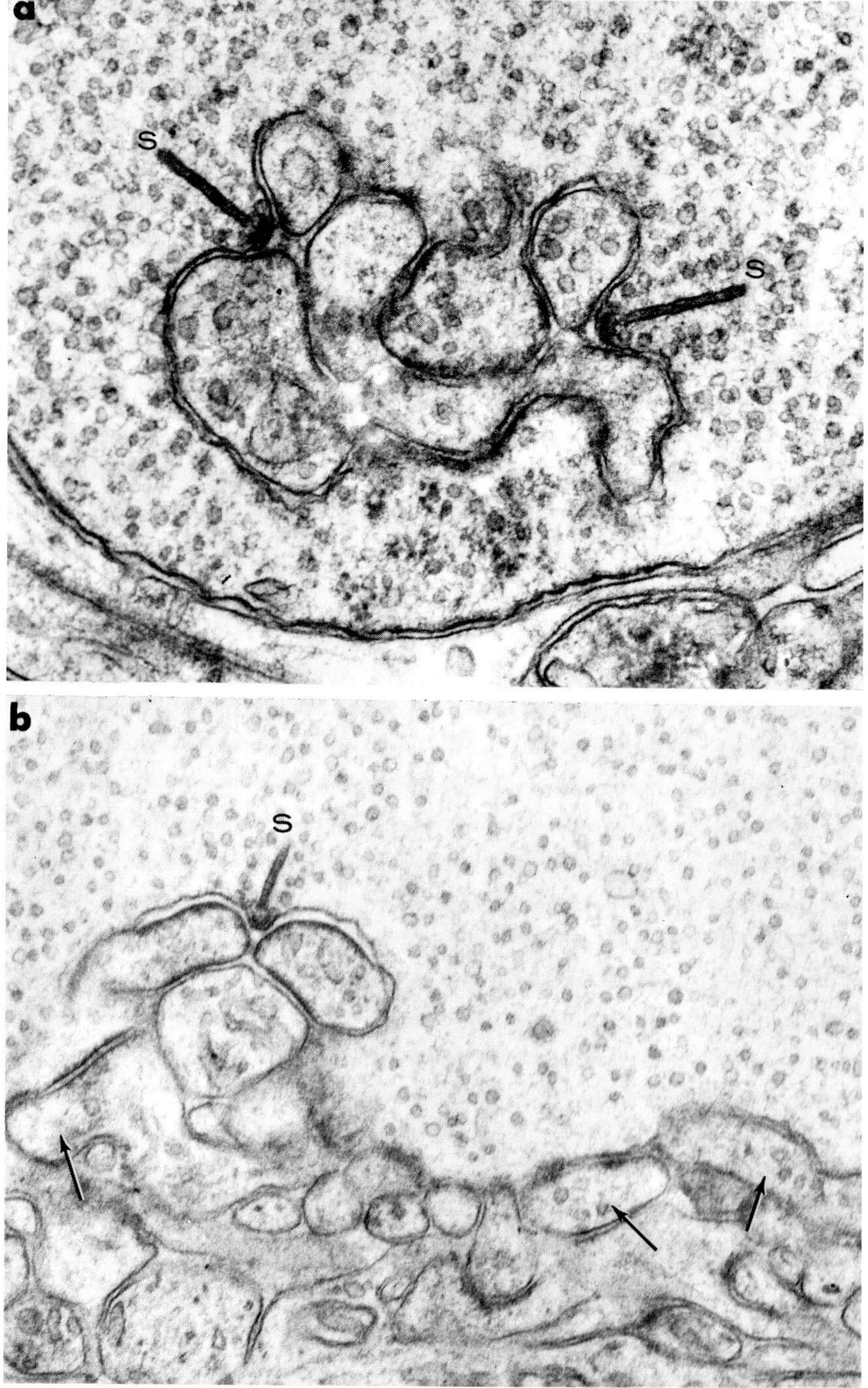

Figure 25 →

supported by the recent work of Stell (106), who carried out electron microscopy on Golgi impregnated retinas; this author, however, believes he has traced the dendrites of the horizontal cell to a lateral position. Missotten has termed the synaptic arrangements of cones "triads" because of the involvement of one central and two lateral neurites. Numerous reconstructions from serial sections in my laboratory show that the central neurites of cone synapses, as in rod synapses, are not contiguous with the cell membrane adjacent to the synaptic lamella; this applies to human material and may not be true in other species.

The tracing of fine neurites in serial sections is most unwieldy; some of the difficulties have been discussed by Pedler & Tilly (88). In general, the problem is that neurites may be thinner than 0.2 μ, change course often, and tend to smear and fuse in the electron micrographs when they parallel the section plane. The recent combined use of the Golgi and serial reconstruction methods by Stell (106) offers great promise for circumventing some of these obstacles, but the known capriciousness of the Golgi method has still to be overcome, particularly with mature nervous tissue. The Golgi procedure may also result in imperfect fixation of the background cells for electron microscopic study. Finally, the number of cells studied by these methods is so very small in comparison with the possible variations, that the question of sampling errors must be continually in mind.

Areas Needing Exploration

There are clearly a great many gaps in those morphological parameters which might pertain to the receptor function of rods and cones. With reference to the outer segments, it is necessary to explore by a variety of means whether the lumina of rod saccules and most saccules of mammalian cones are isolated from the extracellular space; an attempt should be made to confirm the observation of De Robertis & Lasansky (33) that rod saccules show osmotic expansion and shrinkage, which would indicate that they are sealed from the extracellular compartment. The manner and level of termination of the ciliary microtubules in the outer segments warrants further attention; this has not been studied at all in cones, for example. More rod outer segments should be observed in cross-section to see if the scalloping of rod saccules is a constant feature. Needless to say, it would be important to locate the pigment molecules in the saccule membrane.

More attention must be paid to the endoplasmic reticulum, microtubular, and ciliary rootlet systems to see whether any of these consistently span the receptor length in rods and cones of different species.

With reference to the receptor terminals, an attempt should be made to determine if the synaptic end organs contain a neurohumor; this could be investigated

Figure 25. *a:* Synaptic complex in a human rod spherule; note the synaptic lamellae (S) and the U-shaped densities interposed between them and the receptor membrane, also that a gel seems to hold the small vesicles in the cytoplasm off the lamella surface; it is possible that the two lamellar sections shown are portions of the same organelle; ×63,500. *b:* One of the many synaptic complexes in the pedicle of a human cone, illustrating the typical "triad" of neurites opposite each synaptic lamella (S); note the cell processes (arrows) externally contacting the pedicle; occasional vesicles may be seen in these; ×46,000.

by means of chemical assays following the isolation of the terminals, or by comparative chemical studies utilizing normal versus experimental or genetic "rodless" retinas. Further attention must be given to the identification of the neurites terminating on receptors. A particular gap in current thinking involves the identity of neurites ending superficially on cone pedicles; those interested in this problem are urged to explore serial sectioning of Golgi material for electron microscopy as a means to its solution.

SUMMARY

This review deals with those aspects of receptor morphology which may contribute to our understanding of the necessary events between light stimulation of receptors and the transmission of this information to second order neurons. The following areas are discussed: receptor structure as related to wave guiding; distinctions between rods and cones; the localization of visual pigment and the possible relation of the pigment location to polarized light studies and fast electrical potentials; the possible significance of structures within the inner segment and axon for signal transmission; the electrical significance of the absence of tight junctions between receptors and glial cells at the external limiting membrane; the occurrence of interreceptor contacts and an evaluation of whether these are of synaptic significance; a description of the receptor terminals and the contacts with second-order neurons. Among the observations cited are the absence of evidence that most outer segment saccules in rods are connected to the cell membrane or to each other, as well as some evidence to the contrary; also noted is the occurrence of extensive interreceptor contacts involving cones, or rods and cones (in humans and other species) mediated by processes from cone pedicles. The difficulty involved in trying to deduce from morphology whether these are of significance in information transmission—a conclusion which would be contrary to current physiological evidence—is also noted. Finally, deficiencies in our knowledge of receptor structure are detailed in the form of suggestions for future investigation.

REFERENCES

1. Arden, G. B., Bridges, C. D. B., Ikeda, H., and Siegel, I. M., Isolation of a new fast component of the early receptor potential. *J. Physiol.* (London), 1966, **186**: 123–124*P*.
2. Arden, G. B., and Silver, P. H., Visual thresholds and spectral sensitivities of the grey squirrel (*Sciurus carolinensis leucotis*). *J. Physiol.* (London), 1962, **163**: 540–557.
3. Barets, A., and Szabo, T., Appareil synaptique des cellules sensorielles de l'ampoule de Lorenzini chez la torpille, *Torpédo marmorata*. *J. Microscopie*, 1962, **1**: 47–54.
4. Barr, L., and Alpern, M., Photosensitivity of the frog iris. *J. Gen. Physiol.*, 1963, **46**: 1249–1265.
5. Bell, A. L., and DiStefano, H. S., Comparative fine structure of two photosensitive irises. *Anat. Rec.*, 1966, **154**: 498.

6. Blasie, J. K., Dewey, M. M., Blaurock, A. E., and Worthington, C. R., Electron microscope and low-angle X-ray diffraction studies on outer segment membranes from the retina of the frog. *J. Molec. Biol.*, 1965, **14**: 143–152.

7. Bonting, S. L., Caravaggio, L. L., and Canady, M. R., Studies of sodium-potassium-activated adenosine triphosphatase. X. Occurrence in retinal rods and relation to rhodopsin. *Exp. Eye Res.*, 1964, **3**: 47–56.

8. Brindley, G. S., and Gardner-Medwin, A. R., The origin of the early receptor potential of the retina. *J. Physiol.* (London), 1966, **182**: 185–194.

9. Brown, K. T., An early potential evoked by light from the pigment epithelium-choroid complex of the toad. *Nature* (London), 1965, **207**: 1249–1253.

10. Brown, K. T., and Watanabe, K., Isolation and identification of a receptor potential from the pure cone fovea of the monkey retina. *Nature* (London), 1962, **193**: 958–960.

11. ———, Rod receptor potential from the retina of the night monkey. *Nature* (London), 1962, **196**: 547–550.

12. Brown, P. K., Gibbons, I. R., and Wald, G., The visual cells and visual pigment of the mudpuppy, *Necturus*. *J. Cell Biol.*, 1963, **19**: 79–106.

13. Brown-Sequard, E., Recherches expérimentales sur l'influence excitatrice de la lumière, du froid, et la chaleur sur l'iris dans les cinq classes d'animaux vertébrés. *Physiol. de l'Homme et des Animaux*, 1859, **2**: 281–294; 451–460.

14. Bruecke, E., Ueber die physiologische Bedeutung der stabförmigen Körper und der Zwillingszapfen in den Augen der Wirbelthiere. *Archiv Anat. Physiol. wiss. Med.*, 1844: 444–451.

15. Bysov, A. L., and Hanitzsch, R., Die elektrischen Eigenschaften und die Struktur der R-Membran. *Vision Res.*, 1964, **4**: 483–492.

16. Carasso, N., Étude au microscope électronique des synapses des cellules visuelles chez le têtard d'*Alytes obstetricans*. *C. R. Acad. Sci.* (Paris), 1957, **245**: 216–219.

17. Carr, R. E., Ripps, H., Siegel, I. M., and Weale, R. A., Rhodopsin and the electrical activity of the retina in congenital night blindness. *Invest. Ophthal.*, 1966, **5**: 497–507.

18. Cohen, A. I., The ultrastructure of the rods of the mouse retina. *Am. J. Anat.*, 1960, **107**: 23–48.

19. ———, The fine structure of the extrafoveal receptors of the Rhesus monkey. *Exp. Eye Res.*, 1961, **1**: 128–136.

20. ———, The fine structure of the visual receptors of the pigeon. *Exp. Eye Res.*, 1963, **2**: 88–97.

21. ———, Vertebrate retinal cells and their organization. *Biol. Rev.*, 1963, **38**: 427–459.

22. ———, Some observations on the fine structure of the retinal receptors of the American gray squirrel. *Invest. Ophthal.*, 1964, **3**: 198–216.

23. ———, New details of the ultrastructure of the outer segments and ciliary connectives of the rods of human and macaque retinas. *Anat. Rec.*, 1965, **152**: 63–80.

24. ———, A possible cytological basis for the 'R' membrane in the vertebrate eye. *Nature* (London), 1965, **205**: 1222–1223.

25. ———, Some electron microscopic observations on inter-receptor contacts in the human and macaque retinae. *J. Anat.*, 1965, **99**: 595–610.

26. ———, An electron microscopic study of the modification by monosodium glutamate of the retinas of normal and "rodless" mice. *Am. J. Anat.*, 1967, **120**: 319–356.

27. Cone, R. A., The early receptor potential of the vertebrate eye. *Sympos. Quant. Biol.*, 1965, **30**: 483–490.
28. Crosby, E. C., Humphrey, T., and Lauer, E. W., *Correlative Anatomy of the Nervous System*. Macmillan, New York, 1962.
29. Dartnall, H. J. A., Visual pigment from a pure-cone retina. *Nature* (London), 1960, **188**: 475–479.
30. Denton, E. J., The contributions of the oriented photosensitive and other molecules to the absorption of whole retina. *Proc. Roy. Soc. London B.*, 1959, **150**: 78–94.
31. De Robertis, E., Electron microscope observations on the submicroscopic organization of the retinal rods. *J. Biophys. Biochem. Cytol.*, 1956, **2**: 319–330.
32. De Robertis, E., and Franchi, C. M., Electron microscope observations on synaptic vesicles in synapses of the retinal rods and cones. *Ibid.*: 307–318.
33. De Robertis, E., and Lasansky, A., Ultrastructure and chemical organization of photoreceptors. In: *The Structure of the Eye* (G. K. Smelser, Ed.). Academic Press, New York, 1961: 29–49.
34. Dowling, J. E., Visual adaptation: its mechanism. *Science*, 1967, **157**: 584–585.
35. Dowling, J. E., and Boycott, B. B., Neural connections of the retina: fine structure of the inner plexiform layer. *Sympos. Quant. Biol.*, 1965, **30**, 393–402.
36. Dowling, J. E., Brown, J. E., and Major, D., Synapses of horizontal cells in rabbit and rat retinas. *Science*, 1966, **153**: 1639–1641.
37. Dowling, J. E., and Gibbons, I. R., The effect of vitamin A deficiency on the fine structure of the retina. In: *The Structure of the Eye* (G. K. Smelser, Ed.). Academic Press, New York, 1961: 85–99.
38. ———, The fine structure of the pigment epithelium in the albino rat. *J. Cell Biol.*, 1962, **14**: 459–474.
39. Dowling, J. E., and Wald, G., Vitamin A deficiency and night blindness. *Proc. Nat. Acad. Sci. USA*, 1958, **44**: 648–661.
40. Droz, B., Synthesis and migration of proteins in the visual cells of rats and mice. *Anat. Rec.*, 1961, **139**: 222.
41. ———, Dynamic condition of proteins in the visual cells of rats and mice as shown by radioautography with labeled amino acids. *Anat. Rec.*, 1963, **145**: 157–168.
42. Edsall, J. T., and Wyman, J., *Biophysical Chemistry* (Vol. I). Academic Press, New York, 1958.
43. Enoch, J. M., Waveguide modes: are they present, and what is their role in the visual mechanism? *J. Opt. Soc. Amer.*, 1960, **50**: 1025–1026.
44. ———, The use of tetrazolium to distinguish between retinal receptors exposed and not exposed to light. *Invest. Ophthal.*, 1963, **2**: 16–23.
45. ———, Validation of an indicator of mammalian retinal receptor response: density of stain as a function of stimulus magnitude. *J. Opt. Soc. Amer.*, 1966, **56**: 116–123.
46. Eränkö, O., Niemi, M., and Merenmies, E., Histochemical observations on esterases and oxidative enzymes of the retina. In: *The Structure of the Eye* (G. K. Smelser, Ed.). Academic Press, New York, 1961: 159–171.
47. Falk, G., and Fatt, P., Photoconductive changes in a suspension of rod outer segments. *J. Physiol.* (London), 1963, **167**: 36–37*P*.
48. ———, Rapid hydrogen ion uptake of rod outer segments and rhodopsin solutions on illumination. *J. Physiol.* (London), 1966, **183**: 211–224.

49. Fatt, P., and Katz, B., An analysis of the end-plate potential recorded with an intra-cellular electrode. *J. Physiol.* (London), 1951, **115**: 320–370.
50. Feeney, L., Grieshaber, J. A., and Hogan, M. J., Studies on human ocular pigment. In: *The Structure of the Eye; II. Symposium* (J. W. Rohen, Ed.). Schattauer, Stuttgart, 1965: 535–548.
51. Fine, B. S., and Zimmerman, L. E., Observations on the rod and cone layer of the human retina; a light and electron microscopic study. *Invest. Ophthal.*, 1963, **2**: 446–459.
52. Frank, R. N., and Goldsmith, T. H., Adenosine triphosphatase activity in the rod outer segments of the pig's retina. *Arch. Biochem. Biophys.*, 1965, **110**: 517–525.
53. Goldstein, E. B., Early receptor potential of the isolated frog (*Rana pipiens*) retina. *Vision Res.*, 1967, **7**: 837–845.
54. Gouras, P., Duplex function in the gray squirrel's electroretinogram. *Nature* (London), 1964, **203**: 767–768.
55. Granit, R., Retina and optic nerve. In: *The Eye, Vol. 2: The Visual Process* (H. Davson, Ed.). Academic Press, New York, 1962: 541–574.
56. Hagins, W. A., Electrical signs of information flow in photoreceptors. *Sympos. Quant. Biol.*, 1965, **30**: 403–418.
57. Hagins, W. A., and Jennings, W. H., Radiationless migration of electronic excitation in retinal rods. *Faraday Soc. Disc.*, 1959, **27**: 180–190.
58. Hara, T., The effect of illumination on the electrical conductance of rhodopsin solutions. *J. Gen. Physiol.*, 1958, **41**: 857–877.
59. Hellner, K. A., Das adaptive Verhalten der Mäusenetzhaut. *Graefe Arch. klin. exp. Ophthal.*, 1966, **169**: 166–175.
60. Hendrickson, A., Landolt's club in the amphibian retina: a Golgi and electron microscopic study. *Invest. Ophthal.*, 1966, **5**: 484-496.
61. Karli, P., Les dégénérescences rétiniennes spontanées et expérimentales chez l'animal. *Progr. Ophthal.*, 1963, **14**: 51–89.
62. Karli, P., Stoeckel, M. E., and Porte, A., Dégénérescence des cellules visuelles photoréceptrices et persistance d'une sensibilité de la rétine a la stimulation photique. Observations au microscope électronique. *Zschr. Zellforsch.*, 1965, **65**: 238–252.
63. Kuffler, S. W., and Potter, D. D., Glia in the leech central nervous system: physiological properties and neuron-glia relationship. *J. Neurophysiol.*, 1964, **27**: 290–320.
64. Kühne, W., *On the Photochemistry of the Retina and on Visual Purple.* Macmillan, London, 1878.
65. Kuwabara, T., Microtubules in the retina. In: *The Structure of the Eye; II. Symposium* (J. W. Rohen, Ed.). Schattauer, Stuttgart, 1965: 69–84.
66. Laatsch, R. H., and Cowan, W. M., Electron microscopic studies of the dentate gyrus of the rat. I. Normal structure with special reference to synaptic organization. *J. Comp. Neurol.*, 1966, **128**: 359–396.
67. Ladman, A. J., The fine structure of the rod-bipolar cell synapse in the retina of the albino rat. *J. Biophys. Biochem. Cytol.*, 1958, **4**: 459–466.
68. Lanzavecchia, G., Ultrastruttura dei coni e dei bastoncelli della retina di *Xenopus laevis. Arch. Ital. Anat. Embriol.*, 1950, **65**: 417–435.
69. Lasansky, A., Functional implications of structural findings in retinal glial cells. *Progr. Brain Res.*, 1965, **15**: 48–72.

70. Lasansky, A., and de Fisch, F. W., Studies on the function of the pigment epithelium in relation to ionic movement between retina and chorioid. In: *The Structure of the Eye; II. Symposium* (J. W. Rohen, Ed.). Schattauer, Stuttgart, 1965: 139–144.

71. Lettvin, J. Y., Platt, J. R., Wald, G., and Brown, K. T., General discussion: early receptor potential. *Sympos. Quant. Biol.*, 1965, **30**: 501–504.

72. Martin, A. R., and Pilar, G., Dual mode of synaptic transmission in the avian ciliary ganglion. *J. Physiol.* (London), 1963, **168**: 443–463.

73. McConnell, D., and Scarpelli, D. G., Rhodopsin: an enzyme. *Science*, 1963, **139**: 848.

74. Missotten, L., L'ultrastructure des tissus oculaires. *Bull. Soc. Belg. Ophtal.*, 1964, **136**: 1–204.

75. ———, *The Ultrastructure of the Human Retina*. Arscia, Brussels, 1965.

76. Missotten, L., Appelmans, M., and Michiels, J., L'ultra-structure des synapses des cellules visuelles de la rétine humaine. *Bull. Soc. Franc. Ophtal.*, 1963, **76**: 59–82.

77. Missotten, L., deHauwere, E., and Guzik, A., L'ultrastructure de la rétine humaine. A propos des cellules bipolaires et leur synapses. *Bull. Soc. Belg. Ophtal.*, 1964, **137**: 277–293.

78. Moody, M. F., Photoreceptor organelles in animals. *Biol. Rev.*, 1964, **39**: 43–86.

79. Moody, M. F., and Robertson, J. D., The fine structure of some retinal photoreceptors. *J. Biophys. Biochem. Cytol.*, 1960, **7**: 87–92.

80. Mountford, S., Effects of light and dark adaptation on the vesicle populations of receptor-bipolar synapses. *J. Ultrastruct. Res.*, 1963, **9**: 403–418.

81. ———, Filamentous organelles in receptor-bipolar synapses of the retina. *J. Ultrastruct. Res.*, 1964, **10**: 207–216.

82. Nilsson, S. E. G., A globular substructure of the retinal receptor outer segment membranes and some other cell membranes in the tadpole. *Nature* (London), 1964, **202**: 509–510.

83. ———, Interreceptor contacts in the retina of the frog (*Rana pipiens*). *J. Ultrastruct. Res.*, 1964, **11**: 147–165.

84. ———, The ultrastructure of the receptor outer segments in the retina of the leopard frog (*Rana pipiens*). *J. Ultrastruct. Res.*, 1965, **12**: 207–231.

85. Noell, W. K., Walker, V. S., Kang, B. S., and Berman, S., Retinal damage by light in rats. *Invest. Ophthal.*, 1966, **5**: 450–473.

86. Nover, A., and Schultze, B., Autoradiographische Untersuchung über den Eiweissstoffwechsel in den Geweben und Zellen des Auges. (Untersucht mit S^{35}-Thio-Aminosäuren, C^{14}-Aminosäuren, H^{3}-Leucin an Maus, Ratte und Kaninchen.) *Graefe Arch. klin. exp. Ophthal.*, 1960, **161**: 554–578.

87. Pak, W. L., and Ebrey, T. G., Visual receptor potential observed at sub-zero temperatures. *Nature* (London), 1965, **205**: 484–486.

88. Pedler, C. M. H., and Tilly, R., The serial reconstruction of a complex receptor synapse. In: *The Structure of the Eye; II. Symposium* (J. W. Rohen, Ed.). Schattauer, Stuttgart, 1965: 29–53.

89. Pirenne, M. H., Visual acuity. In: *The Eye, Vol. 2: The Visual Process* (H. Davson, Ed.). Academic Press, New York, 1962: 175–195.

90. Polyak, S. L., *The Retina*. Univ. of Chicago Press, Chicago, 1941.

91. Porter, K. R., The submicroscopic morphology of protoplasm. *Harvey Lect.*, 1956, **51**: 175–228.

92. Porter, K. R., and Yamada, E., Studies on the endoplasmic reticulum. V. Its form and differentiation in pigment epithelial cells of the frog retina. *J. Biophys. Biochem. Cytol.*, 1960, **8**: 181–205.

93. Robertson, J. D., A possible ultrastructural correlate of function in the frog retinal rod. *Proc. Nat. Acad. Sci. USA*, 1965, **53**: 860–866.

94. ———, Granulo-fibrillar and globular structure in unit membranes. *Ann. N. Y. Acad. Sci.*, 1966, **137**: 421–440.

95. Rosenberg, B., Orlando, R. A., and Orlando, J. M., Photoconduction and semiconduction in dried receptors of sheep eyes. *Arch. Biochem. Biophys.*, 1961, **93**: 395–398.

96. Schmidt, W. J., Polarisationsoptische Analyse eines Eiweiss-Lipoid Systems, erläutert am Aussenglied der Sehzellen. *Kolloid Zschr.*, 1938, **85**: 137–148.

97. Schultze, M., Zur Anatomie und Physiologie der Retina. *Arch. mikr. Anat.*, 1866, **2**: 175–286.

98. Silver, P. H., A Purkinje shift in the spectral sensitivity of grey squirrels. *J. Physiol.* (London), 1966, **186**: 439–450.

99. Sjöstrand, F. S., The ultrastructure of the outer segments of rods and cones of the eye as revealed by the electron microscope. *J. Cell Comp. Physiol.*, 1953, **42**: 15–44.

100. ———, The ultrastructure of the inner segments of the retinal rods of the guinea pig eye as revealed by electron microscopy. *Ibid.*: 45–70.

101. ———, Ultrastructure of retinal rod synapses of the guinea pig eye as revealed by three-dimensional reconstructions from serial sections. *J. Ultrastruct. Res.*, 1958, **2**: 122–170.

102. ———, Fine structure of cytoplasm; the organization of membranous layers. In: *Biophysical Science—A Study Program* (J. L. Oncley et al., Eds.). Wiley, New York, 1959: 301–318.

103. ———, The synaptology of the retina. In: *Colour Vision, Physiology and Experimental Psychology* (A. V. S. de Reuck and J. Knight, Eds.). Churchill, London, 1965: 110–151.

104. Smith, C. A., and Sjöstrand, F. S., A synaptic structure in the hair cells of the guinea pig cochlea. *J. Ultrastruct. Res.*, 1961, **5**: 184–192.

105. Stell, W. K., Correlated light and electron microscope observations on Golgi preparations of goldfish retina. *J. Cell Biol.*, 1964, **23**: 89a.

106. ———, Correlation of retinal cytoarchitecture and ultrastructure in Golgi preparations. *Anat. Res.*, 1965, **153**: 389–398.

107. Tomita, T., Electrophysiological study of the mechanisms subserving color coding in the fish retina. *Ibid.*: 559–566.

108. Trujillo-Cenóz, O., Some aspects of the structural organization of the arthropod eye. *Ibid.*: 371–382.

109. Wald, G., Mechanism of vision. In: *Nerve Impulse; Transactions of the Fourth Conference* (D. Nachmanson, Ed.). Josiah Macy, Jr. Foundation, 1954: 11–57.

110. Wald, G., Brown, P. K., and Gibbons, I. R., Visual excitation: a chemo-anatomical study. *Symp. Soc. Exp. Biol.*, 1962, **16**: 32–57.

111. Walls, G. L., *The Vertebrate Eye and Its Adaptive Radiation.* Cranbrook Press, Bloomfield Hills, 1942.

112. Weale, R. A., Molecular and fine structure of receptors; discussion secretary's report. In: *Recent Progress in Photobiology* (E. J. Bower, Ed.). Blackwell, Oxford, 1965: 153–157.

113. Webster, H. deF., and Ames, A., Reversible and irreversible changes in the fine structure of nervous tissue during oxygen and glucose deprivation. *J. Cell Biol.*, 1965, **26**: 885–909.

114. Yamada, E., Tokuyasu, K., and Iwaki, S., The fine structure of retina studied with electron microscope. II. Pigment epithelium and capillaries of the choriocapillary layer. *J. Electron Micr.* (Tokyo), 1958, **6**: 42–46.

115. Young, R. W., Renewal of photoreceptor outer segments. *Anat. Rec.*, 1965, **151**: 484.

116. — —, Further studies on the renewal of photoreceptor outer segments. *Anat. Rec.*, 1966, **154**: 446.

THE OUTER PLEXIFORM LAYER AND THE NEURAL ORGANIZATION OF THE RETINA

A Circuit Anatomy Analysis
A New Approach to the Study of Nervous Centers Applied to the Retina

FRITIOF S. SJÖSTRAND
University of California
Los Angeles, California

The Principle of Detailed Circuitry Analysis of Nervous Centers

In order to understand the functioning of an electronic circuit, knowledge of the elements involved and of the connections between them is necessary. A diagram of such a circuit is read by following the wiring pattern and connections of the basic elements—resistors, condensers, diodes, and so on. The type of elements and their physical characteristics provide additional information which further elucidates the behavior of the circuit on a given input signal.

The neuronal centers in the retina and in the brain resemble electronic circuits in that they consist of well-defined elements, the neurons, and of a more or less complicated coupling of neurons through dendrites and axons. An understanding of the functioning of such neuronal circuits could be attained through the knowledge of the circuit diagrams involved. The tracing of the diagrams of nervous centers requires the determination of the numbers of neurons involved and of the connections between them and the input and output sides of the circuit. The circuit could then be imitated by means of computer techniques, and the imitation circuit activated; in the absence of any information regarding the physical properties of the various neurons and interneuronal contacts, it could be made to respond in an almost infinite number of ways—for instance, inhibitory and excitatory connections could be introduced with no restrictions as to their distribution. Knowledge of the electrical behavior of such a circuit at some points (test points) when a defined input signal is activating the circuit would reduce the number of ways in which the imitating circuit could be activated to only those alternatives leading to the proper electrical responses at the analogs of the test points in the imitating circuit. If the electrical events at a sufficient number of test points were known, then only one or very few alternative ways to activate the imitation circuit would remain that would satisfy all the known conditions. In such a situation it should be possible to define the physical properties of the various elements of the circuit; the functioning of the circuit could then be understood.

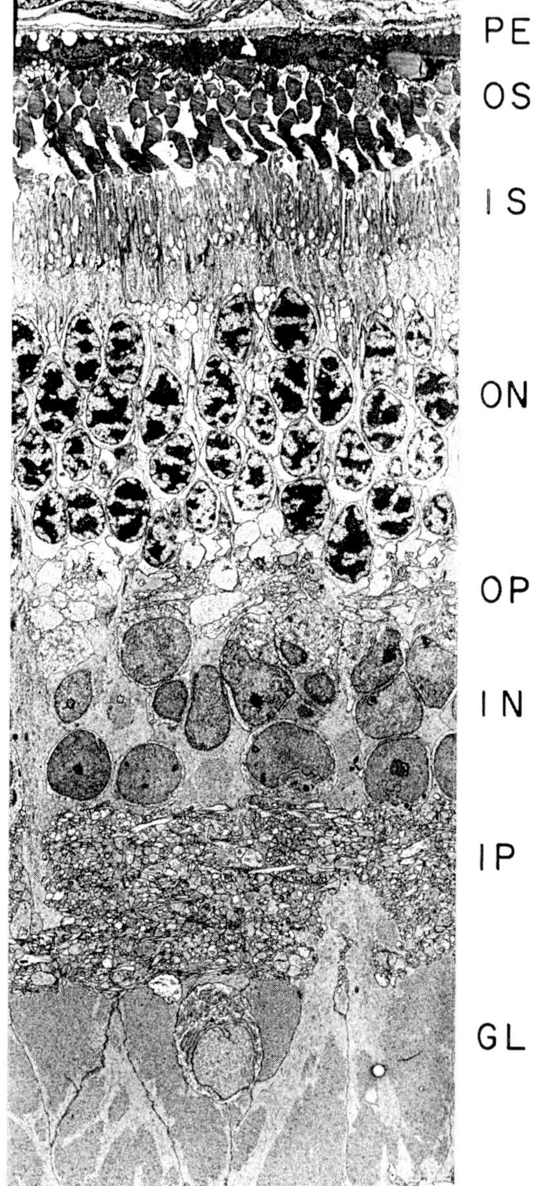

Figure 26. Survey picture of cross section through the rabbit retina. From top to bottom: choroid layer and pigment epithelium (*PE*); layer of the outer segments (*OS*) of the receptor cells; the inner segments (*IS*); outer nuclear layer (*ON*); outer plexiform layer (*OP*); inner nuclear layer (*IN*); inner plexiform layer (*IP*); and ganglion cell layer (*GL*), represented by a single ganglion cell embedded in the foot processes of the Müller cells, the equivalent of the glial cells in the central nervous system. Note the extensive convergence in the retinal circuity in this part of the rabbit retina, reflected in the successive reduction of conducting elements in the direction, receptor cells to ganglion cells. × 1700. (From Sjöstrand & Nilsson, 11.)

Two sets of information are thus needed to construct the circuit diagram—the structural organization of the circuit, represented by the number of neurons as well as the interneuronal contact relations, and the electrical behavior of the circuit at a certain number of points in it. The first set of information can be obtained by means of three-dimensional reconstructions of nervous centers from extensive series of serial sections photographed in the electron microscope. The second can be collected by electrophysiological recordings, using microelectrodes under conditions where the position of the tip of the microelectrode in relation to the elementary components of the circuit is known.

During the last ten years our laboratory has been involved in a project aimed at discovery of the limitations of the technique for revealing the three-dimensional structure of nervous centers. Both the retina and a brain center such as the lateral geniculate body were used as material for this exploratory work. In the case of the retina, the most delicate structural elements—the branches of bipolar and horizontal cells and of the β-type receptor cells—are very thin, and the volume of tissue containing the complete basic circuits is limited. On the other hand, the structural components to be traced in the lateral geniculate body are coarser, and the three-dimensional extension of the circuits is greater than in the retina. The minimum size of a structure that can be traced with exactitude in three dimensions and the total volume of tissue that can be analyzed by this technique are the two basic factors that must be experimentally determined in order to establish whether three-dimensional reconstructions can be applied on a sufficiently large scale to make nervous centers available for more than fragmentary analysis.

Our experience clearly indicates that there are no major technical limitations on the volume of tissue that can be analyzed in three dimensions which would prevent the study of nervous centers with this technique. Time is the main restricting factor, making such studies the task of only particularly devoted researchers. However, modifications in the design of the electron microscope and new techniques for the analysis of the photographic recordings should keep the time factor within reasonable limits.

In addition to the higher resolution of electron microscopy, the great advantage of the three-dimensional reconstruction of nervous centers from electron micrographs, as compared with light microscopic neuroanatomy, is the capability of reconstructing all neuronal and glial elements at the same time. Light microscopic neuroanatomy, on the other hand, allows visualization of isolated elements—neurons or glial cells—but affords no guarantee of the completeness of the presentation and no opportunity to observe the finest neuronal branches nor the situation at the points of interneuronal contact. The diagram published by Polyak (2), based on such information obtained from analysis of the retina, is not a true circuit diagram but a composite picture constructed to illustrate in compact form all the elements that have been observed when analyzing a large number of specimens. The same limitation applies to diagrams—such as the one presented by Dowling & Boycott (1)—constructed on the basis of fragmentary information from electron microscopic analysis of nervous centers. The detailed and precise elucidation of contact relations in nervous centers sought in our

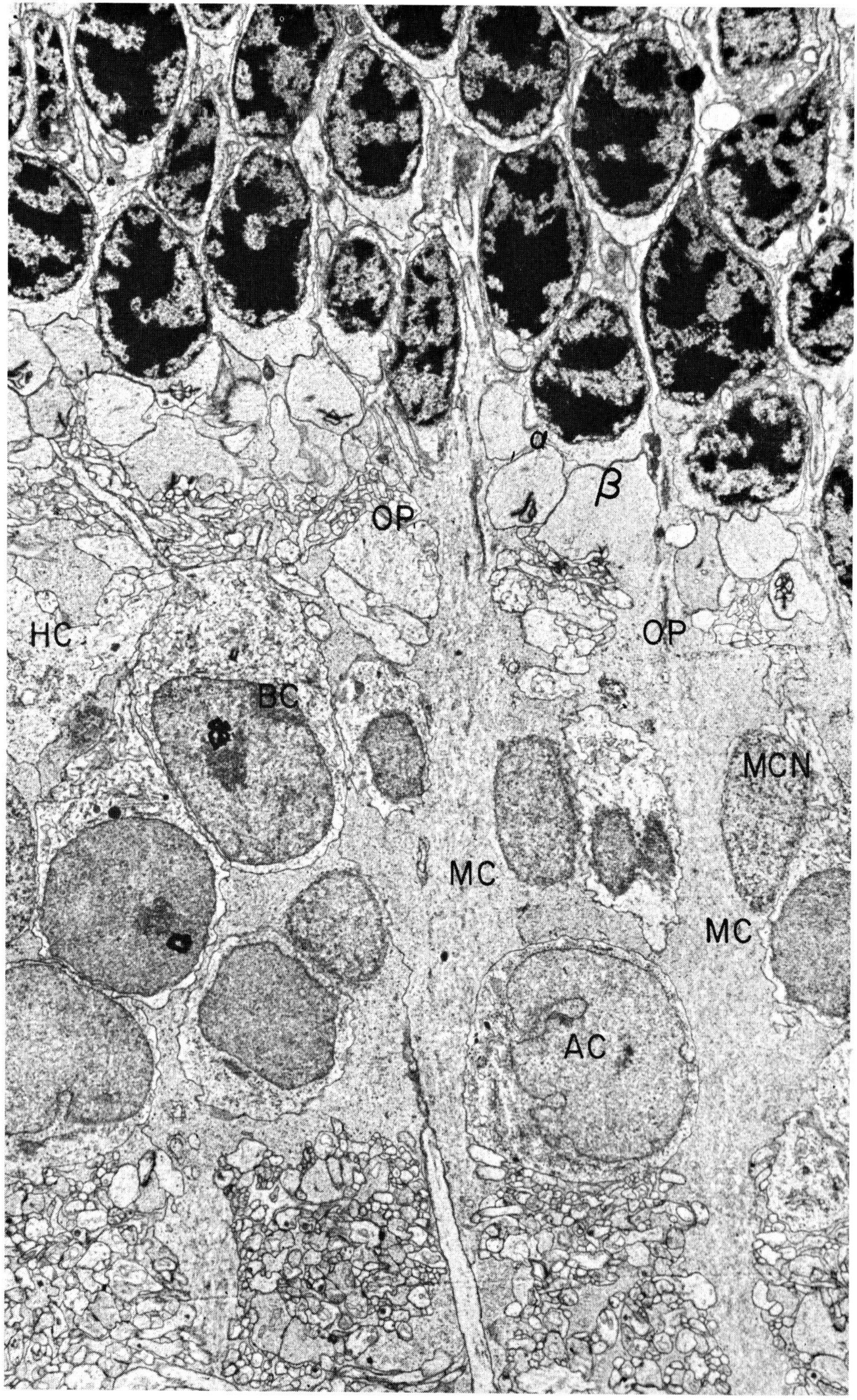

Figure 26 →

studies represents therefore a new approach to the analysis of the central nervous system. Information collected in such studies will be so directly related to function that distinction between physiological and anatomical information will cease to have meaning.

Lateral Connections Between Receptor Cells

Our most extensive three-dimensional analysis of nervous centers has involved the outer plexiform layer of the retina. It was found that the circuitry starts becoming complicated at the receptor cell level, owing to the direct lateral connections between receptor cells, as discovered by Sjöstrand (8). Two types of receptor cells, α and β, (4,6,7) could be identified in the guinea pig retina, assumed to be a pure rod retina. Figures 26–28 show these two types in the rabbit retina.

The α- and β-type receptor cells are distinguished by the shape of their synaptic bodies, which in α-type cells (Figures 28,29) are ovoid in shape. Sometimes the synaptic structures are located close to the cell nucleus when this is positioned at the vitread end of the receptor cell (Figure 28). The β-type receptor cells (Figures 28,29) are characterized by a conical synaptic body, with the base of the cone facing the neuropil of the outer plexiform layer and the top of the cone continuous with the rod fiber. The structure of the synaptic bodies (3–8) is more complex in the β- than in the α-type cells. Other parts of the receptor cells were found to be basically identical in structure in both types of cells in the guinea pig retina.

From the edges of the broad base of the β-type receptor cells, processes extend laterally (Figures 29–31) to make contact with the vitread pole of several surrounding α-type receptor cells, as well as with the dendritic end branches from bipolar cells which make synaptic connections with these receptor cells (8). These processes also make contact with the lateral surface of the synaptic body of the α-type cells (Figures 30,32,33). This contact is restricted to a limited area of the synaptic body, and each α-type synaptic body appears to be contacted by only one β-type receptor cell in this manner, while several β-type cells make contact with each α-type cell at the vitread pole of the synaptic body. Later studies by Sjöstrand and Mountford (9) have shown that some of these lateral branches reached only a short distance to contact some of the more adjacent α-type receptor cells, while other processes passed by several rows of α-type receptor cells to contact those located farther away (Figure 32). One β-type receptor cell sends out a number of such lateral branches, and each α-type receptor cell was found to be contacted by branches from three to four β-type receptor cells (8), located at varying distances and in different directions from the α-type cell (Figures 33,34) (9,10).

Figure 27. Rabbit retina, outer plexiform layer (*OP*) between the inner portion of the outer nuclear layer and the inner nuclear layer; part of the inner plexiform layer is shown. In the outer plexiform layer synaptic bodies of the α- and β-type receptor cells are seen. Below the synaptic bodies, branches from bipolar cells are mixed with branches from horizontal cells and lateral branches from the β-type receptor cell. Bipolar cell with two branches (*BC*), horizontal cell (*HC*); Müller cell (*MC*) with cell nucleus (*MCN*); amacrine cell (*AC*). ×6000.

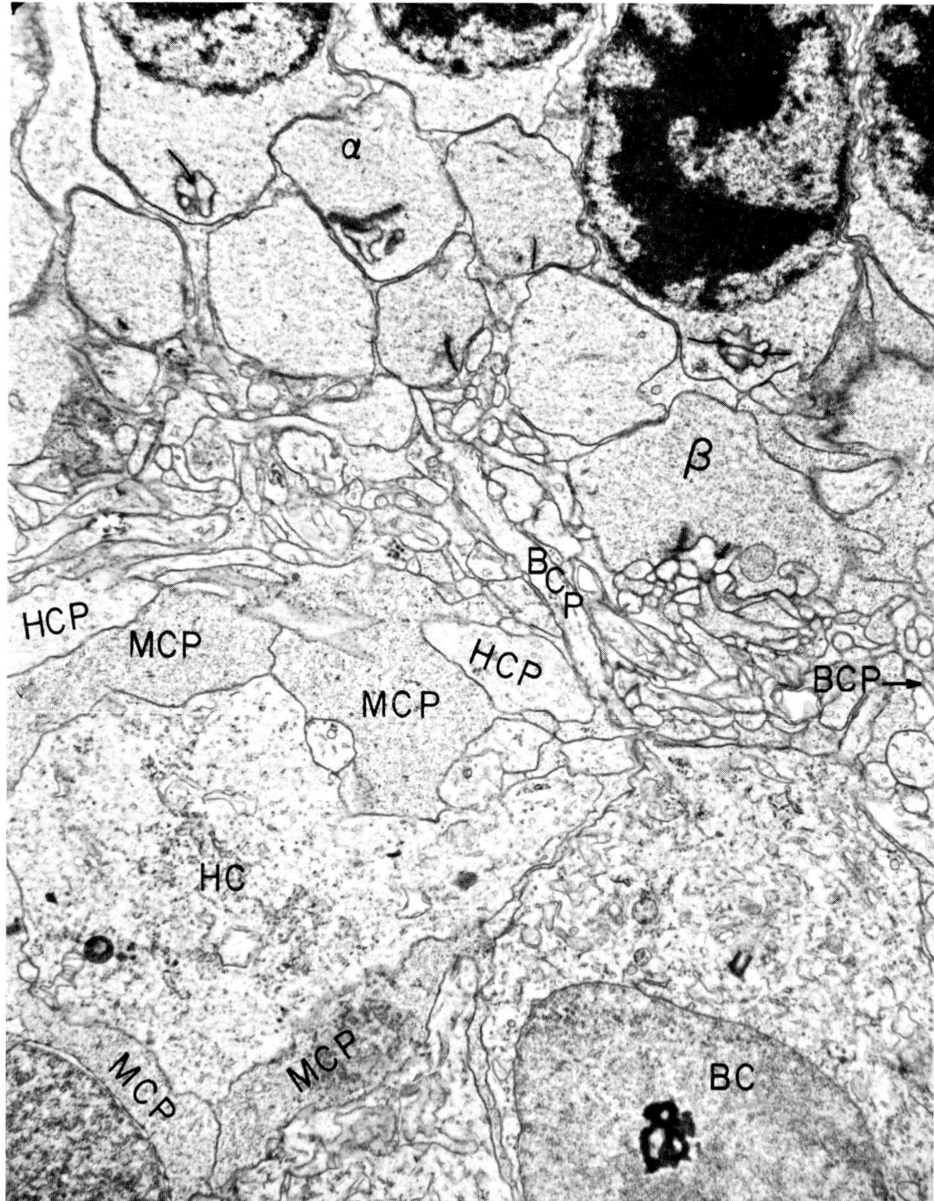

Figure 28. Rabbit retina; higher magnification of outer plexiform layer with its main components: α- and β-type receptor cell synaptic bodies, bipolar cell (*BC*) with processes (*BCP*), horizontal cell (*HC*), horizontal cell processes (*HCP*), Müller cell processes (*MCP*). × 13,000.

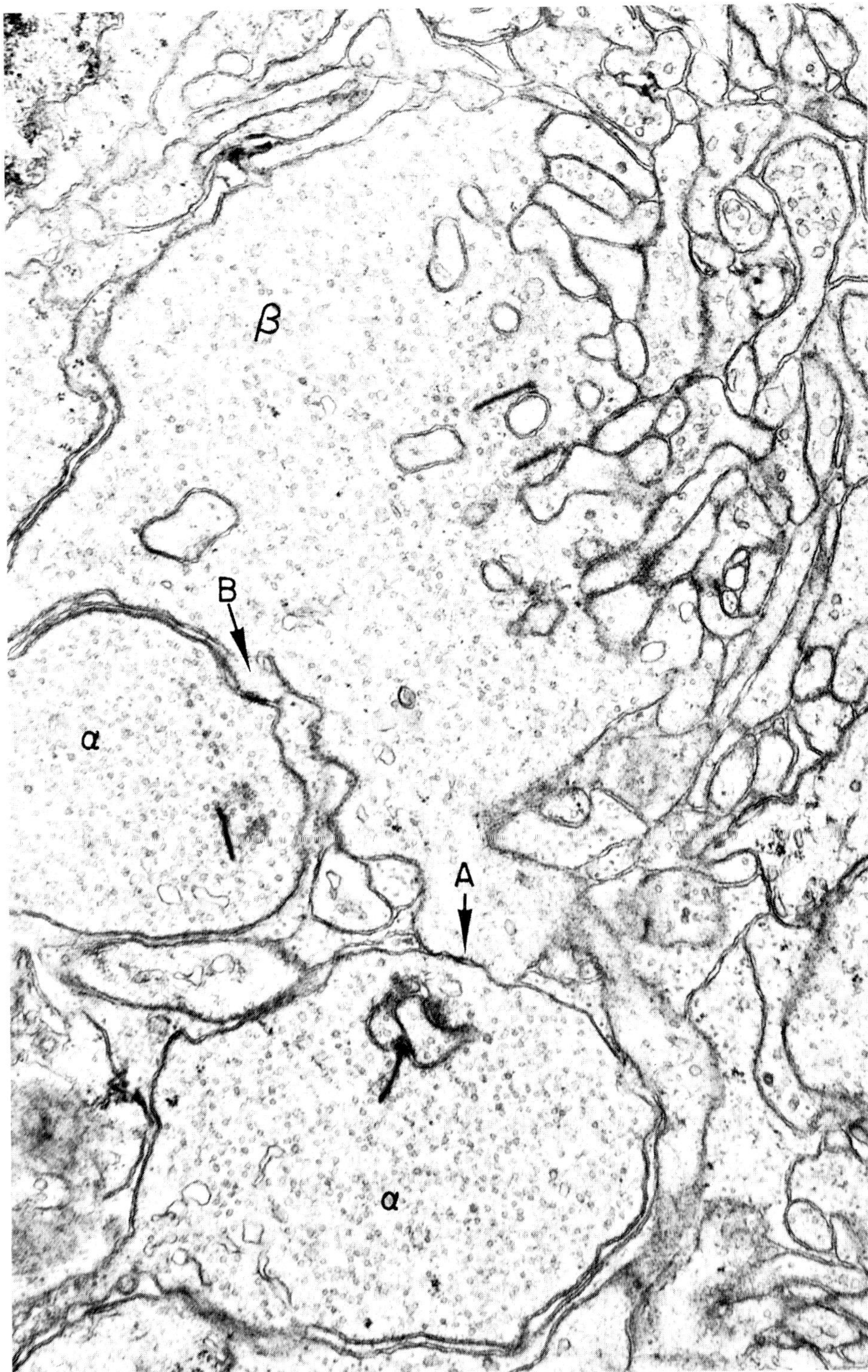

Figure 29. Rabbit retina; one β-type receptor cell synaptic body and two α-type receptor cell synaptic bodies. Lateral process of the β-type cell synaptic body extends laterally to make contact with one of the α-type cell synaptic bodies (arrow *A*). A short process also contacts the other α-type cell synaptic body (arrow *B*). $\times 36{,}000$.

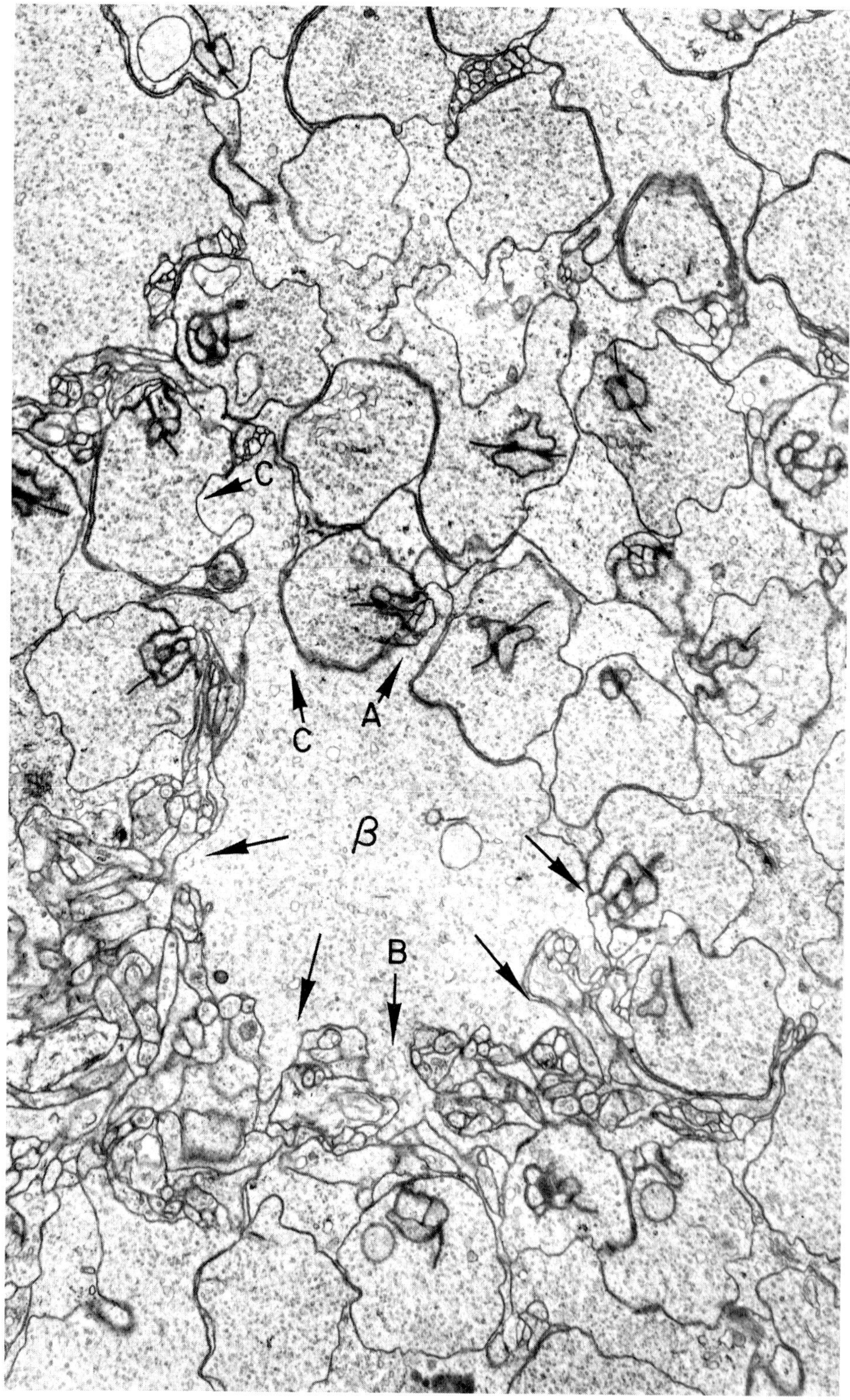

Figure 30 →

In addition to lateral connections between β- and α-type receptor cells, the β-type cells are mutually connected by lateral processes (9,10), thus forming a network of interconnected receptor cells. Furthermore, the β-type cells appear to be arranged in pairs in the area reconstructed in Figure 34. Figure 35 shows a contact between two adjacent β-type receptor cells forming such a pair; in this case, a process extending from the cell to the left is invaginated in the synaptic body of the β-type receptor cell to the right. In Figures 36 and 37 a process from the β-type cell in the lower part of the picture makes contact with two cells—one β-type cell (upper portion of the figure) and one α-type cell. In the latter case the first β-type cell contacts the lateral surface of the α-type synaptic body, from which a process is received in an invagination of the plasma membrane of the β-type cell; only one of the β-type cells enters into this kind of contact relation with the α-type cell—other β-type cells contact the synaptic body of the α-type cell at its vitread pole, where the processes from bipolar cells enter the synaptic body invagination. Figure 38 shows the relationship between these three cells further up in a scleral direction in the series of sections; the β-type receptor cell in the upper part of the picture makes contacts with one α-type receptor cell through a lateral process. One of the processes of this β-type cell extending upward in Figure 36 can be followed in Figure 39, where it passes two α-type receptor cells while making contact with their surfaces close to the area where the bipolar cell processes enter the synaptic invaginations.

The lateral processes from the β-type cells characteristically make contact with the α-type cells within limited areas. The main part of the processes are separated from α-type cell synaptic bodies and from branches of bipolar and horizontal cells by the interposition of a layer formed by Müller cell processes. It is also characteristic that the lateral processes seek their way to the vitread pole of the α-type receptor cells, where the plasma membrane of the synaptic body is invaginated to receive end branches from bipolar and horizontal cells. The only exceptions are the contacts between β-type cell processes and the lateral surface of the α-type cells; these contacts also show striking order and regularity, reflected in the fact that the α-type cells are involved in only one such contact, while they are contacted by several β-type cells at the pole of their synaptic bodies.

We are undoubtedly dealing with a system of lateral connections between receptor cells furnished by the β-type cells, which are arranged in a highly organized and systematic way. The ordered arrangement of these contacts makes it unlikely their being due to occasional defective covering by Müller cell processes of closely packed receptor cells, whether anatomically determined or dependent on artifactual shrinkage of the Müller cells.

The lateral processes of the β-type receptor cells always contain synaptic vesicles at their ends, even though in the long processes a large section between

Figure 30. Rabbit retina; β-type cell synaptic body in cross section (section oriented tangential to the surface of the retina). Several processes (arrows) extend laterally toward surrounding α-type cell synaptic bodies. Two of these processes (*A*, *B*) are seen making contact with the vitread pole of two α-type cell synaptic bodies; one contacts the lateral surface of a third α-type cell synaptic body (*C*). × 16,000.

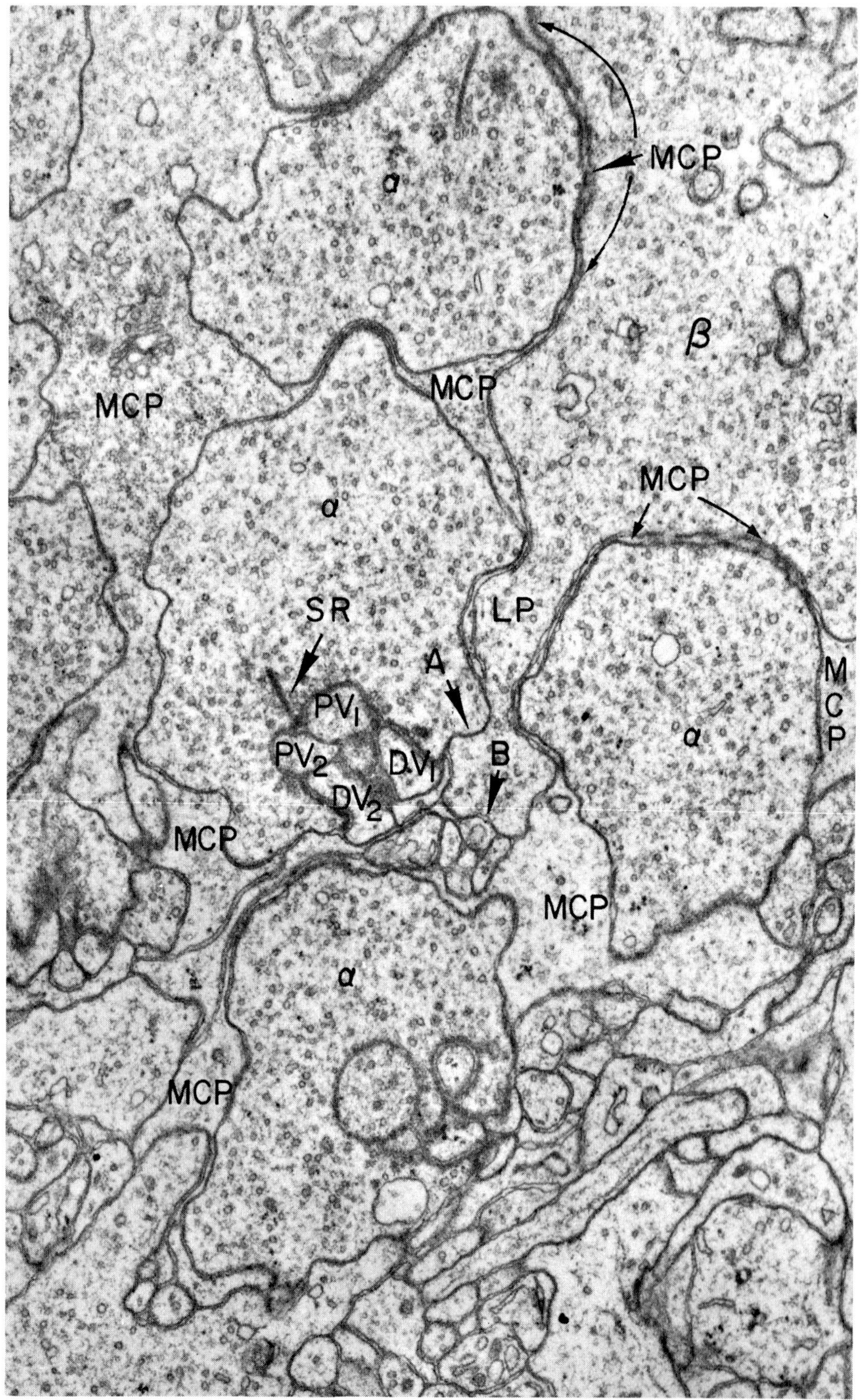

Figure 31 →

the main part of the synaptic body and the ending can be free from typical synaptic vesicles. Indeed, these sections of the lateral processes can be identified as originating from β-type cells only by tracing the processes to their origin.

It would appear strangely nihilistic not to ascribe an important functional significance to this elaborate system of lateral connections at the receptor cell level. It would also seem impossible to assume any function for these connections without accepting their influence on the response of the receptor cells to light stimuli. A mutual influence or a one-directional influence would be a reasonable assumption. The fact that the lateral processes from β-type cells enter into direct contact relations with both the α-type receptor cells and the end branches of the bipolar cells at the vitread pole of the α-type synaptic bodies can be interpreted in favor of the influence of the β-type cells on the other elements.

A possible reciprocal influence by the α-type receptor cells on the β-type cells cannot be excluded. Particularly the considerably larger contact areas between these two types of cells at the lateral surface of the α-type cells might mean functionally a contact where the direction of influence is predominantly from the α- to the β-type cells. These contacts can definitely be differentiated from those at the vitread pole of the α-type cells through their position and their considerably larger surface area.

On the theory that the structural connections between receptor cells have a functional significance, it can be assumed that these contacts are transferring either excitatory or inhibitory influences. The lateral connections between receptor cells was proposed by the author (8) to represent inhibitory connections that would contribute to an enhancement of the image contrast, as illustrated by the case of the image of an edge projected onto the retina by the optical system of the eye: The β-type receptor cells on the bright side of the edge will exert an inhibitory influence on surrounding α-type receptor cells; this inhibition is presumably proportional to the strength of the stimulus of the β-type receptor cells. The α-type cells located just at the edge on the darker side will then be exposed to an inhibitory influence stronger than that affecting α-type cells located further away from the edge on the darker side, since β-type receptor cells located on the bright side of the edge will contribute to the inhibition of the former cells; this additional inhibition of the α-type cells at the edge would serve to increase the contrast by making the brightness of the darker field appear to drop at the edge. The α-type cells located close to the edge of the bright side will be at least partially

Figure 31. Rabbit retina; tangential section through the outer plexiform layer with several α-type receptor cells. From the right upper corner a lateral process (*LP*) from a β-type cell extends down towards the center of the picture and makes contact with one α-type cell at its vitread pole (arrow *A*), where an invagination of the synaptic body plasma membrane receives several end processes from the neuropil of the outer plexiform layer. The typical synaptic complex consisting of two proximal vacuoles (PV_1, PV_2) with one synaptic ribbon (*SR*) and two distal vacuoles (DV_1, DV_2) is shown in this synaptic body. Note that the lateral process from the β-type cell is screened from contact with the α-type cell along the lateral surface of its synaptic body by Müller cell processes (*MCP*), and that the contact is confined to a limited area at the pole of its synaptic body at arrow *A*. The β-type cell process also contacts one end process outside the α-type receptor cell body (cross sectioned and indicated by arrow *B*). $\times$ 37,000.

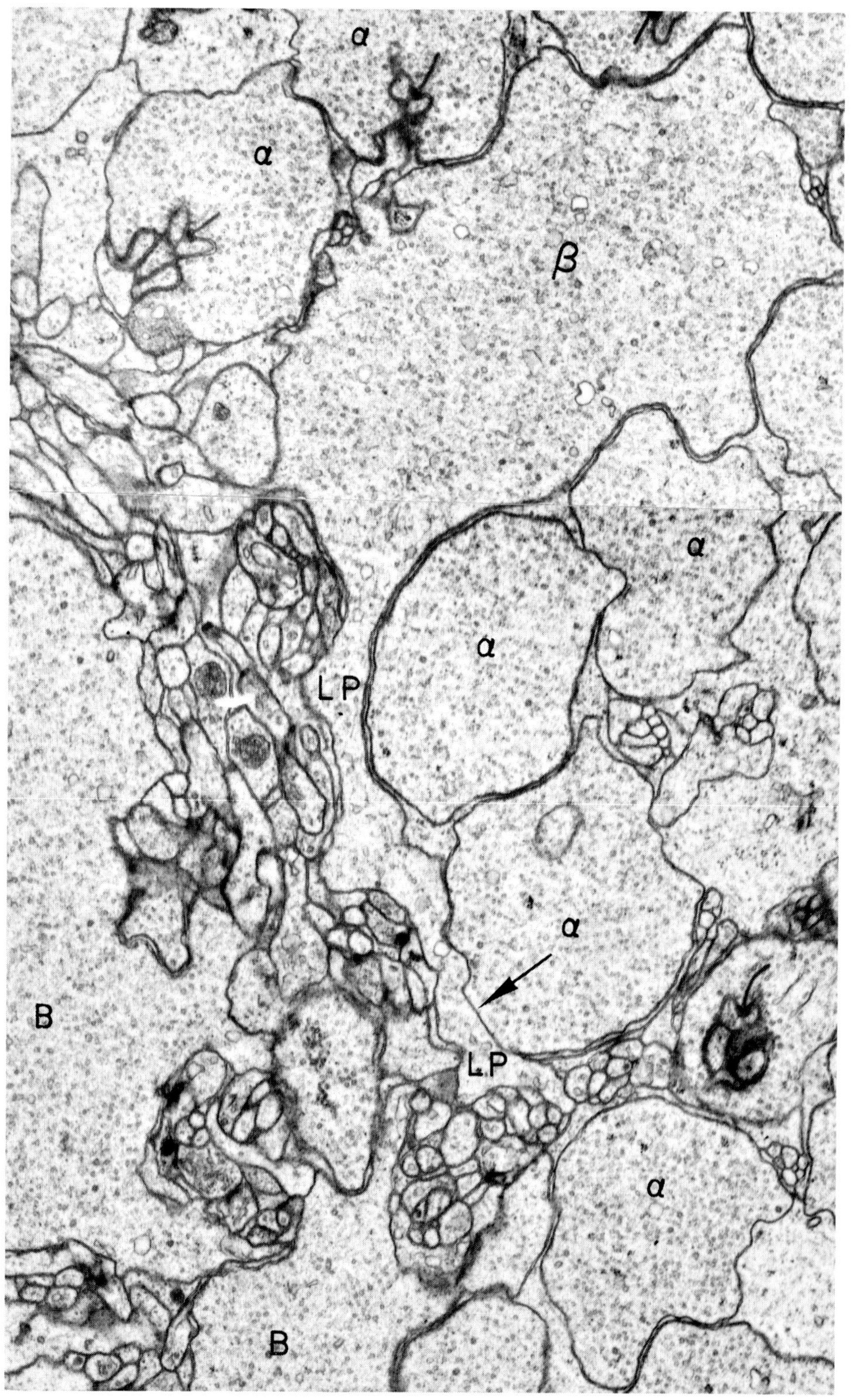

Figure 32 →

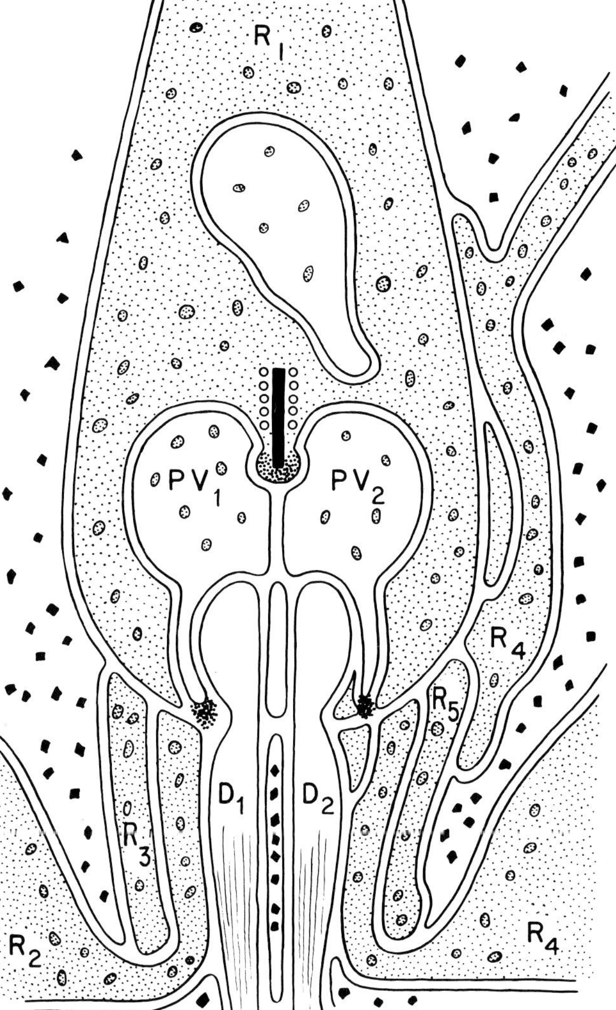

Figure 33. Schematic drawing showing the relationship between the ends of the lateral processes from β-type receptor cells (R_2, R_3, R_4, R_5) and the synaptic body of one α-type cell (R_1), as well as between these processes and the end branches of bipolar cells (D_1, D_2) in the guinea pig retina. In this case the tracing of the proximal vacuoles (PV_1, PV_2) farther than the vitread pole of the synaptic body was unsuccessful. (From Sjöstrand, 8.)

Figure 32. Rabbit retina; long lateral process (*LP*) from β-type cell synaptic body seen in tangential section through the retina. Note the outer portion of a thin layer of Müller cell cytoplasm between the β-type cell and the α-type cell synaptic bodies, with the exception of the one indicated by arrow, where the synaptic body plasma membranes are in direct contact. × 18,000.

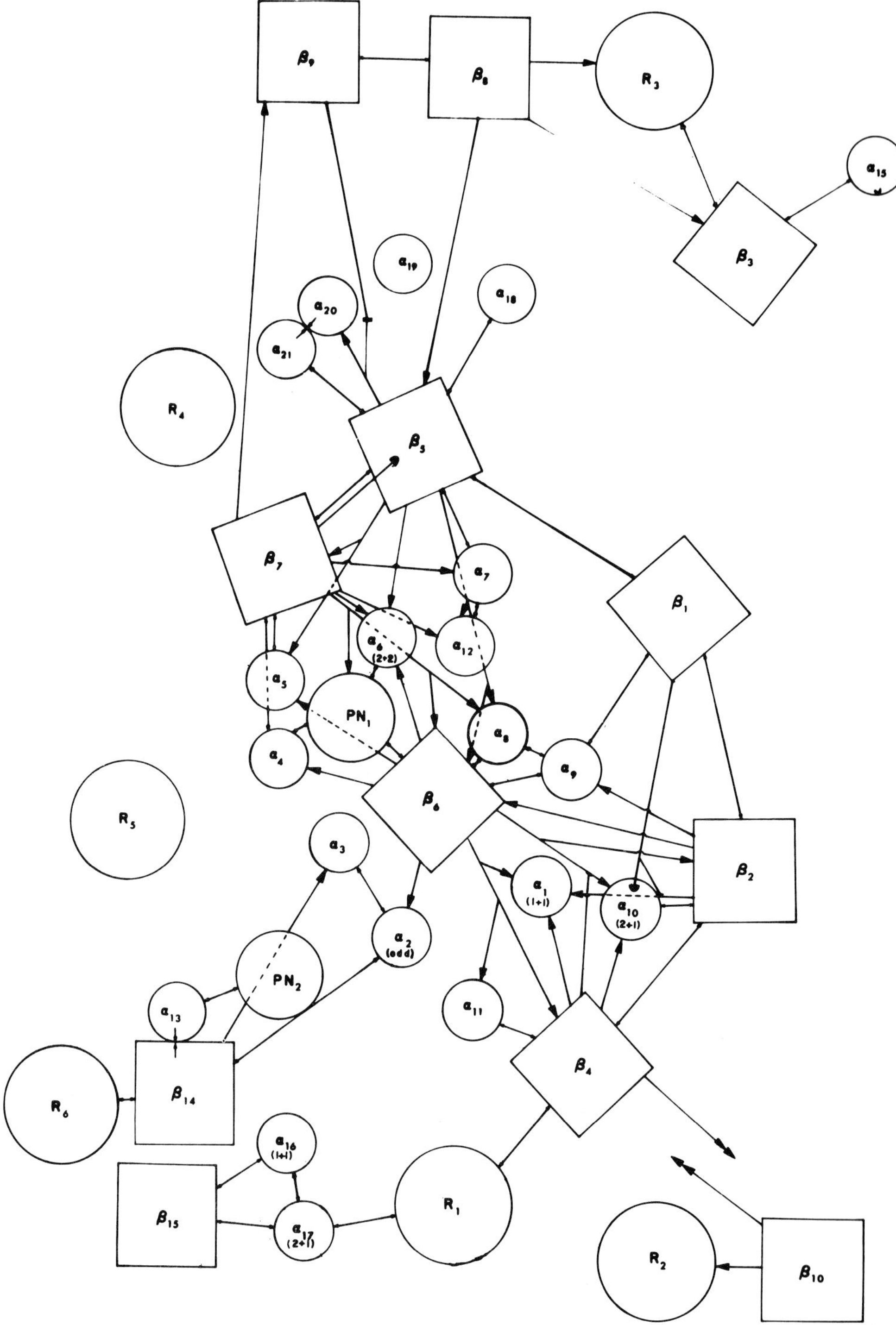
β_9
β_8
R_3
α_{15}
β_3
α_{19}
α_{18}
α_{20}
α_{21}
R_4
β_5
β_7
β_1
α_7
α_6 (2+2)
α_{12}
α_5
PN_1
α_8
α_4
α_9
β_6
R_5
β_2
α_3
α_1 (1+1)
α_{10} (2+1)
α_2 (odd)
PN_2
α_{11}
α_{13}
β_{14}
β_4
R_6
α_{16} (1+1)
β_{15}
α_{17} (2+1)
R_1
R_2
β_{10}

Figure 34 →

affected by β-type cells in the darker field, and the total inhibition of these cells will be less than that of cells located farther away from the edge in the bright field. The result is an apparent exaggeration of the brightness just at the edge.

These direct contacts between the receptor cells would allow the inhibitory effect to be exerted with a minimum of time delay, since only contacts between two cells arranged in series are involved; this seems to be a rather important prerequisite for any contrast-enhancing mechanism.

The system of lateral connections extending from the β-type receptor cells to the α-type cells, is, in fact, the structural feature that distinguishes these two types of cells. It appears justifiable to assume that the β-type receptor cells exert a modifying effect on the responses of the α-type cells or on the transmission between these and the bipolar cells. The lateral branches account for the basic difference in shape of the synaptic bodies of α- and β-type cells and, as already pointed out, is frequently the only structural difference between these two types of cells.

Connections Between Receptor, Bipolar, and Horizontal Cells

In addition to the difference in shape between the α- and the β-type receptor cells, the size of their synaptic bodies and the complexity of the structure of their synaptic endings vary considerably.

The structure of the synaptic bodies is characterized by the reception of end branches from bipolar and horizontal cells in an invagination of the plasma membrane of the receptor cells (Figure 40) extending in a scleral direction from the vitread pole or surface of the synaptic bodies of these cells (4–8). In individual sections through this region, these end branches appear generally as vacuoles, arranged in a regular fashion and at two different levels above the vitread pole of the synaptic body. Most sclerad, a pair of closely arranged vacuoles (proximal vacuoles) are found associated with a dense ribbon-shaped structure, the synaptic ribbon (Figures 41 and 42), which is located in the sclerad furrow between the vacuoles (5–8). Between the proximal vacuoles and the vitread surface of the

Figure 34. Map of the interreceptor contacts established in a 98-section series through the outer plexiform layer in a guinea pig retina. Shown are 22 α-type synapses, two of which are paranuclear (*PN*); 12 β-type synapses; and six other receptors (*R*) whose synaptic regions were below the level of the series and therefore could not be classified. The axes of the cells are placed in approximately accurate locations with respect to one another. Each cell is shown much smaller than its actual diameter, as can be seen by the lines with a small arrowhead at each end, which indicate mutual contact between receptors. The lines with large arrows are processes from βs to other receptors. The two lines with double arrowheads in the lower right corner indicate two of the major processes which were cut off at the end of the series. Two lines ending with rounded heads in β_5 and in α_{10} indicate invaginations of β_7 and of β_1 respectively. Other symbols show processes of β_5 and β_9 contacting one another, a process of β_1 ending on a process of β_2, and a process of β_4 ending on processes of β_2 and β_6; no attempt was made to show the processes in their actual location or true length, as they twisted and overlapped greatly; only the vast number of connections is shown. Many of the α-type synapses had no invaginations at all; those which had real synaptic areas were reconstructed and the invagination pattern type is noted on the map; α_1 and α_{16} were of type $1 + 1$; α_{10} and α_{17} were of type $2 + 1$; α_6 was of type $2 + 2$; α_2 was odd, having a large bulbous invagination accompanied by a swelling of the extracellular space and a peripheral ribbon; α_{15} had a peripheral V-shaped ribbon but no invaginations.

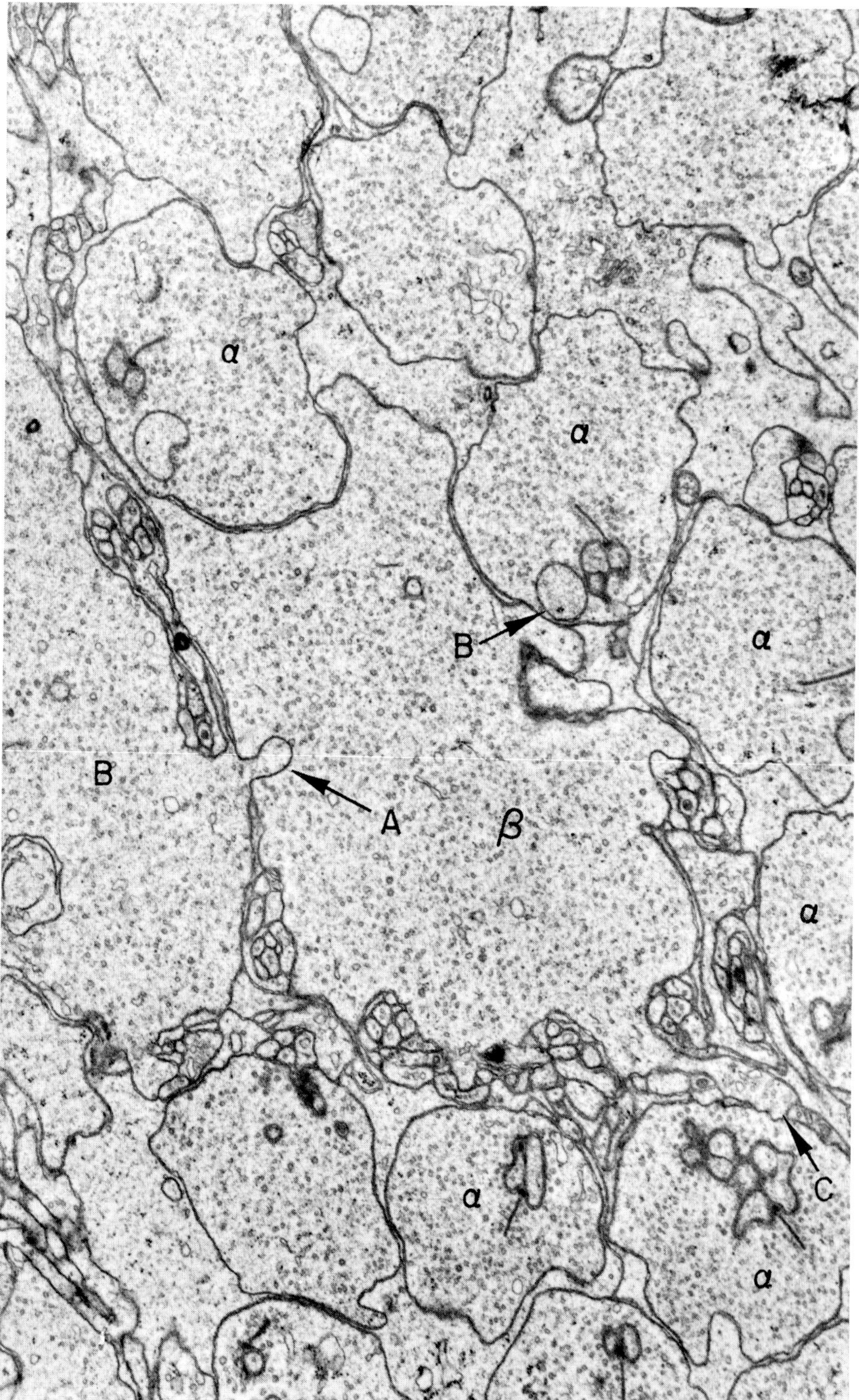

Figure 35. Rabbit retina. Interreceptor contact between two β-type receptor cells (arrow *A*) and between one β-type cell and two α-type receptor cells (arrows *B* and *C*). $\times$ 19,000.

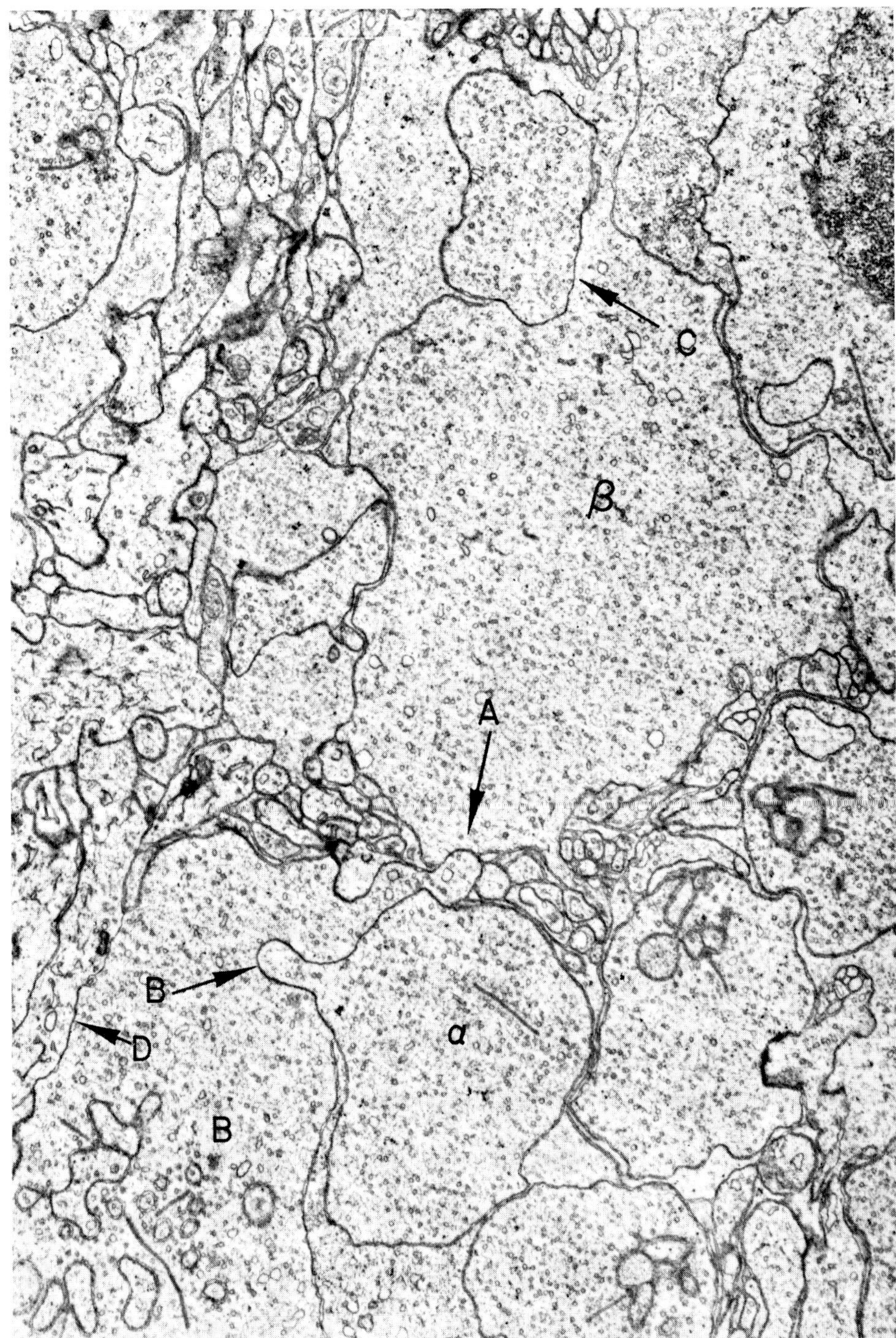

Figure 36. Rabbit retina. Interreceptor contacts between two β-type cells (arrow *A*) and between β-type and α-type cells (arrows *B* and *C*). The latter contacts involve the lateral surface of the α-type cells. A contact area between the β-type cell in the lower part of the picture and a process from a horizontal cell is shown at arrow *D*. × 19,000.

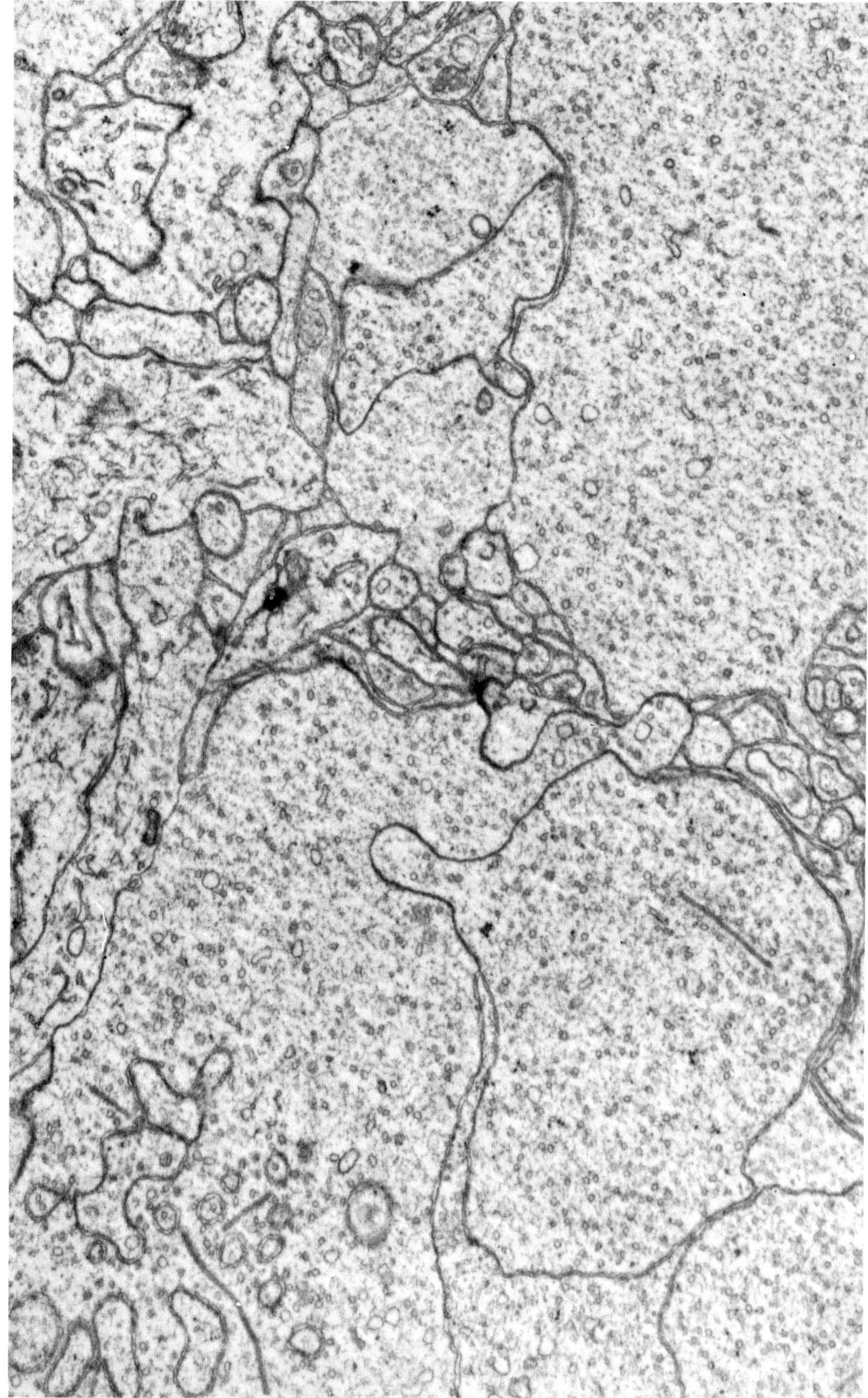

Figure 37. Higher magnification of section adjacent to that shown in Figure 36, showing the same contact areas between the β-type cells and one β-type and one α-type cell (arrows *A* and *B* in Figure 36). ×31,000.

synaptic body, one or two vacuoles (distal vacuoles) are observed to make contact with the vitread surfaces of the proximal vacuoles.

In three-dimensional reconstructions of the synaptic bodies it has been possible to show that all these vacuoles are the endings of branches from either bipolar or horizontal cells. The α-type receptor cells can be classified according to the number and arrangement of the end branches associated with their synaptic bodies. The most elaborate α-type synaptic body is characterized by four end branches entering into the plasma membrane invagination of the synaptic body; two of these end branches form a pair of proximal vacuoles and two form a pair of distal vacuoles; this can be labeled a 2 + 2 type. Another type of synaptic body, the 1 + 2 type, is characterized by one single end process branching to form both proximal vacuoles, with the synaptic ribbon located in the furrow between the widened ends of the two branches (Figure 43); in this case there are two distal vacuoles, corresponding to two end branches.

A third type of synaptic body is characterized by the proximal vacuoles representing two turns of a spiral-shaped single end branch. The end branch forms about one and a half turns of a spiral with its axis parallel to the long axis of the receptor cell (Figure 44). The synaptic ribbon is located between the first and the second turn and its large surface is oriented perpendicular to the long axis of the cell. In this case usually only one process forms a single distal vacuole, and this type of synapse can therefore be labeled a 1 + 1 type. Figure 45 shows schematically the arrangement of the end branches in these three types of receptor cells.

As already mentioned, the lateral processes from the β-type receptor cells make contact both with the surface of the α-type cell synaptic body at its vitread pole and with the surfaces of the bipolar cell end branches as they enter into the plasma membrane invagination of the synaptic body. Figures 32 and 46 show the situation relative to one α-type synaptic body reconstructed in 1957 (8); a circuit diagram describing these connections is shown in Figure 47. This diagram for an α-type receptor cell was the first attempt to construct a circuit diagram of the kind discussed above.

The β-type synaptic body shows the same structural features as the α-type but, instead of a single synaptic ribbon and one pair of proximal vacuoles, several such complexes are present—three to five in the guinea pig retina and ten or more in the rabbit retina (Figure 48). The large number of proximal vacuoles does not, however, reflect an identical number of end branches. In the guinea pig retina, all or almost all proximal vacuoles (Figure 49) were found to be widened parts of one single end branch (9,11); in the rabbit retina, several proximal vacuoles are formed by a single end branch. There is no question, however, that the β-type receptor cells are contacted by a larger number of end branches from bipolar and horizontal cells than are the α-type cells.

The end branches associated with the synaptic bodies of the receptor cells stem either from bipolar cell dendrites or from horizontal cells. The latter cells extend thick branches over long distances in the outer plexiform layer (Figures 40 and 48), and these branches appear to form a network with a rather well-defined angle of about 120° between crossing branches. Minute processes extend directly

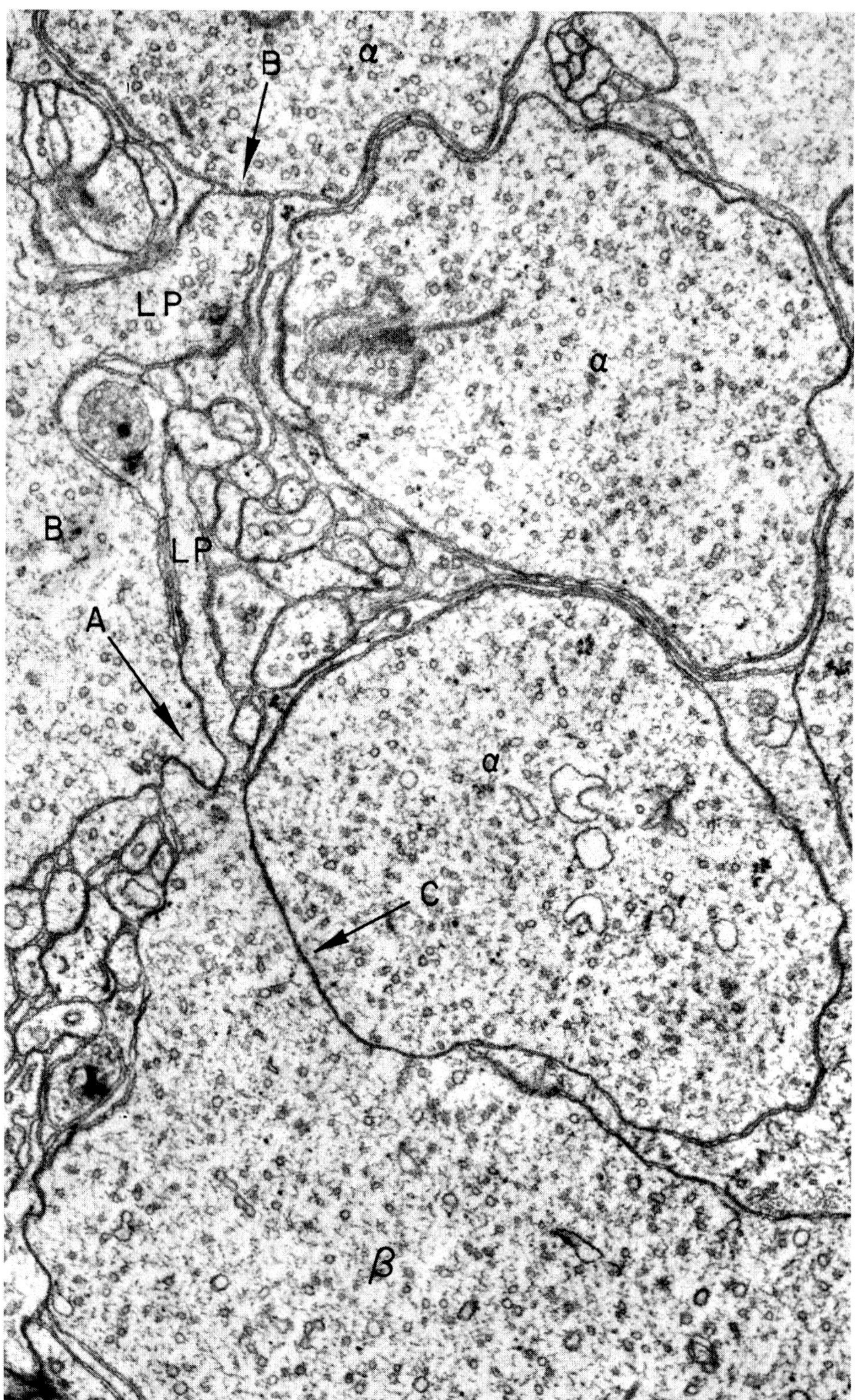

Figure 38 →

from the thick processes (Figure 50) and enter into contact with a receptor cell synaptic body. Medium-sized processes are distributed in a layer more sclerad than that in which the thick processes are located (Figure 40); branches also twig off from these medium-sized processes and enter into contact with the receptor cell synaptic bodies (Figure 51).

In order to trace the synaptic relations of the receptor cells to such an extent that the contacting cells can be identified as either bipolar or horizontal, it is necessary to reconstruct a perfect series of at least 100 consecutive sections, with the plane of sectioning oriented tangentially to the surface of the retina. A series of 400 to 500 sections is required to ensure that it will contain a perfect sequence of 100 sections through the proper zone. Two such series of sections through the rabbit retina are presently being analyzed in our laboratory; this study is aimed particularly at a three-dimensional reconstruction of the β-type receptor cells.

The system of long-range lateral connections in the outer plexiform layer appears to be more elaborate in the rabbit retina than in the guinea pig's. Numerous large horizontal cells are responsible for these connections. Upon tracing the end branches associated with β-type receptor cells in the rabbit retina, it was found that the proximal vacuoles could be identified as the endings of horizontal cell processes. On the other hand, most of the distal vacuoles were identified as endings of dendritic branches from the bipolar cells.

In the β-type receptor cells of the rabbit retina, the proximal vacuoles of the 10 to 15 synaptic complexes consisting of a pair of proximal vacuoles, a synaptic ribbon, and one or two distal vacuoles (Figure 48) are formed by three to five separate processes. Thus, while each process from a horizontal cell forms several proximal vacuoles, these are distributed among different synaptic complexes; of the pair of proximal vacuoles associated with a synaptic ribbon, the two vacuoles are therefore usually formed by separate horizontal cell processes.

In the great complexity of the structure of receptor cell synaptic bodies there seems to be a certain regularity and a definite order. The basis for detection of this order is the distinction between proximal and distal vacuoles, proximal vacuoles being defined as those associated directly with the synaptic ribbons. A pair of such vacuoles, the associated synaptic ribbon, and one or two distal vacuoles form a synaptic complex. The proximal vacuoles appear always to be the end branches of horizontal cells. In most cases in the guinea pig retina, a single branch forms all proximal vacuoles of the β-type receptor cells. In the rabbit retina several processes contribute to the large number of proximal vacuoles, and each process is associated with two or more synaptic complexes. The distal vacuoles appear to be formed by endings of dendritic branches from bipolar cells.

Figure 38. Interreceptor contact between the two β-type cells (arrow *A*) shown in Figures 36 and 37, from sections located further up in a sclerad direction. In this figure, contact has been established between the upper β-type cell and another α-type (arrow *B*) at the latter's vitread pole through a lateral process (*LP*) from the β-type cell. The picture suggests the difference in area of contact as compared to contacts at the lateral surface (arrow *C*) and at the vitread pole of the α-type receptor cells. Note the close association of the plasma membrane at the area of contact. $\times$ 37,000.

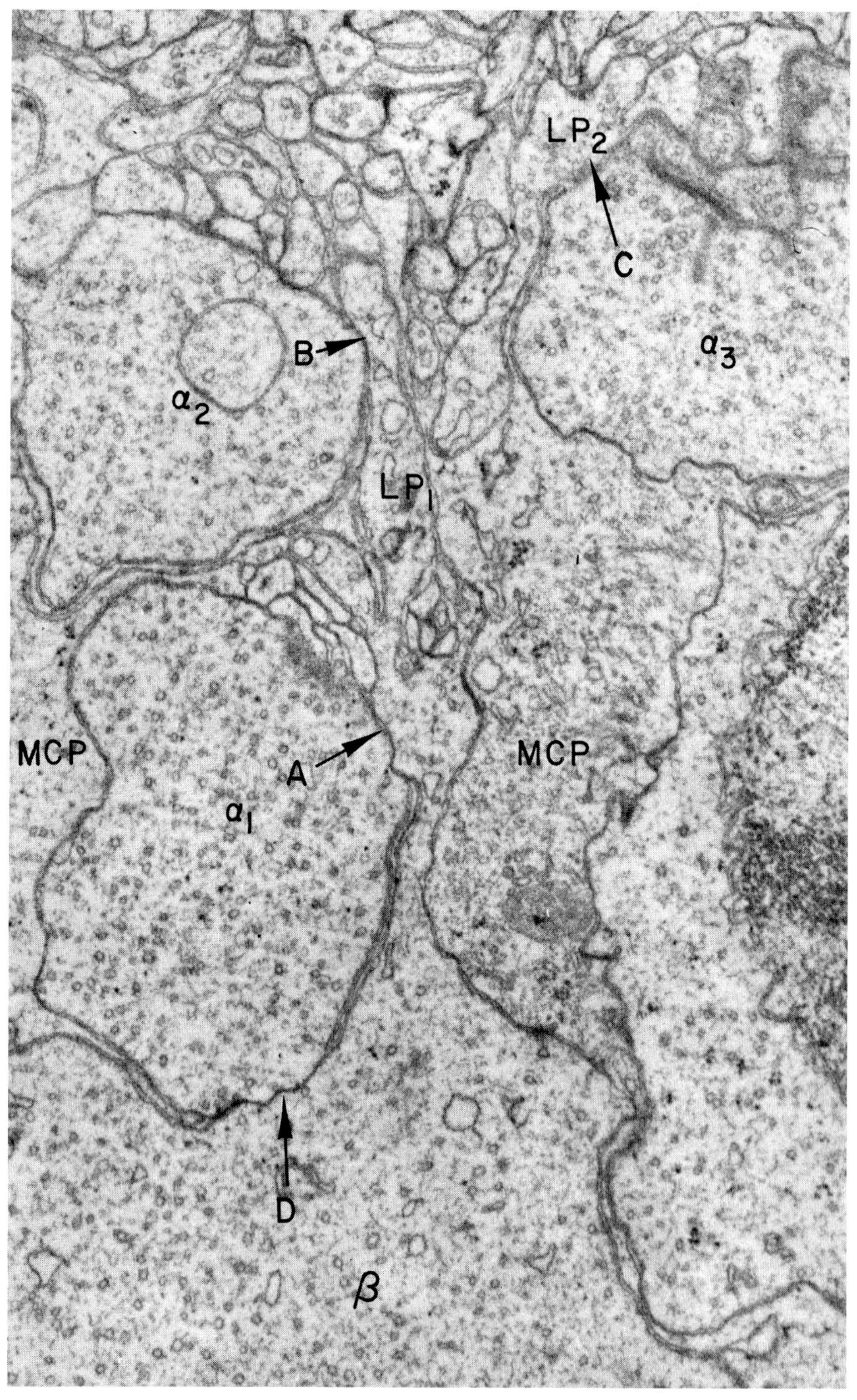

Figure 39 →

A larger number of β-type receptor cells must be analyzed by means of three-dimensional reconstructions before these rules can be accepted as generally valid. However, the observations made so far justify these tentative conclusions.

Functional Significance of the Outer Plexiform Layer

It appears quite clear that the outer plexiform layer is primarily associated with lateral connections between receptor cells. These lateral connections are of two kinds, depending upon the distance and number of synaptic contacts involved. The direct interreceptor contacts through lateral branches from the β-type receptor cells connect the β-type cells with adjacent α-type cells as well as with other β-type cells. These connections are either very short or of an intermediate range of up to 40–50 μ, and all are monosynaptic.

The lateral connections through the horizontal cells extend over long distances, perhaps a millimeter. The receptor cells are contacted by minute processes, either from medium-sized horizontal cell branches or branching off directly from the thickest horizontal cell processes. The medium-sized branches gradually taper off as they split up into the end branches, while the thick branches do not appear to be reduced in width as they send off the small processes. These two types of horizontal cell branches might be functionally different, with one type of end process receiving impulses from, and the other type transmitting impulses to, the receptor cells.

It has been proposed that the direct interreceptor connections from the β- to the α-type cells exert an inhibitory influence on the latter, thereby enhancing contrast (8). This contrast enhancement could affect the resolution and therefore become an important mechanism in connection with the high visual acuity of foveal vision. As has been demonstrated by Dr. Cohen,* the receptor cells of the human fovea are interconnected through such direct contacts between the synaptic bodies.

Assuming this functional significance of their lateral processes, the β-type receptor cells appear as contrast-enhancing elements in the receptor cell population. Since the rabbit retina cannot discriminate colors, the contrast enhancement is confined to the mechanism increasing the black-and-white contrast.

The cone cells are characteristically equipped with a synaptic body identical to that of the β-type receptor cells. The color-discriminating cells are primarily contrast-enhancing elements. The enhancement of contrast by the introduction of color contrast is combined with the mechanism of contrast enhancement through lateral inhibition, as illustrated by the simultaneous contrast phenomenon. The

---

* Cf. pages 31–62.

Figure 39. Higher magnification of the process extending upwards in Figure 36 from the upper β-type receptor cell; picture from the same section as that shown in Figure 38. This process (LP_1) passes two α-type cells (α_1 and α_2) and makes contact with their surfaces within limited areas (arrows *A* and *B*). Another process (LP_2) from a β-type cell is seen contacting a third α-type cell (α_3) (arrow *C*). Arrow *D* points to contact area between the β-type cell and the lateral surface of the α_1 synaptic body. *MCP:* Müller cell processes. $\times$ 37,000.

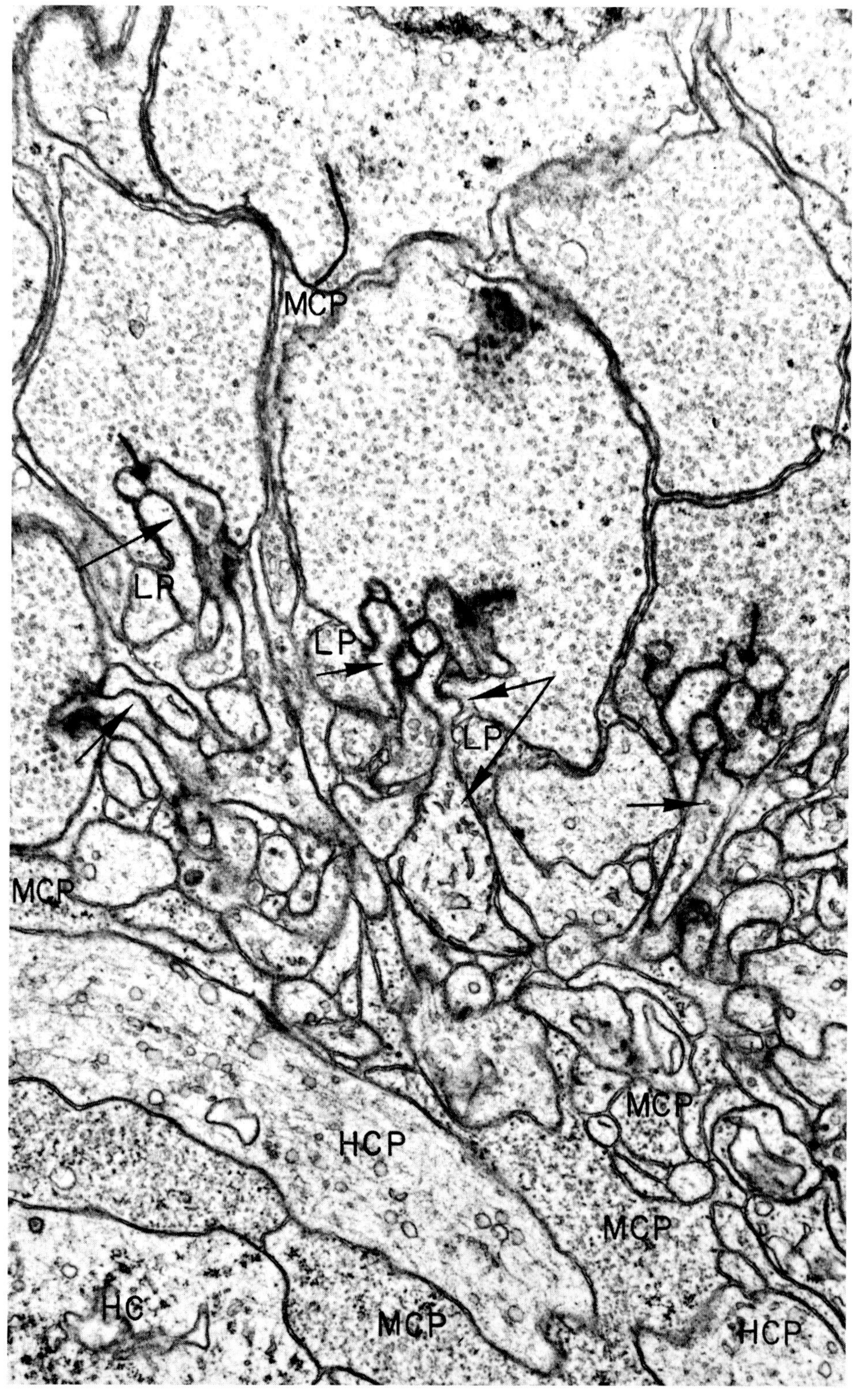

Figure 40 →

β-type synaptic body with its lateral interreceptor connections offers an anatomical background for this phenomenon, as proposed by Sjöstrand (8). In addition to enhancing contrast by the introduction of color contrast, the color-discriminating cells might also affect the black-and-white contrast through lateral inhibition of the α-type cells or rods, since they extend lateral processes to the "non-color"-discriminating rod cells as well as to the color-discriminating cells. Thus it would be understandable that the mechanism of color discrimination is associated with cells equipped with the β-type synaptic body. The contrast enhancement due to color discrimination is combined with the black-and-white contrast enhancement in the receptor cell type, the function of which is contrast enhancement. The color-discriminating cells can then, in fact, be considered β-type cells equipped with the proper photopigment in the outer segment to assure selective sensitivity for a certain wavelength range. Considering color discrimination at the receptor cell level as primarily a mechanism for contrast enhancement, it appears quite reasonable to consider the possibility that color discrimination can be confined to the receptor cell level and that color perception is not necessarily associated with color discrimination at this level.

It is conceivable that the size and shape of the outer segment (whether a small cone, a large cone, or a rod) have no relevance to the color-discriminating mechanism per se, but pertain rather to the threshold for excitation (9). The typical cones with a small conical outer segment are characterized by a higher threshold than the rod cells.

The fact that the lateral processes of the β-type synaptic bodies represent a basic structural feature that must be associated functionally with lateral interaction at the receptor cell level justifies the use of this structural feature as a main basis for distinguishing between different types of retinal receptor cells. This type of synaptic body is found in receptor cells with an outer segment identical to or smaller than the outer segment of the α-type receptor cells, as well as in receptor cells with an outer segment of conical shape. The size and shape of the outer segments can be considered less decisive for the classification of cell types than the structural feature that leads to the establishment of interreceptor contacts; such differences in the appearance of the outer segments reflect most probably different thresholds for excitation. Smaller outer segments, presumably representing a higher threshold, are frequently characteristic of the β-type receptor cells. This structural feature could well represent an adjustment of the level of stimulation intensity at which lateral interference between receptor cells is fully activated.

It is thus proposed that the controversial classification of receptor cells as rods and cones should not be given the significance generally ascribed to it. This characterization, so intimately associated with the phenomenon of color discrimination, has led to great confusion, since there is no strict parallelism between

Figure 40. Rabbit retina. Several α-type receptor cell synaptic bodies with end processes from the plexus entering into the invaginated vitread pole of their synaptic bodies (arrows). *LP:* Lateral processes of β-type cells contacting vitread pole of the synaptic bodies; *HC:* part of a horizontal cell cellbody; *HCP:* horizontal cell processes; *MCP:* Müller cell processes. × 30,000.

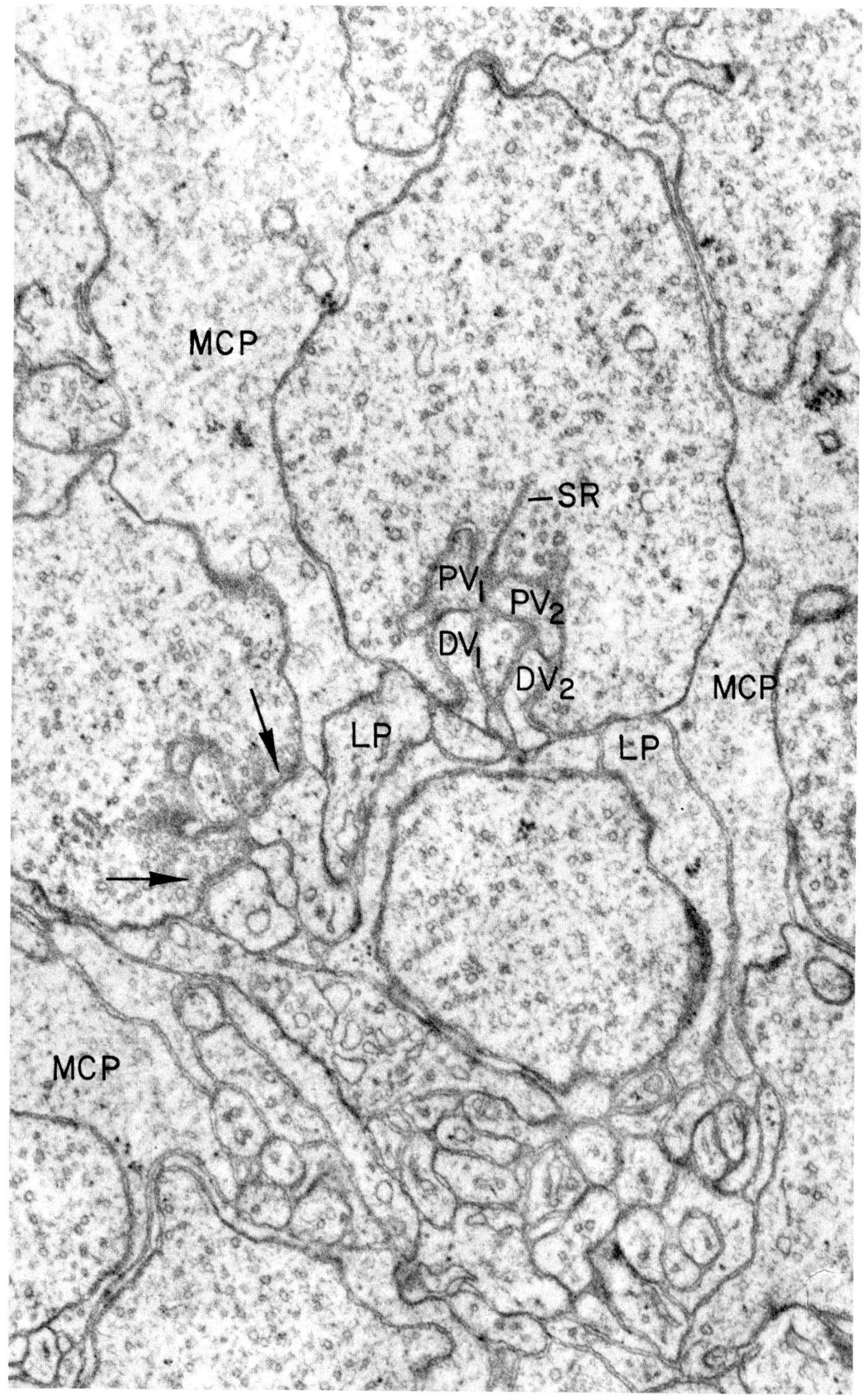

Figure 41 →

shape and color-discriminating function of the cells. Receptor cells that have been shown to be associated with color discrimination have been thus classified as cone cells even when they lacked the structural characteristics of cone cells. It appears more logical to distinguish between color-discriminating and non-color-discriminating receptor cells, and to base this classification entirely on physiological criteria. Whatever shape a receptor cell might have, it cannot be used as a rigorous criterion for color discrimination; even a structurally typical cone cell should be tested physiologically before any color-discriminating function is attributed to it.

A more satisfactory classification of retinal receptor cells, in which structural and functional features are likely to be most intimately coupled, would be one based on the structural features characterizing the α- and β-types. It is very likely that the β-type cells are functionally contrast-enhancing elements, while the α-type cells are simple light recording cells. The β-type cells reach the full capacity of their contrast-enhancing function when equipped with a color-discriminating mechanism located at their outer segments. The contrast enhancement achieved by lateral inhibition makes the perceived image excel the quality of the image projected onto the retina by the optical system of the eye.

If the β-type receptor cells are equipped with a color-discriminating mechanism, this will be reflected in their structure only if this mechanism is associated with a low threshold for stimulation; in that case the outer segments would be smaller than the rod outer segments. The variation in the molecular structure of the photopigment responsible for color discrimination does not necessarily impose variation in the basic structure of the receptor cells at the resolution of the electron microscope.

The functional significance of the long lateral connections through the horizontal cells can be conjectured: these connections may well represent the structural basis for retinal perception of movement and of shape (9), and could be involved in the mechanism of neural adaptation through inhibitory effects on receptor-bipolar cell transmission.

Figure 41. Rabbit retina. An α-type synaptic body with the pair of proximal vacuoles (PV_1, PV_2), synaptic ribbon (*SR*), and a pair of distal vacuoles (DV_1, DV_2) separated by interposed receptor cell cytoplasm. Processes from adjacent β-type receptor cells (*LP*) make contact with the vitread pole of the synaptic body; several such processes are also seen contacting the vitread pole of an adjacent α-type receptor cell (arrows). *MCP:* Müller cell processes. $\times$ 37,000.

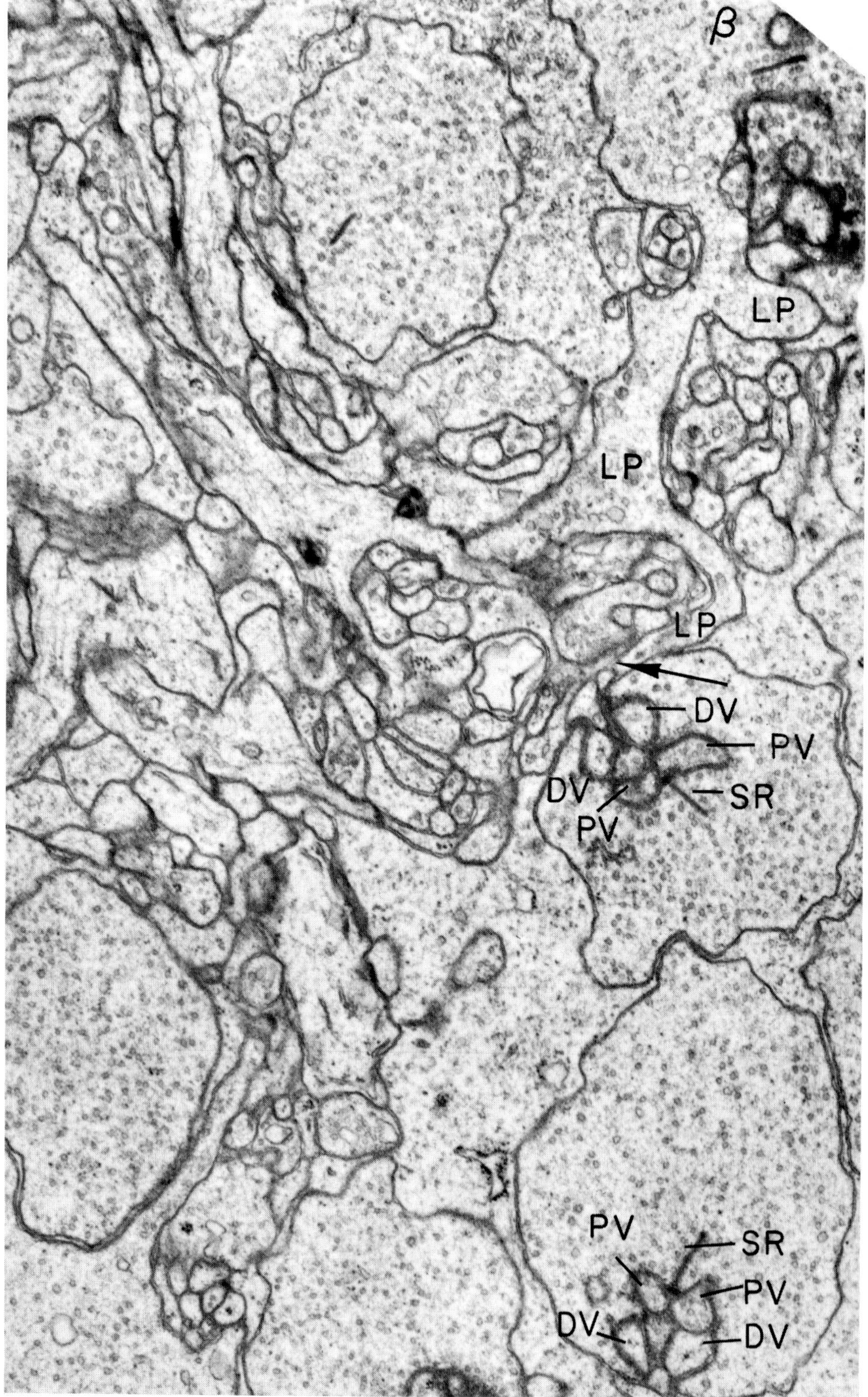

Figure 42. Two α-type receptor cells in the rabbit retina, showing the typical synaptic body complex with a pair of proximal vacuoles (*PV*), a synaptic ribbon (*SR*), and a pair of distal vacuoles (*DV*). A fairly long process from a β-type cell (*LP*) contacts the upper α-type cell at its vitread pole (arrow). ×25,000.

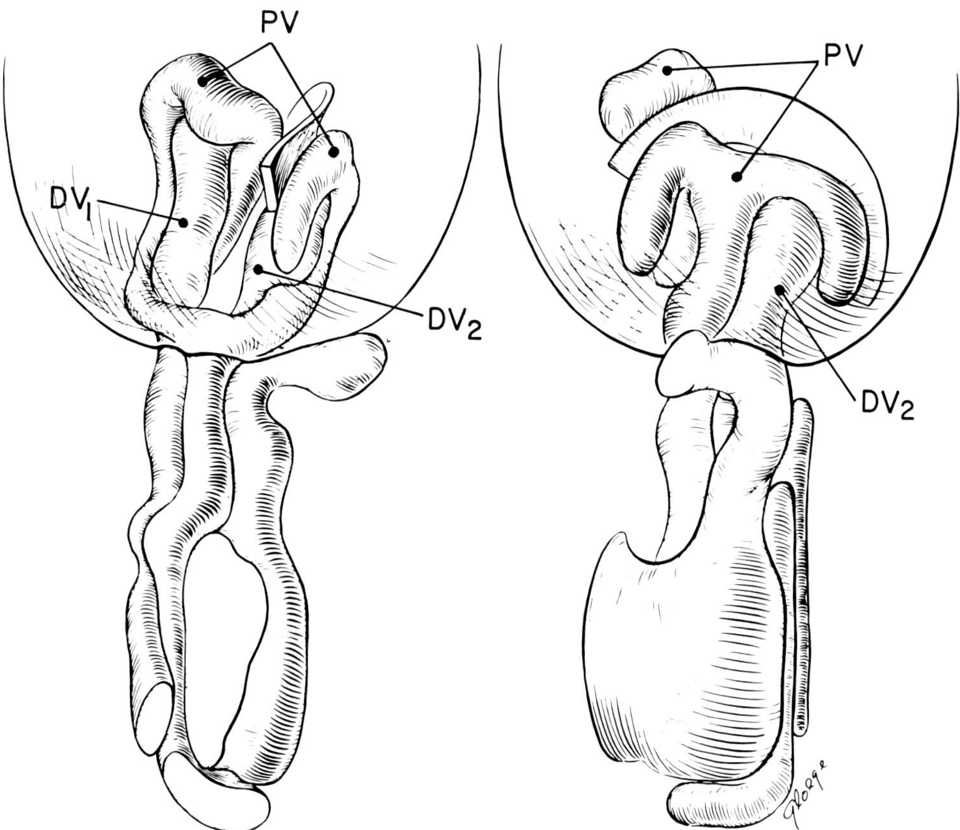

Figure 43. Three-dimensional reconstruction of synaptic contacts of α-type receptor cells, the 1 + 2 type. Proximal vacuoles (*PV*) are branches of a single process entering through the vitread pole of the synaptic body. Two other processes enter independently and end as distal vacuoles (DV_1, DV_2) in contact with the proximal vacuoles. *SR:* Synaptic ribbon. (F. S. Sjöstrand and S. Mountford, unpublished material.)

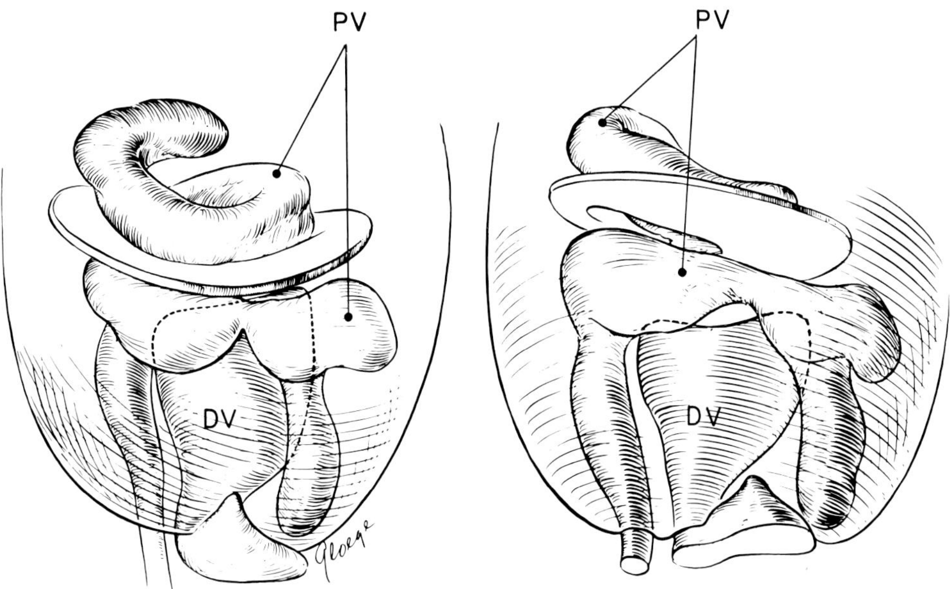

Figure 44. Three-dimensional reconstruction of an α-type receptor cell synaptic body of the 1 + 1 type. The proximal vacuoles (*PV*) are formed from a process entering the vitread pole of the synaptic body and assuming a spiral course. One single process of a different type forms a single distal vacuole (*DV*). (F. S. Sjöstrand and S. Mountford, unpublished material.)

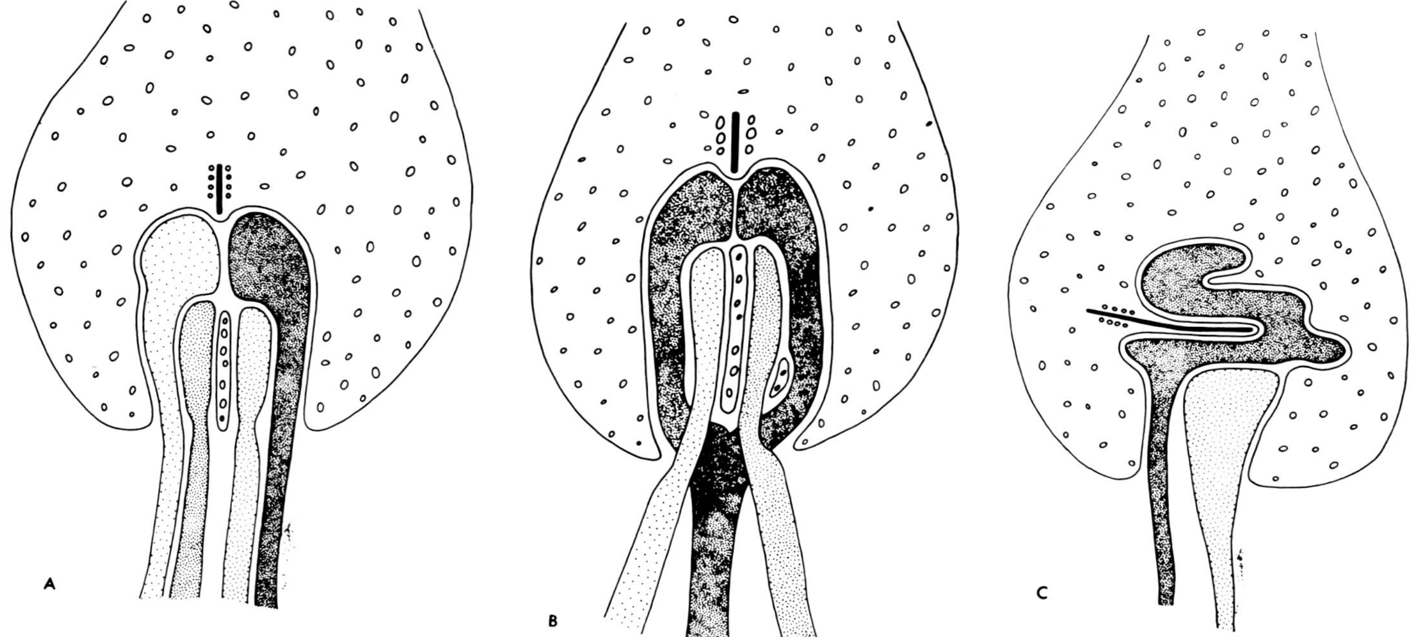

Figure 45. Types of 2-receptor cells. *A*: 2 + 2 type, with two separate processes forming a pair of proximal vacuoles and two other separate processes forming a pair of distal vacuoles. *B*: 1 + 2 type, with one process contributing to both the proximal vacuoles, and two separate processes forming a pair of distal vacuoles. *C*: 1 + 1 type, with one process forming the proximal vacuoles and another contributing a single distal vacuole. (From Sjöstrand, 9.)

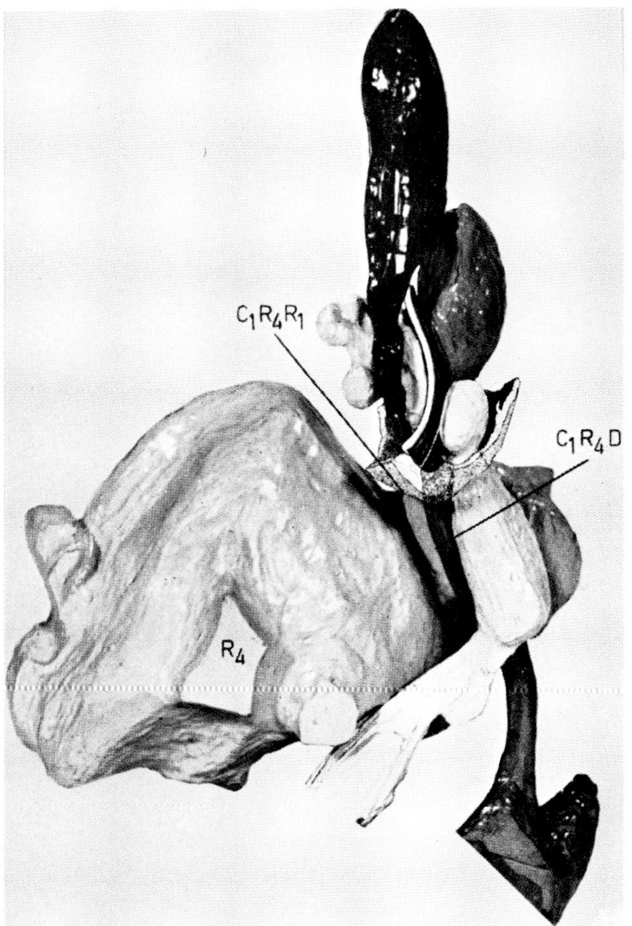

Figure 46. Plastic model of the synaptic body of an α-type receptor cell in the guinea pig retina, with part of the synaptic body of an adjacent β-type cell (R_4). C_1 R_4 R_1: Contact No. 1 between the β-type cell (R_4) and the α-type cell (R_1); C_1 R_4 D_1: contact area No. 1 between R_4 and the dendrite from bipolar cell No. 1 at the vitread pole of the α-type cell. The plasma membrane of the latter cell has been removed, with the exception of a small area at the vitread pole, in order to show the synaptic vacuoles and the synaptic ribbon. (From Sjöstrand, 8.)

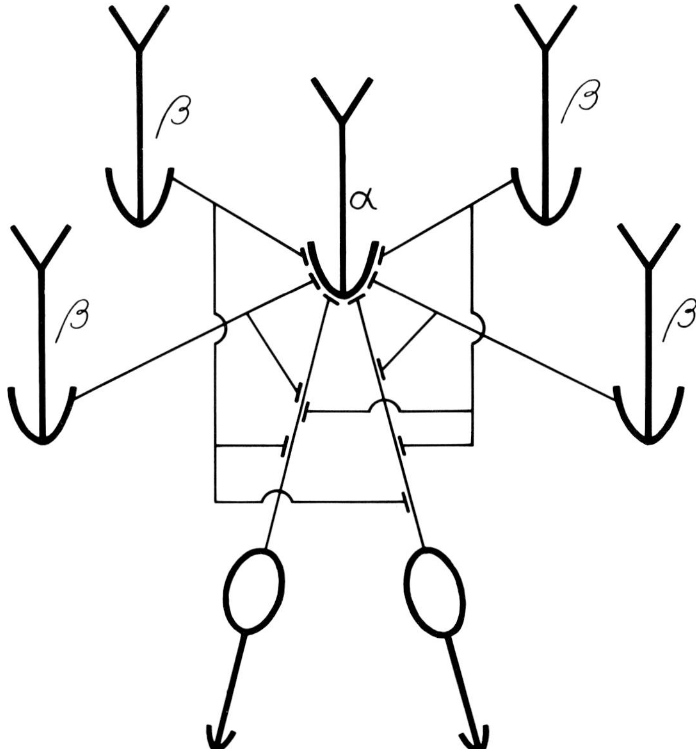

Figure 47. Circuit diagram illustrating the lateral connections between receptor cells associated with one α-type cell and the two bipolar cells contacting this cell in the guinea pig retina. Note that all lateral branches from the β-type cell contact the surface of the α-type cell at its vitread pole and also the end branches of the dendrites from the bipolar cell just beyond the vitread pole of the α-type cell. (From Sjöstrand, 8.)

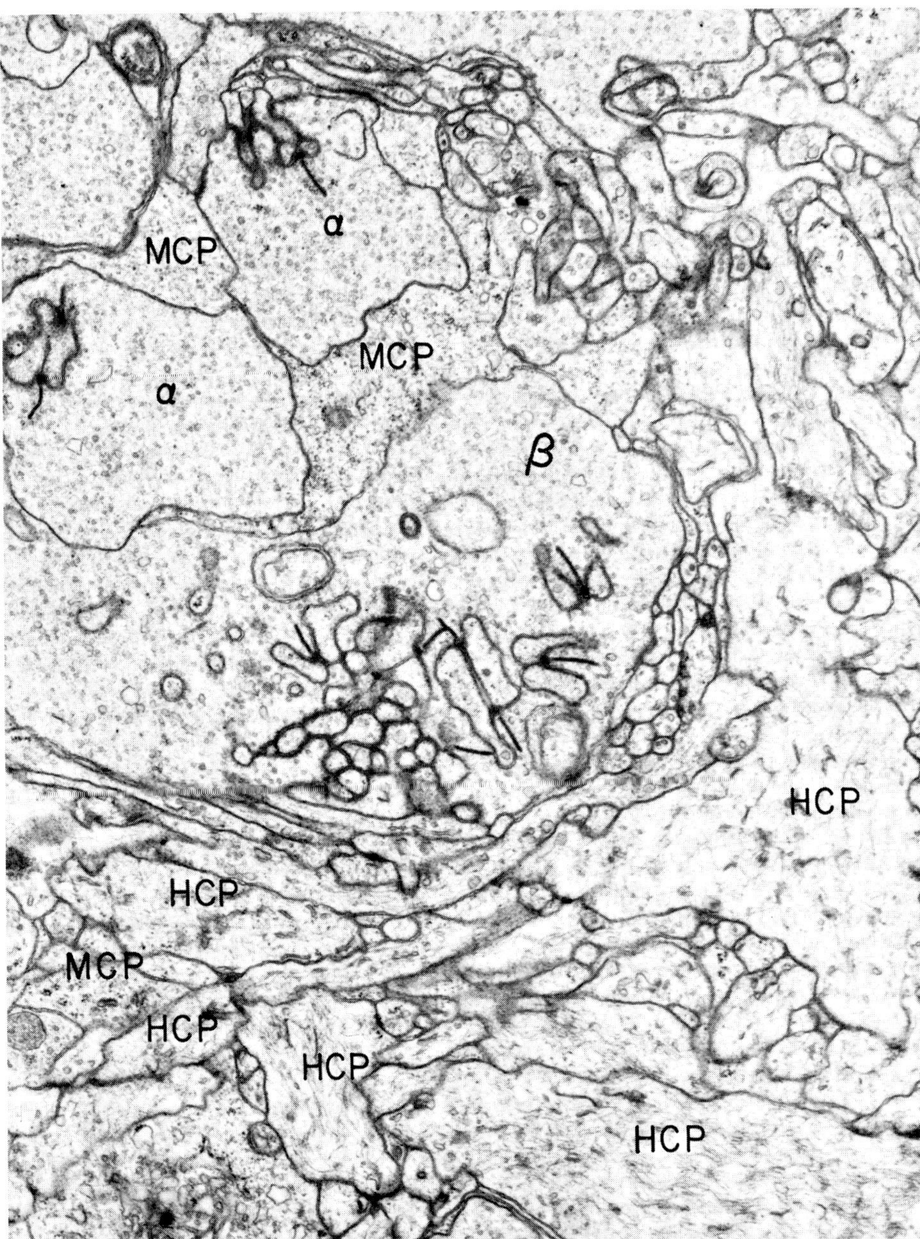

Figure 48. Tangential section through the outer plexiform layer of the rabbit retina, showing one β-type cell cut across close to its vitread surface. The complicated system of vacuoles and synaptic ribbons is illustrated. Processes from horizontal cells (*HCP*) of different thicknesses are shown in the lower part of the figure. *MCP:* Müller cell processes. × 19,000.

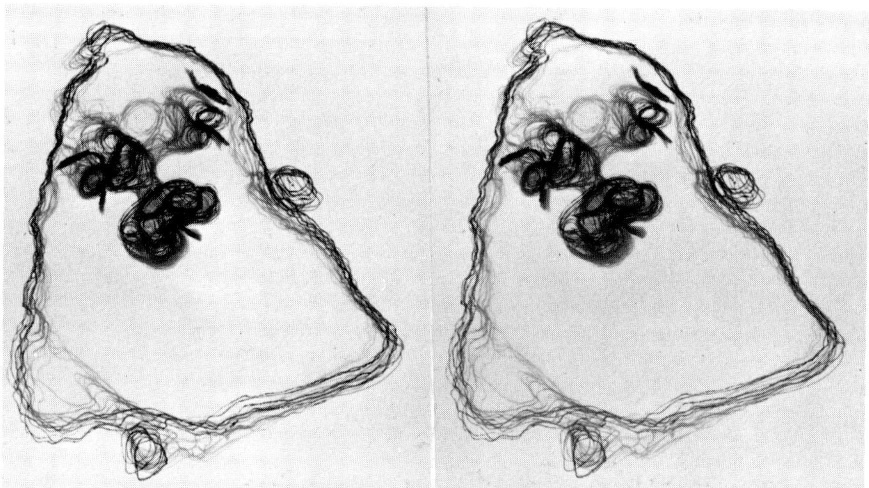

Figure 49. Stereo pair of pictures of part of β-type receptor cell synaptic body in the guinea pig retina as it appears during three-dimensional analysis. The drawings, made from consecutive sections on transparent sheets of plastic, have been piled on top of each other and photographed in two camera positions illuminated from below. These pictures show piles of 20 sheets, which represent only a part of the series of sections used for reconstruction of one β-type synaptic body. (From Sjöstrand & Mountford, 10.)

Figure 50. Tangential section through the outer plexiform layer of the rabbit retina. The section cuts through a layer located outside on the vitread side of one β-type receptor cell which has been reconstructed in three dimensions. A thick process from a horizontal cell is shown sending a thin branch (arrow) toward the neuropil associated with the reconstructed β-type receptor cell. This branch could be followed when entering the invagination of the synaptic body and could be shown to end by forming several proximal vacuoles. × 19,000.

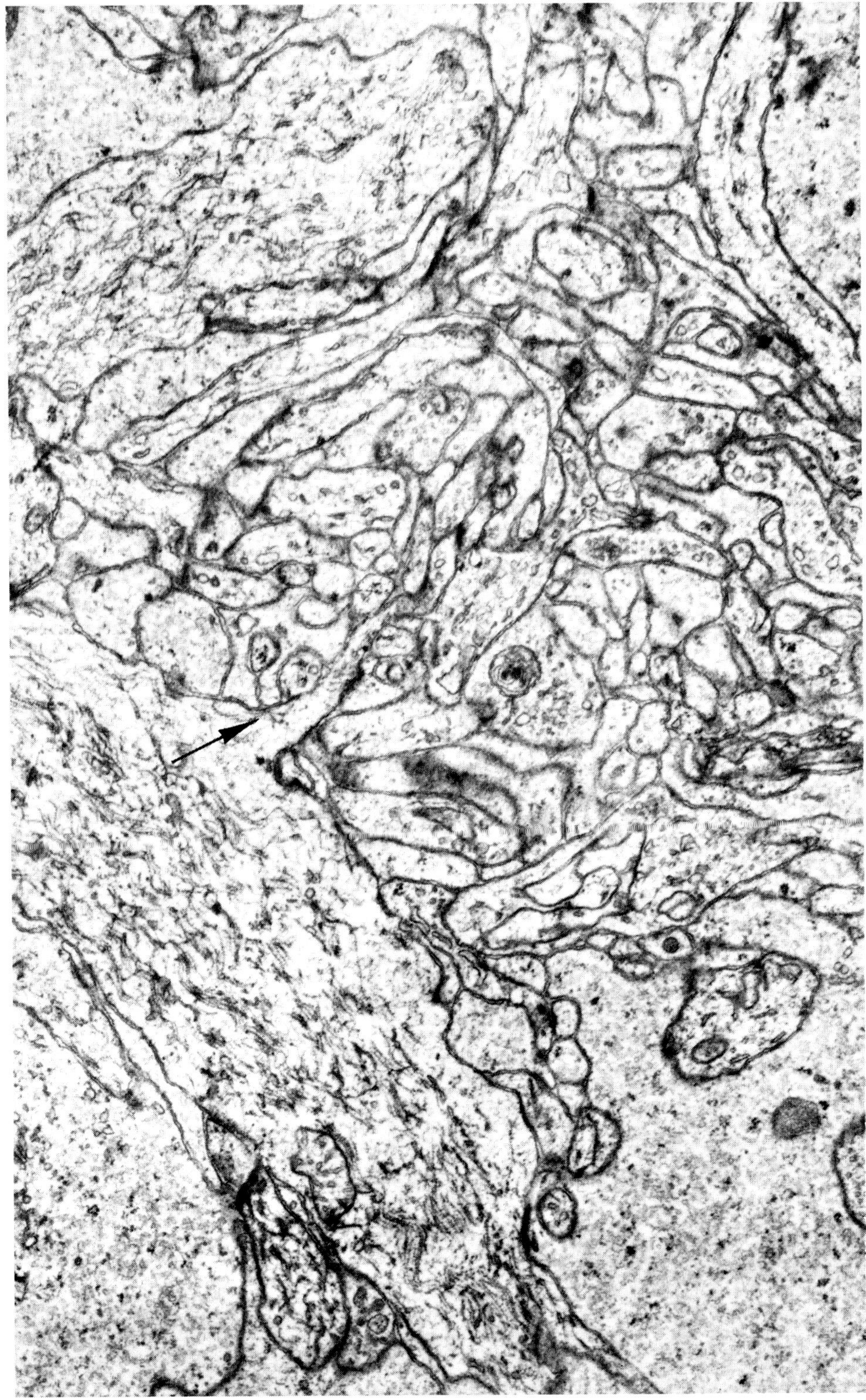

← **Figure 50**

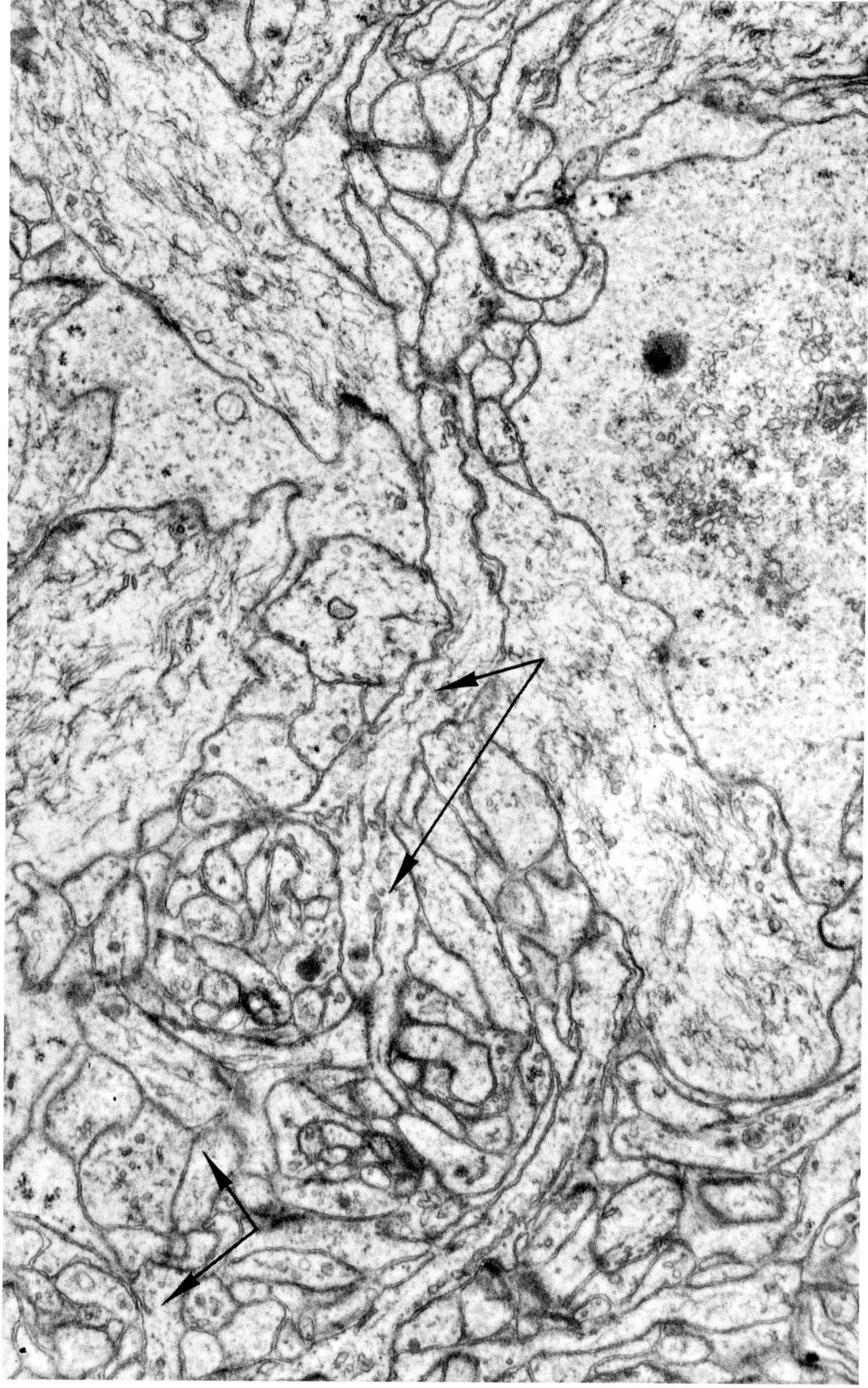

Figure 51. Section close to that illustrated in Figure 50. Two medium-sized processes (arrows) from horizontal cells are shown, both of which enter the invagination of the reconstructed β-type receptor cell, each forming several proximal vacuoles. $\times$ 19,000.

SUMMARY

Three-dimensional reconstructions of nervous centers such as the retina aim to reveal their circuitry in a precise way. Such a revealing of the circuitry together with electrophysiological recordings at known points in the circuits would provide information for the imitation of the circuit by means of computer techniques, and for finding circuit-activating conditions which would correspond closely to its physiological behavior.

The outer plexiform layer is characterized by short- and medium-range lateral connections extending from the β-type receptor cells to the α-, as well as to the β-type receptor cells. Furthermore, long-range lateral connections are furnished by the horizontal cells. The structural organization is interpreted as reflecting lateral inhibitory influence of the β-type receptor cells on both α- and β-type cells. The lateral inhibition at the receptor cell level is assumed to result in contrast enhancement. According to this concept, the β-type cells can be characterized as contrast-enhancing elements acting on the α-type receptor cells, which are purely intensity-recording elements. Color-discriminating cells, whether of the cone or of the rod type, have one property in common—they are of the β-type with respect to structure of the synaptic body, with lateral processes making contact with surrounding receptor cells.

Color discrimination can be considered an improvement in contrast enhancement as compared to that involving intensity modulation imposed by non-color-discriminating β-cells. Both contrast-enhancing mechanisms, i.e., accentuation of differences in intensity and color discrimination, are associated with the same type of receptor cells, the β-type. It appears fundamental to distinguish between contrast-enhancing elements and intensity recording elements in the retina and to consider color discrimination as merely an improvement of the contrast-enhancing mechanism of the β-type receptor cells.

REFERENCES

1. Dowling, J. E., and Boycott, B. B., Neural connections of the retina: fine structure of the inner plexiform layer. *Sympos. Quant. Biol.*, 1965, **30**: 393–402.
2. Polyak, S. L., *The Retina.* Univ. of Chicago Press, Chicago, 1941.
3. Sjöstrand, F. S., The ultrastructural organization of retinal rods and cones. *J. Appl. Physics*, 1953, **24**: 117.
4. ———, The ultrastructure of the inner segments of the retinal rods of the guinea pig eye as revealed by electron microscopy. *J. Cell. Comp. Physiol.*, 1953, **42**: 45–70.
5. ———, The ultrastructure of the retinal rod synapses of the guinea pig eye. *J. Appl. Physics*, 1953, **24**: 1422.
6. ———, Die routinenmässige Herstellung von ultradünnen (ca. 200 Å) Gewebeschnitten für elektronenmikroskopische Untersuchungen der Gewebszellen bei hoher Auflösung. *Zschr. wiss. Mikr.*, 1954, **62**: 65–86.
7. ———, Synaptic structures of the retina of the mammalian eye. In: *The Proceedings of the Third International Conference on Electron Microscopy* (R. Ross, Ed.). Royal Microscopical Society, London, 1956: 428–431.

8. Sjöstrand, F. S., Ultrastructure of retinal rod synapses of the guinea pig eye as revealed by three-dimensional reconstructions from serial sections. *J. Ultrastruct. Res.*, 1958, **2**: 122–170.

9. ———, The synaptology of the retina. In: *Colour Vision; Physiology and Experimental Psychology* (A. V. S. de Reuck and J. Knight, Eds.). Churchill, London, 1965: 110–151.

10. Sjöstrand, F. S., and Mountford, S., Three-dimensional revealing of lateral connections between receptor cells in the rabbit retina. In preparation, 1968.

11. Sjöstrand, F. S., and Nilsson, S. E., The structure of the rabbit retina as revealed by electron microscopy. In: *The Rabbit in Eye Research* (J. H. Prince, Ed.). Thomas, Springfield, 1964: 449–513.

THE RETINAL BIPOLAR CELLS AND THEIR SYNAPSES IN THE INNER PLEXIFORM LAYER *

RAYMOND A. ALLEN †
UCLA School of Medicine
Los Angeles, California

The retina has long held special fascination for anatomists (37): nowhere else in the central nervous system (in the strict sense) are the cells more highly ordered, nor does structure seem so clearly related to function. Earlier investigators sought important clues to more general neural relationships in the ordered simplicity of the retinal layers; thus a wealth of detailed information relating to retinal histology has been accumulated.

The studies of the earlier workers, and of Ramón y Cajal in particular, dealt extensively with the retinas of mammals, birds, and fish (52,53,54). Present retinal anatomical concepts, with comparatively minor modifications, are still those of Ramón y Cajal.

It remained, however, for Polyak, the most devoted of all retinal histologists, to compile the main body of information concerning various retinal cell types and, with his own detailed studies, to work out presumptive synaptic connections between them. This was achieved mainly through application of the silver impregnation techniques of Golgi. *The Retina* (49), Polyak's monumental work published in 1941, and *The Vertebrate Visual System* (50), the culmination of his life's labors, published posthumously in 1957, contained a great wealth of detailed information, much of which remains unexploited. Even before Polyak's latter work was published, the electron microscope had extended the range of observation to entirely new dimensions. It is fortunate that so broad and sound a foundation had been laid, for it is unlikely that such an exhaustive study by those methods will be repeated.

Of the various retinal neuronal types, those of the outermost cell layer (the photoreceptors) and those of the innermost layer (the ganglion cells) are fairly accessible for direct functional measurements. The cells of the middle neuronal layer, and particularly the processes which together comprise the inner plexiform

* This study was supported in part by USPHS Research Grant NB-2866. Grateful appreciation and acknowledgement is due Mr. Walter Miyamasu, Miss Monica Guthrie, and Miss Alice Arvin for outstanding technical assistance, Miss Kathryn Torvik for her artistic skill, and Mr. Peter Kleinert and Mr. Herman Kabe for photographic assistance.

† Presently with the Mayo Clinic, Rochester, Minnesota.

layer, pose special problems to anatomists and physiologists alike (22). The inner retinal neuropil is perhaps the least accessible of all the retinal layers for direct study: the feltwork of neural processes with supporting glia and blood vessels was aptly termed "plexiform"—a tangle. The intimate cellular relationships and the synaptic connections between cells in this layer remain but little known. The processes of one of the main classes of retinal neurons, the bipolar cells, are among the most numerous of those which comprise this layer. The importance of these cells in the general retinal architectural scheme has been recognized since the earliest investigations, and their critical role in retinal function has been deemed no less important. As yet few reports have dealt with detailed structural features of bipolar telodendrites at the electron microscopic level (13,14,33,35,36,40,63,65,66).

This study of individual bipolar cells, utilizing serial section techniques with electron microscopy, has the following main objectives: (*a*) To define the three-dimensional form of perikaryon, axon, and telodendron; (*b*) to determine the exact cellular topography, and the size, number, and distribution of interneuronal contacts and differentiated synaptic regions over the neuron; (*c*) to ascertain synaptic relationships between bipolar telodendrons and surrounding processes; (*d*) to determine whether synaptic relationships occur between the individual processes which synapse with a particular bipolar telodendron.

Materials and Methods

The material was taken from normal human eyes removed surgically as orbital exenteration specimens. The specimens were obtained within two or three minutes after blood flow in the central retinal artery was interrupted.

The eyeball, freed as quickly as possible from attached tissues and with least possible manipulation, was cut coronally anterior to the ora serrata. Most of the vitreous body came away with the anterior portion of the eye. The posterior portion, with retina attached at ora serrata, was put into chilled isotonic 1 per cent osmium tetroxide buffered with veronal acetate. The specimens were fixed entire, with occasional moderate agitation and in several changes of generous quantity of fixative. In some instances, meridional slits in the retina were made just posterior to the ora serrata, and the retina was gently lifted to permit fixative to flow beneath. After fixation the specimen was placed in chilled 70 per cent alcohol and, with the aid of a dissecting microscope, segments of retina were cut, identified by location, and oriented for embedding.

The specimen was dehydrated in alcohol and embedded in "Vestopal" (Martin Jaeger). Serial sections cut with the LKB Ultrotome were mounted on copper discs 3.1 mm in diameter with a single slot measuring 1.0 × 2.0 mm. The loops on which the sections were collected were previously coated with 0.1 per cent or 0.2 per cent Formvar. This thin film served as sole support for the sections. The specimens were stained with an alkaline solution of lead hydroxide after brief staining in uranyl acetate. The sections were approximately 250 Å in thickness as calculated by measurements of apparently spherical structures within cells which were followed through consecutive sections. Repeated measurements of many specimens have shown consistent results. The sections were cut perpendicular to the retinal layers. The techniques for cutting and mounting serial sections were essentially those developed by Sjöstrand and workers in his laboratory (20,31,61).

Survey micrographs were taken at 4000 magnification, so that orientation of the total cell could be achieved in the serial montages of higher magnification which were used for the detailed analyses. The micrographs of the cell analyzed in detail were made from original magnifications of 16,000 and printed at ×46,000. Selected portions of the cell were studied from micrographs originally made at 40,000 magnification. Each section was studied in overlapping micrographs

TABLE 1

Ribbon Synapses and Their Relationships

Extent of Individual Ribbon Synapses of a Primary Bipolar Cell Through Consecutive Serial Sections and the Number and Types of Postsynaptic Processes

Ribbon Synapse		Number of Sections	Postsynaptic Processes	
No.	Extent*		No.	Type
2′	4–12	9	41	Axon
			44	Axon
			50	Axon
3′	22–28	7	47	Axon
			80	Dendrite
10′	8–13	6	40	Axon
			44	Axon
11′	14–19	6	44	Axon
			47	Axon
13′	2–9	8	34	Axon
			36	Axon
			37	Axon
17′	8–14	7	42	Axon
			44	Axon
18′	6–10	5	42	Axon
			43	Axon
			38	Axon
22′	24–28	5	48	Axon
23′	24–31	8	38	Axon
			47	Axon
			48	Axon
27′	31–43	13	24	Axon
			38	Axon
			39	Axon
28′	32–34	3	38	Axon
			39	Axon
30′	24–37	14	12	Axon
			18	Axon
			56	Axon
			58	Dendrite
37′	43–49	7	17	Axon
			72	Dendrite
38′	42–46	5	20	Axon
			72	Dendrite
40′	36–43	8	20	Axon
			73	Dendrite
43′	48–53	6	5	Axon
			20	Axon
			60	Dendrite
46′	53–61	9	3	Dendrite
			4	Axon
			17	Axon
53′	33–39	7	64	Axon
			65	Dendrite
			68	Axon
			76	Dendrite
56′	20–30	11	61	Axon
			62	Axon
			31	Axon
65′	16–22	7	20	Axon
			36	Axon
			74	Dendrite
66′	15–21	7	30	Axon
			31	Dendrite
			74	Dendrite
89′	45–48	4	64	Axon
			65	Dendrite
			96	Axon
			76	Dendrite
91′	47–51	5	65	Dendrite
			69	Axon
			77	Axon

* Numbered consecutive serial sections (inclusive) in which ribbon appeared.

mounted in montage (see Figures 53,54)* and composite drawings were made from tracings of each of the micrograph montages. Colors, numbers and, when necessary, letter combinations were used to identify neural processes and synaptic sites as these numerous structures were followed through serial micrographs. In this study of individual synapses, a series of micrographs was considered satisfactory for analysis only if it included all consecutive sections, with each one complete, and if foreign material, breaks, folds, or wrinkles did not preclude taking micrographs or analysis of detail in micrographs of any portion of the cell under study.

From the mounted montages of serial electron micrographs printed at 46,000 magnification, the following were done: (*a*) The three-dimensional form of the cell and some of the synapsing processes (those at the edge of the cell) were depicted as composite artist's drawings from detailed serial tracings (Figure 52); (*b*) a topographic projection of the telodendritic surface was made in order to show the number, type, and distribution of surface synapses, to find the number and types of neural processes which formed contacts, and to determine the approximate surface area occupied by each (Figure 55); (*c*) the number, type, and distribution of synaptic ribbons within the bipolar telodendron were determined, and the dimensions of each (with respect to number of consecutive serial sections) was charted (Figure 55,a,b; Table 1); (*d*) diagrammatic representations of individual synapses and direction of synapses were made, so as to depict the synaptic circuitry with respect to the primary bipolar cell and to selected synapsing processes which were included in the montages (Figures 56 and 57).

The terminology is that pertaining to nerve cells generally (2,4,6,31), but with respect to special retinal structures and cellular relationships, an attempt was made, where possible, to follow the usage of Polyak (49,50).

Observations

General Assumptions Used in Interpretations

Determination of precise cellular origin of the intertwining processes of the retinal neuropils is a formidable obstacle to the study of retinal cellular relations and synaptic connections. The starting point in this study was positive identification of a bipolar telodendron with a parent cell in a series of consecutive sections of sufficient number, length and width, oriented to include the perikaryon, axon and most of the telodendritic expansions.

There are still no definite criteria for morphologic classification of many neural processes in electron micrographs of random sections (23,31,47,48,67,68). Recognizing the lack of positive neurophysiologic confirmation, two commonly held assumptions relating to the morphology of the structures of the central nervous system were used in these analyses: (*a*) Axons and dendrites may be differentiated by their ultrastructural characteristics (8,9,23,44,46,47,55,56,69,70); (*b*) synaptic contacts may be identified and, further, certain features indicating direction of the synapse may be distinguished (9,10,23–26,44,46,51,55,69,70).

---

* Figure section, pp. 124–143.

The features believed to distinguish axons from dendrites in the central nervous system at the electron microscopic level have been well described (8,23,24,44,67); these distinctions have also been applied to the neural elements of the inner neuropil of the retina (13,14,35,36,40,41,63–66). The smaller dendrites generally contain ribosomes, have a more irregular contour, and follow a more sinuous course through the neuropil. Axons typically do not contain ribosomes; however, the most important single difference is the presence of synaptic vesicles within the cytoplasm of the axon (48,68). This critical feature may only appear within an axon at a synaptic junction, and the combination of synaptic vesicles and ribosomes occurs very rarely (48); retinal amacrine processes constitute one exception to this general statement. Thus, the presence of synaptic vesicles characterizes a given process as axonal; the presence of ribosomes is suggestive, but not positive, evidence that a small process is dendritic.

Serial section techniques seem to support these assumptions by making it generally possible to follow a process of indeterminate type until characteristic features appear. In numerous instances in this and parallel studies, where cell processes have been followed to parent cell through serial sections, the findings have agreed with assertions of Palay and others (8,47,48). The finding that analyses of bipolar synaptic relationships through serial sections yield consistent patterns could probably be considered additional supporting evidence.

Morphologic criteria for synaptic contacts in the inner neuropil are generally those described elsewhere in the central nervous system (3,8,24–26,32,33,40, 42–44,46). The plasma membranes of the synapsing neural processes come into apposition in such a way as to lie parallel to each other, and are further characterized by an accumulation of electron-dense material along the membranes and in the adjacent cytoplasm; it may appear symmetrical, but is not necessarily so (25). Vesicles within the cytoplasm of one of the components at the junction may represent the presynaptic side of the synapse (8,10,11,23–25,28,42,43). When vesicles were found within both processes, closely related to the contact, the synapse was regarded as bidirectional or axoaxonal (7,48). Contacts with no associated synaptic vesicles have been considered adhesive (26,27,48). Thus, both the characteristic apposition and specialization of plasma membranes with associated synaptic vesicles at that site were considered essential components of a synaptic contact. The synaptic apparatus of bipolar cells also includes a synaptic ribbon of characteristic location and appearance. Minor variations of individual synapses include electron-dense material, often with fairly distinct periodicity within the synaptic cleft or within the cytoplasm of the postsynaptic member adjacent to the synaptic site (38). Interneuronal specialized areas of the "tight junction" type (13,17,57,58) were not found in this material.

Applying these assumptions to the analysis of serial micrographs, it is possible to define the number and types of synapses and their general distribution over the cell, the number and general types of cell processes which apparently form the synaptic relationships, and the relative areas of the cell surface with which individual cell processes and glia are in contact.

In individual micrographs of the inner plexiform layer, bipolar axons may generally be identified by their size and radial course and by their round and regular contour in profile. The telodendrons may be distinguished by their characteristic balloon shape and by their cytoplasmic organelles and synaptic apparatus (13,32,33,35,40,41,63,65). Tentative identification of the remaining neural components of this layer is far less certain and in many instances impossible in single micrographs. Amacrine cell processes are generally characterized by fairly large size, sinuous course and, at synaptic sites, the occurrence of large clusters of synaptic vesicles. In this report, according to forementioned criteria, individual cell processes were considered simply axonal or dendritic in character where they could not be positively identified by joining to their cell of origin, or where features apparently characteristic of bipolar or of amacrine cell processes were not clearly evident.

General Aspects of Inner Retinal Neuropil

The inner retinal neuropil in primates consists principally of the following neural elements: axonal extensions of bipolar and amacrine cells, dendrites of ganglion cells, and glial matrix. Other neural components, less well studied, include processes of associational neurons in the ganglion cell layer and exogenous centrifugal fibers to the retina (12,49,50). Blood vessels course across the entire thickness and ramify within the inner nuclear layer.

The layer is thickest at the macula, where the neurons are most numerous and their processes most thickly set. In this area both the dendritic and the axonal processes of the bipolar cell are longest and extend over relatively great distances; they course obliquely with respect to the retinal layers, and hence also to the perikarya of the respective cells of their origin.

Towards the retinal periphery the layer is thinner, the cell processes are less numerous and less closely crowded together. Although individual cells in this area are probably no less complex in their ramifications, their cellular extensions are easier to follow and specialized interneuronal relationships are easier to define. The axons of the bipolar cell are oriented radially to the retinal layers, so that, in small samples of retinal tissue, the likelihood of including the bipolar cell body with its telodendritic extensions is greater if sections are cut in this direction. Thus, in a study aimed at defining the ramifications of single cell processes within the inner plexiform layer, there are important advantages in selecting for study the more peripheral portions of the retina.

As in neuropils elsewhere in the nervous system, the neural elements of the inner plexiform layer are packed together with little free space beyond the narrow clefts measuring 150–200 Å which separate the plasma membranes of the adjacent components. Ramifying among the various processes are exceedingly complicated and irregular sheet-like extensions of glia. The blood vessels which traverse the inner plexiform layer of the peripheral retina are comparatively sparse.

This report is mostly related to the bipolar axonal and telodendritic extensions and the specialized interneuronal relationships which were found over these portions of the cell. So that the interneuronal and synaptic relationships of the bipolar cell may be better defined, the other cellular processes of the neuropil will be briefly described.

Amacrine Cells. These are characterized by numerous processes which extend over broad areas within the inner plexiform layer (49,50). "Amacrine", a term used originally by Ramón y Cajal to denote cells supposedly lacking axons, has been rendered even more incongruous by electron microscopic studies. Previous such studies have shown that the amacrine processes are clearly axonal in structure (61) in that they contain large clusters of synaptic vesicles, but their organelles resemble those more commonly associated with dendrites (13). In this report, the amacrine processes which contain synaptic vesicles are considered axonal; thus, amacrine cells are considered simply as a general class of retinal neurons, and no attempt is made to classify them into subtypes.

The amacrine perikaryon, of flask or urn shape, is usually tilted slightly from the radial axis and is notably larger than that of the bipolar neuron. In the peripheral retina most of the cell bodies along the inner edge of the inner nuclear layer are those of amacrine neurons (Polyak zone 6d). The nucleus of the amacrine neuron is typically located nearer the outer edge of the perikaryon, and is nearly round in profile, in contrast to the elliptical outline of bipolar and glial cells. Nuclear infoldings are ordinarily more prominent than in other retinal neurons of the inner nuclear layer (13).

The amacrine cell cytoplasm, more abundant than that of neighboring bipolar or glial cells, lies mostly at the inner side of the perikaryon, and contains numerous large mitochondria, abundant rough-surfaced endoplasmic reticulum (Nissl substance), and numerous variously sized dark spherical bodies, presumably of lipoidal nature. The cytocentrum is at the vitreal edge of the nucleus, and many amacrine cells bear a cilium of interesting internal structure (1). Subsurface cisterns are occasionally found within the perikaryon and processes of amacrine cells (41,59).

From an irregular trunk-like extension of the perikaryon, often protruding well into the neuropil, large processes diverge abruptly. Coursing generally horizontally, the branches curve so sharply that they usually pass almost immediately from the plane of the parent cell body. Even when they are in close proximity to the parent cell, their exact cellular origins are rarely evident in single sections.

The diameter of amacrine cell processes in profile is usually two to three times that of bipolar cells. The cytoplasm of the amacrine processes contain numerous mitochondria, abundant neurofibrils, large vesicles, multivesiculated bodies, and occasional dense bodies. Scattered ribosomes, often arrayed around neurotubules, are also present.

The arborizations of the amacrine processes within the inner neuropil are more complex, extend over far greater distances, and pursue a more sinuous course than those of bipolar cells. By comparison, the thin stem-like axons of the bipolar cell in the peripheral retina course radially almost in a straight line to form the telodendria.

Expanded segments occur at synaptic sites along the course of the amacrine processes and their terminal bulb-like expansions are only slightly larger. Well-defined boutons of the type which characterizes bipolar cells have not been seen. Within the expanded synaptic segments, large clusters of synaptic vesicles occur, and the number and sharply localized distribution of such synaptic vesicles have been found only within amacrine cell processes. Long segments of the ramifying processes may be entirely free of synaptic vesicles, for these large clusters apparently occur only at synaptic sites.

Ganglion Cell Processes within the Inner Plexiform Layer. Numerous processes of ganglion cell origin ramify in all layers of the neuropil. While most of these are known to be dendritic, occasional ganglion cells displaced outwards may present complicating features. The largest ganglion cell dendrites, often several times larger in profile than processes of known amacrine origin, may course over great distances. They may at times sweep directly across entire sections. Smaller dendrites and branchings typically follow a much more sinuous course.

Because of the limited sampling methods of electron microscopy and of the discrepancy in the order of magnification between light and electron micrographs, earlier light microscopic classifications (49,52) have thus far been of little help in analyzing individual ganglion cells and their processes within the inner plexiform layer.

These processes have the appearance of dendrites, and their large size and direct course are characteristic, but so far no truly distinctive features have been recognized which identify them as belonging to ganglion cells. The source of origin of a few processes, usually of larger size, can be verified through serial sections, but in most cases the sampling methods are far too limited to deal with the far-flung extensions of these larger neurons.

Within the human retina, spine-type synapses (32,33) have been encountered in this material only between amacrine cells and large dendritic trunks.* It is the smaller ganglion cell dendritic branches which usually form synaptic complexes with bipolar cells.

The Enveloping Glia. It is generally held that the glia of the peripheral retina consist principally of Müller cells. As yet there is no complete classification of these cells either at the light or at the electron microscopic level (19,30,35,36,49,50,66). The electron micrographic appearance of the glial cell body and main protoplasmic extensions is fairly distinctive, and has been described in general terms by others (13,14,19,30,35,36,66). The finest glial extensions may be difficult to identify in single electron micrographs, but their true nature becomes generally evident as they are traced through serial sections. The neural processes usually have a regular outline and, except where branchings occur, remain relatively constant in size as they are followed from section to section. By contrast, glial processes change rapidly in both size and contour, becoming larger or smaller as they are followed respectively towards or away from the parent cell body.

* Author's unpublished observations.

Perikarya of glial cells in the peripheral retina are mostly located in Polyak zones 6c and 6d. The glial nuclei are oval, generally free of infoldings, and arranged in an uneven layer. The glial cytoplasm is less specialized in appearance than that of the neurons, and the organelles within are more widely dispersed. These organelles include neurofibrils, occasional large mitochondria, neurotubules, small clusters of ribosomes, rough-surfaced endoplasmic reticulum, and vesicles of various kinds, including lipofuscin (60). The cytocentrum is usually at the scleral edge of the nucleus. Cilia have been observed in glial cells in some instances.

In single sections, radial columns of glial cytoplasm extend at intervals across the inner plexiform layer as if dividing the neuropil into compartments. Broader glial extensions ramify irregularly into the closely packed elements of the neuropil, and still finer branches insinuate themselves among the neural branchings, dividing and subdividing among more densely packed neural processes. As the glial column is followed through successive serial micrographs, ascending bipolar processes appear and are lost into the adjacent compartments, and occasional larger neural processes sweep horizontally across it.

Along the course of the glial plasma membranes there are occasional adhesive plaques with neighboring neural processes or, less commonly, with other glial extensions.

The Three-Dimensional Form of Peripheral Retinal Bipolar Cells

The bipolar perikarya, mostly located in Polyak zones 6b and 6c, are occasionally seen along either edge of the inner nuclear layer (Polyak zones 6a and 6d).

In serial reconstructions, the perikaryon is characteristically oval (Figure 52a). The nucleus, eccentrically placed, occupies the broader inner end of the cell body from which the axon extends. The outer narrower pole of the perikaryon tapers to form a blunt trunk which divides to form several main dendritic branches. These in turn branch further, ultimately forming small twigs which weave through the external neuropil.

The nucleus is an ellipsoid, aligned to the long axis of the cell. One or two nucleoli are usually present. Occasional longitudinal infoldings of the nuclear membrane are seen, but these rarely extend the full length of the nucleus. No really distinctive nuclear features of these cells have been recognized. Sections including the edge of the nuclear membrane show prominent nuclear pores.

Abundant Golgi apparatus is found at the scleral edge of the nucleus. The centrioles are usually at the outer edge of the Golgi organelle, often with rootlets extending towards the nucleus. Scattered ribosomes and rough-surfaced endoplasmic reticulum, more plentiful in the region of the cytocentrum, are present in the cytoplasm throughout the perikaryon. Randomly oriented mitochondria are numerous at the outer pole, and are distributed mainly through the broader rim of cytoplasm between cell membrane and nucleus and towards the side of the cell from which the axon extends (Figure 52a). At the axon hillock the mitochondria and neurotubules converge and funnel into the emerging axon.

The axon hillock is situated towards one edge of the inner broader pole of the perikaryon, and with the main body of the cytoplasm forms a broad stream extending almost perfectly vertically from the main dendritic branchings to the axonal telodendron. The main organelles of the perikaryon appear as though tiered, whereas abundant neurotubules and mitochondria extend in orderly fashion from the outer end of the neural cell body to the inner end of the axon at its specialized telodendritic expansion.

From the cell body the stem-like axon courses radially to the inner plexiform layer, weaving slightly as it passes between more vitreally located cell bodies which may be several layers thick. Typically this portion of the axon is enveloped by glia, but as the axon emerges into and within the inner plexiform layer, the neural processes crowd closely about it. The course of the bipolar axon remains nearly radial with respect to the inner plexiform layer and its size does not change appreciably until the abrupt transition of axon to telodendron. No consistent relationship has yet been recognized between location of cell body within Polyak zone 6 and the levels to which the telodendritic expansions occur within the neuropil (Polyak zone 7). In addition to neurotubules and neurofilaments, the cytoplasm of the axon contains occasional mitochondria, and these organelles are arrayed parallel to the course of the axon.

Vesicular structures, many of which appear to be dilated neurotubules, may be seen in fortuitous sections, sometimes beading along the course of a single neurotubule. The neurotubules of the axon are generally prominent, measuring approximately 125 Å in diameter (33,34). Occasional vesicles of much larger size (1000 to 2000 Å) may be present; some of these are clear, others contain multiple vesicles of smaller size (200 Å). Bodies of variable size and composition, resembling lipofuscin (60), may be present within the axon. Ribonucleic acid granules may also be found within the axon, but in fewer numbers than in the dendritic cytoplasm.

General Features of the Telodendron

Bipolar axons form telodendritic expansions at all levels of the neuropil, but those which extend to the inner zones of the inner plexiform layer typically course most of the distance within the broad glial columns. Contrary to stated opinions (14), occasional synaptic contacts occur over the distal axon (Figure 52, arrow). As the axon expands to become telodendron, the individual boutons often assume an oblique or horizontal position with respect to the retinal layers, and the enveloping glia is abruptly replaced by apposing neural processes.

The bipolar telodendron is of characteristic configuration, consisting of several more or less separate pear-shaped boutons, usually positioned at various different levels within the neuropil. The short narrow segment connecting more widely separated boutons resembles the axon in structure. In single micrographs the connecting segments between boutons are usually not evident, being of relatively small diameter, and the separated individual boutons appear only rarely at the same level and plane as the section.

In single micrographs the processes surrounding the telodendron are distributed in a distinctive mosaic arrangement. Typically, the synapsing processes are arrayed in pairs, a pattern often accentuated by the configuration of all the cell processes involved, and also by the position of a synaptic ribbon within the bipolar telodendron nearby. The majority of the processes which contact the primary cell may be shown in serial sections to form synaptic relationships of one or another type with it.

Within the telodendron, neurotubules and neurofibrils are less conspicuous and their arrangement is less ordered than in the axon. Mitochondria are larger, more numerous, and more complicated in form. Synaptic vesicles, scattered generally through the cytoplasm of the telodendrite, are more numerous at the periphery, especially at synaptic sites; they surround the synaptic ribbons as cloud-like masses. In the human retina the synaptic vesicles average approximately 300 Å in diameter. Occasional larger vesicles containing a darker central body may be present. These structures resemble those described in neurosecretory cells (21,45,62).

Bipolar Telodendritic Synapses

The primary bipolar telodendron analyzed in detail was used as a reference point. The emissive (or outgoing) synapses are termed "efferent"; where the bipolar telodendron itself is presumed postsynaptic, the synapse is termed "afferent". The neural elements with which the bipolar cell forms specialized relationships are termed "synapsing processes" regardless of the direction of the synapses assumed to be present.

Two general types of efferent synapses of the bipolar telodendron were recognized. The first type, the "ribbon synapse" (32,33), consisted of the characteristic synaptic ribbon within the bipolar cell, with associated distinctive changes of the plasma membranes of both the primary and the synapsing cell processes, and with a distinct accumulation of synaptic vesicles about the synaptic ribbon and often along the synaptic site within the bipolar telodendron. The second efferent synapse type, termed "conventional" (32,33) or "simple" (31), consisted of the thickened darker plasma membranes of the two neural processes at the synaptic site, with an accumulation of synaptic vesicles distinctly related to the synaptic site. This synapse type was similar to the first, except that the ribbon was not present and the synapse at any one site involved only one postsynaptic member. Although the specialized areas are usually discontinuous at the region of contact, they are ordinarily fewer and closer together than the multiple contact areas of a given process at a ribbon synaptic complex.

The ribbon synapse with the distinctive paired arrangement of postsynaptic processes appears to be characteristic of the bipolar cells (13,18,39,65). There is considerable variation between the individual ribbon synapses over the bipolar cell (Table 1). Serial section analysis has disclosed that an individual ribbon is usually associated with an entire synaptic complex involving as many as four postsynapsing processes, some of which may also be members of other ribbon synaptic complexes.

Within the bipolar telodendron the synaptic ribbon is characteristically directed perpendicularly to the plasma membrane at the synaptic area. It often appears to be pointed between the paired postsynaptic processes which abut upon the bipolar cell. The latter, molded in contour to the closely applied synapsing processes, presents a distinctive faceted appearance at the synaptic sites. In sections which pass through the edge of the telodendron, the ribbon may appear oriented parallel to the plasma membrane, and only a single postsynaptic member may be evident. Three-dimensional reconstructions of selected synaptic ribbons have shown that they are disk-like structures of fairly uniform thickness (240–270 Å), usually curving slightly in several different planes (Figure 58). Hence they may appear in single sections as curved U- or sometimes S-shaped structures; in some thin sections the ribbon may appear laminated (Figure 59).

Clustered about the ribbon and closely aligned at its edges, as well as along the thickened plasma membrane of the primary cell, are numerous synaptic vesicles. Generally fewer vesicles appear in intimate association with the synaptic site with ribbon synapses than with those of the simple or conventional variety. Considerable variation is present with respect to size and shape of individual synaptic ribbons and in the number and types of synapsing processes which comprise the entire ribbon synaptic complexes (Figures 56,57; Table 1).

Individual ribbons within this bipolar cell varied in extent from three to fourteen consecutive serial sections (Table 1), but most ribbons were present through five to ten sections. As a synaptic ribbon with nearby surface synaptic contacts is followed through serial sections, complicated interrelationships between the primary cell and synapsing processes can be determined. As many as four separate synapsing processes were distinctly associated with a single synaptic ribbon, and some processes were associated with as many as four separate synaptic ribbons (Figures 56 and 57).

Each of the synaptic ribbons within the bipolar cell was associated with a complex of individual efferent and afferent synapses. The synapsing processes were predominantly axonal, and the number and distribution of dendrites among the synaptic complexes formed no recognizable pattern. Moreover, most synapsing processes formed synaptic contacts with the primary cell at sites related to several synaptic ribbons (Figures 56 and 57). There was considerable variation in the extent and hence in the area of individual synapses, and also in the number of synapsing processes associated with a synaptic complex. The precise relationship of the synaptic ribbon to the individual synapsing processes remains unclear. In single sections the ribbon appears associated with two or three synapsing members. Analyses of a synaptic ribbon, its associated surface specializations, and related synapsing processes through consecutive serial sections have invariably shown them forming complicated groupings and interrelationships.

The simple synapses, on the other hand, consist of the apposition of the plasma membranes of the synapsing processes with accumulation of electron-dense material along the membranes and in the adjacent cytoplasm. Within the cytoplasm of the presynaptic member there is an accumulation of synaptic vesicles, and these are distinctly associated with the synaptic site. Synaptic junctions with larger neural processes were often localized and discontinuous, and in the analysis these were identified by separate numbers (Figures 56 and 57); these separate specialized areas varied in size and extent, but no other significant differences in appearance of the essential components of the synapse were noted. The synaptic cleft of the simple (or conventional) synapse measured approximately 200 Å in width.

Topographic projection of the telodendron surface was done in order to determine the areas of contact over the primary bipolar telodendron by each of the surrounding processes (Figure 55). The boutons of the telodendron exist at different planes; in the analyses each was shown as it appeared in sequence. The individual apposing processes were identified by number, and were followed through the sections where they were in contact with the primary cell. The areas of contact shown are approximate, for no correction was made for the curvatures of the irregular telodendritic cylindroids, which are depicted in two-dimensions. The projection is thus a flat surface derived from chords tangent to the curves of the surface irregularities of the cell membrane; it depicts only the single plane of the cell surface followed through the consecutive sections, and therefore those few neural processes which curved away from and back to the cell surface can be shown only as forming contacts at separated points. The efferent synapses (with respect to the bipolar cell) are shown as prime numbers in black circles, and the afferent synaptic contacts as prime numbers in squares. This stylized representation of synaptic areas shows the number, type, and distribution of synapses over the cell, but precludes precise representation of the relationships of the individual members of the synaptic complexes.

The synaptic ribbons associated with respective synaptic complexes are within the cell at different planes and at various oblique angles relative to the cell surface, hence their location could not be shown in the projection. The cell processes which comprise a particular synaptic complex usually make contact over a comparatively large area and, since they usually do not converge at a common point, they appear as separated areas in the projection.

The topographic analysis disclosed definite differences in the number, type, and distribution of the synaptic areas over each of the boutons of the telodendron, as well as in number, type, and area of contact of the processes which abut upon the primary cell. The efferent synapses are relatively more numerous over the proximal bouton and are localized towards one area of the cell. The efferent synapses (black circles) of the two inner boutons also appear localized to certain areas of the cell surface, whereas the afferent (with respect to the primary cell) synapses appear fairly evenly distributed over the cell surface (Figure 55,a,b).

The projection demonstrated that most cell processes which are in surface contact with the primary bipolar telodendron form synaptic relationships with it. Although most cell processes remain in apposition only in the region of the synapse, a few neural elements remained in close contact with the cell through many sections. The terminal axons which synapsed with the bipolar cell were bulbous, whereas axons which formed subterminal synapses were less strikingly dilated; this feature may prove helpful in distinguishing axons from dendrites within the neuropil.

The topographic projection also revealed the approximate cell surface area overlain by glia. Proximal to the subterminal bouton, the cell (including most of the axon), the cell body and the proximal dendrites are virtually surrounded by glia. By comparison, only a relatively small proportion of the surface area of the telodendron is in contact with glia.

Direction of Synapses

Seventy-two neural processes formed synaptic contacts with the bipolar telodendron; 61 were axons, 11 dendrites. All but three of the dendrites were associated with ribbon synapses and were members of complex synaptic groupings (Figure 56). There were 18 axons which formed simple afferent synapses with primary telodendron and were unassociated with ribbon synaptic complexes; one axon was associated at a bidirectional synapse. Three individual dendrites were also unassociated with ribbon synaptic complexes; all occurred well within the series of sections and appeared to be completely included.

When individual synapses between synapsing processes and primary bipolar telodendron were diagrammed to show direction, interesting relationships were revealed. The synapsing processes which in single micrographs often appear in groups of two or three at ribbon synapses proved to be members of larger and more complicated synaptic complexes. While the aspect of these synaptic groupings is one of apparent complexity, it results from a fairly simple interlocking system of repetitive pairs or triples joined in series by a common member, and, at fairly regular intervals, with a single member joining smaller groupings into larger complexes. The synapsing members of these more complicated groupings showed serial as well as hierarchical arrangement. A single synapsing member in many instances was related to two or more separate ribbon synapses. In three cases a single synapsing member was associated with four synaptic ribbons.

The number and type of neuronal components varied between individual synaptic complexes. Most of the synapsing processes were axonal in character and formed serial synapses, as described in the retina by Kidd (33). Among the processes forming the synaptic complexes, the relationships of dendrites to axons formed no consistent nor recognizable pattern.

There were 23 ribbon synaptic complexes, and most of the processes at these sites formed serial (33)—reciprocal (13)—synapses with the bipolar cells. It is apparent from the diagram that most bipolar efferent synapses occur in association with the synaptic ribbon organelle.

Many processes, apparently of amacrine cell type, formed more than one afferent synapse with the primary cell. In a few cases such processes (numbered 30A, 21A, 20A, 62A, 39A) formed two separate synapses; one such process (No. 40A) formed three separate afferent synaptic contacts (Figure 56). Although these multiple synaptic contacts were separate and discontinuous, they were located closely together. Thirty processes of axonal nature were involved in ribbon synaptic complexes, and 23 of these formed serial synapses; seven axons did not (Nos. 43, 50, 44, 38, 77, 37, 63). Three processes (Nos. 10d, 15d, 59d) are noteworthy in that they appeared unassociated with any of the other processes in the micrographs and did not fit into any of the interconnecting synaptic groupings.

Of the hierarchically arranged axons, only two (Nos. 44A and 38A), each of which formed synapses related to four separate synaptic ribbons, did not show reciprocal relationships with the primary cell. No significant differences appeared between these and the remaining processes which formed synapses with the primary cell. Available evidence indicates that only one terminal from a given process enters into synaptic relationship with a particular cell. It cannot necessarily be inferred that each synapsing process originated from a different cell, even though accumulated evidence indicates this to be likely. Although uncommonly, a particular neural process may form two widely separated synaptic contacts at different parts of the primary cell.

Of the 13 dendritic processes synapsing at ribbons, six (Nos. 80d, 3d, 58d, 73d, 60d, and 31d) were associated at one ribbon each; three (Nos. 76d, 72d, and 74d) were each associated with two ribbons, and one (No. 65d) with three separate ribbons.

From the topographical projection and from the directional diagram of synapses, it is evident that the synaptic complexes correspond generally to the individual telodendritic boutons or even to portions of boutons, and in this cell they apparently did not extend across connecting segments of the telodendron.

The more complicated synaptic interconnections within groupings comprised of fewer members are located at the innermost or terminal boutons. By comparison, the interrelationships between members of synapsing groupings in the proximal bouton appear less complicated, even though more individual processes are involved (Figure 56, lower left, cf. key by numbered synapses in Figure 55c).

The bipolar efferent synaptic transmission appears predominantly to be by way of the ribbon synaptic complexes. The functional significance of this and the other synaptic types rcmains unknown.

From an anatomical viewpoint, the individual boutons, each with separate, possibly independent circuitry, and their distribution through several zones of the inner plexiform layer, suggest different integrative levels within this layer (6).

Amacrine Cell Synapses

Included in the montages of the sections was a portion of the perikaryon and proximal segments of many large processes of an amacrine cell (Process No. 43). The synapse No. 18′ with the primary bipolar cell (Figure 56) occurred near the beginning of the series, and it was possible to diagram the general pattern of synapses between amacrine cell No. 43 and a nearby bipolar telodendron "G". Process No. 50 (Figure 56) was associated at synapse 16″ with the second bipolar cell "G". Process No. 42A, associated with Process No. 43 at synapse 17′ in Circuit A_1 (box), but formed no further synaptic relationships with processes which appeared in the second diagram (Figure 57). The processes that did not synapse with the primary bipolar cell but did synapse with amacrine cell No. 43

and bipolar "G" were identified by letters as they were followed through serial sections. Portions of bipolar telodendron "G" were present through 61 of the 67 consecutive sections. This cell formed efferent ribbon synapses 13″ and 17″ (Figure 57) with amacrine cell No. 43. Within the montages, processes Ea, Ua, and La could be identified as portions of other bipolar telodendrons; a few of their synaptic relationships are shown. Figure 57 thus represents a small portion of a presumptive second retinal synaptic circuit with respect to the bipolar cell in Figure 54 (see also Figure 56). Although the results are less complete, and hence less conclusive, the similarity between the synaptic connections of this cell and the primary bipolar cell is apparent.

These general relationships have also been found in other bipolar cells similarly analyzed and possibly represent a more general organizational and functional pattern.

The synaptic relationships of the amacrine cell processes are apparently simpler and the number of synaptic contacts of a single process considerably fewer than those of bipolar telodendria. Also of interest, very few of the processes synapsing with the amacrine cell formed serial synapses.

Except for reciprocal synapses between individual processes, it was not possible in these circuit diagrams to achieve completion of the synaptic circuit with respect to the original cell. Indeed, of all the numerous processes analyzed through long series of sections, only Process No. 50A appeared as a common member of the two diagrams. Of the numerous processes which formed synaptic relationships with the primary bipolar cell, none were found to form synapses with each other.

Conclusions

Essential to a more complete understanding of neural connections of the retina is the quantitative determination of the kinds of synapses, their distribution over each of the various cell types, and the number and kinds of cellular processes which enter into these specialized interneuronal contacts. At present, the best method for gaining such information appears to be through application of serial section techniques adequate to include entire cell processes. These methods are difficult and arduous but they yield precise information relating to individual cells and to the number, types and distribution of specialized interneuronal relationships with which each is associated.

The peripheral retina was chosen for this study in order to facilitate the identification of a particular bipolar telodendron with its parent cell: fewer cells and cell processes are found there than in the more central areas of retina; axonal and dendritic extensions of individual cells are shorter and thus can more easily be related to cell of origin. Whether significant differences exist between telodendria and synaptic connections of individual types of bipolar cells of the central and peripheral retina is not known, but studies of Golgi preparations by light microscopy indicate that they do not (49).

Differences are known to exist at both the light and electron microscopic levels between rod and cone bipolar cells (41,49). In the present study, although micrographs were made of the dendritic extensions of the primary bipolar cell, they were not analyzed through the external neuropil; the number and types of receptors with which it formed synapses are therefore not yet known.

The precise origin of most of the processes synapsing with the primary bipolar cell in the sample tissue analyzed remains unknown. However, by tracing individual processes through serial sections, it was possible to distinguish the general types and, by commonly accepted criteria, to characterize the axons and dendrites, to ascertain the specialized areas of synaptic contacts, and to determine at the synaptic site the direction of the neural impulse. From such information simple diagrams of the presumptive synaptic relationships of individual cells can be constructed, representative of tentative neural circuits. As yet, however, the true functional nature of the individual synapses, whether inhibitory or excitatory (15,16,28), cannot be ascertained from their morphologic appearance.

The bipolar cells have traditionally been considered as intermediary or internuncial neurons, receiving the neural impulse from the rods or cones at the outer pole and transmitting it to the ganglion cells and presumably to associational neurons of the inner plexiform layer at the inner pole (49,50).

The three-dimensional form of the bipolar cell (Figure 52) and some of the surrounding processes at the electron microscopic level are of interest in showing the distribution of the intracellular organelles and depicting the spatial relationships between the bipolar cell and the processes by which it is surrounded and with which it forms synaptic contacts within the inner plexiform layer. The number, extent, and types of its dendritic extensions are not yet known, nor are the number and types of receptor cells with which it forms dendritic synaptic connections.

The distinctive and orderly spatial arrangement of the single bipolar telodendron surrounded by the various processes which form synaptic relationships with it appears anatomically to form a fairly distinct organizational unit of possible functional significance, as was believed by Polyak on the basis of his light microscopic studies (49). There is an interesting anatomical resemblance of bipolar telodendria and synapsing processes to the "glomerular unit" described in the lateral geniculate body (48), and also to the pyramidal neurons of Ammon's horn (29). The regional or localized distribution of the efferent synapses over the telodendron as a whole, and even over the individual boutons, is evident. The afferent (or incoming) synapses, however (shown with identifying primed numbers in squares), are fairly uniformly distributed over the cell. The precise orientation of the cell within the retina is not known, and hence it is impossible to relate the distribution of these specialized areas to the direction of the main flow of visual impulses.

Of the cell itself, special mention should be made of the synapses and the associated organelles. The synapses are of two main types, but in the present study considerable variation was found in size and shape between individual synapses.

The ribbon synapses are the most conspicuous of the bipolar synaptic organelles and thus they have attracted most attention (13,14,18,63–66). The results of this study indicate that the ribbon synapses are not associated with a single synaptic area but rather form complicated groupings of interrelated synapsing processes through many specialized areas of contact. Serial section analyses have shown considerable variation in size and extent of these synapses, in the number of synapsing processes comprising a synaptic complex, and in the patterns which are formed when the synapses are diagrammed.

Although synaptic ribbons are most characteristically seen within bipolar axons in the inner plexiform layer, they occur also at other sites in the retina; they are most striking within the light receptor cells (61). Such structures have been found within neuronal perikarya and within cell processes clearly well inside the external neural processes in the outer plexiform layer.*

The bipolar efferent simple (31) or conventional (32,33) synapses numbered only four, three of which involved processes believed to be dendritic (Nos. 10d, 15d, 59d); only one (No. 14A) appeared to conform to the serial synaptic type of Kidd (33). Analysis of synaptic areas through serial sections did not yield clear-cut evidence in the human retina of two distinct types of conventional synapses described by Kidd (32,33) in the inner neuropil of cats and pigeons. Indeed, the changing configuration of the synapsing process through the serial sections often presented unusual appearances of thickenings of all of the synaptic organelles (Figure 59).

Among the more interesting findings which emerged from this study of a particular bipolar neuron in the periphery of the human retina are the following: (*a*) Most by far of the synaptic connections are afferent with respect to the bipolar cell, and they derive from almost as many separate neural processes; (*b*) some neuronal processes formed more complicated synaptic relationships, including both afferent and efferent synapses, and entered into distinctive interrelationships with other neural processes with several bipolar synaptic ribbons (Figures 55,a,b;56;57).

The patterns described here, which apply to a single neuron are, however, only one aspect of a far larger and more complicated problem. The morphological aspects of these cellular organelles, their distribution and their relationships to other cell processes may be presumed to form the structural basis of function, but they do not indicate what the function might have been. Some of the interesting aspects relating to neural electrical activity and the functional implications of some known neural relationships and of obstacles which confront present investigators have been reviewed by Dr. Brazier (5).

Compared to neurons generally, the bipolar neurons are very small. Of those within the eye these are the smallest, their axons the shortest and probably the simplest, and the area of their extent the least. Bullock (6) has postulated that some neurons, probably of very small size, might be found with no capacity for all-or-none impulses, whose axons would carry only graded and decrementally spreading activity; that such neurons might constitute the more complex and finely textured higher centers; further, that such function may depend upon such graded and decremental activity and with nerve impulses in the sense of all-or-none propagated spikes.

When the entire emissive synaptic apparatus of the bipolar cell (i.e., its axon

---

* Author's unpublished observations.

and its telodendritic expansions with complicated synaptic organelles, the numerous synapsing processes of complex synaptic circuitry, and with serial synaptic relationships) is considered, it is not difficult to assume that such elaborate and specialized aspects may well constitute the morphologic basis for cells which function less by the familiar all-or nothing response than by means of graded and decrementally spreading activity. Indeed, this study produced some evidence that not only individual boutons, but various portions (segments) of boutons of the telodendron are anatomically discrete and specialized and may thus function as finer and still finer units, each at a different but not entirely separate integrative level.

In Bullock's statement of the problem with reference to the known nerve cell membrane potentials, he postulated that the different kinds of activity represent specialized kinds of cell surface membranes. Thus, striking differences in properties and localization of each of these properties would occur in restricted regions of the neuron (6).

The findings reported here with respect to the number and types of synaptic contacts of bipolar telodendrons, their distribution over the cell surface, their spatial separation, the number and type of synapsing processes, and the apparent directional orientation of these synapses, are all consistent with, but not necessarily in favor of, Bullock's hypothesis. These highly ordered, anatomically very balanced parts of the cell may indeed be concerned with subtle and finely graded or integrated cellular responses.

The distribution of the synapses over the cell surface, the complex relationships between efferent synaptic contacts, as well as between the afferent ones, the complex relationships between bipolar cells and between various parts of the same cell, and surely more, much more, than we now see or even suspect, bespeak functional subtleties and capabilities within and between cells beyond present imaginings.

These details regarding the bipolar axon and telodendron cannot yet be related precisely to known neurophysiologic data. They may be interpreted as being in accord with but not in direct support of supposed refinements which exist at cellular and even subcellular levels, if neurons can do what they are known to do. As Bullock (6) has so aptly stated the problem of the complexity within unity of the neuron, "The size, number, and distribution over the neuron of these functionally differentiated regions and the labile coupling functions between the successive processes that eventually determine what information is transferred to the next neuron provide an enormous range of possible complexity within this single cellular unit."

SUMMARY

The ultrastructure of the cells of the inner nuclear and inner plexiform layers of the midperiphery of the human retina were studied in electron micrographs of consecutive serial sections, with special emphasis on axonal extensions of the bipolar cells into the inner plexiform layer. The cytoplasmic organelles of the subterminal and terminal boutons were studied, and three-dimensional forms of these processes analyzed. The number, type, and distribution of the synapses of such cells were determined with respect to the primary cell and also to the number, type, and distribution of the synapsing neural processes.

The bipolar synapses are of two main types—ribbon and conventional. Individual synaptic areas of both types vary considerably. Ribbon synapses join neural processes into complicated groupings which can be ranked both serially and hierarchically by means of their members in common. Serial synapses characterize many of these processes. Conventional synapses are simpler, and generally involve single processes of dendritic type.

REFERENCES

1. Allen, R. A., Isolated cilia in inner retinal neurons and in retinal pigment epithelium. *J. Ultrastruct. Res.*, 1965, **12**: 730–747.
2. Bishop, G. H., The dendrite: receptive pole of the neurone. *EEG Clin. Neurophysiol.*, 1958, Supp., **10**: 12–21.
3. Blackstad, T. W., and Dahl, H. A., Quantitative evaluation of structures in contact with neuronal somata; an electron microscopic study on the fascia dentata of the rat. *Acta Morph. Neerl.-Scand.*, 1961, **4**: 329–343.
4. Bodian, D., The generalized vertebrate neuron. *Science*, 1962, **137**: 323–326.
5. Brazier, M. A. B., The electrical activity of the nervous system. *Science*, 1964, **146**: 1423–1428.
6. Bullock, T. H., Neuron doctrine and electrophysiology. *Science*, 1959, **129**: 997–1002.
7. Charleton, B. T., and Gray, E. G., Comparative electron microscopy of synapses in the vertebrate spinal cord. *J. Cell Sci.*, 1966, **1**: 67–80.
8. De Robertis, E. D. P., *Histophysiology of Synapses and Neurosecretion.* Pergamon, Oxford, 1964.
9. De Robertis, E. D. P., and Bennett, H. S., Some features of the submicroscopic morphology of synapses in frog and earthworm. *J. Biophys. Biochem. Cytol.*, 1955, **1**: 47–58.
10. De Robertis, E. D. P., Nowinski, W. W., and Saez, F. A., *General Cytology* (3rd ed.). Saunders, Philadelphia, 1960.
11. Dewey, M. M., and Barr, L., A study of the structure and distribution of the nexus. *J. Cell Biol.*, 1964, **23**: 553–586.
12. Dogiel, A. S., Die Retina der Vögel. *Arch. Mikr. Anat.*, 1895, **44**: 622–648.
13. Dowling, J. E., and Boycott, B. B., Neural connections of the retina: fine structure of the inner plexiform layer. *Sympos. Quant. Biol.*, 1965, **30**: 393–402.
14. ———, Organization of the primate retina: electron microscopy. *Proc. Roy. Soc. London B*, 1966, **166**: 80–111.
15. Eccles, J. C., *The Physiology of Synapses.* Academic Press, New York, 1964.
16. ———, Functional meaning of the patterns of synaptic connections in the cerebellum. *Perspect. Biol. Med.*, 1965, **8**: 289–310.
17. Farquhar, M. G., and Palade, G. E., Junctional complexes in various epithelia. *J. Cell Biol.*, 1963, **17**: 375–412.
18. Fine, B. S., Synaptic lamellas in the human retina: an electron microscopic study. *J. Neuropath. Exp. Neurol.*, 1962, **22**: 255–262.
19. Fine, B. S., and Zimmerman, L. E., Müller's cells and the "middle limiting

membrane" of the human retina; an electron microscopic study. *Invest. Ophthal.*, 1962, **1**: 304–326.

20. Galey, F. R., and Nilsson, S. E. G., A new method for transferring sections from the liquid surface of the trough through staining solutions to the supporting film of a grid. *J. Ultrastruct. Res.*, 1966, **14**: 405–410.
21. Gerschenfeld, H. M., Tramezzani, J. H., and De Robertis, E., Ultrastructure and function in neurohypophysis of the toad. *Endocrinology*, 1960, **66**: 741–762.
22. Granit, R., *Sensory Mechanisms of the Retina.* Hafner, New York, 1960.
23. Gray, E. G., Axo-somatic and axo-dendritic synapses of the cerebral cortex: an electron microscope study. *J. Anat.*, 1959, **93**: 420–433.
24. ———, Electron microscopy of dendrites and axons of the cerebral cortex. *J. Physiol.* (London), 1959, **145**: 25–26*P*.
25. ———, Electron microscopy of synaptic contacts on dendrite spines of the cerebral cortex. *Nature* (London), 1959, **183**: 1592–1593.
26. ———, The granule cells, mossy synapses and Purkinje spine synapses of the cerebellum: light and electron microscope observations. *J. Anat.*, 1961, **95**: 345–356.
27. ———, Ultra-structure of synapses of the cerebral cortex and of certain specialisations of neurologlial membranes. In: *Electron Microscopy in Anatomy* (J. D. Boyd, F. R. Johnson, and J. D. Lever, Eds.). Arnold, London, 1961: 54–73.
28. ———, A morphological basis for pre-synaptic inhibition? *Nature* (London), 1962, **193**: 82–83.
29. Hamlyn, L. H., An electron microscope study of pyramidal neurons in the Ammon's Horn of the rabbit. *J. Anat.*, 1963, **97**: 189–201.
30. Hogan, M. J., and Feeney, L., The ultrastructure of the retinal vessels. III. Vascular-glial relationships. *J. Ultrastruct. Res.*, 1963, **9**: 47–64.
31. Karlsson, U., Electron microscopic studies on the visual pathway. *J. Ultrastruct. Res.*, 1966–1967.
32. Kidd, M., Electron microscopy of the inner plexiform layer of the retina. In: *Cytology of Nervous Tissue*, Proc. Anatomical Society of Great Britain and Ireland. Taylor & Francis, London, 1961: 88–91.
33. ———, Electron microscopy of the inner plexiform layer of the retina in the cat and the pigeon. *J. Anat.*, 1962, **96**: 179–187.
34. Kuwabara, T., Microtubules in the retina. In: *The Structure of the Eye; II. Symposium* (J. W. Rohen, Ed.). Schattauer, Stuttgart, 1965: 69–84.
35. Meller, K., Elektronenmikroskopische Befunde zur Differenzierung der Rezeptorzellen und Bipolarzellen der Retina und ihrer synaptischen Verbindungen. *Zschr. Zellforsch.*, 1964, **64**: 733–750.
36. Meller, K., and Glees, P., The differentiation of neuroglia-Müller-cells in the retina of chick. *Zschr. Zellforsch.*, 1965, **66**: 321–332.
37. Mettler, C. C., *History of Medicine.* Blakiston, Philadelphia, 1947.
38. Milhaud, M., and Pappas, G. D., Postsynaptic bodies in the habenula and interpeduncular nuclei of the cat. *J. Cell Biol.*, 1966, **30**: 437–441.
39. Missotten, L., Étude des synapses de la rétine humaine au microscope électronique. In: *The Proceedings of the European Regional Conference on Electron Microscopy*, Vol. II (A. L. Houwink and B. J. Spit, Eds.). De Nederlandse Vereniging voor Electronenmicroscopie, Delft, 1961: 818–821.
40. ———, L'ultrastructure des tissus oculaires. *Bull. Soc. Belg. Ophtal.*, 1964, **136**: 1–204.

41. MISSOTTEN, L., The synapses in the human retina. In: *The Structure of the Eye; II. Symposium* (J. W. Rohen, Ed.). Schattauer, Stuttgart, 1965: 17–28.
42. PALADE, G. E., Electron microscope observations of interneuronal and neuromuscular synapses. *Anat. Rec.*, 1954, **118**: 335–336.
43. PALAY, S. L., Electron microscope study of the cytoplasm of neurons. *Ibid*: 336.
44. ———, Synapses in the central nervous system. *J. Biophys. Biochem. Cytol.*, 1956, **2**, Supp. 193–202.
45. ———, The fine structure of the neurohypophysis. In: *Progress in Neurobiology, Vol. II: Ultrastructure and Cellular Chemistry of Neural Tissue* (H. Waelsch, Ed.). Hoeber-Harper, New York, 1957: 31–49.
46. ———, The morphology of synapses in the central nervous system. *Exp. Cell Res.*, 1958, Supp. **5**: 275–293.
47. ———, The structural basis for neural action. In: *Brain Function, Vol. II: RNA and Brain Function; Memory and Learning* (M. A. B. Brazier, Ed.). UCLA Forum Med. Sci. No. 2, Univ. of California Press, Los Angeles, 1964: 69–108.
48. PETERS, A., and PALAY, S. L., The morphology of laminae A and A_1 of the dorsal nucleus of the lateral geniculate body of the cat. *J. Anat.*, 1966, **100**: 451–486.
49. POLYAK, S. L., *The Retina.* Univ. of Chicago Press, Chicago, 1941.
50. ———, *The Vertebrate Visual System* (ed. by H. Klüver). Univ. of Chicago Press, Chicago, 1957.
51. PURPURA, D. P., Structure and function of cortical synaptic organizations activated by corticipetal afferents in newborn cat. In: *Brain and Behavior*, Vol. I (M. A. B. Brazier, Ed.). American Institute of Biological Sciences, Washington, D.C., 1961: 95–138.
52. RAMÓN Y CAJAL, S., *Histologie du Système Nerveux de l'Homme et des Vertébrés*, Vol. II (L. Azoulay, Transl.). Maloine, Paris, 1911: Ch. 15.
53. ———, *Degeneration and Regeneration of the Nervous System*, Vol. II (R. M. May, Transl. and Ed.). Oxford Univ. Press, London, 1928.
54. ———, *Studies on Vertebrate Neurogenesis* (L. Guth, Transl.). Thomas, Springfield 1960.
55. ROBERTSON, J. D., Ultrastructure of two invertebrate synapses. *Proc. Soc. Exp. Biol. Med.*, 1953, **82**: 219–223.
56. ———, Electron microscope observations on a reptilian myoneural junction. *Anat. Rec.*, 1954, **118**: 346.
57. ———, The occurrence of a subunit pattern in the unit membranes of club endings in Mauthner cell synapses in goldfish brains. *J. Cell Biol.*, 1963, **19**: 201–221.
58. ROBERTSON, J. D., BODENHEIMER, T. S., and STAGE, D. E., The ultrastructure of Mauthner cell synapses and nodes in goldfish brains. *Ibid.*: 159–199.
59. ROSENBLUTH, J., Subsurface cisterns and their relationship to the neuronal plasma membrane. *J. Cell Biol.*, 1962, **13**: 405–421.
60. SAMORAJSKI, T., ORDY, J. M., and KEEFE, J. R., The fine structure of lipofuscin age pigment in the nervous system of aged mice. *J. Cell Biol.*, 1965, **26**: 779–796.
61. SJÖSTRAND, F. S., Ultrastructure of retinal rod synapses of the guinea pig eye as revealed by three-dimensional reconstructions from serial sections. *J. Ultrastruct. Res.*, 1958, **2**: 122–170.
62. SJÖSTRAND, F. S., and WETZSTEIN, R., Elektronenmikroskopische Untersuchung der phäochromen (chromaffinen) Granula in den Markzellen der Nebenniere. *Experientia*, 1956, **12**: 196–199.

63. VILLEGAS, G. M., Electron microscopic study of the vertebrate retina. *J. Gen. Physiol.*, 1960, **43** (6), Supp. 2: 15–43.

64. ———, Comparative ultrastructure of the retina in fish, monkey and man. In: *The Visual System: Neurophysiology and Psychophysics* (R. Jung and H. Kornhuber, Eds.). Springer, Berlin, 1961: 3–13.

65. ———, Ultrastructure of the human retina. *J. Anat.*, 1964, **98**: 501–513.

66. VILLEGAS, G. M., and VILLEGAS, R., Neuron-glia relationship in the bipolar cell layer of the fish retina. *J. Ultrastruct. Res.*, 1963, **8**: 89–106.

67. WESTRUM, L. E., and BLACKSTAD, T. W., An electron microscopic study of the stratum radiatum of the rat hippocampus (regio superior, CA 1) with particular emphasis on synaptology. *J. Comp. Neurol.*, 1962, **119**: 281–292.

68. WOLFE, D. E., Electron microscopic criteria for distinguishing dendrites from preterminal nonmyelinated axons in the area postrema of the rat, and characterization of a novel synapse. *Am. Soc. Cell Biol.*, 1961: 228.

69. WYCKOFF, R. W. G., and YOUNG, J. Z., The nerve cell surface. *J. Anat.*, 1954, **88**: 568.

70. ———, The motoneurone surface. *Proc. Roy. Soc. London B*, 1956, **144**: 440–450.

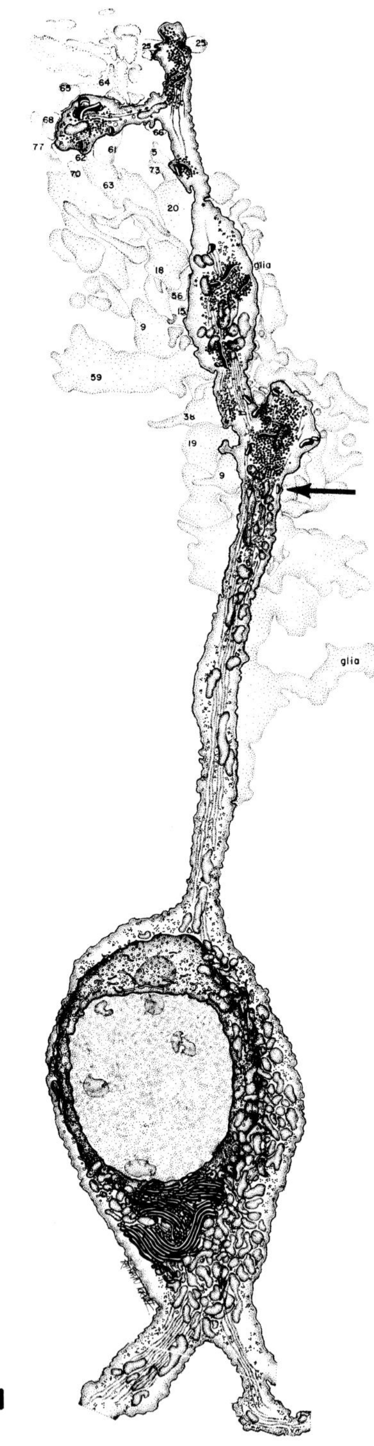

Figure 52. Three-dimensional drawing of primary retinal bipolar telodendron, perikaryon, and proximal segments of dendrites. *b:* Enlargement of upper portion of *a*. The reconstruction was made from montages of each of 67 consecutive serial sections believed to have included almost the entire cell. The lighter area over the nucleus represents cut edge. The Golgi apparatus (lower edge of nucleus) obscures centrioles which lay nearby. The mitochondria are accurately represented in number, shape, and distribution within the cell. Towards the upper edge of nucleus (shown as semitransparent) there is an oval nucleolus; several scattered mitochondria in cytoplasm surrounding the nucleus on opposite side of cell

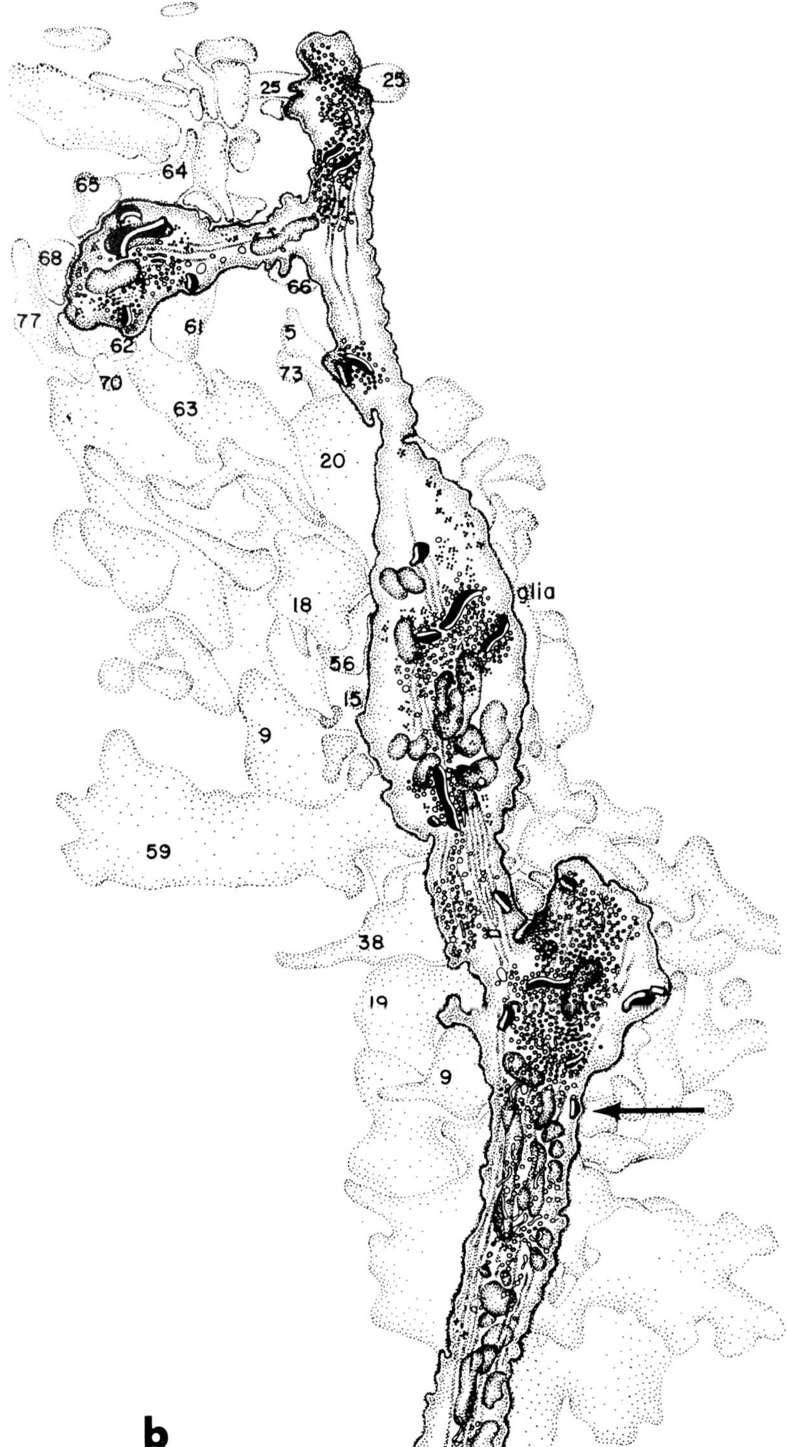

are shown. Locations of neurotubules and ribosomes are represented at sites of occurrence, but not in exact number present in the cell. The cell processes shown as surrounding the telodendron are those present at the level included in the first five sections. The numbered processes are those which formed synaptic contact with the cell or were glial and in extensive intimate association. The approximate size, orientation, and location of the synaptic ribbons are shown (synaptic ribbon in distal axon shown at arrow). Synaptic vesicles are also shown in the locations where they occurred but are not drawn precisely to scale. Original magnification ×46,000.

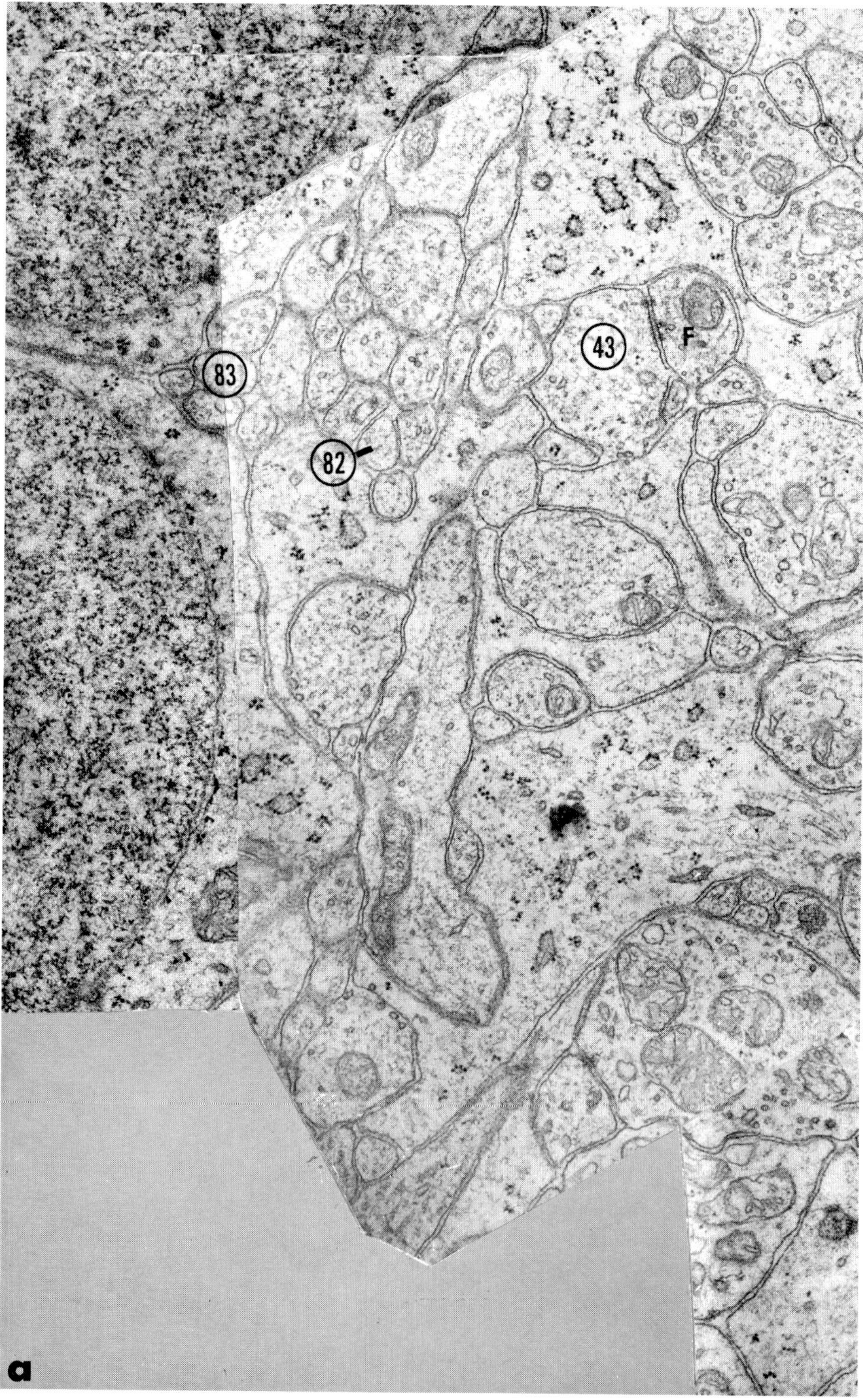

Figure 53, *a–f.* A portion of the montage of Section 24, which includes much of the inner plexiform layer with the portions of the bipolar axon and telodendron which were analyzed. The primary bipolar cell ① and the processes which formed surface contacts with it are

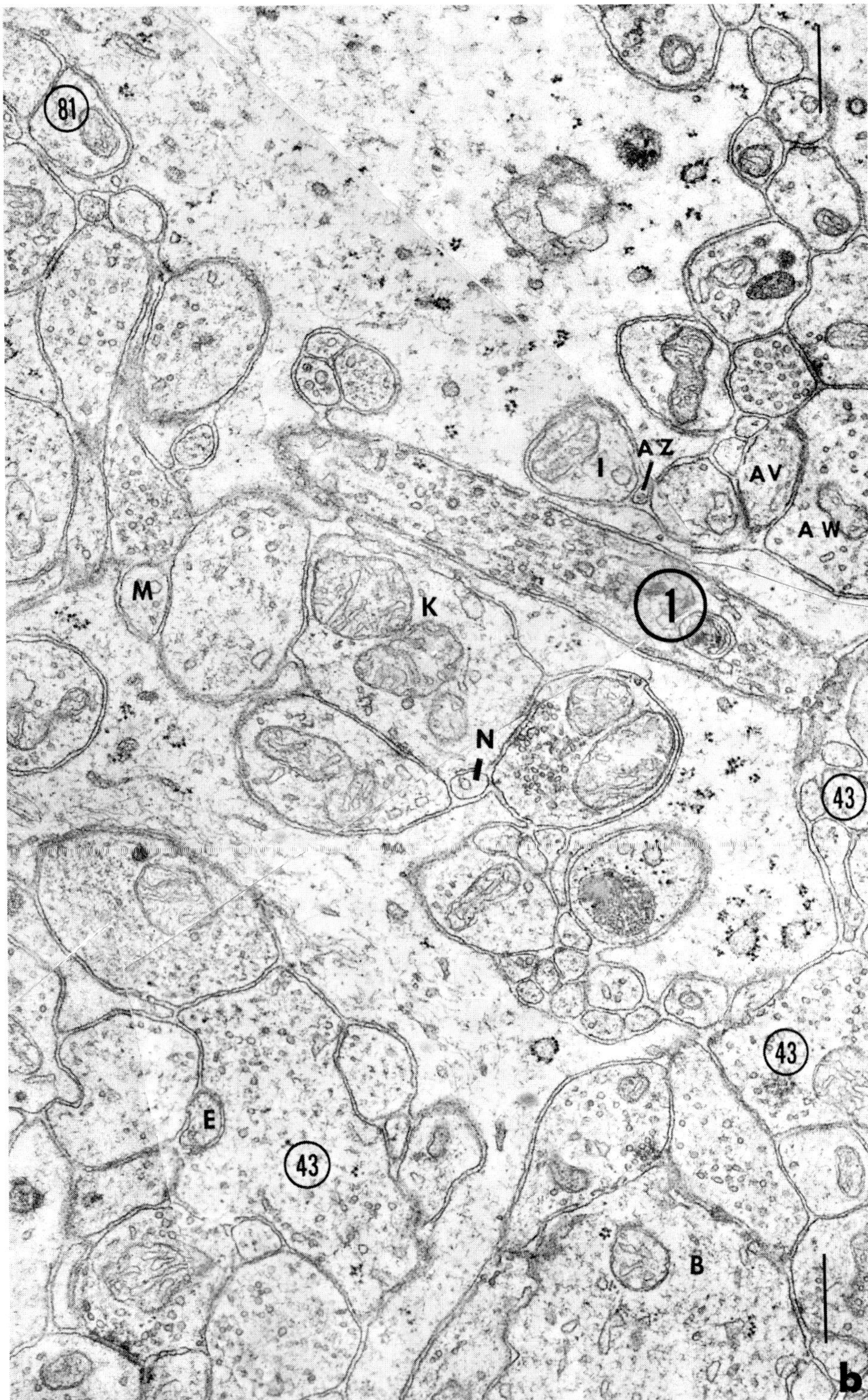

identified by number. Portions of an amacrine cell (Process No. 43) are seen in the montages. The individual processes which entered into synaptic relationships with this cell are identified by capital letters. In consecutive plates extending inward (towards vitreous) from the

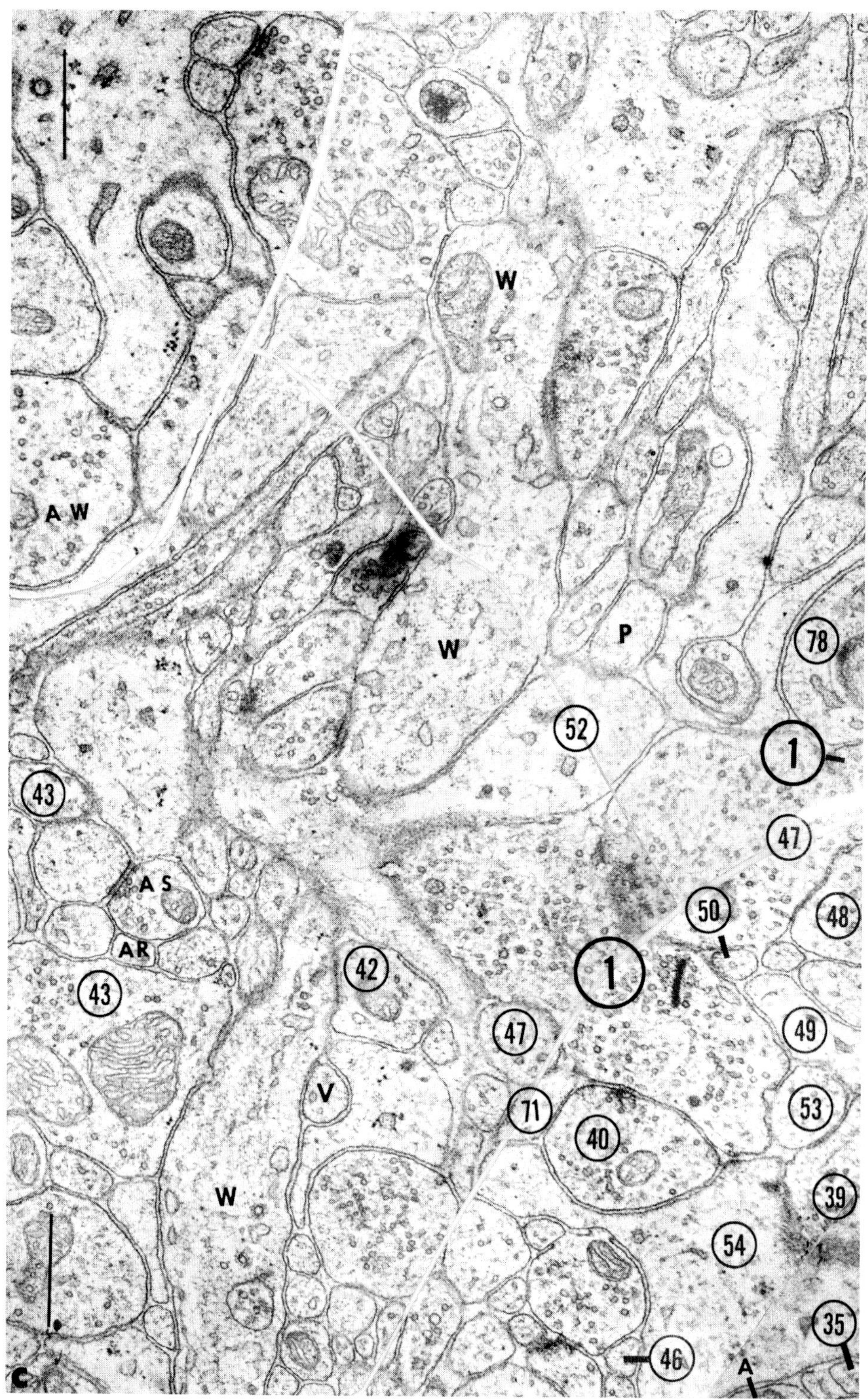

inner edge of the inner nuclear layer, left, there is a slight overlap between each plate and the one following (lines near edge). While all synapses involving the primary cell were also numbered in the analysis, these are not shown in the micrographs. The identifying numbers

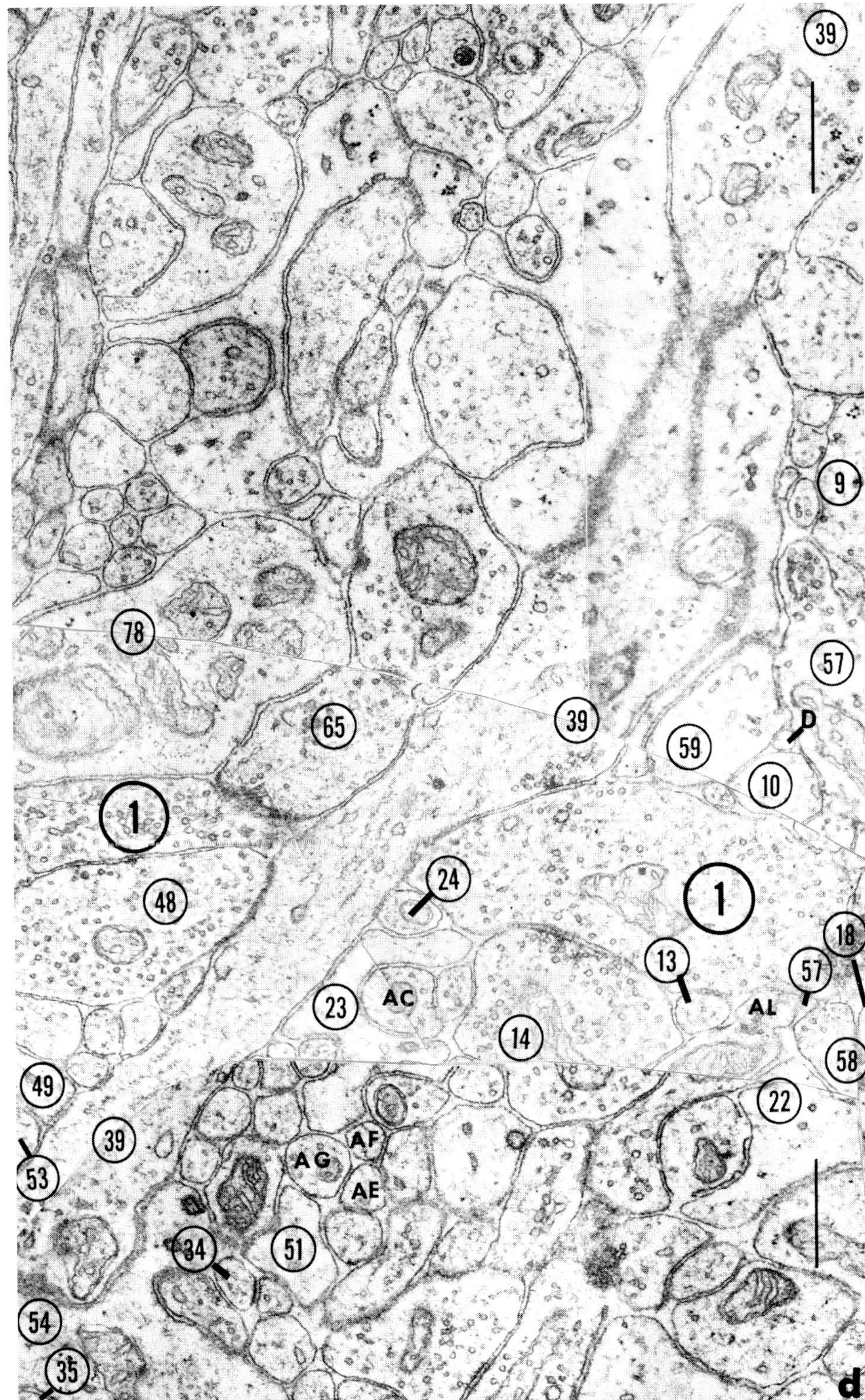

in this and all the following charts and diagrams are keyed to the same structures. (See text for full explanation.) × 36,000.

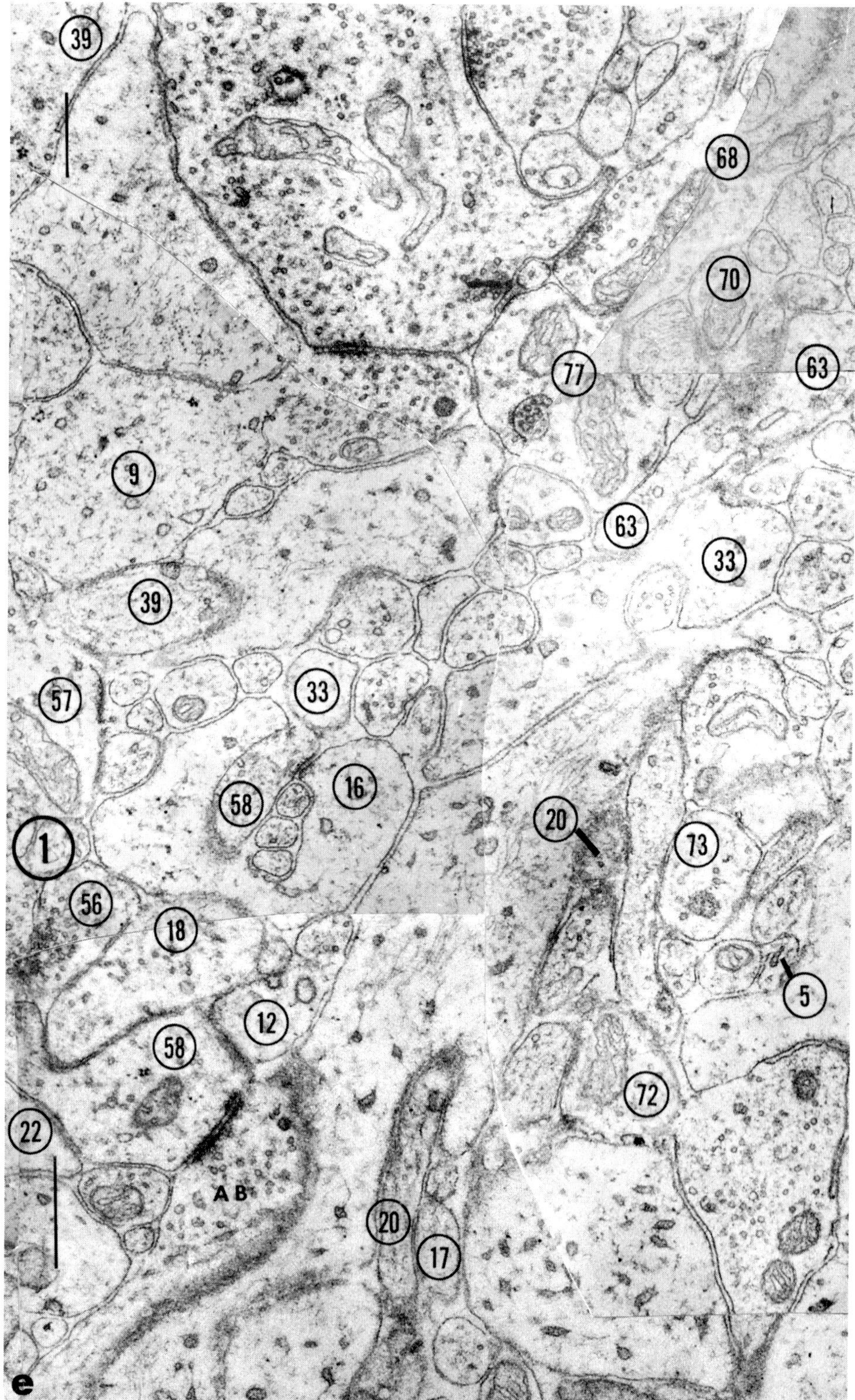
39
68
70
63
77
9
63
33
39
57
33
16
58
1
20
73
56
18
5
12
58
72
22
A B
20
17
e

Figure 53*e*

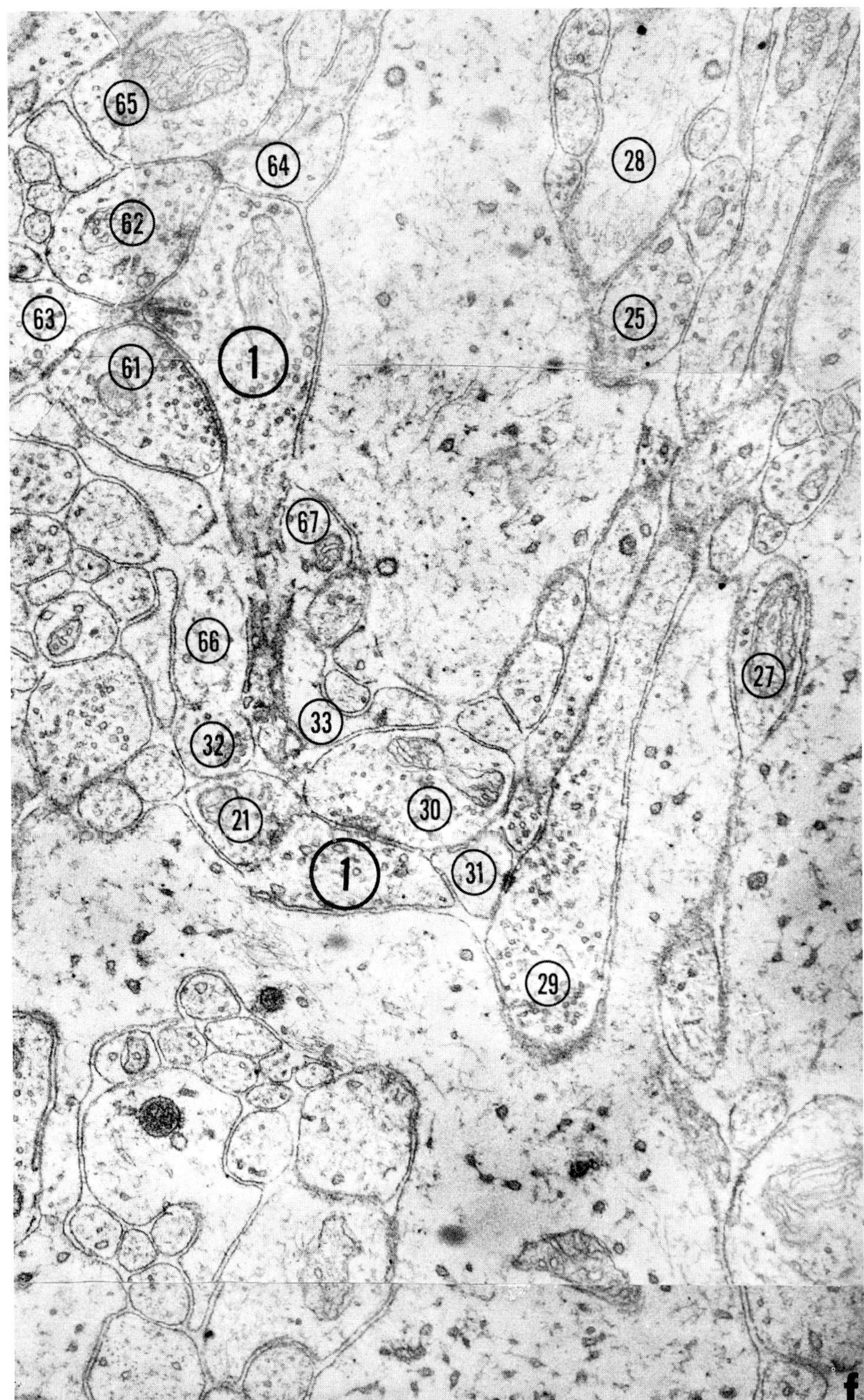

Figure 53*f*

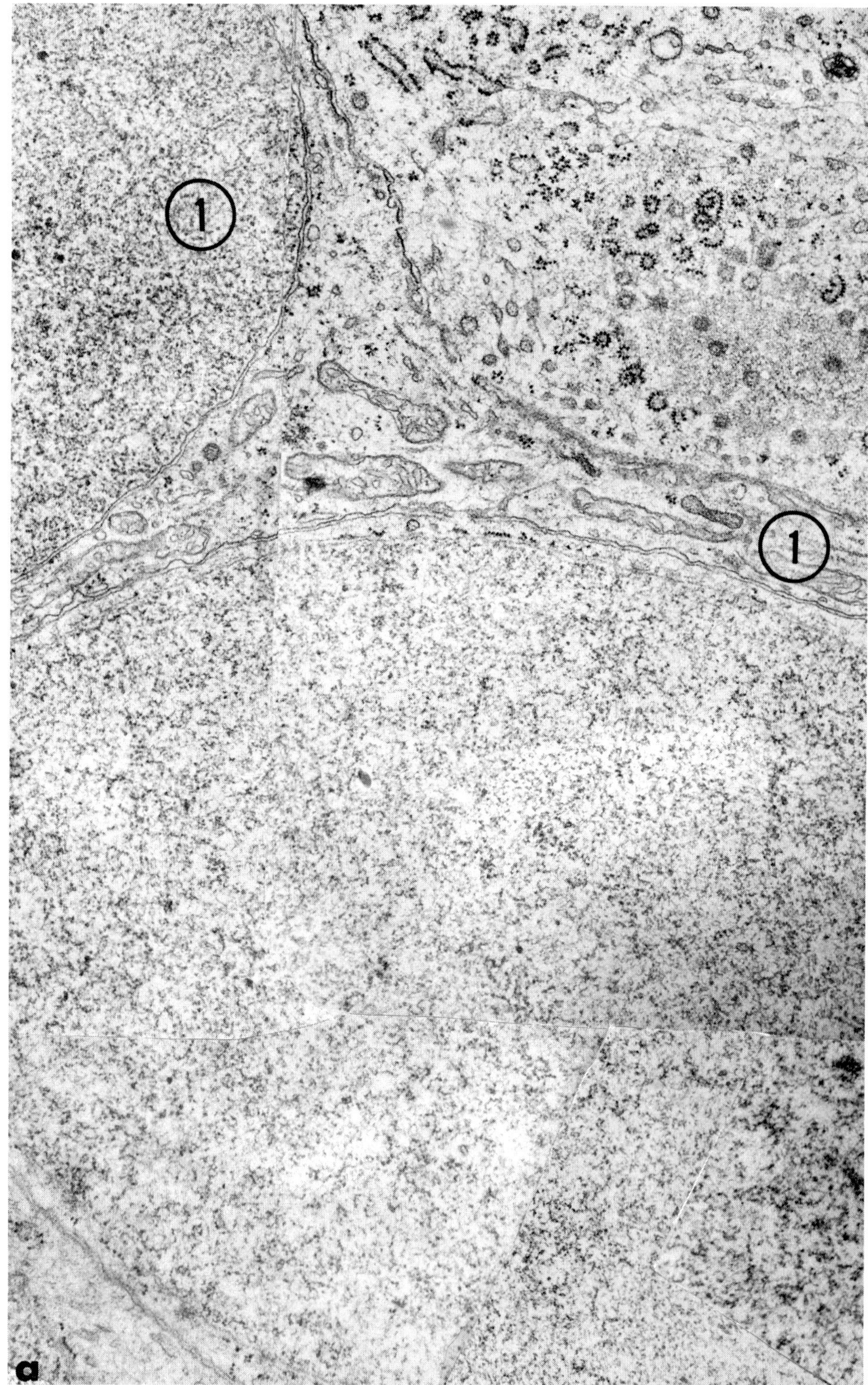

Figure 54, *a–f.* A portion of the montage of Section 52 is shown in six plates, each with a slight overlap as in Figure 53, and including portion of perikaryon with the connecting axon. The processes of the neuropil which formed synaptic connections with the primary bipolar

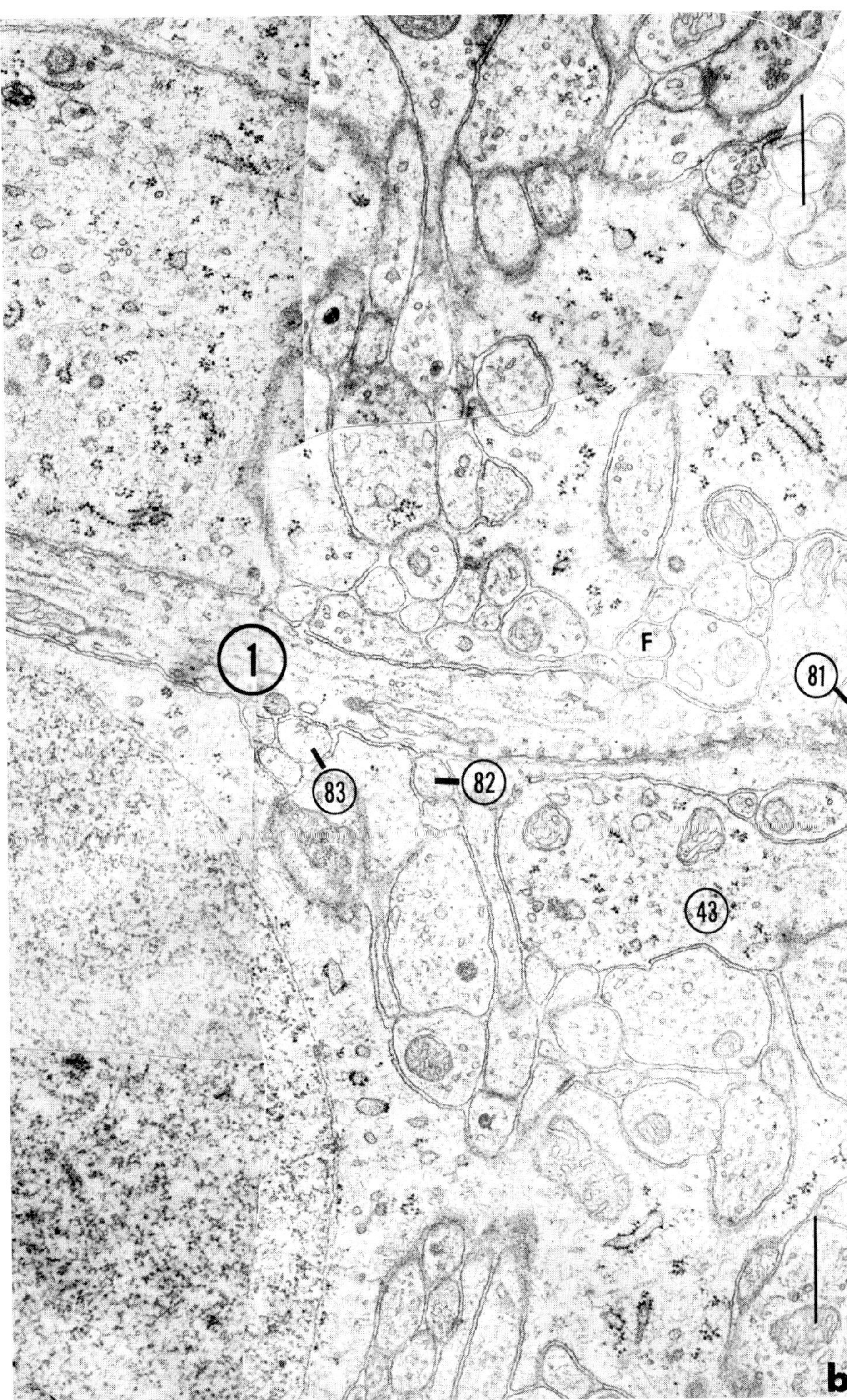

cell or with amacrine cell (Process No. 43) are designated as in Figure 52 for identification. × 33,600.

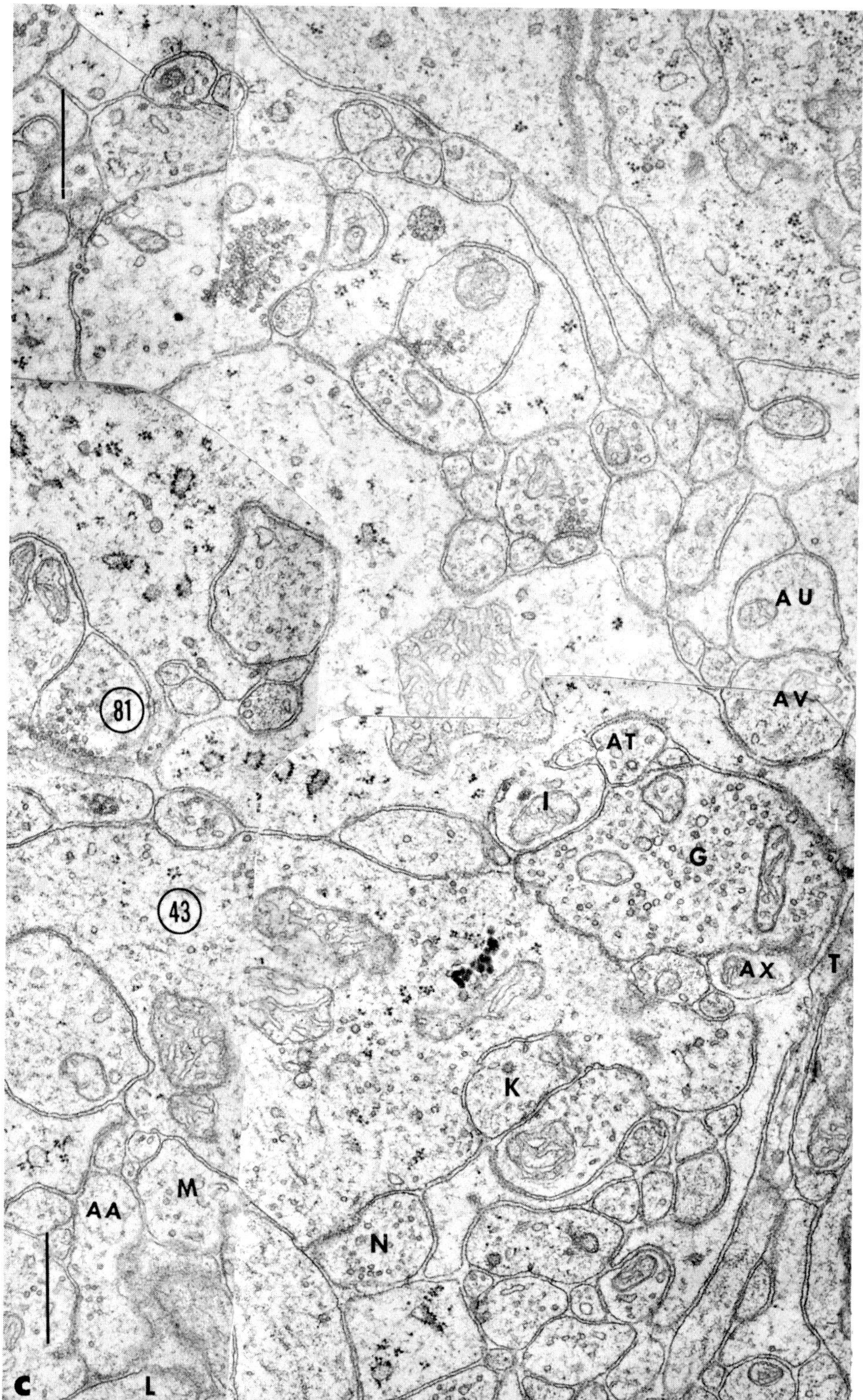

Figure 54*c*

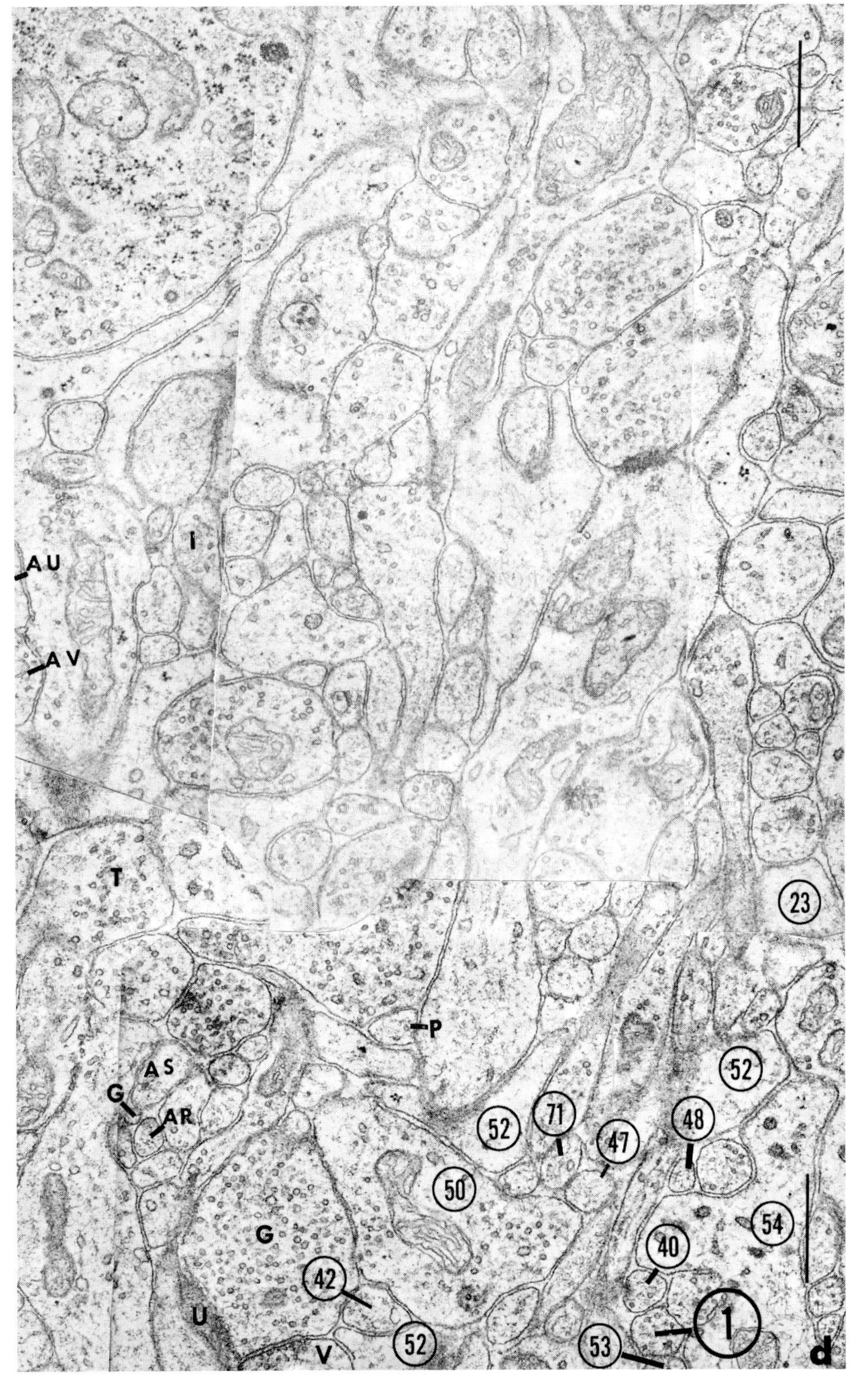

Figure 54*d*

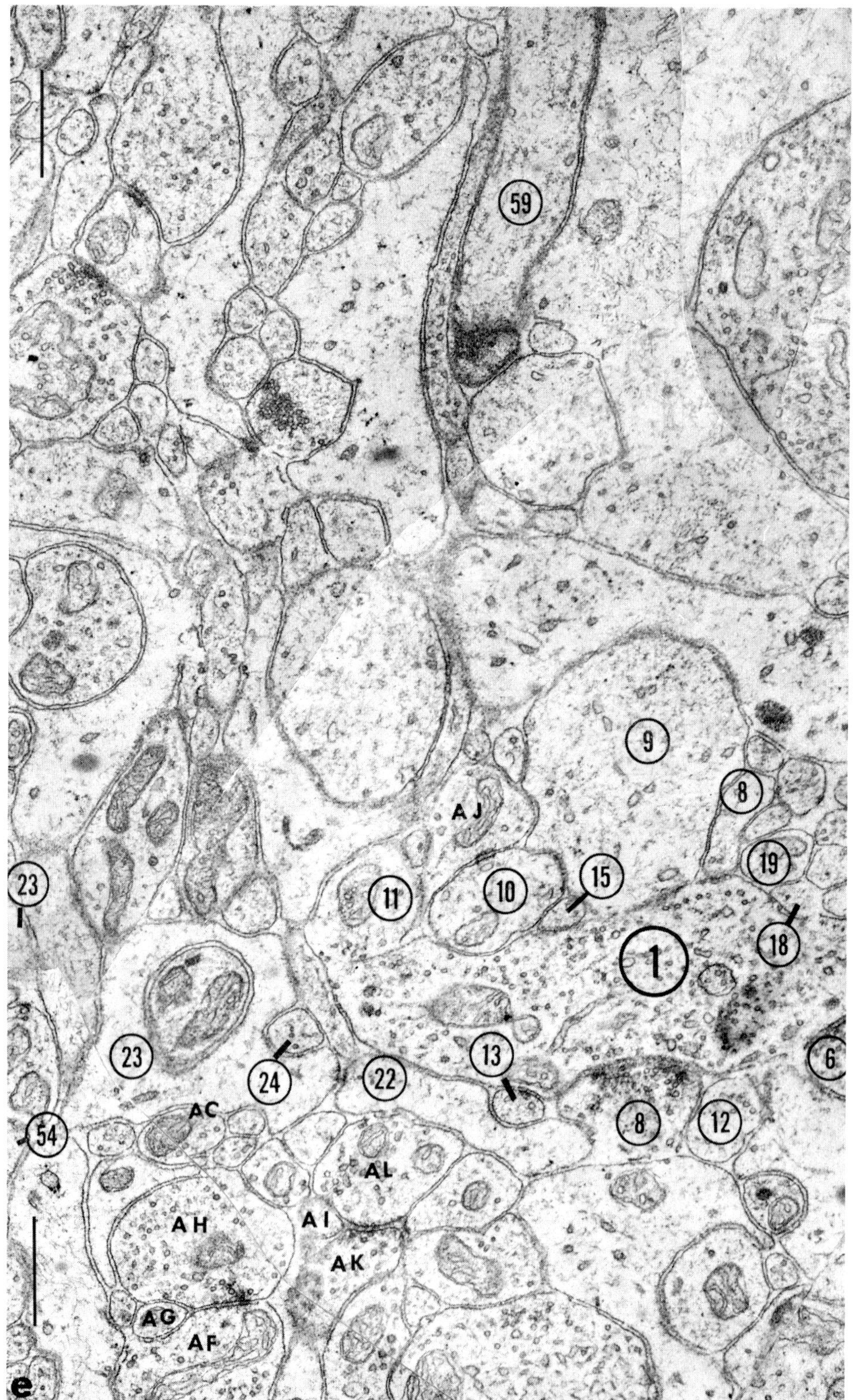

Figure 54*e*

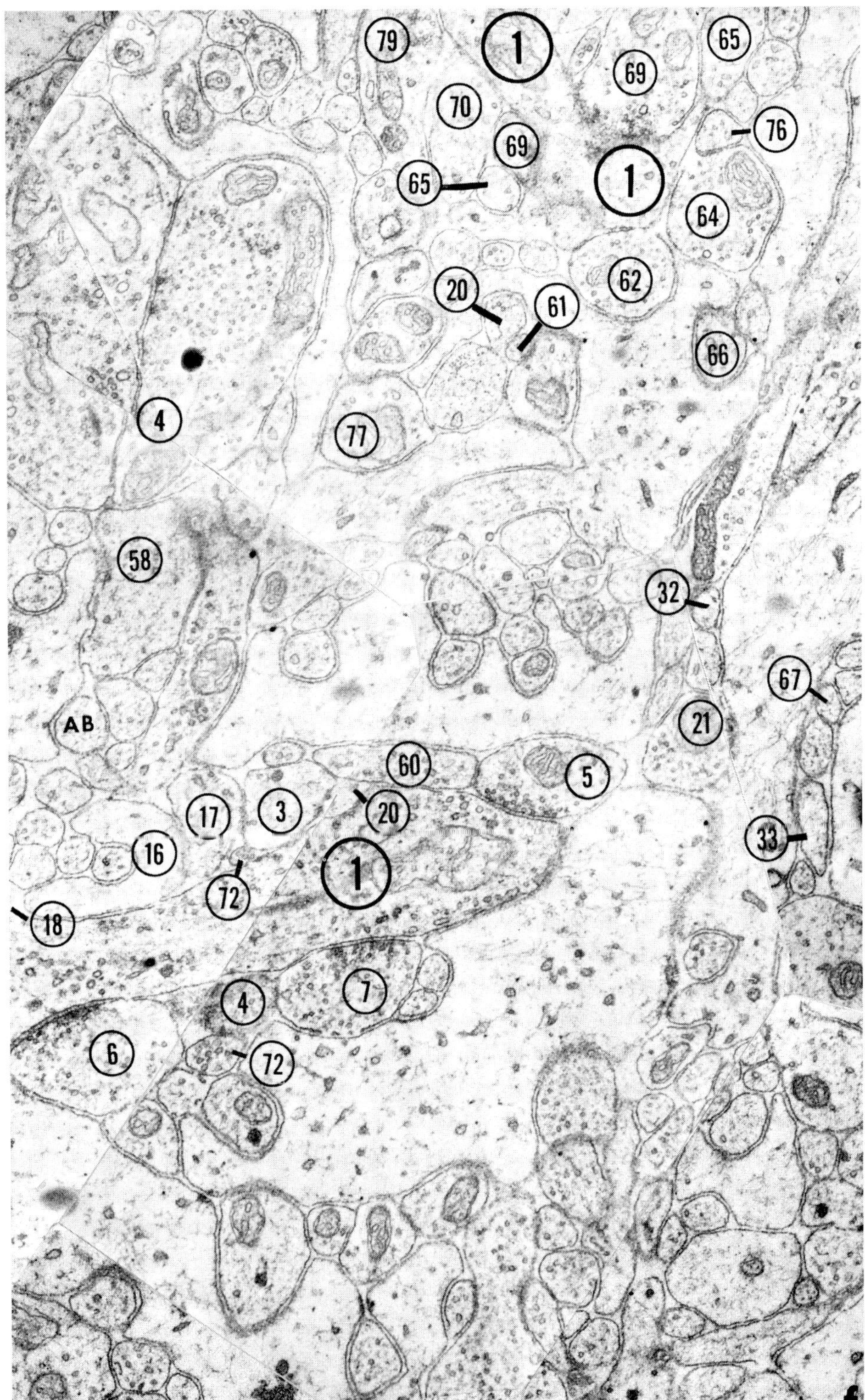
79
1
65
69
70
69
76
65
1
64
62
20
61
66
4
77
58
32
67
AB
21
60
5
17
3
20
33
16
1
72
18
4
7
6
72
f

Figure 54*f*

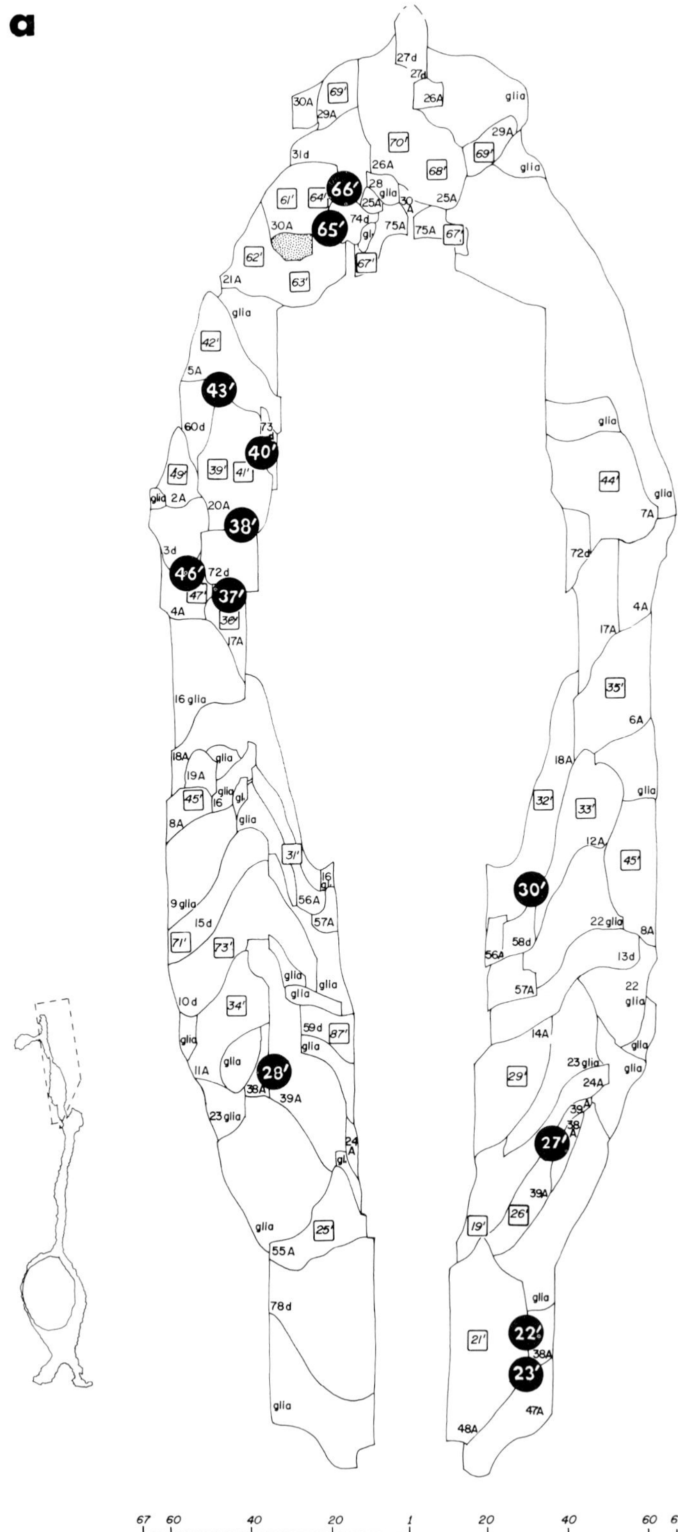

Figure 55, *a–c.* Topographic projection of the surface of each of the boutons of the bipolar telodendron, depicting areas of contact of the various surrounding processes (identified by number). Each ribbon synaptic complex is represented by a black circle and a primed number. The simple efferent synapses are shown in squares, each identified by a primed number as well. The projection was made from montages of micrographs printed at × 46,000

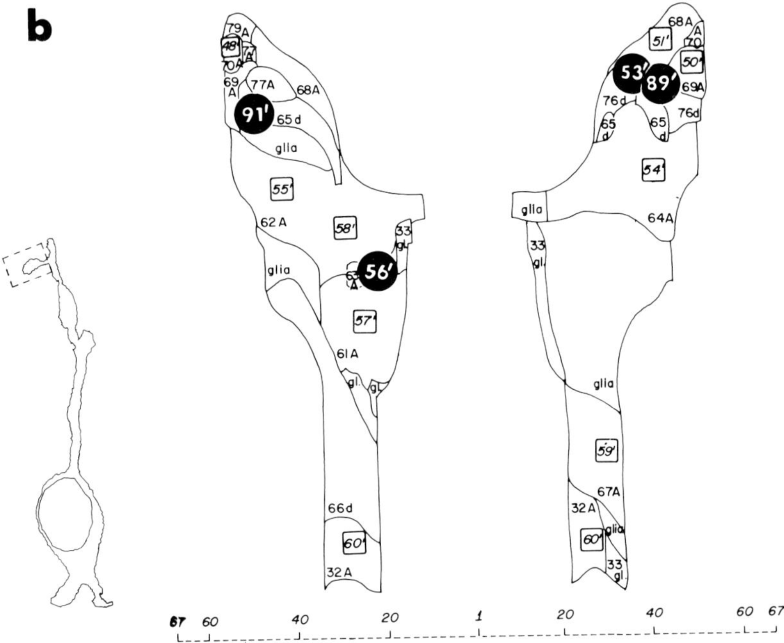

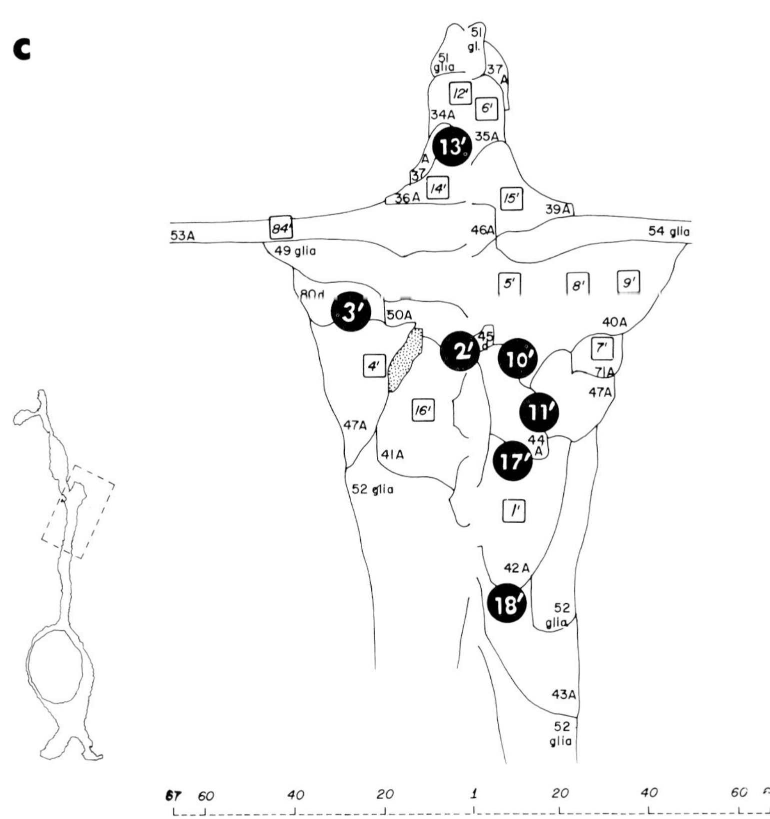

and was drawn in the same scale. The boutons of the telodendron exist at different planes; each is shown as it appeared in the sequence of the numbered serial sections of the series (1–67 shown as dotted lines at scale at bottom). The orientation of the boutons with respect to the main cell body is shown within the enclosed segments of the outline drawing of the entire cell. The stippled small areas indicate sites at which boutons are connected. In most cases glial processes were not numbered separately, but all glial contacts are identified.

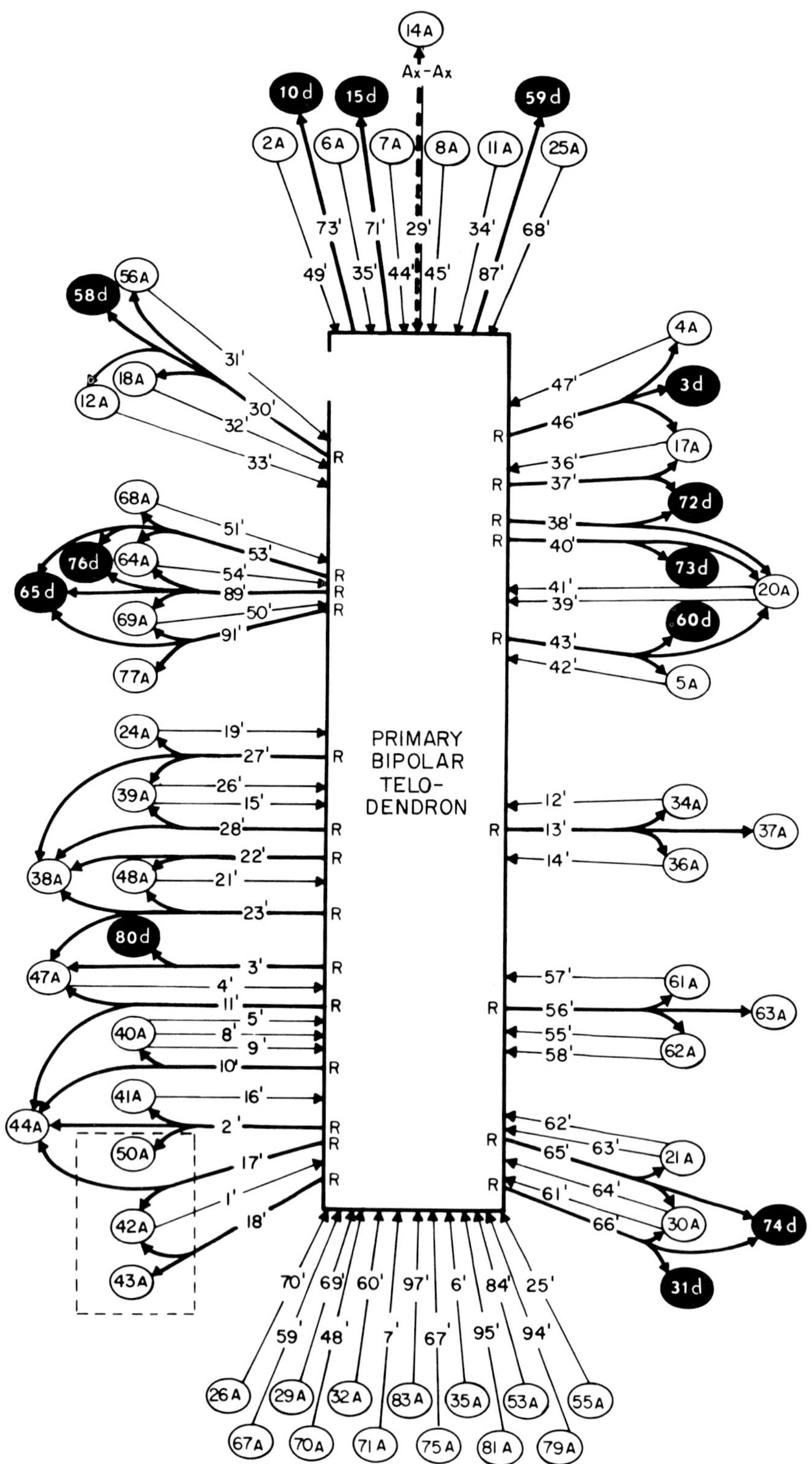

Figure 56 →

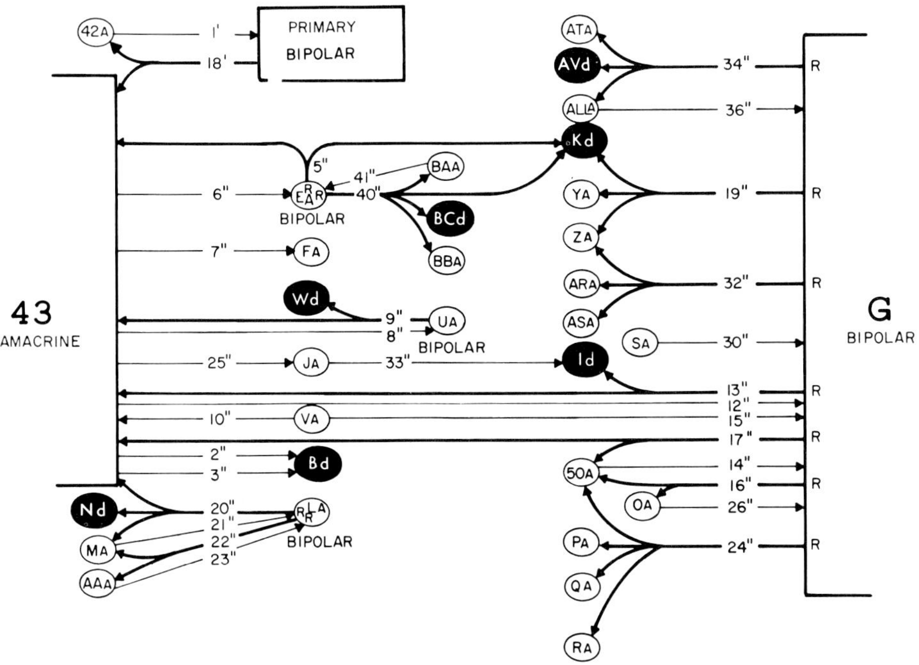

Figure 57. The synaptic relations of a large amacrine process (No. 43, which connected to parent cell body in the series) and a second bipolar telodendron (*G*). Large portions of both processes were present in the series, though original micrographs were not intended to include these cells. The diagram thus represents a small portion of the synaptic circuit beyond that shown in Figure 56 (connected at synapse 18′ upper left, primary bipolar shown as box). The synapses are represented as double-primed numbers, with direction indicated by arrow; line weight indicates direction with respect to bipolar telodendria, each of which is labeled. The individual processes are identified by letters and combinations of letters. R within bipolar processes indicates ribbon synapse. Processes believed to be dendrites are black with *d*; those believed to be axons are white with A.

Figure 56. Schematic diagram to show direction of individual synapses (primed numbers) and individual processes involved. The individual synapsing processes are identified by numbers, labeled *d* for those considered dendrites (black circles), and A for those believed to be axons (light circles). Efferent synapses from the primary bipolar cell are shown as heavy arrows; those associated with ribbons are marked by Rs within the large box. Only one synaptic site (top 29′ to 14A) appeared clearly bidirectional (vertical double arrow with both heavy dashed and fine lines). The large box is shown as incomplete (upper left) to indicate portion of telodendron not included at one edge of sections. The small rectangle (lower left, dashed line) indicates cellular processes that had large portions present in montages and which were analyzed (see Figure 57).

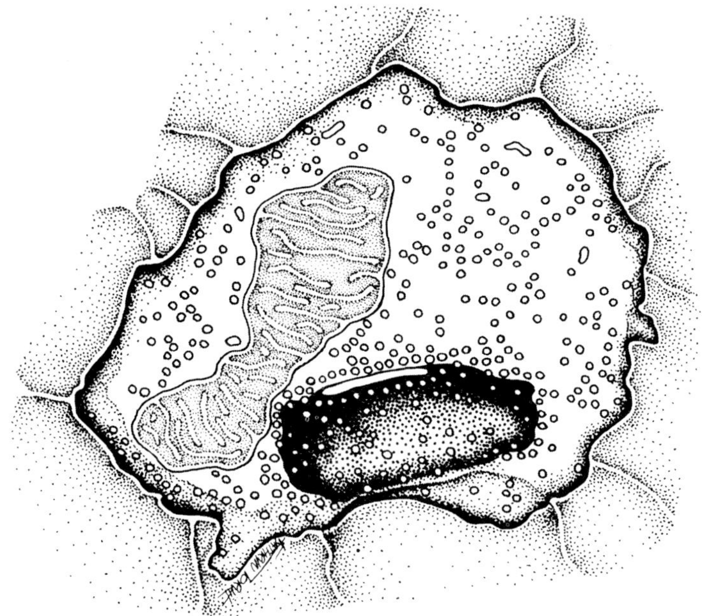

Figure 58. Three-dimensional drawing of a synaptic ribbon which appeared through 16 consecutive sections of a small telodendritic projection of a bipolar neuron. The structure, which in curvature and shape resembles a discus, is surrounded by synaptic vesicles (white area at top represents cut edge). (This cell was not part of that shown in Figures 52–57.) Original drawing $\times$ 143,000.

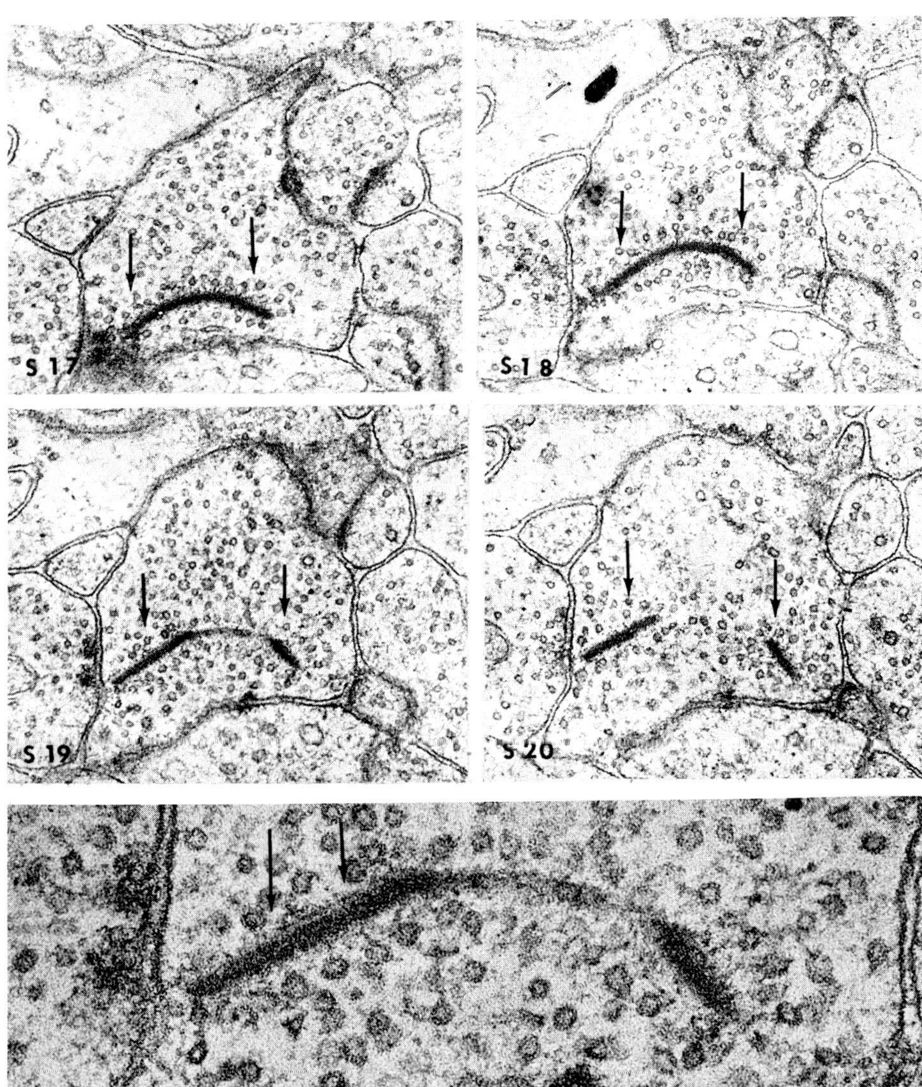

Figure 59. *Above:* Four consecutive sections (S17, S18, S19, S20) of a synaptic ribbon near the edge of a bipolar ribbon photographed through 22 sections; widely separated parts are shown, which in S20 simulate two separate ribbons. The synaptic complexes shown in Figure 57 and described in Table 1 were obtained by tracing such structures serially; this structure resembles but is not the same as that shown in Figure 58. × 36,800. *Below:* Laminated appearance of synaptic ribbon within bipolar telodendron (arrow); the structure is the same as that shown above in S19. × 112,800.

RETINAL GANGLION CELLS: A CORRELATION OF ANATOMICAL AND PHYSIOLOGICAL APPROACHES*

JOHN E. DOWLING
Johns Hopkins University School of Medicine
Baltimore, Maryland

BRIAN B. BOYCOTT
University College London
London, England

Experiments carried out during the past decade have substantially determined the nature of the "data processing" occurring at or before the level of ganglion cells of the vertebrate retina. Distal to the ganglion cells are four cell types: receptors, bipolars, amacrines, and horizontals, with synaptic connections located in the two plexiform layers of the retina. Because of its structural regularity, the vertebrate retina is very suitable for anatomical analysis, and offers a unique opportunity for correlating structure and function in a complex piece of nervous tissue. Understanding the physiology of the various types of retinal neurons has proved difficult, however, and only the ganglion cells have yielded reliable single-cell recordings.

Numerous studies have provided considerable information regarding the responses of ganglion cells when the retina is stimulated by light; we shall attempt here to correlate some aspects of the ganglion cell physiology with retinal anatomy. We have examined recently the primate retina by both light and electron microscopy, and we shall draw extensively on these observations (3,8,9).

Light Microscopy

Polyak (22) described two major classes of ganglion cells in the primate retina, which he further subdivided into at least six varieties, mainly on the basis of the differences in their shapes as observed in Golgi-stained material. Our Golgi-stained material shows these six varieties, but it also reveals many types apparently intermediate between them. It is often not possible for us to categorize convincingly a cell as belonging to any of Polyak's varieties. Thus, for the present account,

* The research reported in this paper was supported in part by the U.S. Public Health Service (NB-05336), U.S. Air Force (AF-49 (638)-1011), and Research to Prevent Blindness, Inc. The authors thank Mrs. Patricia Sheppard for excellent technical assistance and for preparation of the drawings. Publication No. 13 from the Augustus C. Long Laboratories, Alan C. Woods Research Building, Wilmer Institute.

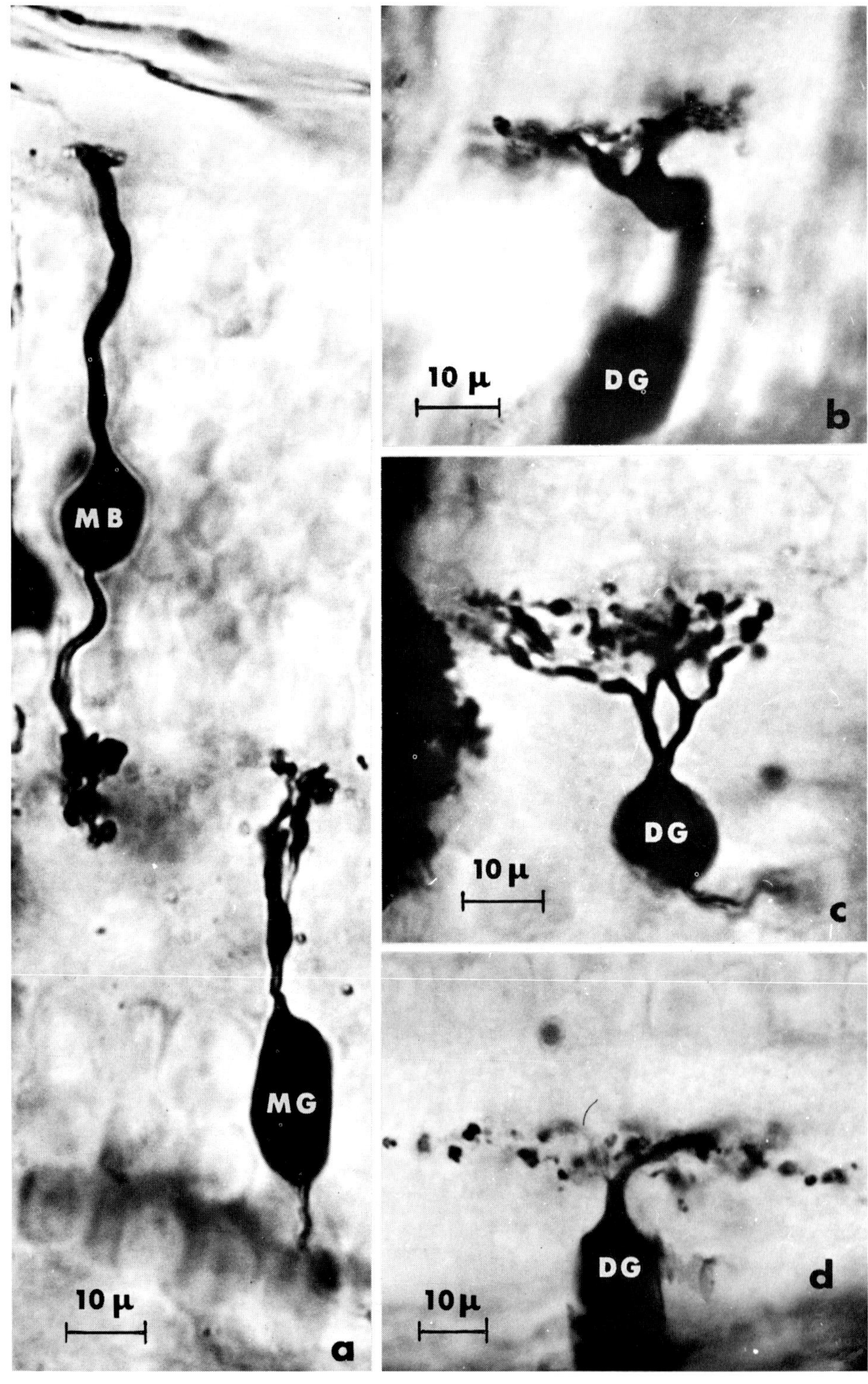

Figure 60 →

we shall classify ganglion cells only as belonging to one or the other of Polyak's two major classes: those that collect information over a large area we shall call "diffuse ganglion cells", and those that collect information from a very restricted area, perhaps from a single bipolar, we shall call "midget ganglion cells".*

The diffuse ganglion cells are found throughout the retina and have dendritic diameters of about 50 to 750 μ (or even more) (22). The midget ganglion cells stain most numerously in the foveal region, where they have very narrow dendritic spreads of only 10–15 μ; very near the fovea these dendritic spreads are sometimes even less. Midget ganglion cells are also found several millimeters away from the fovea, but they usually have a wider dendritic spread of about 25–40 μ, corresponding to the wider spread of the midget bipolar terminals in this retinal region. In these circumstances it becomes difficult to distinguish them from small diffuse ganglion cells.

Figure 60 shows typical diffuse and midget ganglion cells from the parafoveal region of the monkey retina. In Figure 60a, a midget bipolar cell is seen above and to one side of the midget ganglion cell; the spread of the axon terminals of the midget bipolar almost exactly matches in size the dendritic spread of the midget ganglion cell, suggesting that a midget ganglion cell probably contacts only one midget bipolar. This is occasionally illustrated in Golgi-stained material when a midget bipolar and the corresponding midget ganglion cell are stained together. Similarly, the dendritic spread of the midget bipolar is about 5–7 μ, which corresponds closely to the diameter of a cone pedicle in the foveal region (6).

Thus, the midget system in the central part of the primate retina is (as Polyak said) capable of mediating a *direct* private pathway from a single cone to a midget ganglion cell, and from there to the brain. That is not to say that a midget ganglion cell is influenced by only one cone, but rather that a midget ganglion cell may perhaps be in *direct* contact with only one bipolar terminal, which in turn has its dendrites in *direct* contact with just one cone pedicle. The interneurons of the retina (amacrine and horizontal cells) clearly provide lateral interconnections between the retinal cells, and in this way numerous receptors can affect any particular midget ganglion cell.

To summarize: the midget ganglion cell probably contacts directly only one midget bipolar, which in turn contacts directly only one cone. However, other cones and bipolars are connected indirectly with the midget ganglion cell via the amacrines and horizontal cells, which are the retinal interneurons (see physiology discussion below). Diffuse ganglion cells, on the other hand, receive direct input from numerous bipolars and, probably, most of the diffuse ganglion cells connect directly with both rod and cone bipolars (3).

---

* See footnote on p. 157.

Figure 60. Micrographs of Golgi-stained cells from the monkey retina. *a:* A midget bipolar (MB) and midget ganglion cell (MG); note that the dendritic spread of the midget ganglion cell is about the size of the spread of the axon terminals of the midget bipolar cell, suggesting that the midget ganglion cell receives its primary input from only one midget bipolar; × 1200. *b, c, d:* Small diffuse ganglion cells (DG); their dendritic spread is of sufficient size to contact numerous bipolars directly; *b,* × 1200; *c,* × 1200; *d,* × 1000.

Electron Microscopy

Electron micrographs of primate retinal ganglion cells show them to be typical neurons (12); they contain abundant particle-studded endoplasmic reticulum (Nissl substance), as well as other cytoplasmic organelles such as mitochondria and free ribosomes (Figure 61). Dendrites from the ganglion cells extend throughout the inner plexiform layer and make numerous synaptic contacts. Occasionally, bipolar axon terminals extend to the ganglion cell perikarya and make direct axosomatic contacts with the ganglion cells; the axodendritic contacts of the ganglion cells are much more common, however.

Axodendritic Contacts

In the central portion of the retina, the processes of the small ganglion cells are particularly stout and easy to follow from the cell body into the inner plexiform layer, where they contact the bipolar terminals (Figure 62). These bipolar terminals are readily recognizable by the numerous evenly distributed synaptic vesicles and dense synaptic ribbons they contain. The ribbons indicate the sites of presynaptic contact of the bipolar terminals, and ganglion cell dendrites are often seen making specialized contacts with the bipolar terminals at sites adjacent to a ribbon (Figure 62). The ribbons in the bipolar terminals are usually associated with two postsynaptic processes, and typically the ribbon is orientated to point between them; one of these postsynaptic elements is usually a ganglion cell dendrite and the other an amacrine cell process. Ganglion cell dendrites are recognizable, even when they cannot be traced back to the perikaryon, because they ordinarily show clusters of ribosome-like particles in their cytoplasm. The amacrine cell processes usually contain some synaptic vesicles, and the processes can often be seen making a synaptic contact back onto the bipolar terminal at a point as close as 0.5–1.0 μ distance from a synaptic ribbon. This arrangement is suggestive of a reciprocal contact between bipolar terminals and amacrine cell processes, and allows for the possibility of a feedback from the amacrine process to the bipolar terminal. The implications of this arrangement for mechanisms of visual adaptation, for example, have been discussed elsewhere (7).

Figure 63 is a diagram of the typical synaptic complex between the bipolar terminals and amacrine and ganglion cell processes; these synaptic complexes have been called "dyads" (9) because of the consistent presence of two postsynaptic elements in single sections. In all vertebrate retinas we have examined —including those of mammals, birds, fish, and amphibia—dyads have been

Figure 61. Ganglion cell (*G*) from the monkey retina. The cytoplasm of the cell is filled with numerous ribosomal-like particles, vesicular profiles of endoplasmic reticulum, and mitochondria. One dendritic process of the cell (dashed line) extends well into the inner plexiform layer (*IPL*). Glial (Müller) cell cytoplasm (*M*) surrounds much of the ganglion cell perikaryon and the proximal portion of the ganglion cell dendrite. An axonal terminal is seen making an axosomatic contact on the ganglion cell body (arrow). O_SO_4 fixation, × 9000.

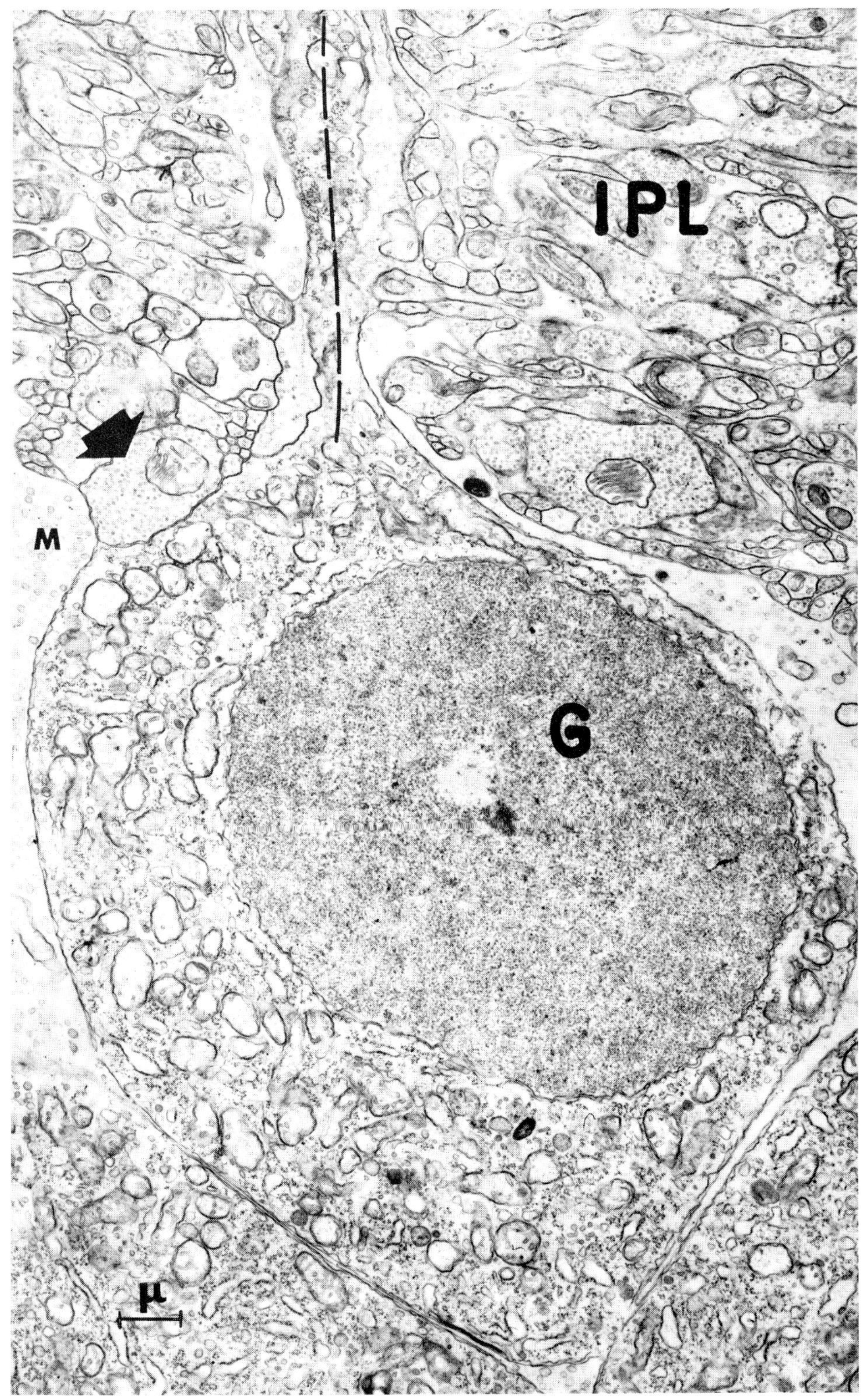

← Figure 61

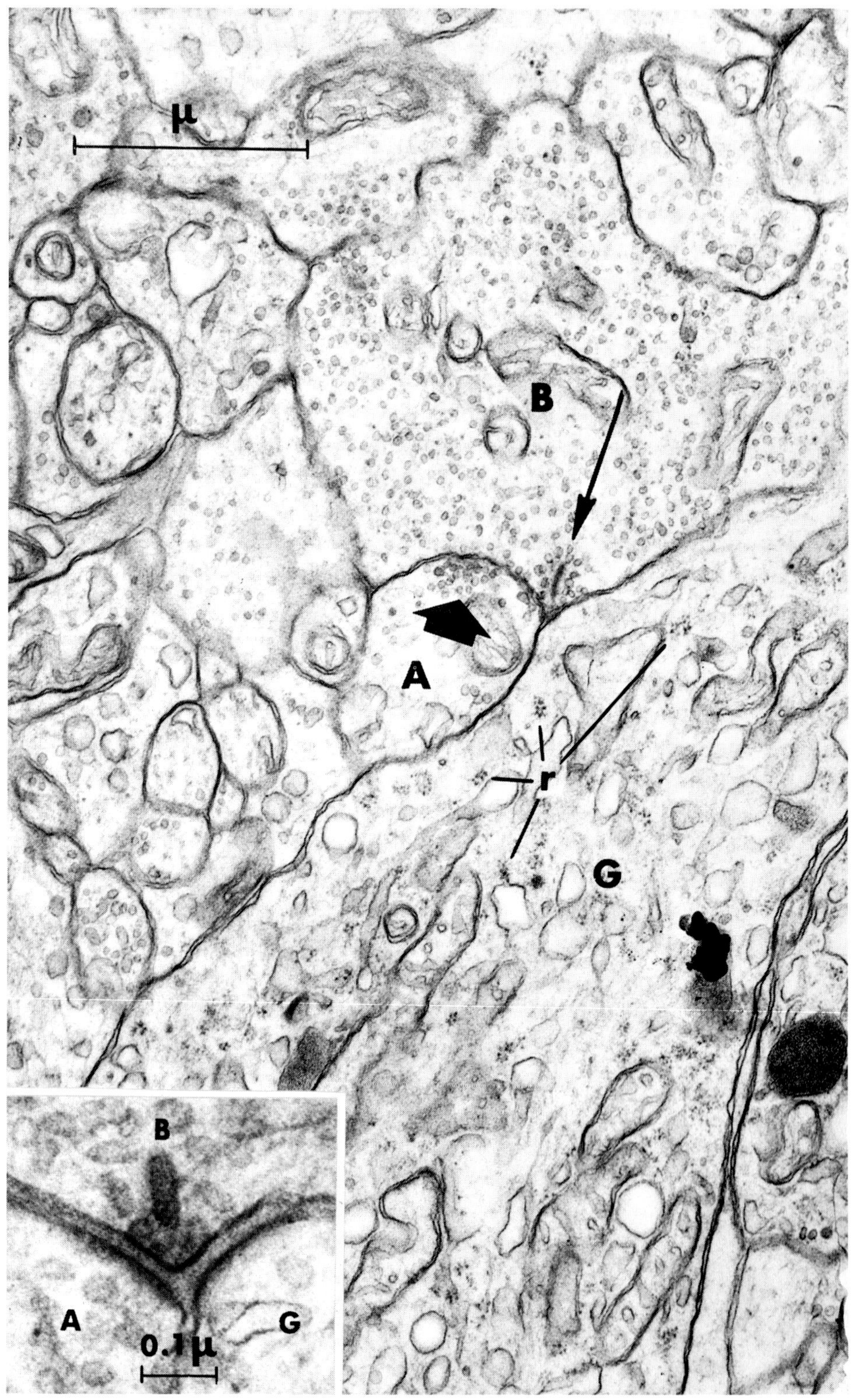

Figure 62 →

recognized in the inner plexiform layer. With certain fixatives, such as glutaraldehyde, membrane thickenings are delineated at the synaptic contacts in the primate retina (inset, Figure 62); these thickenings are indicated in Figure 63. In other retinas—e.g., frog's or bird's—such membrane thickenings are seen with all fixatives commonly used with these tissues. It is particularly noteworthy that the membrane thickenings associated with the synaptic ribbon junctions are found on both of the postsynaptic elements, and that these thickenings are greater than those on the presynaptic (bipolar) membrane. In accordance with currently

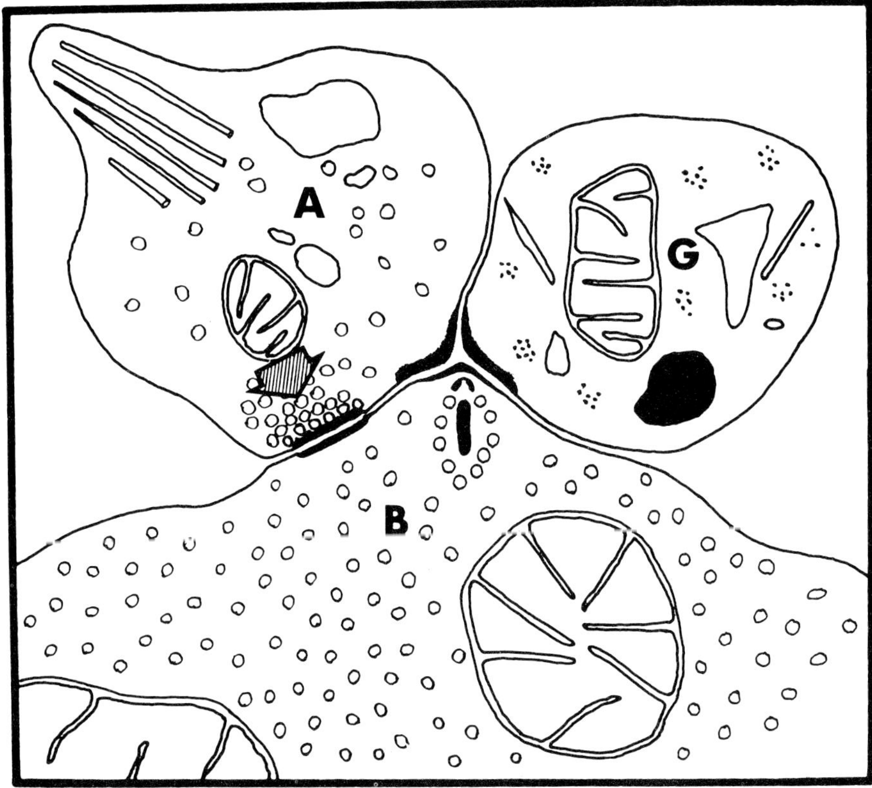

Figure 63. Diagram of the "dyad" synaptic contact of the bipolar terminal (*B*) with ganglion cell dendrite (*G*) and amacrine cell process (*A*). Frequently, the amacrine cell process makes a synaptic contact back onto the bipolar terminal, with the formation of a reciprocal contact between the two (arrow). Membrane thickenings are drawn as seen in glutaraldehyde-preserved material.

Figure 62. A ganglion cell dendrite (*G*) contacting a bipolar terminal (*B*). The synaptic ribbon in the bipolar terminal (thin arrow) is believed to indicate the site of synaptic contact. At the ribbon, the bipolar probably contacts both the ganglion cell dendrite and amacrine cell process (*A*); just adjacent to the ribbon contact of the bipolar terminal, the amacrine process appears to make synaptic contact back onto the bipolar terminal (thick arrow). Ganglion cell dendrites are readily identified by the clusters of ribosomal-like particles they contain (r); human retina, O_SO_4 fixation; × 36,000. *Inset* shows ribbon synaptic contact of a bipolar terminal in glutaraldehyde-fixed material; the membrane thickenings associated with the synapse are clearly delineated; monkey retina, × 90,000.

accepted criteria for synapses (14), this substantiates the idea that the sites of synaptic contact of the bipolar terminals are at the synaptic ribbons, and emphasizes that the polarity of the junction is from bipolar terminal to amacrine process and ganglion cell dendrite.

Besides the dyad synaptic complexes in the inner plexiform layer, synapses of amacrine cell processes are found directly with the ganglion cell dendrites, and also between amacrine cell processes. These contacts, which morphologically look similar to the reciprocal amacrine cell contacts "back onto" the bipolar cell terminals (Figure 63), are characterized by a dense aggregation of synaptic vesicles clustered close to the presynaptic (amacrine cell) membrane, along with some membrane thickenings that are seen on both the pre- and postsynaptic membranes when suitable fixatives are used.

Axosomatic Contacts

Occasionally, processes from the inner plexiform layer extend to the ganglion cell perikarya and make axosomatic synaptic contacts with the ganglion cells. Some of the processes are from amacrine cells, and these synaptic contacts are morphologically similar to the amacrine cell contacts with the bipolar terminals and ganglion cell dendrites described above (Figure 64). The other axosomatic contacts are made by bipolar terminals and are quite rare (Figure 64); these contacts are also quite unusual and deserve special comment.

First, the bipolar axosomatic contacts have never been seen in the all-cone portion of the retina, which suggests that they are made only by the rod bipolars; this is confirmed by light microscopy, which shows that only the rod bipolar terminals extend to the ganglion cell perikaryon (a conclusion reached by Ramón y Cajal). A second feature of these contacts is that they are usually large, but along the extensive junction zone one does not observe any of the morphological characteristics of chemical synapses such as those associated with the amacrine cell synapses onto the ganglion cell somata (Figure 64) or the other synapses in the inner plexiform layer: no aggregations of synaptic vesicles, nor synaptic ribbons or membrane thickenings are seen at these contacts, although such specializations may be clearly seen elsewhere in the same bipolar terminal (Figure 64). High-resolution electron micrographs show that the membrane of such a terminal and the membrane of the ganglion cell soma are occasionally in apposition, forming a series of "tight junctions" (5,10,11) along the contact zone. Such areas of membrane fusion are known in many instances to mediate electrical interactions between cells (2,5,23), suggesting that the axosomatic contacts

Figure 64. Axosomatic contacts on the ganglion cell perikaryon. No typical synaptic specializations are seen along the contact zone between the bipolar terminal (*B*) and ganglion cell soma (*G*), although such specializations may be seen elsewhere in such bipolar terminals (note the synaptic ribbons in the terminal—thin arrow). At various places along this contact region the two plasma membranes are fused, forming a series of "tight junctions" between the terminal and cell body (circles and inset). The smaller process (*A*), probably an amacrine process, also makes an axosomatic contact with the ganglion cell body, a contact which is typical of a chemical synapse with an aggregation of vesicles clustered close to the presynaptic membrane (thick arrow); human retina, O_sO_4 fixation; ×20,000. *Inset* shows a tight junction at high magnification; human retina, ×300,000.

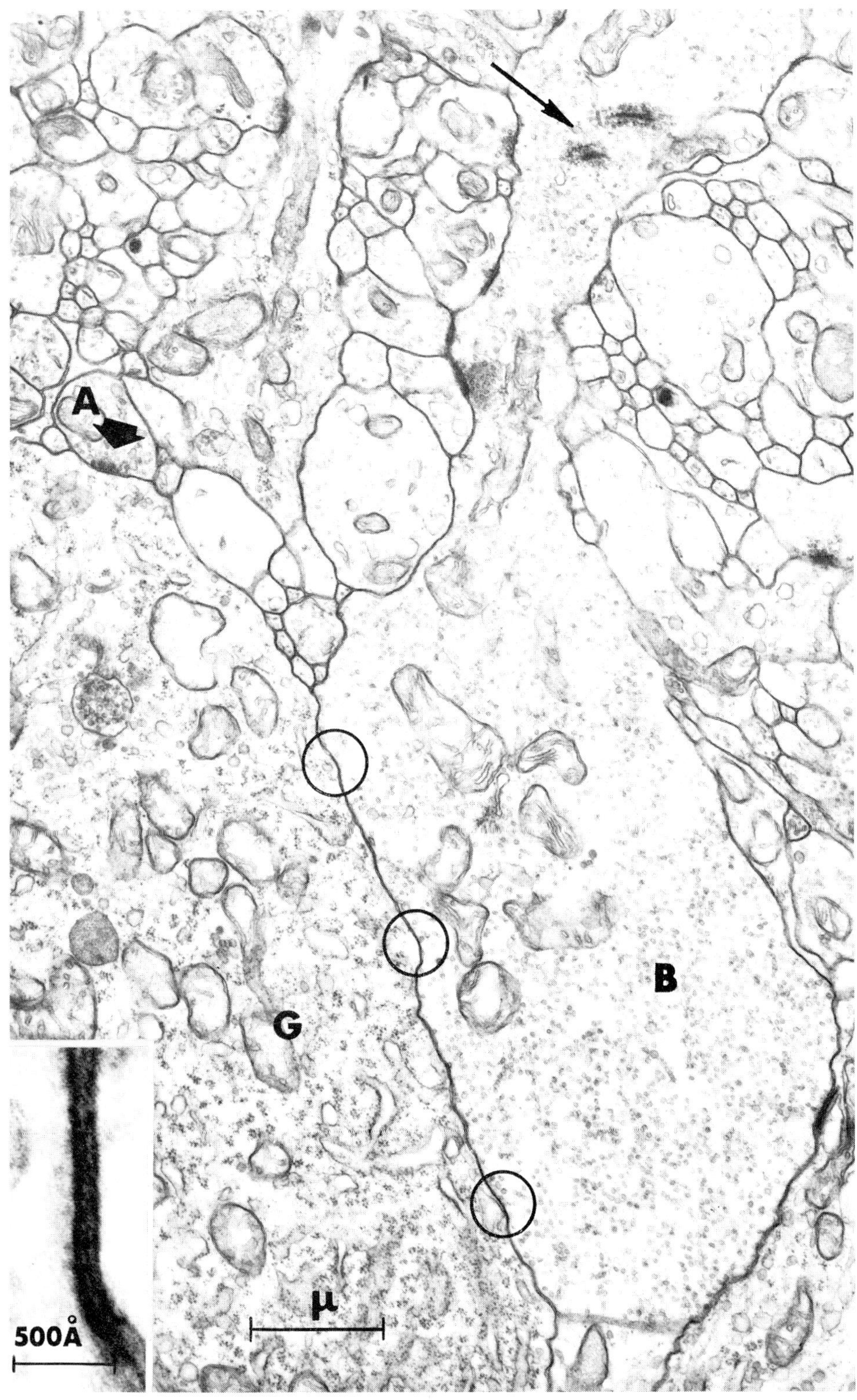

← Figure 64

between the rod bipolars and ganglion cell perikarya may be electrical synaptic contacts. However, recent work showing that "tight junctions" can be produced throughout the mammalian nervous system by certain fixation procedures cautions against fully accepting this suggestion until further evidence is presented (16). Future work must determine not only whether or not these contacts are electrical, but also whether or not they are synaptic.

Summary of Ganglion Cell Contacts

Figure 65 is a summary diagram of the contacts in the inner plexiform layer of the primate retina. Ganglion cell dendrites extend throughout the inner plexiform layer, where they contact bipolar terminals adjacent to the synaptic ribbons. At

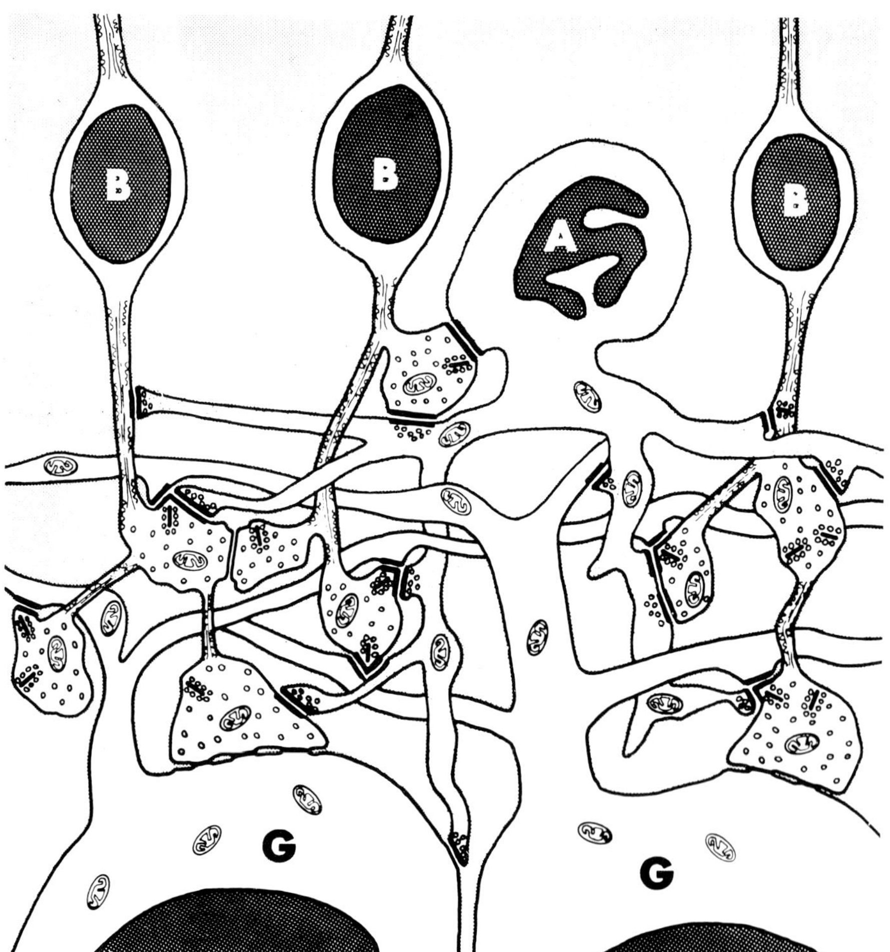

Figure 65. Synaptic contacts in the inner plexiform layer of the retina. The bipolar terminals make synaptic junctions at the synaptic ribbons, where they contact two postsynaptic elements, one usually a ganglion cell dendrite, the other an amacrine process. The amacrine processes extend laterally in the inner plexiform layer and make synaptic contacts on bipolar terminals, ganglion cell dendrites and perikarya, and with each other. The bipolar terminals also make direct axosomatic contacts with the ganglion cell somata; these contacts appear as if they might be electrical junctions. *B*: Bipolar cell; *A*: amacrine cell; *G*: ganglion cell.

the ribbons the bipolar terminals contact two postsynaptic elements: one is usually a ganglion cell dendrite and the other an amacrine cell process. These synaptic complexes (dyads) are by far the most common synaptic arrangement found in the inner plexiform layer of primates. Often the amacrine process involved in a dyad is seen to make a reciprocal synaptic contact back onto the receptor terminal just adjacent to the ribbon.

Other synaptic contacts seen frequently in the inner plexiform layer are those between amacrine cell processes and those between the amacrine cell processes and the dendrites and perikarya of the ganglion cells. Occasionally, axosomatic contacts between rod bipolar terminals and ganglion cell perikarya are seen; these junctions show areas of membrane fusion (tight junctions), suggesting that they could be synapses that work by electrical rather than chemical transmission.

Physiology and Anatomy

The electrical responses of single ganglion cells have been examined in a variety of vertebrates. In retinas of mammals such as the cat or the monkey, the ganglion cell responses are quite similar from cell to cell (15,17). In amphibia (19) and in birds (18) the retinal responses are much more varied, and a given ganglion cell will respond best to a quite specific stimulus such as a moving or a convex edge. In a few mammalian species, such as the ground squirrel (21) or rabbit (1), there may also be more varied responses than are at present known for primates or cats; for example, in the rabbit there are units which are directionally selective. Fundamentally, however, the responsiveness of most of the ganglion cells of the mammalian retina is based on two circular and concentric zones antagonistic to each other; these are the responses we shall attempt to interpret anatomically.

The area of the retina which affects a ganglion cell upon stimulation is called the receptive field of that cell. In general, the receptive field in the light-adapted mammalian retina is arranged into two circular and concentric zones, which are antagonistic to each other (17) (Figure 66). Illumination of the field center with a spot of light causes a ganglion cell to discharge either when the light comes on or when it goes off, whereas illumination of the field periphery gives a response antagonistic to that obtained from the center. That is, for an on-center cell, illumination of the periphery causes an off-response; for off-center cells, illumination of the field periphery gives an on-response. In animals with well-developed color vision, such as the monkey or goldfish (25), the antagonistic zones of the receptive fields may also be differentially sensitive to color; that is, the center of the field would respond best to light of a particular wavelength, whereas the periphery would respond maximally to light of a second wavelength.

An obvious problem raised by physiological observations is the anatomical organization of the receptive fields of the ganglion cells. An important clue is provided by the recent work of Wiesel & Hubel (26), who showed that near the fovea in the monkey the receptive field centers are very small, compared to those in the peripheral retina. The foveal receptive field centers are often too small to measure, and Wiesel & Hubel suggest that the smallest receptive field centers may be only the size of a single cone. This physiological observation appears to

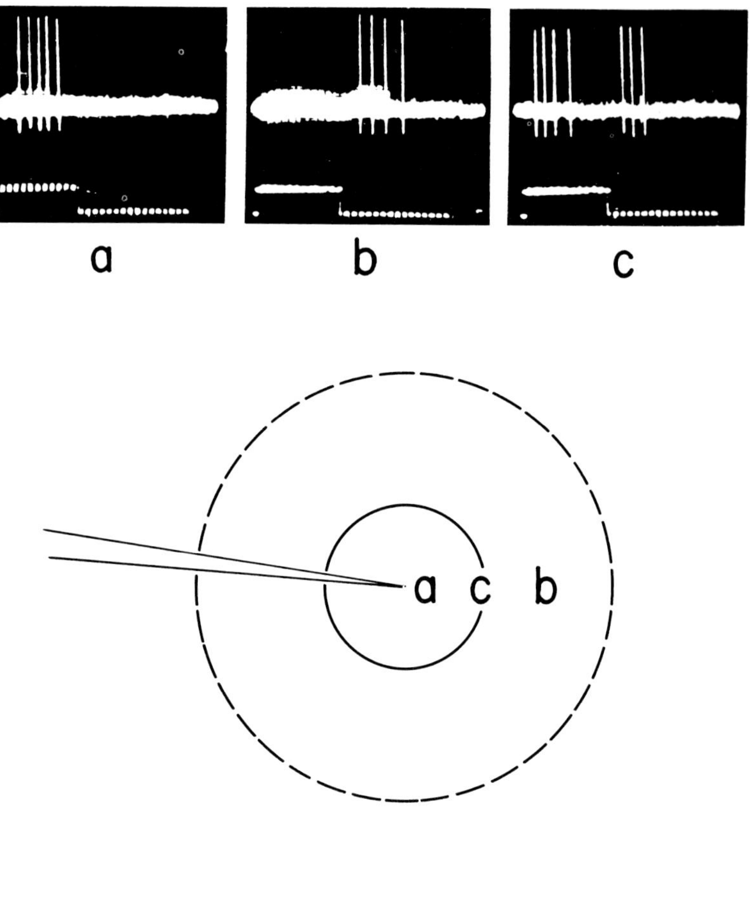

Figure 66. Ganglion cell responses of the on-center type from the cat retina. A schematic representation of the receptive field with a microelectrode positioned in the center of the field is shown below the records. With spot illumination presented to the center of the field (*a*), the ganglion cell fires when the light comes on; with illumination of the field periphery (*b*), the cell fires when the light goes off; when the zone between center and periphery is illuminated (*c*), the cell fires at both on and off. (Records from Kuffler, 17.)

correlate with the anatomical finding of numerous midget bipolars and midget ganglion cells near the fovea in the primate retina; the system of midget cells, as was suggested above, appears to mediate a direct pathway from single cones through to the brain which could explain the smallness of the receptive field centers of the ganglion cells in the foveal region of the primate retina.

On the other hand, the antagonistic peripheral "surrounds" of the receptive fields do not become correspondingly small as one approaches the fovea; they remain substantial in size regardless of the receptive field's location in the retina. This behavior of the antagonistic surround correlates anatomically with that of the retinal interneurons, which do not vary substantially in size or lateral extent within a radius of at least 8 mm from the foveal center. Thus, these findings suggest that the center of a receptive field is mediated by the direct vertical pathways to the ganglion cell, whereas the antagonistic (peripheral) surround is connected to a ganglion cell via the interneurons of the retina.

Further evidence that only the center of a receptive field is mediated by a direct receptor-bipolar-ganglion cell pathway has come from the work of Gallego (13) and of Brown & Major (4). These investigators measured the dendritic spreads of the ganglion cells in the cat retina and found that they closely match the size of the receptive field centers, and not the entire fields. Wagner (24) also has pointed out that the sizes of whole receptive fields in cats, monkeys, rabbits, and fish are considerably larger than the direct receptor-bipolar-ganglion cell relationship. Observations and deductions from a variety of sources thus show that only the receptive field center corresponds to the ganglion cell dendritic spread; therefore, the activity from the antagonistic surround must be transmitted to the ganglion cell indirectly, via the retinal interneurons.

Of the two types of retinal interneurons, the amacrines seem best suited for mediating the peripheral responses of the receptive fields (9). Amacrine cells in the primate retina make synaptic contacts with bipolar terminals, ganglion cell dendrites and somata, and with each other. Thus, they provide a pathway between a bipolar cell and the dendrites of a ganglion cell that would otherwise be beyond the reach of the bipolar cell terminals. Since amacrine cells also synapse with each other, it seems likely that lateral information might be conveyed over considerable distances in the retina via the amacrines. Recently, McIlwain (20) showed that the discharges of ganglion cells in the cat retina can be affected by presenting moving stimuli as far away as 10 mm from the receptive field center; McIlwain provides evidence that these far-peripheral effects are mediated by intraretinal pathways, and it seems most likely that these influences are mediated by the amacrines (9).

In the primate, we distinguish three varieties of amacrine cells on the basis of their processes' extent of spread, density, and location in the inner plexiform layer (Figure 67).* The *large* amacrine cells extend over a diameter of 500–1000 μ, show almost no spines or branches, and have relatively few processes, perhaps only four to six, which run along the inner nuclear layer. *The intermediate-sized* amacrines have a dendritic spread of 200–500 μ, many more processes than the large amacrines, and relatively profuse branching; their processes usually run in the upper (distal) half of the inner plexiform layer, but occasionally extend deeper. The *small* amacrines often have quite knobby processes, and the cells branch more frequently than either of the other two kinds of amacrines; their processes spread laterally for about 30 to 100 μ but, unlike the others, they extend through the entire thickness of the inner plexiform layer and may form axosomatic junctions with the ganglion cells.

* *Added by Dr. Dowling after the Conference:* Since this paper was prepared, we have made further observations which suggest that the classifications of both amacrine and ganglion cells presented in this account are somewhat oversimplified. A more thorough discussion of these cell types will appear shortly (3).

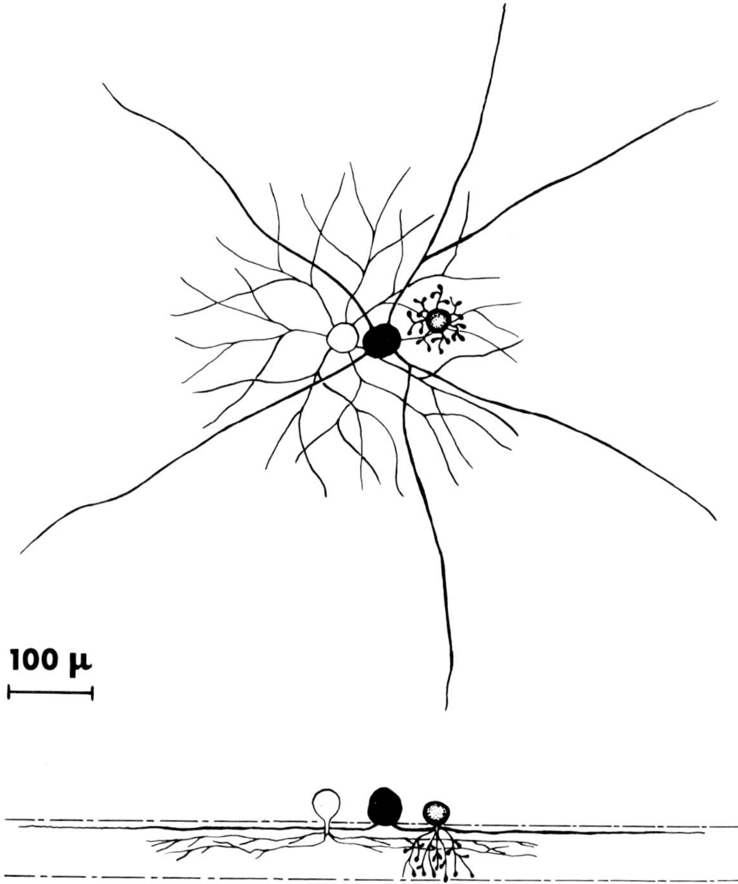

Figure 67. Three varieties of amacrine cells seen in the primate retina when stained by the Golgi method. The cells, described in the text, are shown in flat view (top) and in longitudinal sections (bottom). The dashed line indicates the relative width of the inner plexiform layer.

All varieties of the amacrines overlap with one another and form such a dense network in the inner plexiform layer that every bipolar terminal and ganglion cell dendrite must be in very close association with the processes of at least one amacrine cell and quite probably several different ones. This is confirmed by electron microscopy of the inner plexiform layer.

Figure 68 shows a simple "wiring diagram" for the retina, based on our anatomical findings, that may explain many of the observations of receptive fields of ganglion cells. In this scheme, the ganglion cells connect directly with bipolars only in the center of the receptive field; the other bipolars connect with the ganglion cell through the amacrines. Stimulation of the field center would cause excitation or inhibition of the ganglion cell through the direct receptor-bipolar-ganglion cell junctions. Stimulation of the receptive field periphery would cause an antagonistic response in the ganglion cell via a receptor-bipolar-amacrine-ganglion cell pathway. The amacrine-ganglion cell synapses are presumably

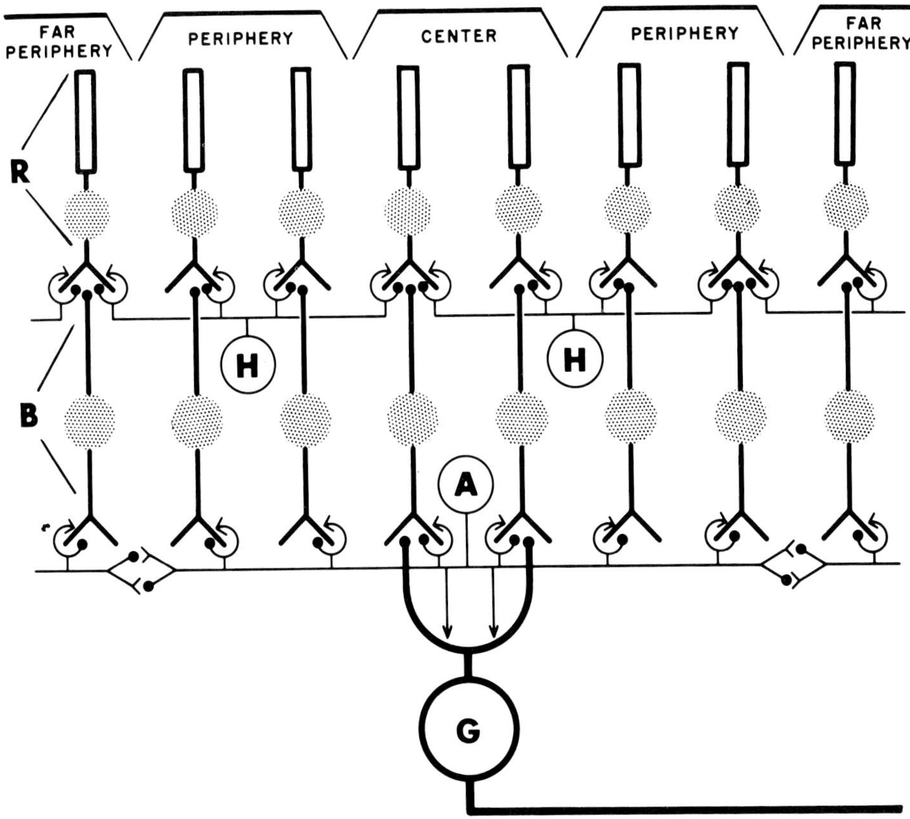

Figure 68. A "wiring diagram" for a ganglion cell (*G*) receptive field. The synaptic contacts between horizontal cells (*H*) and receptor terminals (*R*), and between amacrine processes (*A*) and bipolar terminals (*B*) are thought to be reciprocal, and the others are considered one-way junctions (9). See text for details. ⅄: Excitatory synapse; ↓ : inhibitory synapse.

antagonistic to the bipolar-ganglion cell synapses, so that, if center and periphery are stimulated simultaneously, a weak response of the ganglion cell results, as has been observed experimentally (17). Stimulation of the far periphery could also affect a ganglion cell via amacrine-amacrine synapses.

A slight modification of this scheme could explain other receptive field features such as color coding of the receptive field zones. For color-coded cells, it is postulated that a given ganglion cell connects with bipolar cells that are in contact with only one class of cones (e.g., red-sensitive receptors). However, the amacrines of that receptive field would connect with bipolars of another class (e.g., bipolars that connect with green-sensitive receptors). One feature of this arrangement is that the amacrines could extend throughout the whole field, both center and periphery, to connect with the appropriate bipolars; it would thus be possible to elicit the antagonistic peripheral response from the field center if the appropriate light wavelength were used as a stimulus. This has been demonstrated in the goldfish retina (24).

SUMMARY

This paper has undertaken to correlate structure and physiology in the primate retina. The synapses of the ganglion cells with the bipolar terminals and the amacrine cell processes have been described, with the suggestion that the responses of the centers of the physiologically determined receptive fields of the ganglion cells are mediated via the direct bipolar-ganglion cell synapses, whereas the antagonistic peripheral responses of the receptive field are mediated by bipolar-to-amacrine-to-ganglion cell pathways. However, only the simpler kinds of receptive field organization of mammals such as monkey or cat were considered; in vertebrates such as frogs and birds, the retinal ganglion cell responses are probably more selective, but at present little is known of synaptic connections in these retinas.*

REFERENCES

1. Barlow, H. B., Hill, R. M., and Levick, W. R., Retinal ganglion cells responding selectively to direction and speed of image motion in the rabbit. *J. Physiol.* (London), 1964, **173**: 377–407.
2. Bennett, M. V. L., Aljure, E., Nakajima, Y., and Pappas, G. D., Electrotonic junctions between teleost spinal neurons: electrophysiology and ultrastructure. *Science*, 1963, **141**: 262–264.
3. Boycott, B. B., and Dowling, J. E., Organization of the primate retina: light microscopy. *Phil. Trans. Roy. Soc. London B*, in press.
4. Brown, J. E., and Major, D., Cat retinal ganglion cell dendritic fields. *Exp. Neurol.*, 1966, **15**: 70–78.
5. Dewey, M. M., and Barr, L., Intercellular connection between smooth muscle cells: the nexus. *Science*, 1962, **137**: 670–672.
6. Dowling, J. E., Foveal receptors of the monkey retina: fine structure. *Science*, 1965, **147**: 57–59.
7. ———, The site of visual adaptation. *Science*, 1967, **155**: 273–279.
7a. ———, Synaptic organization of the frog retina: an electron microscopic analysis comparing the retinas of frogs and primates. *Proc. Roy. Soc. London B*, 1968, **170**: 205–228.
8. Dowling, J. E., and Boycott, B. B., Neural connections of the retina: fine structure of the inner plexiform layer. *Sympos. Quant. Biol.*, 1965, **30**: 393–402.
9. ———, Organization of the primate retina: electron microscopy. *Proc. Roy. Soc. London B*, 1966, **166**: 80–111.
10. Farquhar, M. G., and Palade, G. E., Tight intercellular junctions. *First Annual Meeting of American Society of Cell Biology*, 1961: 57.
11. ———, Junctional complexes in various epithelia. *J. Cell Biol.*, 1963, **17**: 375–412.
12. Fine, B. S., Ganglion cells in the human retina; with particular reference to the macula lutea: an electron microscopic study. *Arch. Ophthal.* (Chicago), 1963, **69**: 83–96.
13. Gallego, A., Connexions transversales au niveau des couches plexiformes de la rétine. *Actualités Neurophysiol.*, 1965, **6**: 5–27.

* *Added by Dr. Dowling after the Conference:* A detailed description of the synaptic contacts in the frog retina, along with a discussion of the differences in synaptic organization between frog and primate retinas, has recently appeared (7a).

14. GRAY, E. G., and GUILLERY, R. W., Synaptic morphology in the normal and degenerating nervous system. *Int. Rev. Cytol.*, 1966, **19**: 111–182.
15. HUBEL, D. H., and WIESEL, T. N., Receptive fields of optic nerve fibres in the spider monkey. *J. Physiol.* (London), 1960, **154**: 572–580.
16. KARLSSON, U., and SCHULTZ, R. L., Fixation of the central nervous system for electron microscopy by aldehyde perfusion. I. Preservation with aldehyde perfusates versus direct perfusion with osmium tetroxide with special reference to membranes and the extracellular space. *J. Ultrastruct. Res.*, 1965, **12**: 160–186.
17. KUFFLER, S. W., Discharge patterns and functional organization of mammalian retina. *J. Neurophysiol.*, 1953, **16**: 37–68.
18. MATURANA, H. R., and FRENK, S., Directional movement and horizontal edge detectors in the pigeon retina. *Science*, 1963, **142**: 977–979.
19. MATURANA, H. R., LETTVIN, J. Y., MCCULLOCH, W. S., and PITTS, W. H., Anatomy and physiology of vision in the frog (*Rana pipiens*). *J. Gen. Physiol.*, 1960, **43**: 129–175.
20. MCILWAIN, J. T., Receptive fields of optic tract axons and lateral geniculate cells: peripheral extent and barbiturate sensitivity. *J. Neurophysiol.*, 1964, **27**: 1154–1173.
21. MICHAEL, C. R., Receptive fields of directionally selective units in the optic nerve of the ground squirrel. *Science*, 1965, **152**: 1092–1094.
22. POLYAK, S. L., *The Retina.* Univ. of Chicago Press, Chicago, 1941.
23. ROBERTSON, J. D., BODENHEIMER, T. S., and STAGE, D. E., The ultrastructure of Mauthner cell synapses and nodes in goldfish brains. *J. Cell Biol.*, 1963, **19**: 159–199.
24. WAGNER, H. G., The spatial summation of light stimuli in the retina as revealed by neuron response patterns. In: *The Physiological Basis for Form Discrimination.* Walter S. Hunter Laboratory of Psychology, Brown University, Providence, 1964: 57–69.
25. WAGNER, H. G., MACNICHOL, E. F., JR., and WOLBARSHT, M. L., The response properties of single ganglion cells in the goldfish retina. *J. Gen. Physiol.*, 1960, **43**(**6**): 45–62.
26. WIESEL, T. N., and HUBEL, D. H., Spatial and chromatic interactions in the lateral geniculate body of the rhesus monkey. *J. Neurophysiol.*, 1966, **29**: 1115–1156.

BLOOD VESSELS IN THE NORMAL RETINA*

TOICHIRO KUWABARA
Harvard Medical School
Boston, Massachusetts

The structure and function of retinal vessels might be expected to be basically similar to that of other microcirculatory systems. A number of studies, however, has shown that the retinal vascular system differs in that it has no sphincter control of its circulation, and there is little or no evidence of fluid passage out of its capillaries. Retinal vessels do show considerable variation in different species and are totally absent in some species—yet those retinas which are vascularized show prompt and severe damage when circulation fails. The purpose of this paper is to present a résumé of the anatomy of retinal vessels as demonstrated by the trypsin digestion technique and by electron microscopy, and to discuss some of the paradoxical differences from a general microcirculatory point of view.

Vascularity

The vascularity in the retinas of different species is surprisingly varied, in contrast with the striking uniformity in histological structure and function of nonvascular components of the retinas in these same species. Human beings and monkeys have well-developed vessels, which originate from the central arteries of the optic nerves; these vessels are remarkably abundant in the posterior portion of the eye, although absent in the fovea itself. Cat, dog, hamster, mouse, and rat have similarly well-developed vasculature throughout the retina, but these vessels originate from several of the ciliary arteries. Guinea pig and rabbit retinas have no vessels in the retinal tissue itself. Birds and reptiles have pectens instead of retinal vessels. Some fish have vessels in the vitreous but not in the retina. This great variation of vascularity is not reflected in other retinal structures which are almost identical in all animals.

The only apparent cytological difference between the vascularized and nonvascularized retinas is the amount of glycogen in the Müller cell. The reciprocal relationship between the amount of stored glycogen and the degree of vascularity seems to guarantee a constant supply of glucose to the retina (5,6).

---

* This investigation was supported by U.S. Public Health Service Research grants NB-03015 and HE-04051 from the National Institutes of Health, U.S. Public Health Service.

On the other hand, a massive plexus of choroidal vessels is regularly found in all animals and the species difference is extremely small. The choroidal vessels of all species have thin endothelial linings. The endothelium on the side of the pigment epithelium has numerous pores and the active passage of fluid has been demonstrated in various conditions. These findings suggest that the retinal tissue may be heavily dependent on the choroidal circulation, and this raises the question of significance and purpose of retinal vessels in some animals.

Vascular Pattern

The blood vessels found in the retinal tissue are different from ordinary vessels in their vascular pattern and cytology. Those seen in the vitreous, or in front of the retina (as in the rabbit eye) are almost identical to those in the vascular system elsewhere.

In contrast to most microvessels, arterioles and venules of the retina do not run parallel courses in close proximity to each other. The dichotomous branching of the arteriole is relatively rare in the posterior portion of the retina, although it increases progressively towards the periphery (Figure 69); this type of branching appears to be necessary to maintain uniform blood pressure throughout the capillary bed. Retrograde branching of the secondary arteriole is found in the central portion of the retinas of several species in both normal and pathological conditions, and is especially noteworthy in hypertensive human retinas (Figure 70); this pattern may serve to reduce the capillary pressure in certain areas of the retina.

Arterioles and venules are connected through elaborate networks in which the capillaries are suspended from two arterioles situated in the superficial layers (Figure 71). Venules are also found in the superficial layer in the center of clusters between the two feeding arterioles. The periarteriolar capillary-free zone, often

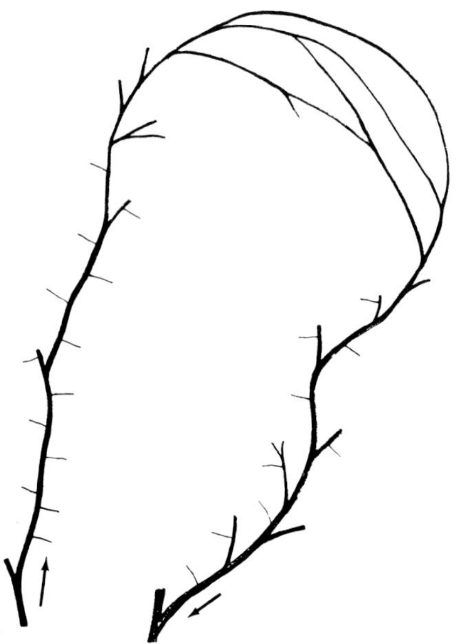

Figure 69. Schematic drawing of the retinal vasculature in man. Dichotomous branching is infrequent in the artery and common in the vein; many small arterioles branch out directly from the main artery at right angles. Artery and vein are connected with relatively large shunting vessels at the peripheral area.

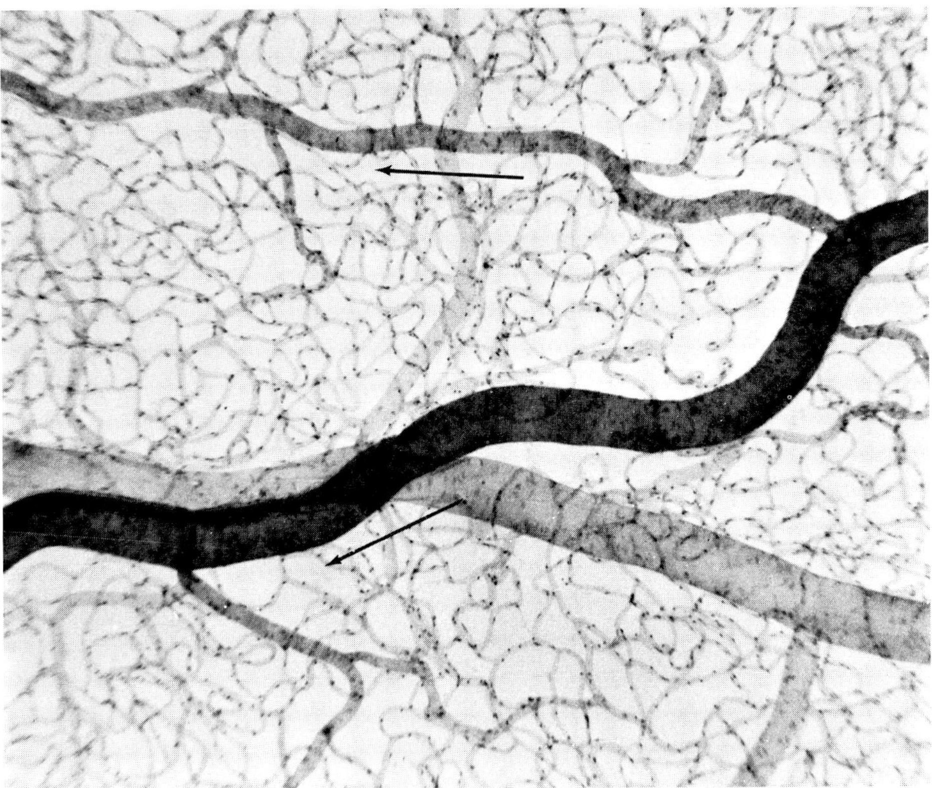

Figure 70. Arteriolar branchings in the retinal vessel of a 40-year-old hypertensive patient, pointing in the retrograde direction. Arrows indicate the direction of the blood flow. PAS-hematoxylin; ×46.

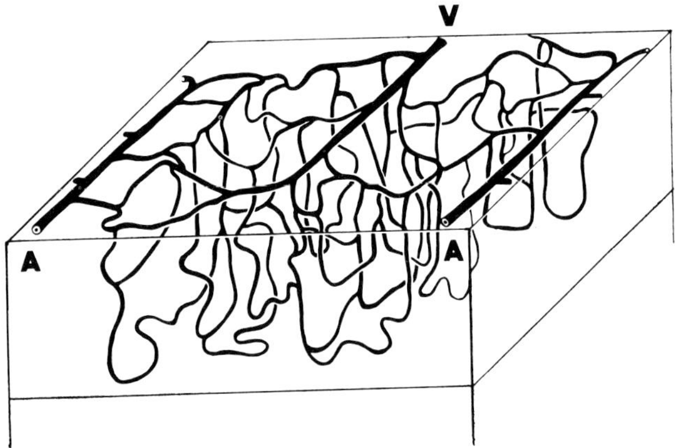

Figure 71. Schematic drawing of the retinal capillary bed. Capillaries are suspended in hammock fashion from two arterioles (*A*); the collecting venule (*V*) is seen between the arterioles.

described as an oxygen-rich area, appears to be formed merely by having a little distance between the arterioles and the territorial capillary clusters; the dependence of this free zone on oxygenation, as claimed, is highly questionable.

There are no shunt vessels in most of the retina. However, the capillaries in the extreme peripheral zone form shunt-like connections by vessels with larger diameters between the artery and the vein (Figure 69); this is most conspicuous in the retinas of the cat and dog. Although no substantial evidence of skimming off the red blood cells from the central capillary plexus has been demonstrated, Thuranszky's theory of skim circulation in the retinal vessels (9) very convincingly matches the anatomical findings of the retinal vascular pattern.

Cytology of the Capillary

The retinal capillaries are very small and uniform in size (Figure 72). The outer diameter is usually 4–5 μ in all animals, or about one-third of the diameter of the capillaries in the conjunctive, and about one-tenth that of the smallest capillaries in the choroid. All capillaries are patent in their normal condition. Although red blood cells are infrequently found in flat preparations, capillary lumens are filled with serum, which is clearly demonstrated in the flat preparations made after glutaraldehyde fixation. Glutaraldehyde fixes not only the capillary wall but also

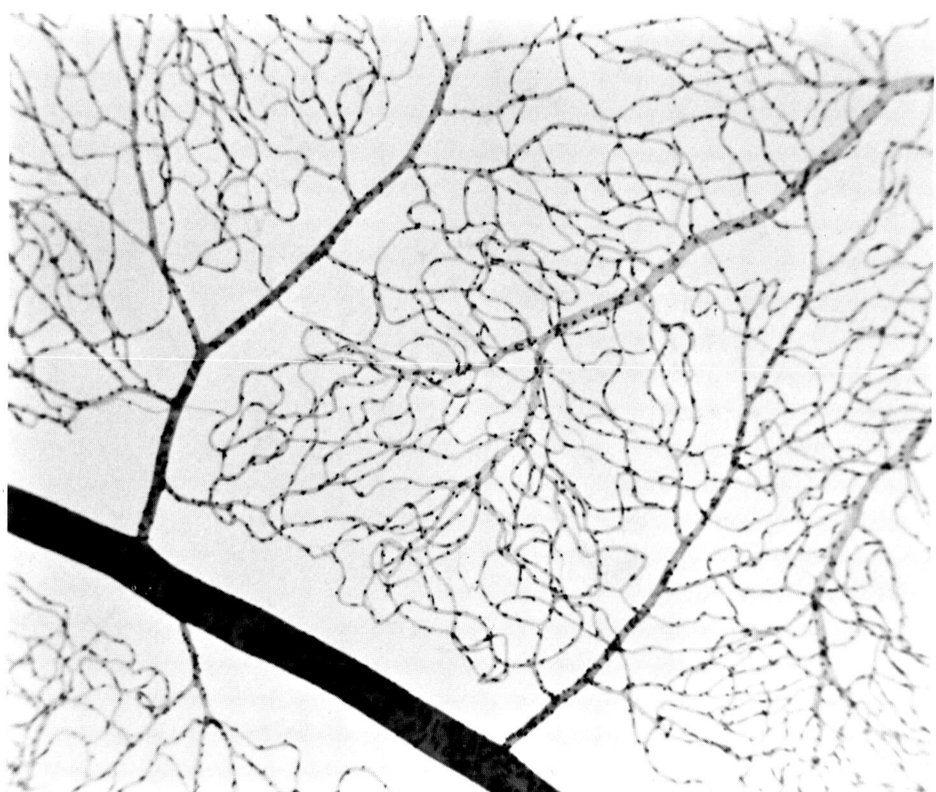

Figure 72. Normal retinal capillary bed of an adult man. Arterioles and venules are interdigitated; capillaries are strikingly uniform in size. PAS-hematoxylin; ×46.

the serum and red blood cells in the lumen; this well-fixed capillary content appears to resist the trypsin digestion and persists as a PAS-positive substance (Figure 73). The diameter of the lumen is strikingly uniform, although the thickness of the wall varies according to the branching and nuclear sites of the endothelium. The site of the right-angle branching in some animals shows annules of PAS-staining substance. No sphincter cell, as described for other vessels, is demonstrable at these branches.

Two kinds of cells, the endothelial and the mural, are found in equal numbers in the wall of the retinal capillary (Figure 74). The cytoplasm of the lining endothelium is always substantial and continuous (Figure 75), with tight junctions and junctional infoldings being consistently found in the inner surface. The number and nature of the various microorganelles are almost identical in all endothelia; large vacuoles are often seen in the area close to the inner surface, but pinocytotic vesicles are normally infrequent. While inclusion bodies of various kinds and degenerative products of the cell are also regularly demonstrated, evidence of active intake, or of passage of fluid or particles through the cytoplasm, seems difficult to substantiate.

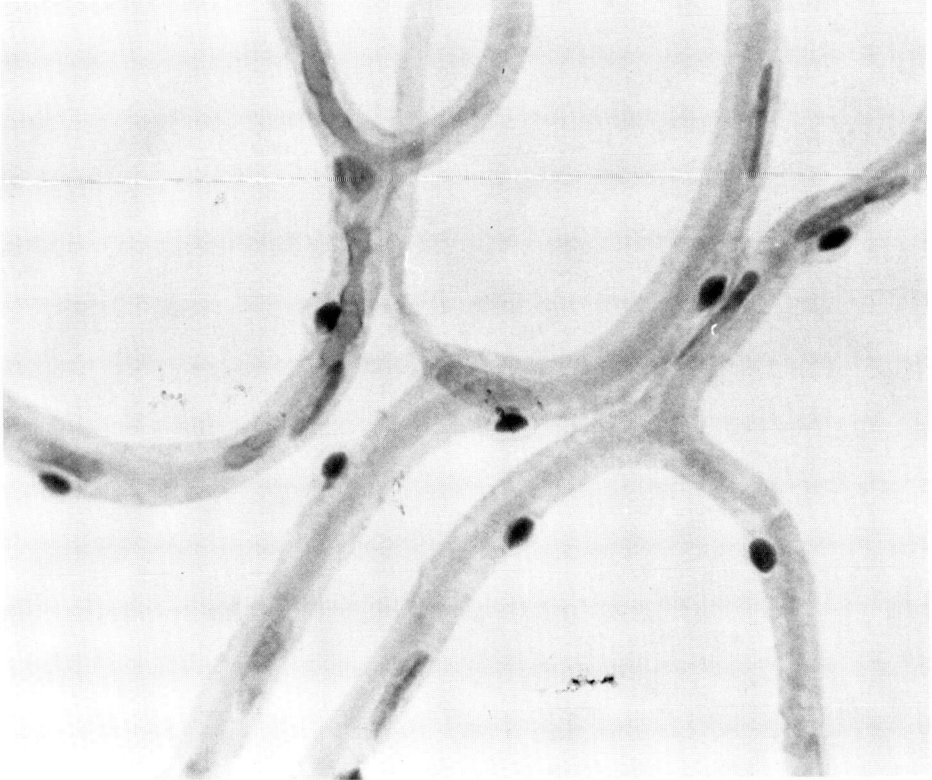

Figure 73. Vessel preparation after glutaraldehyde fixation of the retinal tissue. The endothelial and mural cells are clearly distinguishable; the lumen of the capillary is seen as the PAS-positive core in the vessel. PAS-hematoxylin; ×440.

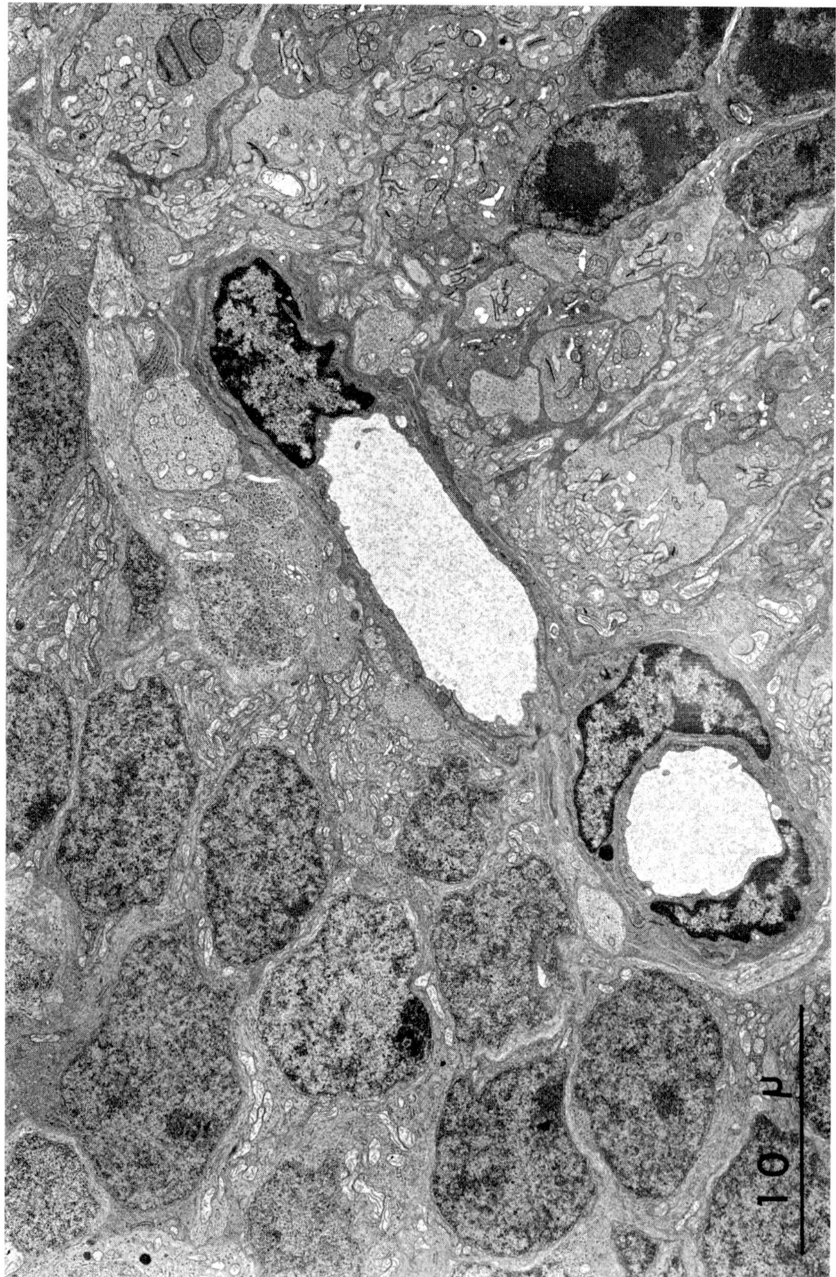

Figure 74. Low-magnification electron micrograph of the outer plexiform layer of a normal monkey, showing two types of cells in the capillary wall. The blood vessel has no perivascular space. ×3300.

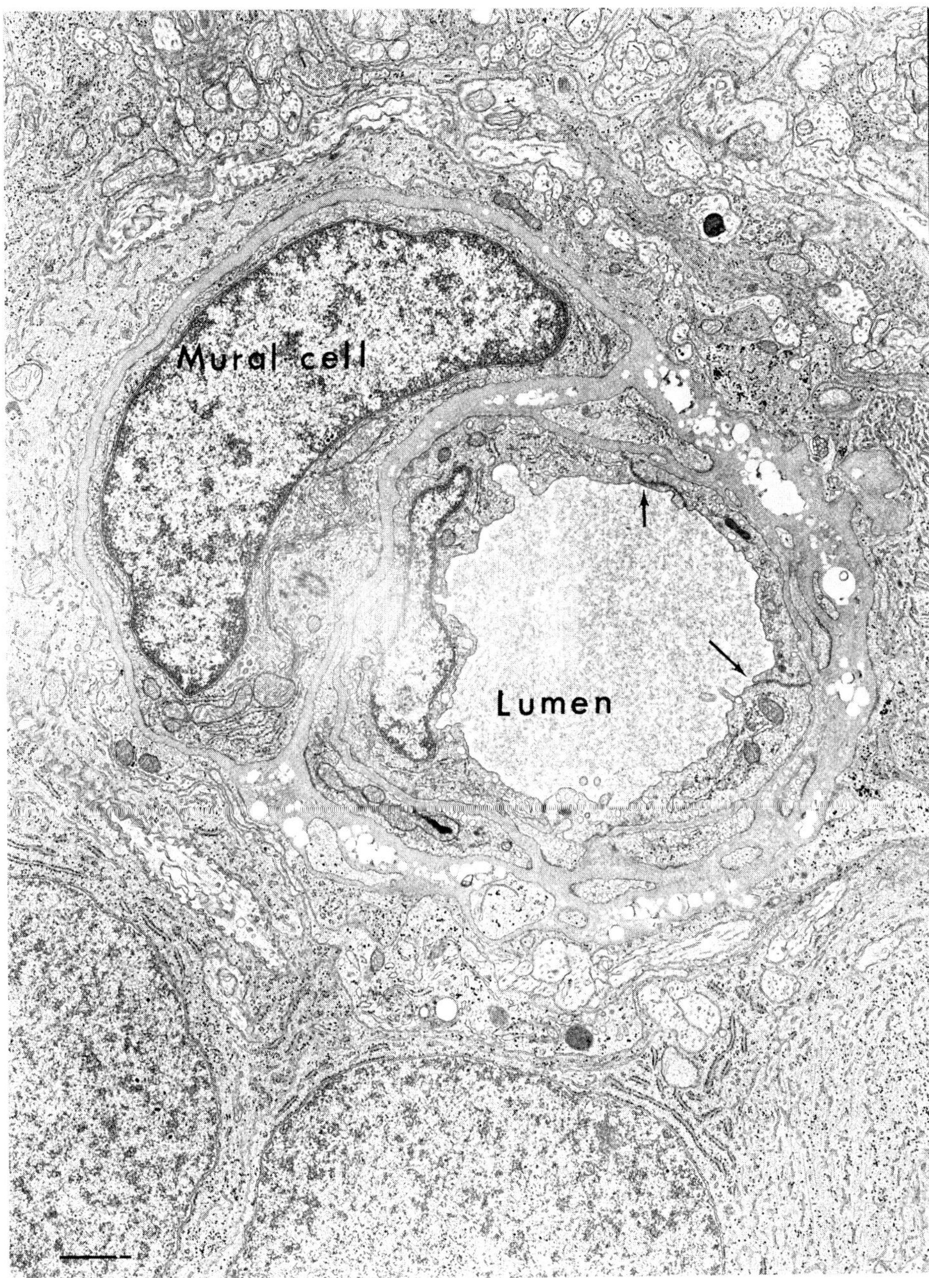

Figure 75. Cross section of a retinal capillary in the inner plexiform layer of an old person. The capillary lumen is lined with unbroken endothelial cytoplasm. Tight junctions are seen (arrows). The basement membrane around the capillary lumen is thickened and vacuolated because of senescence, while the basement membrane around the mural cell retains its healthy appearance. ×9700.

The mural cell, discussed in earlier papers (4,7) by Dr. D. G. Cogan and myself, is believed to be one of the most important factors in the understanding of retinal circulation. While its cytological features are not very different from those of the pericytes of other vessel systems, its regular and intimate situation within the capillary wall is significant.

Basement Membrane and Permeability

A thick and continuous basement membrane is one of the characteristic features of retinal vessels (Figure 76). This membrane begins to form as a fine amorphous substance around the developing vessels and increases in thickness with age. Thick basement membrane may be formed simply by the accumulation of basal lamina substance in the limited space available between the plasmic membranes of the surrounding compact retinal cells and the capillary, but it is not connected to any free perivascular space; permeability may be unaffected by this, however, since the thickness of the basement membrane itself is not a definite hindrance to easy transport of fluid.

In experiments in which animals were fed silver nitrate in their drinking water for a long period of time, marked deposition of silver particles was demonstrated in all capillary basement membranes except those of the retinal and brain capillaries. Basement membranes of the choroidal and meningeal vessels showed an abundant deposition of silver (Figure 77); the kidney glomerules showed the greatest amount. Other experiments in which various fluids (methylene blue, fluorescein, calcium chloride, ferric chloride and sodium chloride solutions) and particles (ferritin, thorotrast and carbon) were injected into the artery, showed no signs of active transport of these materials through the capillary wall. Pathologically and experimentally damaged capillaries were also impermeable from the lumen to the outside (2); in these experiments the thick endothelial cytoplasm rather than the basement membrane may have been the main barrier. It is quite certain that the retinal capillaries are relatively impermeable in normal and in certain pathological conditions.

Pathological changes of the basement membrane are not very different from those of other vessel systems. Vacuole formation and deposition of lipidic material in the basement membrane are common in the aged vessel and in nonspecific pathological vessels.

Perivascular Space

Retinal capillaries have no perivascular space. The cytoplasm of the Müller cell, or of other glial cells, closely attached to the vessel wall, and their plasmic membranes, form the outer border of the basement membrane of the capillary (Figure 78). Under no circumstances has separation or loosening of these connections been observed. Electron-dense particles injected into the vitreous are occasionally seen in these intercellular spaces; the outnumbered particles are present in the Müller cell, however, with the majority accumulating at this cell's outer end. No significant pattern of deposition in relation to the blood vessels has been shown.

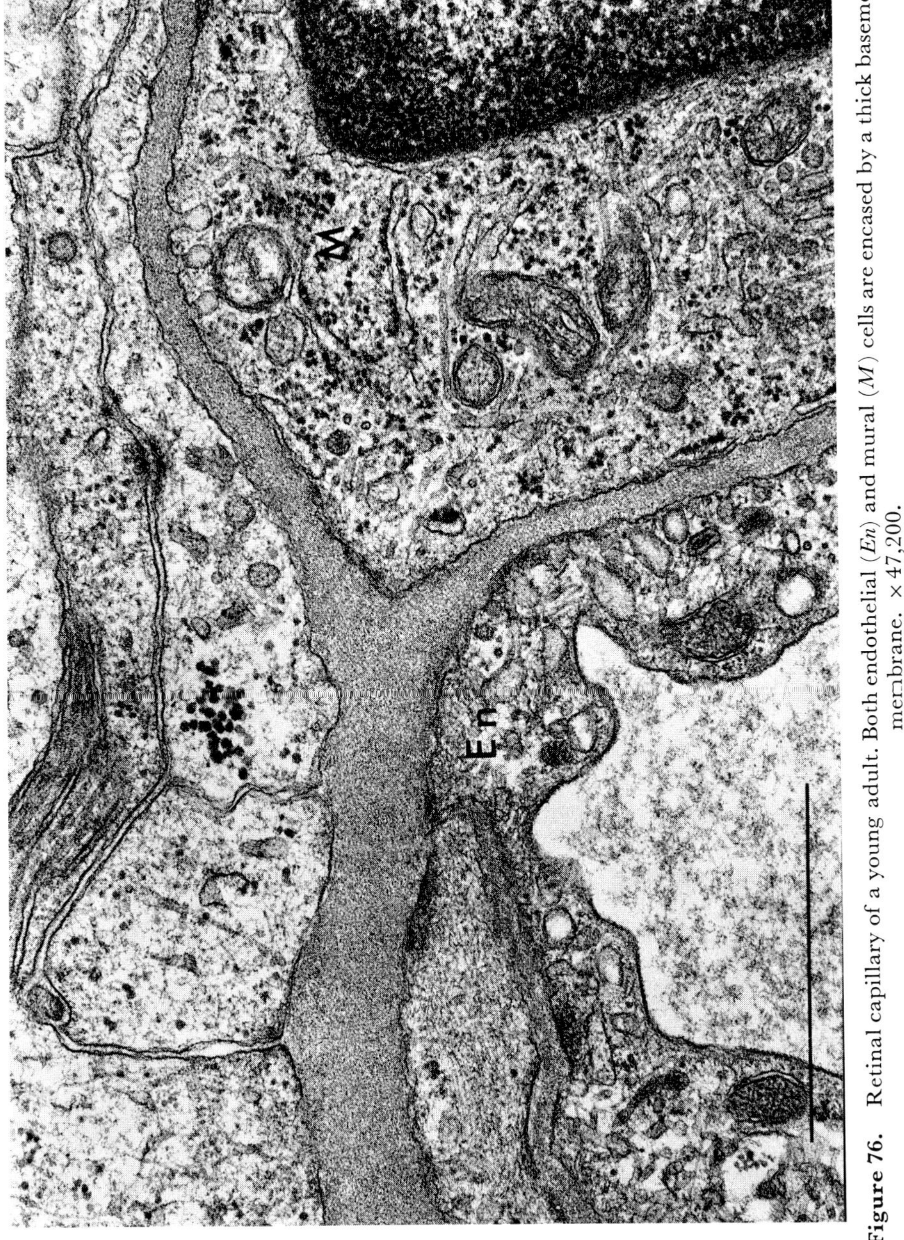

Figure 76. Retinal capillary of a young adult. Both endothelial (*En*) and mural (*M*) cells are encased by a thick basement membrane. ×47,200.

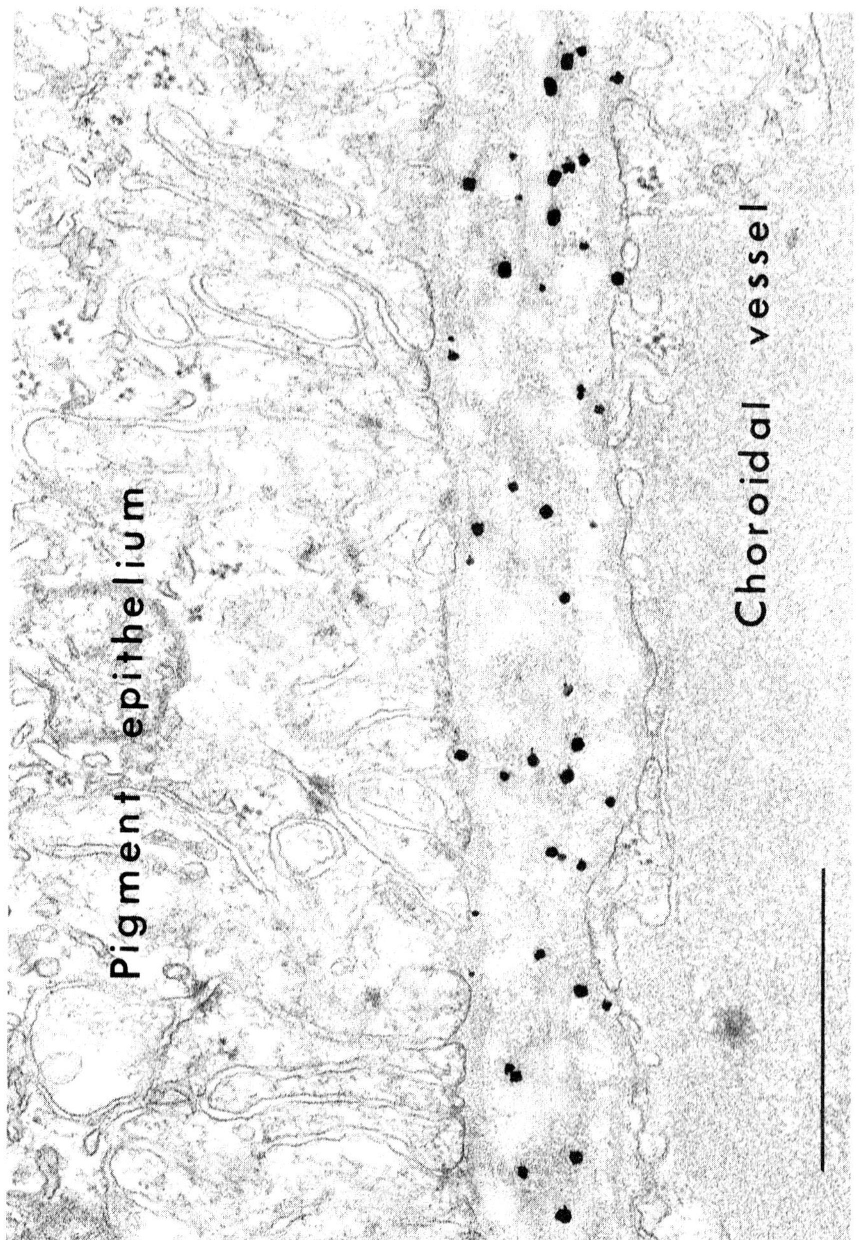

Figure 77. Heavy silver precipitations seen in the Bruch's membrane of a rat fed silver nitrate for one month, indicating free passage of silver ion through the choroidal capillary toward the pigment epithelium. No deposit was detectable in the retinal capillary wall. ×40,500.

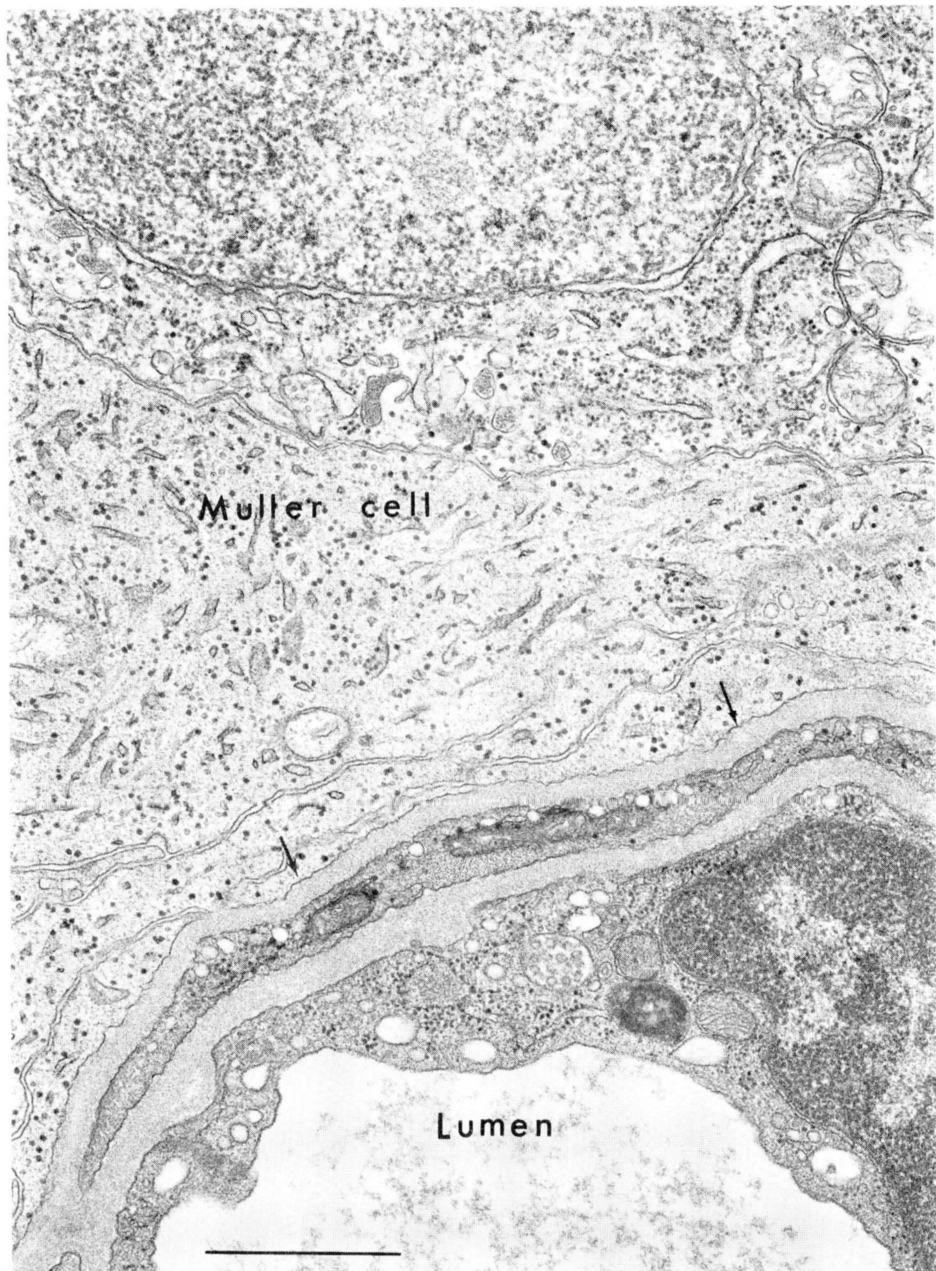

Figure 78. The outer limit of the basement membrane of the capillary wall, consisting of cytoplasmic membrane of glia, mainly Müller cells (arrows). There are intercellular spaces between the processes of the neuronal and glial cells, but none between the capillary basement membrane and the surrounding cells. × 27,000.

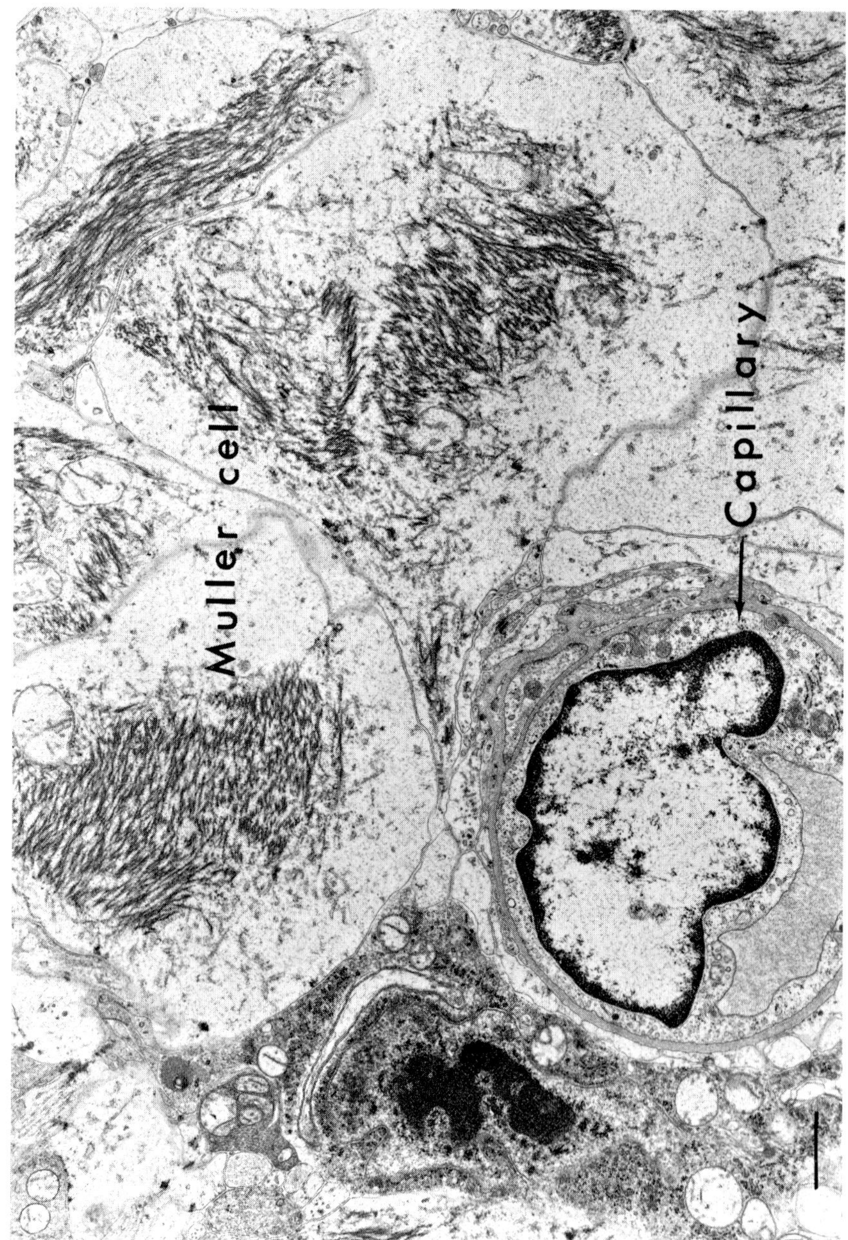

Figure 79. Monkey retina incubated in a tissue culture medium for one hour before fixation in glutaraldehyde. The Müller cell cytoplasm shows marked swelling, whereas the neuronal cells show shrinkage; no perivascular space was formed in this experimental condition. ×9200.

When swelling is induced in the retinal tissue by either soaking the tissue in artificial media *in vitro* or damaging the retina *in vivo*, no separation of the intercellular space is noted. Conspicuous swelling occurs in the Müller cell cytoplasm (Figure 79).

SUMMARY

The cytological construction and the vascular pattern of the retinal blood vessels are different from those of other vascular systems. Some significant aspects of these differences are pointed out by means of electron microscopy and flat preparation technique. The fine structure of the cells of the retinal capillaries and the extravascular components are also discussed.

Discussion

Michaelson: Dr. Kuwabara, you have done so much work on the retina's basement membrane. Is there a diagnostic difference between diabetic retinopathy and other conditions, relative to the basement membrane?

Kuwabara: It is quite characteristic for the basement membrane to thicken in diabetes, but it thickens even more in other conditions, such as hypertension. The changes in diabetes indicate that something is happening in the capillary cells, but the basement membrane change itself may be secondary to some pathological change or to pathological activity of some cells, probably mural cells.

Michaelson: Can basement membrane substances decrease as well as increase?

Kuwabara: In the case of the retina, the basement membrane always increases with age.

Michaelson: Although Dr. Kuwabara's mechanical explanation for the capillary-free zone around the arterioles may appear to be tenable for the definitive eye, there is developmental and experimental evidence that oxygen does in fact play a part in determining this zone (8). In the developing retina, the capillary vessels evolve solely from the venules, and not from the arterioles, which develop pre-capillaries only. The capillaries develop faster from the side of the venule remote from the neighboring venule. Therefore, even in development there is, so to speak, the incipience of a capillary-free zone around the arteriole which cannot be explained in any mechanistic manner. Moreover, by changing the oxygen content of the environment, Dr. Campbell (3) was able to change the width of the capillary-free zone.

Kuwabara: We found that the development of the retinal tissue is quite independent from the retinal capillary system and from most of the retinal organization. The capillary-free zone looks very obscure; the posterior portion reveals no arterioles, so that the capillaries must be distributed around the artery and the vein, but the peripheral area also shows a capillary-free zone around the vein, although very often there are hard-to-see small capillaries passing underneath the galaxy. I thought that was merely an anatomical topographic relationship, but I am no longer sure.

Ashton: I would like to support Dr. Michaelson's views on the nature of the periarterial capillary-free zone. Although Dr. Kuwabara's explanation of these appearances might be tenable in the fully vascularized retina, where there are several networks of capillaries, it clearly cannot apply to the developing retina (as seen perfectly in the rat, for instance), where very definite periarterial free zones are evident at a stage when only one layer of vessels is present. The role of oxygen has perhaps not been conclusively proved, but supporting evidence is very strong, especially as we know that growing retinal capillaries can be destroyed by oxygen. In disputing this hypothesis, Dr. Kuwabara should explain why this clear zone is much more evident around the arteries, and why in the developing retina it can be narrowed by reducing ambient oxygen levels (3) and widened by increasing them (1).

REFERENCES

1. Ashton, N., Retinal vascularization in health and disease. *Am. J. Ophthal.*, 1957, **44**(IV/2): 7–17.
2. Ashton, N., and Cunha-Vaz, J. G., Effect of histamine on the permeability of the ocular vessels. *Arch. Ophthal.* (Chicago), 1965, **73**: 211–223.
3. Campbell, F. W., The influence of a low atmospheric pressure on the development of the retinal vessels in the rat. *Trans. Ophthal. Soc. UK*, 1951, **71**: 287–300.
4. Cogan, D. G., and Kuwabara, T., The mural cell in perspective. *Arch. Ophthal.* (Chicago), 1967, **78**: 133–139.
5. Hutchinson, B. T., and Kuwabara, T., Phosphorylase and uridine diphosphoglucose glycogen synthetase in the retina. *Arch. Ophthal.* (Chicago), 1962, **68**: 538–545.
6. Kuwabara, T., and Cogan, D. G., Retinal glycogen. *Arch. Ophthal.* (Chicago), 1961, **66**: 680–688.
7. ———, Retinal vascular patterns. VI. Mural cells of the retinal capillaries. *Arch. Ophthal.* (Chicago), 1963, **69**: 492–502.
8. Michaelson, I. C., *Retinal Circulation in Man and Animals.* Thomas, Springfield, 1954.
9. Thuranszky, K., *Der Blutkreislauf der Netzhaut; intravitalmikroskopische und histologische Studien an der Katzenretina.* Ungarische Akademie der Wissenschaften, Budapest, 1957.

THE ORGANIZATION OF VERTEBRATE PHOTORECEPTOR CELLS

RICHARD W. YOUNG*
UCLA School of Medicine
Los Angeles, California

The vertebrate photoreceptor is a remarkably specialized cell which responds to the stimulus of light and transmits this response to adjoining neurons for ultimate relay to the visual centers of the brain. The cell detects light by absorbing it within a mass of densely packed pigment molecules. This energy-absorption process alters these molecules, setting off a complex sequence of intracellular events which amplifies the signal, displaces it from one end of the cell to the other, and there conveys it to second-order neurons.

After the visual pigment molecules have been bleached by light, the cell can rapidly reconstitute them at a rate of thousands of molecules per second. In addition, these long-lived cells continually maintain, repair, and renew practically every component of their metabolic machinery (only the genetic material appears to be stable). The retention of vision throughout a lifetime (which may exceed a century in man) attests to the efficiency of this self-maintenance. Nevertheless, there is a delicate balance between continuing function and blinding degeneration, for these exquisitely organized cells are highly vulnerable to serious or fatal injury from a broad spectrum of causes.

The structural basis for these highly coordinated functions is most unusual. The visual cell is elongated, polarized, and segmented (Figure 80). Within each segment, cellular constituents are compartmentalized, yielding a localization of metabolic processes seldom exceeded within the entire realm of vertebrate cell systems.

The vertebrate photoreceptor cell has an elongated cylindrical or slightly tapered *outer segment*, in which the photosensitive pigment molecules are concentrated. At the base of the outer segment, the cell is sharply constricted to a diameter of

---

* The author wishes to thank the following individuals who kindly supplied original photomicrographs for inclusion in this review: Dr. Adolph I. Cohen, Washington University School of Medicine, St. Louis, Missouri; Dr. S. E. G. Nilsson, Karolinska Sjukhuset, Stockholm, Sweden; Dr. A. Bairati, Jr., Universitá di Milano, Milan, Italy; Dr. B. S. Fine, Armed Forces Institute of Pathology, Washington, D.C.; and Dr. D. Bok, UCLA School of Medicine, Los Angeles, California. The technical assistance of Mrs. Mirdza Berzins is gratefully acknowledged. Figures were drawn by Miss Jill Penkhus. The author's research is supported by U.S. Public Health Service Grant NB-03807.

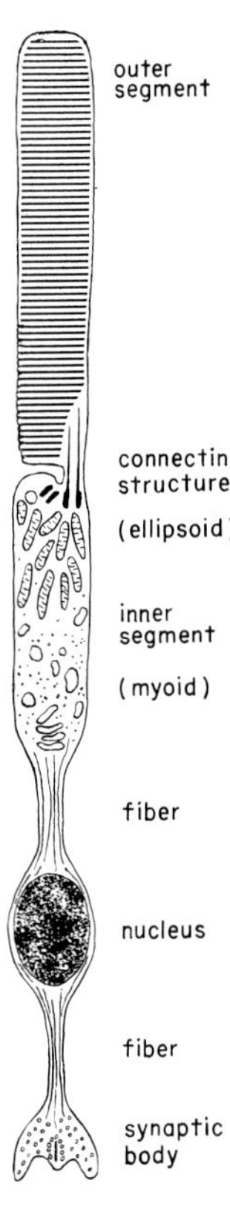

Figure 80. Schematic representation of a typical vertebrate photoreceptor cell. The elongated cell is organized in segmental fashion, each segment having a specialized structure and function.

less than one-half micron. Immediately beyond this *connecting structure* lies the *inner segment* of the cell, within which resides a completely different accumulation of cytoplasmic constituents. The inner segment itself is segmentally arranged into two (or more) zones. Outermost, adjacent to the connecting structure, is a dense aggregation of mitochondria, specialized for the production of energy-yielding molecules; this is the *ellipsoid.* Proximal to it is another zone, the *myoid*, containing apparatus for the synthesis of protein, lipid, and other macromolecules. These organelles also terminate abruptly, giving way to an axon-like *fiber*, a cytoplasmic extension which bulges regionally to contain the cell nucleus, repository of the cell's genetic material. The fiber ultimately terminates in a highly specialized *synaptic body*, in intimate and complex association with second-order neurons.

This segmental organization is reproduced with remarkable regularity in every vertebrate photoreceptor cell which has been studied to date. Nevertheless, it is generally possible to distinguish two general classes of photoreceptors, the rods and cones, using morphological or physiological criteria. According to the "duplicity" theory, vision in dim light is carried out by rods, whereas color vision in bright light is mediated by cones. In different animals, rods and cones may occur as homogeneous (pure-rod or pure-cone) or mixed populations (as in the "duplex" human retina).

Although the known vertebrate photoreceptors are similarly organized, there are minor variations on the common theme. In some lower vertebrates, for

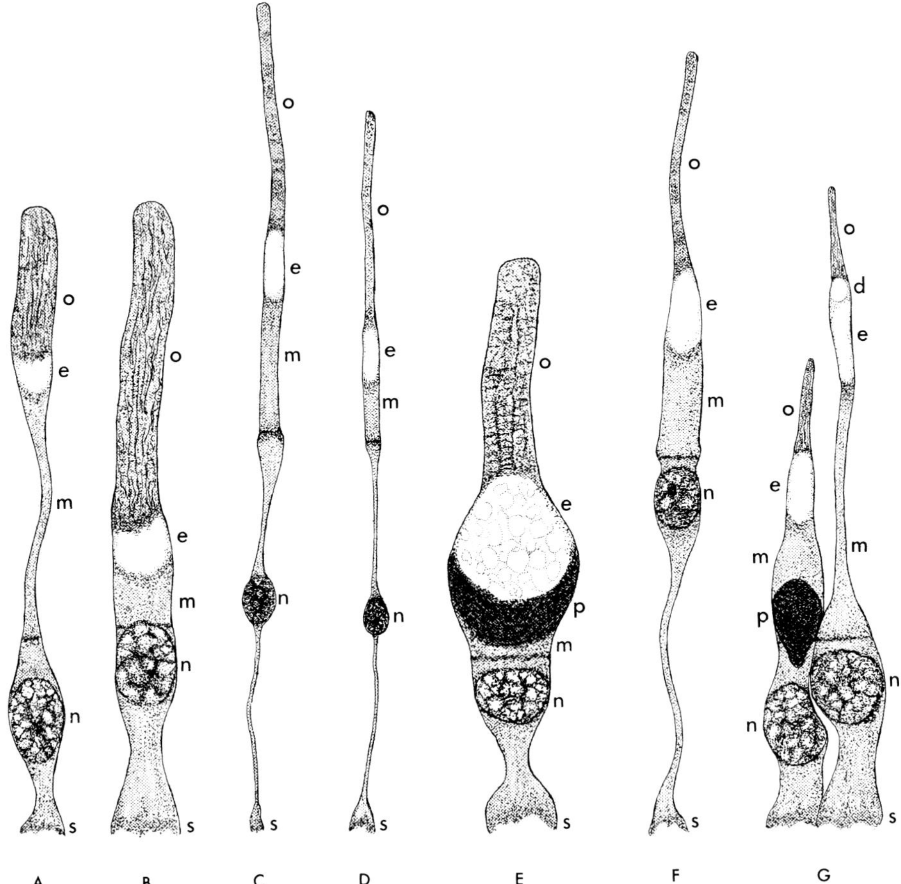

Figure 81. Diagram illustrating the basic similarities in the organization of vertebrate photoreceptor cells of different types and in different species. The cells are drawn to scale, so that differences in relative size may be appreciated. *A:* a green rod, and *B:* a red rod from the frog; *C:* a human rod; *D:* a rod from the rat; *E:* one type of rod found in the retina of the lizard, *Gecko gecko* (cf., Figure 84A); *F:* a human cone. *G* depicts a double cone from the frog; the accessory cone (left) contains a paraboloid (*p*), and the principal cone (right) contains an oil droplet (*d*). Other abbreviations: *o*, outer segment; *e*, ellipsoid; *m*, myoid; n, nucleus; s, synaptic body.

example, the myoid is contractile, responding to changes in retinal illumination; in others, additional segmental specializations are found, such as droplets of oil and clumps of glycogen (paraboloids) (Figure 81).

The Photoreceptor Cell Microenvironment

Cell behavior is continually and significantly modified through interaction with the immediate surroundings. By these unending physical and chemical "conversations", cells are influenced by and in turn influence their microenvironment. The photoreceptor cell is no exception (Figure 82).

The major source of tissue fluid sustaining the photoreceptors is the extensive capillary network in the choroid. Some animals have no retinal blood vessels at

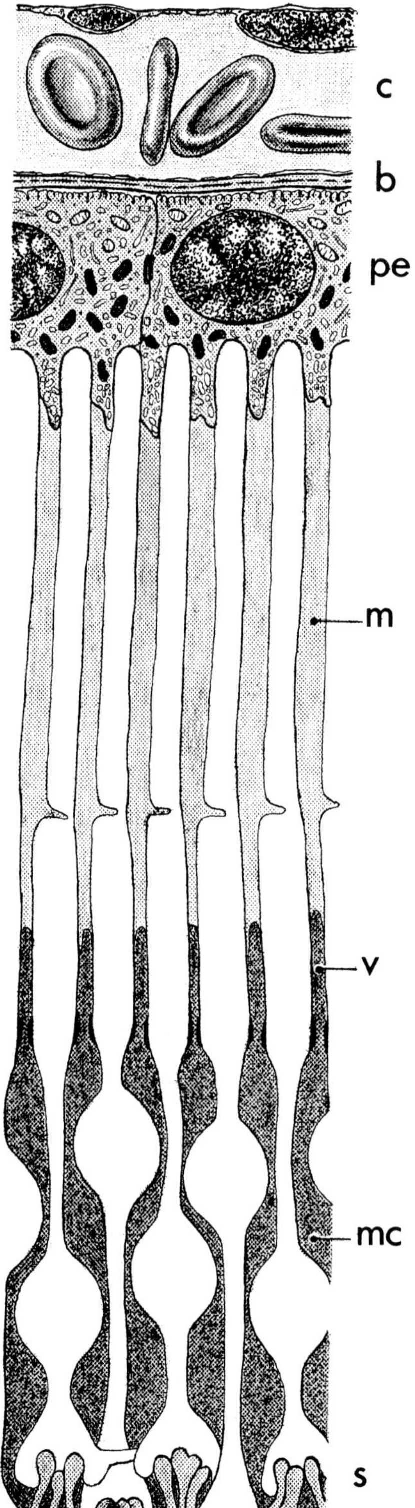

Figure 82. Diagram illustrating the microenvironment of the photoreceptor cell. *c:* Choriocapillaris; *b:* Bruch's membrane; *pe:* pigment epithelium; *m:* mucopolysaccharide; *v:* villous processes of Müller cells; *mc:* Müller cell cytoplasm; *s:* synaptic zone.

all, and in no case is there any vascularization of the layers in which the visual cells are situated. The exchange of tissue fluid between the retina and the choroidal capillaries is facilitated by cytoplasmic thinning and porosities on the retinal side of these vessels (16,97), and influenced by the retinal pigment epithelium and Bruch's membrane. The multilayered membrane exhibits a selective permeability which suggests that it may be the primary site of the physiological "blood-retinal barrier" (7,149), to which the pigment epithelium may also contribute (124).

The retinal pigment epithelium is a single layer of cells reciprocally attached by terminal bars. Passage of material through these cells has been visualized autoradiographically (Figure 83). In fact, the microstructure of the pigment epithelium is specifically modified for this purpose (16,97,143). Pinocytotic vesicles abound at both outer and inner surfaces of the cells, which are further characterized by numerous basal infoldings, and by an extensive vesicular and tubular system extending into the delicate apical processes intimately surrounding the photoreceptor outer segments (3,19,34,35,118). Depending on the species, the scleral ends of as few as five or as many as 300 photoreceptors may be superficially embedded in a single pigment epithelial cell.

In addition to its role as a living fluid filter, the pigment epithelium exerts many other influences on the photoreceptors. In some lower vertebrates, pigment flows down the epithelial cell processes which shroud the visual cell outer segments to screen them in bright light. The local metabolism of vitamin A and the renewal of photoreceptor outer segments involve the mutual participation of both cell types, as will be considered later. The critical nature of the interaction between these two cells is perhaps epitomized by the failure of the photoreceptors to survive if the pigment epithelium is severely damaged (68).

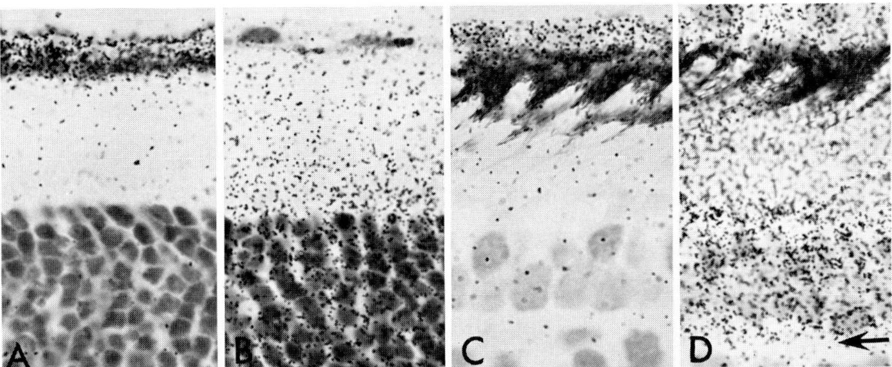

Figure 83. Passage of material through the pigment epithelium on its way to the photoreceptor cells. Adult rats (*A*, *B*) and frogs (*C*, *D*) were injected with taurine-H^3. The location of the radioactive material at different intervals after injection was then determined by autoradiography. One hour after injection (*A*, *C*), practically all of the radioactive material is confined to the pigment epithelium (above). At later intervals (*B*: 4 days; *D*: 10 days), the labeled material is present in the photoreceptor cells; note that in *D* the heavy labeling stops midway through the outer plexiform layer (arrow) at the vitreal end of the visual cells. Taurine is present in high concentration in the retina; its function in retinal metabolism is unknown. Glutaraldehyde fixation, autoradiograms, stained with hematoxylin, × 770.

The space between the photoreceptor outer segments is completely occupied by cytoplasmic extensions of the pigment epithelium in some species (Figure 84A,B). In mammals, however, it is filled with a mucoid material. This substance, identified as mucopolysaccharide by its staining properties (85,111,155), is found in particular abundance in the human retina (49) (Figure 84H).

Along their basal (vitreal) extremities, the densely packed visual cells are almost completely insulated one from the other by the processes of the specialized retinal neuroglia, the Müller cells. Near the base of the visual cell inner segments, the contiguous cell membranes of the photoreceptors and Müller cells are mutually thickened, creating a system of terminal bars which constitutes the external limiting membrane (47,97,137). Extremely delicate and numerous microvillous processes of the Müller cells project slightly beyond the limiting membrane to surround the base of the inner segment (17,48,140). Although the role played by Müller cells in photoreceptor metabolism is poorly understood, circumstantial evidence suggests that they may perform a nutritive or " nursing " function (83,84). The evidence is strongest in avascular retinae, where the Müller cells are loaded with glycogen (82). Concentrations of mitochondria often occur just below the brush border surrounding the photoreceptor inner segments

Figure 84. The preparations depicted in *A* through *G* were prepared by freeze-substitution. All are × 1000.

A: Retinal rods from *Gecko gecko* (cf., Figure 81E) stained with PAS-hematoxylin. PAS stains the outer segments weakly. The glycogen-containing paraboloid is colored a deep red. The ellipsoid is unstained. Note that the scleral ends of the photoreceptor cells are enclosed within pigment-containing processes of the retinal pigment epithelium.

B: Retinal rods from *Gecko gecko* stained with hematoxylin and eosin. The outer segment and ellipsoid contain acidophilic protein, stained reddish pink with eosin. The paraboloid cannot be distinguished.

C: Red rods from the retina of a frog (cf., Figure 81B) killed one half-hour after injection of cytidine-H^3, an RNA precursor. Labeling is concentrated in the nuclei of the photoreceptors and pigment epithelial cells, demonstrating the nuclear synthesis of RNA. A later interval is shown in *F*. PAS-hematoxylin, autoradiogram. (Courtesy of D. Bok.)

D: Frog photoreceptor cells, stained with PAS. Abundant PAS-positive material is present in the cytoplasm surrounding the (unstained) nuclei, in the myoid zone, and in the outer segments. A double cone is shown near the center of the field (cf., Figure 81G). The accessory member contains a deeply stained paraboloid.

E: Frog photoreceptor cells, stained with PAS after extraction with diastase to remove the glycogen. Only the outer segments show significant staining. Most of the PAS-positive material present in the unextracted control (*D*) has been removed.

F: Red rods from the retina of a frog killed 1 week after injection of cytidine-H^3. Most of the labeled RNA has been displaced from the nucleus to the myoid region of the photoreceptor cells, and from the nucleus to the cytoplasm of the pigment epithelial cells (compare with *C*). PAS-hematoxylin, autoradiogram. (Courtesy of D. Bok.)

G: Frog photoreceptor cells stained with the methyl green-pyronin sequence for nucleic acids. DNA, restricted to the cell nucleus, is stained blue. RNA, stained red, is largely concentrated in the myoid portion of the inner segment. (Courtesy of D. Bok.)

H: Photoreceptor cell outer segment region in the human retina, stained with PAS, counterstained with the Hale colloidal iron technique for acid mucopolysaccharides. The outer segments, shown in cross section, are PAS-positive, whereas the material in which they are embedded gives the MPS reaction. The dark granules at the top are in the pigment epithelium. × 2800. (From Fine & Zimmerman, 49.)

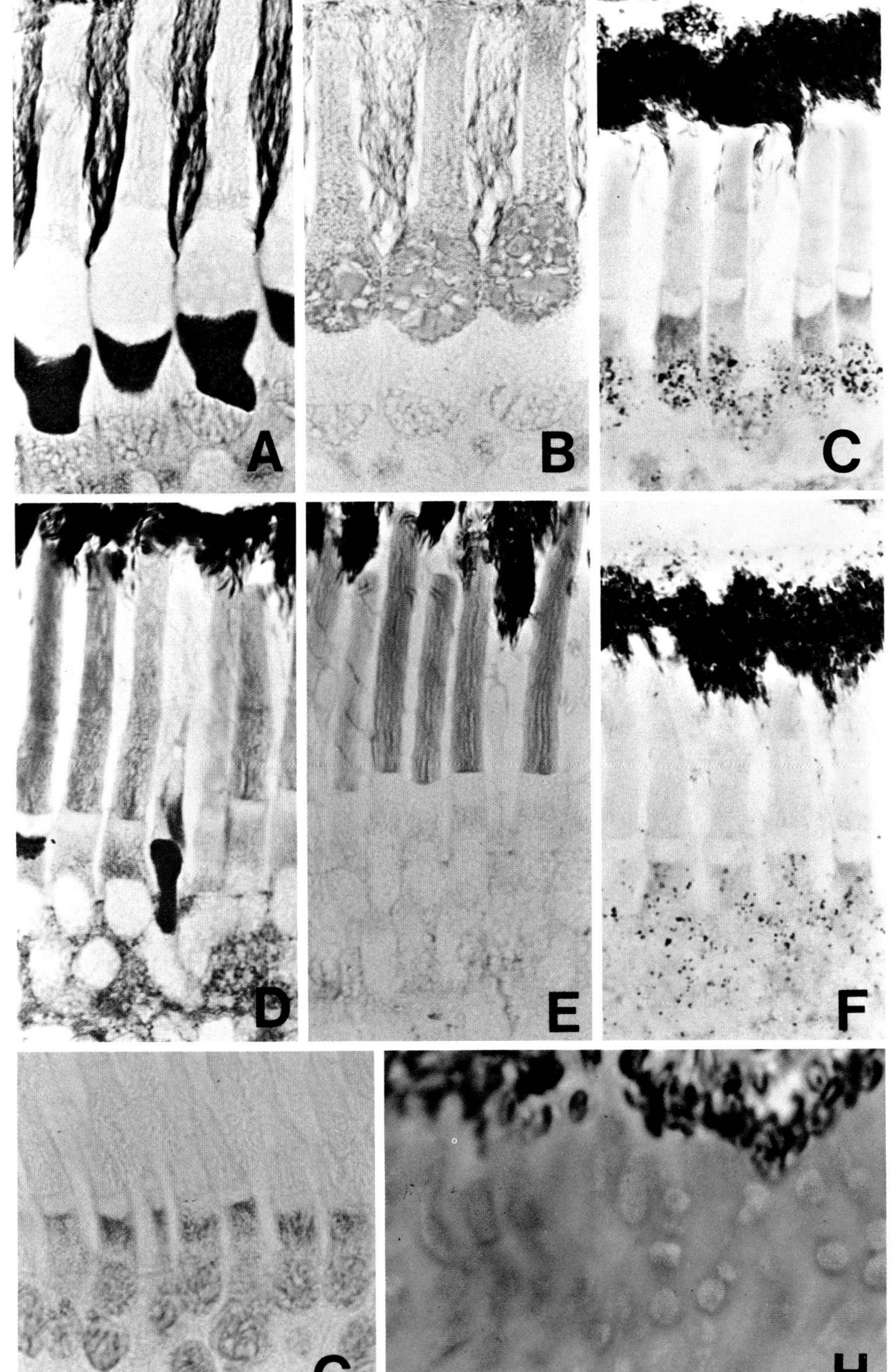
A
B
C
D
E
F
G
H

(41,116,140). In some lower vertebrates there is even a gear-like interdigitation of the base of the inner segments and the Müller cell extensions (18,116,152), which further suggests an active trans-membrane exchange. In vascularized retinae, such as the human, this part of the Müller cell tends to be rather watery and devoid of organelles (48,97); in this case it might serve as an intraretinal supply line for conducting materials to and from the retinal vessels.

At the level of the synaptic body, the photoreceptor endings are separated by thin portions of intervening glial cytoplasm (136,143). The Müller cell insulation is not complete, however, and interreceptor contacts are common (99,105,139) The visual cells are also in intimate contact with two additional cell types at their synaptic surface—the bipolar neurons, which receive and transmit light-induced impulses initiated within the photoreceptors, and the horizontal cells, which are believed to interconnect groups of visual cells.

Anatomy of the Photoreceptor Cell

The outer segment of the vertebrate photoreceptor is a stack of many hundreds of closely packed membranous disks, oriented at right angles to the long axis of the cell, and enclosed within the cell membrane, which is continuous over the inner segment. The most remarkable features of this part of the cell are the regularity of its lamellar organization and the density with which the lamellae are compacted (see Figures 86 and 89). The proportional content of solids in the outer segments is among the highest ever observed in any biological material (133). In effect, the outer segment is a "membranous crystal", consisting largely of transverse alternating layers of lipid and protein. The lipids are longitudinally arranged films, and the protein molecules are transversely oriented (126). The visual pigment molecules, as well as the intermediate and final products of their bleaching, are also oriented (28,146). Even the constituent water may be present in an organized, ice-like state (31,46). This quasi-crystalline structure is clearly designed as an efficient light-trapping device, in which the visual pigment molecules are compacted, stabilized, and precisely aligned. This degree of organization is achieved through exclusion of all other cellular organelles from this part of the cell.

The outer segment disks are formed during cellular development by successive and repeated infoldings of the cell membrane at the level of the connecting structure (Figure 85), followed by fusion of the outer membrane layers to yield a five-layered disk, about 100–150 Å thick (31,101,138,140). New invaginations are repeatedly formed at the basal end of the growing outer segment, gradually displacing the older disks in a scleral direction (106). Depending on its length (107), the mature outer segment may contain from 200 to 2000 of these units. As newly formed disks mature, one or more aligned, lateral incisions may develop. Simultaneously, the region of attachment to the outer membrane contracts and may completely disappear, leaving the disk apparently "free-floating" and unconnected to the cell membrane from which it was derived. Often only the newest disks at the base of the outer segment show clear attachments to the cell membrane. The more distal disks might retain a devious connection through

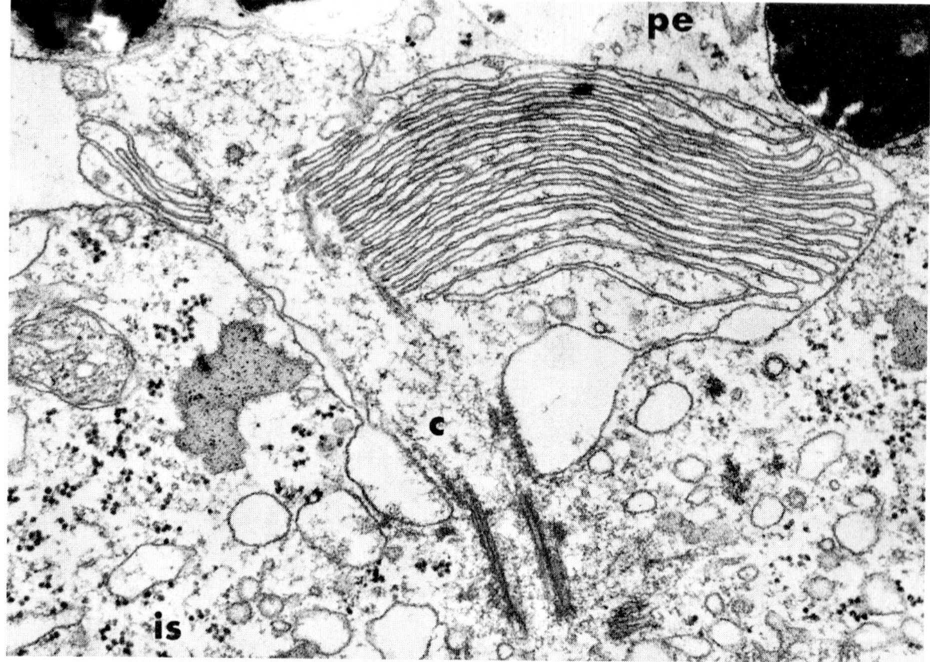

Figure 85. Developing rod outer segment from a 6-day-old tadpole (*Rana pipiens*). This electron micrograph demonstrates that the outer segment disks are derivatives of the cell membrane. Note that many of the disks are mutually continuous, and continuous with the plasma membrane opposite the connecting structure (*c*). *pe:* Pigment epithelium; *is:* inner segment. ×49,000. (From Nilsson, 106.)

microtubules (138) or overlapping lamellae (123), but in the primate retina they definitely seem to be free of such attachments (20,96,97).*

The connecting structure, which links the inner and outer segments of the photoreceptor cell, is an extremely narrow stalk (about 0.3 μ in diameter) enclosed by the cell membrane (Figure 86). Passing through the stalk is a cilium which terminates in the apex of the inner segment in a complex basal body, a modified centriole anchored by a cross-striated rootlet (20,97,142). The cilium consists of nine double filaments arranged in a ring and extending partway into the outer segment in a strand of cytoplasm near the cell membrane. The two central filaments, characteristic of motile cilia, are missing. Thus, the "core" of the connecting structure is apparently hollow (20,30,137). As the sole connection between the site of light absorption and the remainder of the cell, the connecting structure must play a critical role in impulse conduction, as well as in the transfer of materials between the inner and outer segments.

The base of the connecting structure is embedded in the apex of the ellipsoid portion of the inner segment, which generally extends delicate fingerlike projections to surround the base of the outer segment. The ellipsoid is packed with mitochondria (Figure 86). In some photoreceptors, *all* the cell's mitochondria

* See also Dr. Cohen's paper, pp. 31–62.

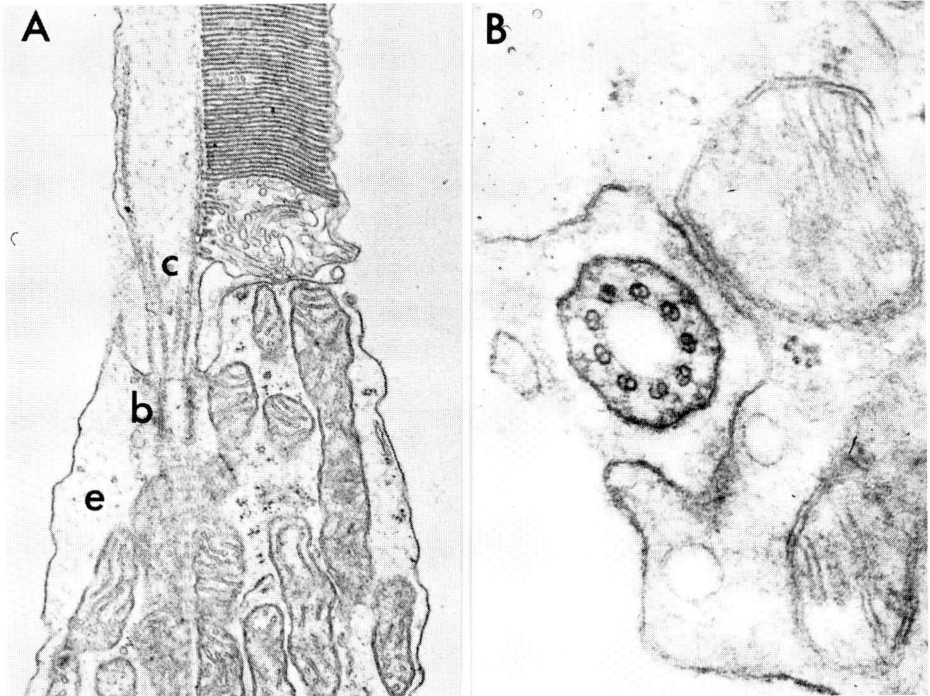

Figure 86. Electron micrographs of vertebrate photoreceptor cells, showing the region of the junction of inner and outer segments. *A:* Longitudinal section of a human rod; note the dense packing of the outer segment disks (top); the irregular arrangement of the membranous structures at the base of the outer segment probably reflects the continued formation of new disks; the filaments of the connecting structure (*c*), which protrude partway into the outer segment, arise from a basal body (*b*) anchored by a cross-striated rootlet in the ellipsoid (*e*) part of the inner segment; mitochondria and scattered ribosomes are found in the sparse cytoplasm of the ellipsoid; ×22,500 (courtesy of Dr. A. Bairati, Jr.). *B:* Cross section of the connecting structure of a rod from the macaque monkey; note the nine pairs of filaments; the cilium appears to have an empty core, whereas the filaments are embedded in a more dense cytoplasm; ×78,000. (From Cohen, 20.)

occur in this region. These organelles are generally arranged parallel to the cell's longitudinal axis, except at the base of the cilium, where they are radially oriented about that structure (104,152). The second centriole of the diplosome, unconnected with a cilium, is found in this region. Scattered granular and vesicular elements are present in the scanty cytoplasm between the mitochondria. These are much more prominent in the myoid zone, which is characterized by larger vesicles and accumulations of ribosomes, both free and membrane-bound. The collapsed, vacuolar clusters of the Golgi complex are situated deep within the myoid, just outside the external limiting membrane (17,49,131,140).

At the junction of the inner segment and the fiber, the characteristic myoid organelles are largely replaced by delicate, longitudinally arranged filaments which resemble the neuroprotofibrils of neuronal axons (29). In human photoreceptors, occasional mitochondria are seen in this region (97). The nuclei of individual visual cells occur at different levels along this "neuronal" part of the cell (so as to provide room for all in the outer nuclear layer). The neuroprotofibrils pass around the nucleus and continue within the fiber, which ultimately terminates in the synaptic body.

The photoreceptor nucleus is generally oval or spherical, sometimes indented or irregular, and usually contains one or more dense masses which may be nucleoli. The nucleoplasm ranges from dense to moderately watery, depending on nuclear size, and is enclosed in a two-layered, porous membrane.

The synaptic body is a highly complicated structure. Generally ovoid (rods) or conical (cones), the synaptic surface is deeply or superficially indented at its base by the dendrites of two or more neurons, commonly identified as bipolar cells.* It contains large numbers of the tiny vesicles which are characteristic of presynaptic terminals elsewhere. In addition, peculiar dense ribbons covered with vesicles are present, disposed perpendicularly to the presynaptic membrane and separated from it by an arciform density. One or more mitochondria may occur in this part of the cell in some species (97,143). Photoreceptor endings may send out lateral processes containing neuroprotofibrils, which make desmosome-like contacts with other synaptic bodies (99,136,143).†

Nucleic Acids

The limits of cellular capabilities are determined by the genetic information coded in the deoxyribonucleic acid (DNA) of the cell nucleus. These instructions are stored in chromosomal DNA by a coding system based on the sequential arrangement of the four DNA building blocks (nucleotides), linked together in a long chain. In parallel with the distribution of chromosomes, DNA occurs in equal amounts in all diploid somatic cells. However, only a particular group of genes is active in each cell; most of these code information for individual proteins. The information in these "structural" genes is transcribed into protein structure through an intermediary molecule, "messenger" ribonucleic acid (RNA). A molecule of messenger RNA is synthesized by a copying mechanism in association with a discrete portion of a DNA chain. The newly formed gene-copy then carries its genetic message to an intracellular site of protein synthesis, usually a ribosome in the cytoplasm. Ribosomes themselves contain ("ribosomal") RNA, as well as protein.

Specific protein structure, determined by the content of amino acids and their sequential arrangement, is controlled by messenger RNA, which serves as a template during protein synthesis. It accomplishes this by moving across the surface of one or more ribosomes, successively exposing 3-nucleotide sequences, to which appropriate amino acids are attached by specific adaptor molecules (a third type of RNA, "transfer" RNA). When the protein is complete, it is detached from the messenger RNA, which may then be used again. Messenger RNA molecules are unstable, however, so that the cell must continually synthesize RNA in order to survive.

---

* *Dr. Young's note after the Conference:* An important analysis of this region in the human retina has recently appeared (98).

† See also Dr. Sjöstrand's paper, pp. 63–100.

DNA

In photoreceptors, as in other vertebrate cells, DNA is confined to the nucleus (40,153) (see Figure 84G). The synthesis of this nucleic acid by cells preparing to divide may be studied by autoradiography, using the specific precursor, thymidine-H^3. In the mature retina, there is no utilization of thymidine (127,134), due to the fact that the genetic material is stable and cell division has ceased. During differentiation of the retina, however, cells may be labeled selectively while DNA is being synthesized (134) in the nucleus. Since the nuclear marker is stable, the subsequent fate of the labeled cells can be followed. In the retina of the mouse, incorporation of thymidine-H^3 (synthesis of DNA) takes place deep within the developing retina, whereas cell division occurs at the outer retinal surface. This spatial separation of DNA synthesis and mitosis involves rapid to-and-fro nuclear migrations (134). After completion of DNA synthesis, the nuclei quickly move to the outer surface, divide, then migrate back into the retina. They may then resume DNA synthesis, or specialize as one of the mature retinal cell types (which do not divide). Cell division ceases last near the ora serrata, and the photoreceptors whose nuclei are most sclerally situated are among the last cells to specialize (134). Work in progress (8) on the terminal stages of development in the rat retina indicates that it follows a similar course (Figure 87).

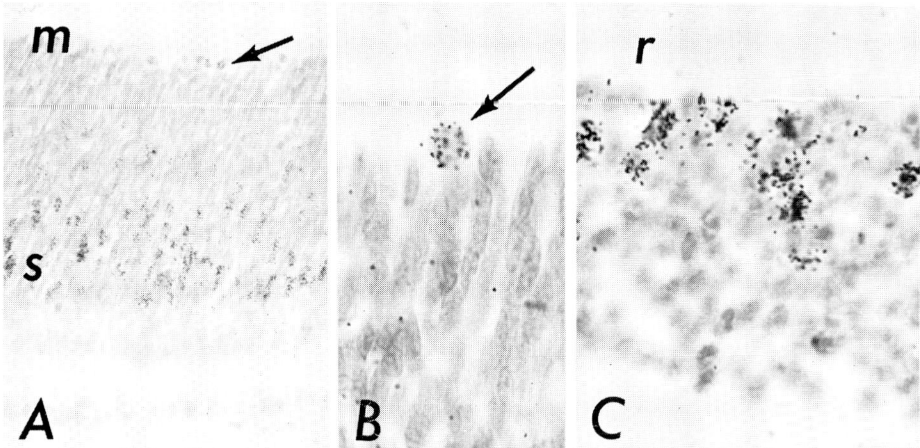

Figure 87. Cell proliferation and specialization in the developing rat retina. One-week-old rats were injected with thymidine-H^3, a precursor used only by cells engaged in DNA synthesis prior to mitosis. *A:* The zone of DNA synthesis (*s*) is deep within the developing retina, as demonstrated by the presence of radioactive nuclei in this region shortly after injection; the zone of mitosis (*m*) is at the scleral border of the retina; the arrow indicates dividing cells; ×240. *B:* From an animal killed 9 hours after injection; by this time, many of the radioactive nuclei have migrated to the zone of mitosis and are undergoing cell division; the arrow indicates a labeled metaphase figure; ×1150. *C:* From a rat killed 3 weeks after injection; some of the cells labeled at 1 week of age have specialized as photoreceptors; the nuclei of the last-formed visual cells are situated in the outermost layers of the outer nuclear layer; *r*: layer of rods and cones; ×1150. Autoradiograms, stained with nuclear fast red. (Courtesy of D. Bok.)

As in most cell systems, proliferation and specialization in the retina are mutually exclusive; that is, a cell which has organized its metabolic machinery for the performance of a specialized function is not able to reproduce itself. The onset of photoreceptor specialization signals the permanent cessation of DNA synthesis in the cell. Furthermore, activation of the particular constellation of genes which underlies the photoreceptor specialization is apparently irreversible. There is no evidence that these cells can subsequently change their specialization.

RNA

In photoreceptor cells, RNA is largely concentrated in the ribosome-rich myoid region of the inner segment, as shown by its content of basophilic material which can be hydrolyzed by ribonuclease (40,119,150). When retinal sections are stained with pyronin, the visual cell myoids bind the dye (see Figure 84G). If the sections are extracted with ribonuclease prior to staining, the stainable material in the myoid is removed.*

Autoradiographic studies have demonstrated that RNA is synthesized in the nucleus of mature photoreceptor cells (8,90) (see Figure 84C). Current research using cytidine-H^3 as the RNA precursor in the rat and frog shows that labeled RNA begins to leave the nucleus within an hour. It progressively accumulates in the myoid region (see Figure 84F), then gradually disappears over a period of several days. The radioactive material is removed by incubation with ribonuclease, demonstrating that it is indeed RNA.* Although it is not yet known what type of RNA is being visualized in these experiments, it is probable that at least part is messenger RNA, which is known to be unstable.

There is some evidence that when animals are subjected to prolonged periods of darkness there is a decrease in the level of cytoplasmic RNA in the visual cells (120), which implies that the metabolism of RNA is related to the functional stimulation of the cell by light. A similar suggestion has been derived from studies of protein metabolism in these cells.

Protein

The cell's protein content represents the direct expression of the gene-complex that has been activated. It is at the protein level that genetic information is translated into coordinated cell metabolism. For example, the innumerable synthetic and catabolic reactions within the cell are mediated by enzymatic protein. Other protein species may also serve a structural role, for instance as components of membranes.

Protein is ubiquitous in the cell. However, it is particularly concentrated in the membranous disks of the outer segments in photoreceptors (37). Much of this is apparently opsin, the visual pigment protein. Both the ellipsoid and outer segment contain acidophilic protein (see Figure 84B), but the outer segment alone gives a strong positive reaction for protein-bound sulfhydryl groups (40,135,150).

The concentration of ribosomes and RNA in the photoreceptor inner segment,

---

* D. Bok, unpublished material.

particularly in its myoid portion, suggests that protein synthesis is largely restricted to this part of the cell. This has been confirmed by autoradiography: shortly after the administration of labeled amino acids, radioactivity is concentrated in the inner segment (37,92,110,154) (Figure 88).

Droz (37) observed that a small portion of the labeled material remained in the inner segment in rat and mouse retinae, presumably consisting of protein destined to participate in the metabolic processes indigenous to this part of the cell. However, most of the protein-bound radioactivity was subsequently displaced from the inner to the outer segments. The author has confirmed these interesting findings in the rat, mouse, and frog (154). When special precautions were taken to ensure good preservation of the photoreceptor outer segments, the radioactive protein was seen to be gradually displaced along the outer segments as a discrete reaction band, which neither increased in width nor decreased in intensity during its migration (Figure 88), and disappeared when it reached the distal extremity of the outer segment, at its junction with the pigment epithelium.

These findings are believed to indicate that the outer segments are continually renewed in mature photoreceptor cells (154). Double-membrane disks are repeatedly assembled at the base of the outer segments. The protein constituents of these membranous units (presumably including opsin) are synthesized in the myoid portion of the inner segment. After synthesis, they are displaced through the ellipsoid zone of concentrated mitochondria. The radial alignment of mitochondria around the base of the connecting structure may provide cytoplasmic channels through which the membrane components are guided to the hollow cilium. These constituents then evidently pass through the connecting structure to reach the base of the outer segment, where they are incorporated into the infolding cell membrane. The new disks are gradually displaced sclerally as a result of the subsequent addition of newer disks.* Thus, the mechanism of outer segment renewal is simply a continuation of the process by which the outer segments are formed, under balanced conditions of synthesis and removal of material.

As noted above, the disposal of old disks appears to occur at the distal extremities of the outer segments, which are in contact with the pigment epithelium. Does the pigment epithelium participate actively in the removal process? The evidence is still somewhat circumstantial. Lysosomes, residual bodies (3,34), acid phosphatase (40,129), lipase (135), and membrane-bound inclusions resembling groups of outer segment disks (16,18,34,45,97) have been noted in pigment epithelial cells of various species. All of these characteristics are indicative of intracellular digestive processes. In rats, outer segment-like inclusions first appear in the pigment epithelium when the outer segments are formed (34), disappear when the outer segments degenerate through vitamin A deficiency, and reappear when these are caused to regenerate by administration of vitamin A (33). Furthermore, electron micrographs of the normal human retina seem to show the

---

* *Note from Dr. Young after the Conference:* Work in progress, using electron microscope autoradiography, has revealed that this process does not occur in cones in the frog.

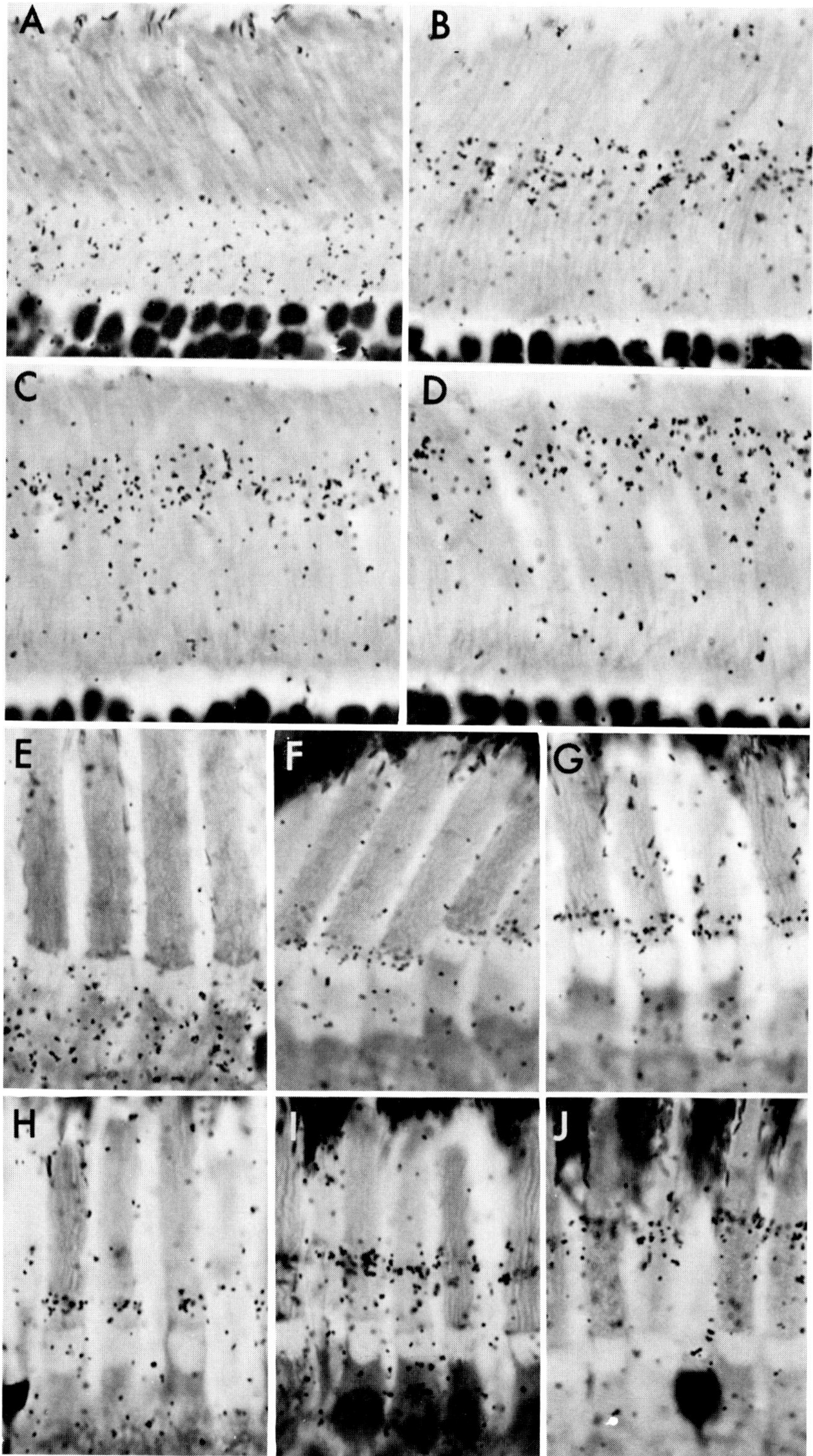

Figure 88 →

detachment of groups of disks from the apex of the photoreceptor outer segment, followed by phagocytosis and gradual absorption of these disks within the pigment epithelium (3)* (Figure 89). It therefore appears likely that the pigment epithelium is involved in the disposal phase of visual cell outer segment renewal.

The photoreceptor outer segments are completely renewed in the rat and mouse in about nine days. In frogs, outer segment renewal requires approximately five to six weeks in green rods, and six to seven weeks in red rods (at room temperature) (154); this difference is due in part to the greater length of the outer segments in red rods. The rate of disk formation (displacement of the reaction band), which is slightly less in green rods, also influences the renewal rate (154). Differences in the disk formation rate seem to imply that the rate of disposal of old disk material at the level of the pigment epithelium may also be unequal for red and green rods. Since five or more rods may be embedded in the apical cytoplasm of a single pigment epithelial cell in the frog, it is suggested that the pigment epithelium has the capacity to "recognize" the difference between photoreceptors of different types and adjust its activities accordingly.

In the frog, the rate of outer segment renewal approximately doubles with each 10° C rise in ambient temperature. The renewal rate also accelerates in animals (rats and frogs) maintained for several days in very bright light at visible wavelengths,† and decelerates in those kept in total darkness (154). Bleaching of the visual pigment probably influences the lipoprotein synthetic machinery of the cell, which affects the rate of production of outer segment disks. Temperature changes in the photoreceptor microenvironment due to absorption of light energy in the pigment epithelium (62) might participate in such a feedback system.

It is perhaps to be expected that the renewal of photoreceptor cell constituents is related to the functional demands made upon this cell type. The observations that RNA content and outer segment renewal rate may be modified by light

*Bairati & Orzalesi (3) suggested that loss of membranous disks at the apex of the outer segment might be balanced by the apposition of newly formed disks at the base of the segment; this hypothesis now appears to have been substantiated, at least in rods.

†The intensity of the light used in these experiments may have been near physiological limits, as indicated by the fact that exposure of albino rats (Sprague-Dawley) to the same conditions of illumination resulted in the rapid death of the photoreceptor cells (Figure 90), a phenomenon first reported by Noell (109).

Figure 88. Synthesis and displacement of radioactive protein (following injection of methionine-H^3) in the photoreceptor cells of the rat (*A–D*) and frog (*E–J*). The outer nuclear layer is at the bottom of the fields, the apical end of the photoreceptors is near the top. *A:* One half-hour after injection, radioactivity is concentrated in the inner segment of the rat retinal rods; during the following day, the radioactive protein is displaced to the base of the outer segments, where it accumulates as a reaction band; the band then gradually moves along the outer segments, disappearing at the apical end of the cell 9–10 days after injection. *B:* 3 days; *C:* 5 days; *D:* 7 days. A comparable course of events occurs in the frog. *E:* One hour after injection, radioactivity is concentrated in the myoid portion of the inner segment. *F:* One day after injection, most of the labeled protein has accumulated as a reaction band at the base of the outer segment. This band of labeled material is then gradually displaced sclerally. *G:* 2 days; *H:* 4 days; *I:* 8 days; *J:* 21 days after injection (part of a cone paraboloid appears in the myoid zone in *J*). *A–D* fixed in 4% formaldehyde; *E–J* prepared by freeze-substitution. Autoradiograms, stained with PAS-hematoxylin; ×1100.

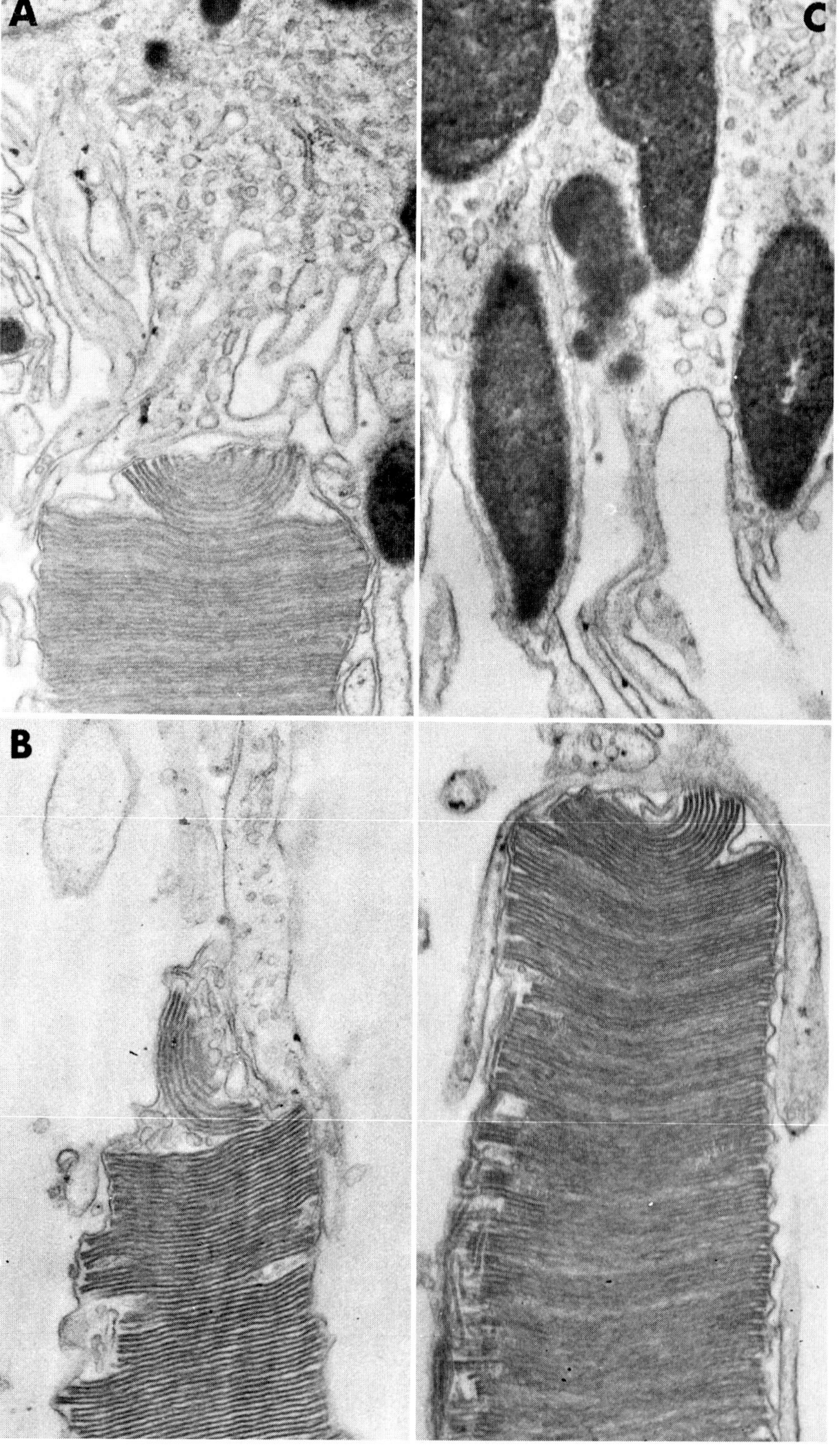

Figure 89 →

stimulation are consistent with this supposition. However, there are conflicting reports. In rats with one eye sealed for six months, deprivation of light stimulation did not appear to change the uptake of labeled amino acid by the deprived retinal cell population, compared to that in the control eye (both examined 1.5 hours after injection) (91). Furthermore, light stimulation of previously dark-adapted mice *decreased* the amount of amino acid incorporated by photoreceptors and other retinal cells examined 30 minutes after injection (38), which seems to be the reverse of what might be predicted. Perhaps the intense stimulation of dark-adapted photoreceptors temporarily diverts cellular energy away from protein synthetic activities and into competing processes of signal conduction and transmission. This might later be readjusted upward through intracellular feedback mechanisms during prolonged light stimulation.

Lipids

Lipids, like protein, are found throughout the cell. They constitute some 10–30 per cent of the weight of intracellular organelles (4), and are a basic constituent of cellular membrane systems (predominantly as phospholipids). So far, there is

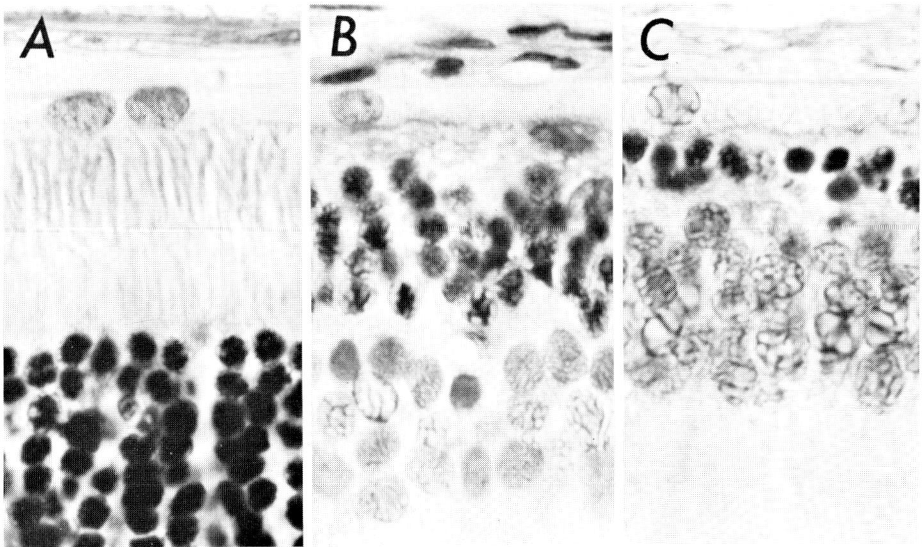

Figure 90. The effect of high-intensity light at visible wavelengths on retinal photoreceptor cells in the albino (Sprague-Dawley) rat. *A:* Normal population of rods; the outer nuclear layer is at the bottom of the field; two pigment epithelial cell nuclei are visible (top center). *B:* After 5 days in bright light (approximately 600 foot-candles), the outer and inner segments of the visual cells have degenerated. *C:* After 10 days in bright light, all that remains of the photoreceptors are one or two rows of degenerating nuclei in contact with the pigment epithelium. Prepared by freeze-substitution, stained with PAS-hematoxylin; × 1150.

Figure 89. Region of the junction of photoreceptor cells within the pigment epithelium in the human retina. The pigment epithelium is at the top in these fields. Note that delicate processes from the pigment epithelium envelop the apical ends of the visual cells, from which groups of outer segment disks are apparently being detached. Electron micrographs, × 30,700. *A*, from Bairati & Orzalesi (3); *B* and *C*, courtesy of Dr. A. Bairati, Jr.

no clear understanding of the functional significance of phospholipids, although it is suggested that they may act as structural elements, assuring the proper orientation of other "active" molecules (such as enzymes), or providing a medium for the passage of lipid-soluble materials (4).

The heavy concentration of lipids in the photoreceptor outer segment has been demonstrated by histochemical analysis of retinal tissue sections. With lipid stains, the outer segment colors intensely, a moderate to heavy binding of dye occurs in the ellipsoid, less in the myoid and fiber, and very little in the nucleus (40,51,121,135,150). The staining characteristics of the outer segments agree well with those for phospholipids generally, and for the lecithins in particular (85). A carbohydrate-containing lipoprotein is also histochemically demonstrable in this part of the cell (85).

Chemical analyses of outer segment preparations generally support these findings. Phospholipid constitutes some 30–35 per cent of the dry weight of the outer segment (24,95,137), a concentration of lipid at least twice that found in mitochondria. The visual pigment itself is apparently a lecithin-containing lipoprotein (80). Lecithin and cephalin are the major lipid constituents of guinea pig and cattle visual cell outer segments; cholesterol and sphingomyelin are also present (137). Lipid extracts of partially purified frog outer segment preparations contain a complex mixture of phospholipids, including lecithin, cephalin, phosphatidyl serine, and sphingomyelin.*

We have begun the analysis of the metabolism of phospholipids by photoreceptor cells, using choline-H^3 as precursor. Preliminary results are consistent with the conclusion that the lipid constituent of the outer segment is continually renewed by synthesis in the myoid region, and subsequently displaced within the cell according to the sequence previously traced for the protein component.

Carbohydrates

Glucose

The main substrate of retinal metabolism, glucose is the principal energy source for a wide variety of processes. It is a very dependable source because its level in the blood is well regulated. In the cell, energy is stored in the form of adenosine triphosphate (ATP), which is generated during the enzymatic breakdown of glucose. This energy is subsequently released at the site of utilization by splitting off phosphate, yielding adenosine diphosphate (ADP).

Anaerobic catabolism of glucose to two molecules of lactic acid (glycolysis) yields a profit of only two molecules of ATP per molecule of glucose. Aerobic oxidation of carbohydrate, fatty acids, or amino acids by oxygen in the mitochondrial citric acid cycle is more efficient. The complete aerobic breakdown of glucose yields 38 molecules of ATP. A series of electron-transferring enzymes (the respiratory chain), embedded in the mitochondrial membranes, represents the final common pathway by which all electrons derived from different cell fuels flow to oxygen, the ultimate electron acceptor in aerobic oxidation. Electrons

---

*J. Freedman and R. W. Young, unpublished observations.

flowing down the chain give up their energy, which is conserved in the generation of ATP. An alternative pathway of glucose degradation, the hexose monophosphate (HMP) shunt, serves to generate ribose phosphate, required for the synthesis of nucleic acids, as well as NADPH (reduced nicotinamide adenine dinucleotide phosphate), a hydrogen donor for synthetic processes.

The investigation of these pathways in the retina has generally followed two different approaches: biochemical analysis of the metabolism of the isolated retina, and microchemical or histochemical analysis of enzymes present in tissue sections.

The isolated retina rapidly converts glucose to lactic acid, even in the presence of oxygen. It also consumes oxygen more rapidly than other tissues (22). Although lactic acid is the prevalent end product of glucose metabolism *in vitro*, the citric acid cycle is also operative. About 35 per cent of the CO_2 produced in the citric acid cycle is derived from substrates other than glucose (21,60). Proportionately little of the glucose utilized *in vitro* is metabolized by the HMP shunt (21,60,66).

These studies on the behavior of retinal cells in an artificial environment deal with the "average" metabolism of a very heterogeneous cell population. In an effort to isolate the photoreceptor cell contribution, differences in the metabolism of young and mature retinae (before and after development of the photoreceptors) have been sought. At the time of visual cell differentiation, there is a sharp increase in glucose oxidation in the citric acid cycle (respiration) and in glycolysis (22,63,65,108), as well as a decrease in the activity of the HMP shunt (9,122). If these age-associated changes are due largely to the special activities of the photoreceptor cells, they should be reversed in animals in which these cells have degenerated. In general, this seems to be the case. Following loss of the visual cells, glycolysis and respiration both decline (63,64,148), whereas the activity of the HMP shunt tends to rise, at least temporarily (9,122).

According to microchemical work (86,87,125), enzymes of the glycolytic pathway are most concentrated in the neuronal end of the photoreceptor cells. An exception is hexokinase, the first enzyme in this pathway (and in the HMP shunt), which was found in high concentration in the inner segments, especially the ellipsoid portion. Lactate dehydrogenase, another glycolytic enzyme, has been detected in the synaptic end of the cell by histochemical techniques (43,113)—this enzyme may also occur in the inner segment (102,113).

Since the end product of glycolysis is lactate, this metabolite would be expected to be present in relatively high amounts near the vitreal end of the cell. This was indeed found to be the case for lactate, as well as for glucose-6-phosphate, the product of the hexokinase reaction (93). Perhaps glucose-6-phosphate, like RNA, accumulates where it is utilized, rather than where it is synthesized.

In visual cells, the citric acid cycle is largely restricted to the ellipsoid. Evidence of a lesser activity of this oxidative sequence in the more vitreal parts of the cell has also been obtained in species in which mitochondria occur in the myoid, fiber, and synaptic body (5,40,86,102,113).

There is no convincing evidence that the citric acid or glycolytic pathways are operative in the photoreceptor outer segments, although there have been reports that outer segment preparations take up molecular oxygen (55,70,72). The significance of this phenomenon is unknown.

Microchemical analysis of the retinal distribution of glucose-6-phosphate dehydrogenase has indicated that this HMP shunt enzyme is largely restricted to the myoid and fiber portion of the photoreceptor cells (87). It has also been detected histochemically in photoreceptors (102,113). In the rat, it appears to be concentrated in the outer segments (113). A preparation of bovine outer segments also gave evidence of the operation of the HMP shunt pathway (57). These findings show inconsistencies both among themselves and with the biochemical studies cited above, but appear at least to indicate that the HMP shunt is active in the cytoplasm of the visual cells, and perhaps in the outer segments as well.

Available evidence consistently documents the active utilization of glucose by photoreceptor cells. Glucose metabolism, like other metabolic pathways, shows signs of intracellular compartmentalization. The anaerobic breakdown of glucose is largely restricted to the neuronal end of the elongated cell, which is farthest removed from the choroidal blood supply. Neither the glycolytic pathway nor the citric acid cycle—the sources of energy-bearing ATP—appear to operate at the other end of the cell, in the outer segment. The oxidative pathway is almost entirely restricted to the ellipsoid, where mitochondria are concentrated close to the major source of oxygen and glucose (the choriocapillaris), and critically situated to serve the energy needs of the outer segment. The outer segment contains enzymes capable of splitting phosphate from ATP (10,52,95,128). If ATP flows from the ellipsoid through the connecting structure to the outer segments, perhaps ADP returns to the ellipsoid by the same route for regeneration. The HMP shunt appears to be distributed throughout the myoid and fiber portions of the cell. One of the products of this pathway, ribose, is presumably used in the synthesis of RNA in the nucleus. The shunt may also be present in the outer segments, where another of its products, NADPH, has been implicated in the visual process (57).

Glycogen

The polymerized storage form of glucose, glycogen, has been detected in retinal tissue sections by the periodic acid Schiff (PAS) staining technique, controlled by digestion with diastase or salivary amylase. The photoreceptor outer segments also stain with PAS, but this staining (unlike that caused by glycogen) is not abolished by the enzymes, and is believed to be due to a glyco-lipoprotein component in the membranous disks (see Figure 84D,E).

Retinal glycogen varies considerably in different species. It is particularly abundant in avascular retinae, where the largest amount occurs in the Müller fibers (82). Glycogen deposits occurring in the region of the photoreceptor nuclei and synaptic bodies are generally attributed to these glial fibers (41,132). Small amounts of glycogen have been detected in the inner segments of the visual cells in many species (41,85,121,150) (see Figure 84D,E). The paraboloid, a specialized zone in the inner segment of certain vertebrate photoreceptors, contains a large deposit of glycogen of unknown function (see Figure 84A,D). Radioactivity is temporarily concentrated in the paraboloid of the frog cones during the first day after injection of choline-H^3. During diastase digestion, the labeled material is removed along with the glycogen.

Paraboloid glycogen does not appear to be mobilized in the frog during starvation (89). Temperature, however, seems to have a pronounced effect in this species. In winter, retinal glycogen is increased, particularly in the plexiform layers, but is diminished in the cone paraboloids. In summer, the situation is reversed (89). A similar effect occurs in frogs raised in the laboratory for 10 days at 13° and 34° C.*

Glycogen is probably synthesized *in situ*, where it is to be stored, but there is little evidence to support this. In the rabbit, an enzyme in this pathway is more concentrated in the outer plexiform layer than in the inner segments, as is glycogen itself (87,93).

Mucopolysaccharides

The presence of mucopolysaccharides (MPS) in the region of the visual cell outer segments has been demonstrated in several mammalian retinae. As noted earlier, this material is particularly abundant in the human retina (see Figure 84H). In the rabbit and in man, these MPS are believed to be nonsulfated, and resistant to digestion with testicular hyaluronidase (49,141). In the cattle retina, however, there is a mixture of MPS, including neutral nonsulfated acid and sulfated acid components, part of which can be broken down by hyaluronidase (53,151). In the rat, a complex mixture of MPS is also present; some are sulfated and some are sensitive to hyaluronidase digestion (69,111). In this species, MPS also occur in the plexiform layers. The different classes of sulfated MPS are not uniformly distributed in the retina, the hyaluronidase-labile fractions being predominant in the layer of photoreceptors (111).

The origin of the MPS in the photoreceptor zone has been variously attributed to the Müller fibers, the pigment epithelium, and the photoreceptors themselves. In human photoreceptors, the presence in the myoid zone of vesicles which contain material resembling the MPS between the outer segments suggests that the MPS may be synthesized in the rod and cone inner segments (49). This appears to be the case in the rat, as shown by autoradiography using sulfate-S^{35} as precursor (111) (Figure 91). Sulfated MPS in the photoreceptor zone of the adult rat are rapidly renewed (111). Thus, not only the outer segments, but the extracellular material in which they are embedded, may undergo continued replacement in the mature retina. Both processes utilize materials synthesized in the visual cell inner segments.

In the frog, in which the intercellular space between the outer segments is occupied by prolongations of the pigment epithelium, MPS content as determined by histochemical staining is low or negligible. Nevertheless, sulfate-S^{35} uptake is evident as a diffuse reaction in this zone.* Perhaps the sulfur-containing

---

* Author's unpublished observations.

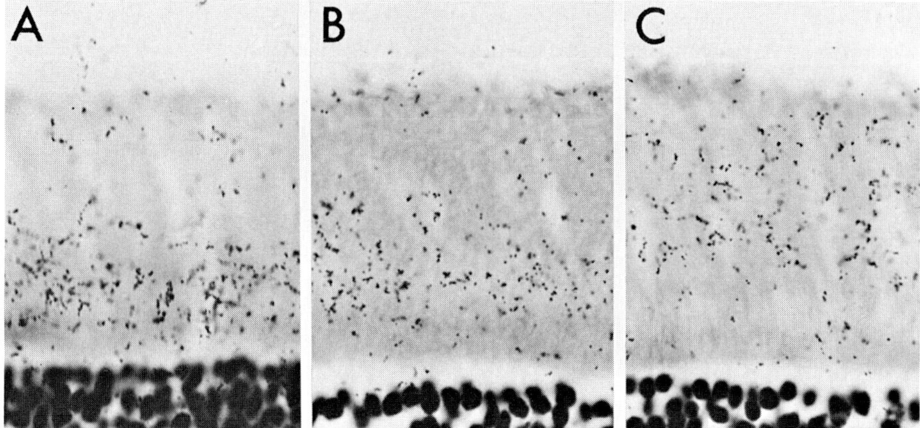

Figure 91. Synthesis and displacement of sulfated mucopolysaccharides in the photoreceptor zone of rats injected with sulfate-S^{35}. *A:* Eight hours after injection, the concentration of labeling is most intense in the inner segments. *B:* At 3 days, the labeled material has been displaced sclerally, and is now most heavily concentrated near the junction of the inner and outer segments. *C:* At 1 week, the reaction is most intense in the outer segment region. Autoradiograms, PAS-hematoxylin; ×620. (From Ocumpaugh & Young, 111.)

material is synthesized by (and retained within) the pigment epithelium, which appears to have the capacity for MPS synthesis in some animals (6).

Bleaching and Regeneration of Visual Pigment

All known vertebrate visual pigments are built on the same general pattern, consisting of a protein (opsin) combined with a particular isomer of vitamin A_1 aldehyde (retinene$_1$) or vitamin A_2 aldehyde (retinene$_2$). All mammalian and most vertebrate pigments utilize retinene$_1$. The wavelength absorbed maximally by the A_1 group of pigments ranges from 430 mμ to 562 mμ (27), whereas the maximum absorption of retinene$_1$ is 387 mμ. Evidently, the variability among visual pigments in the wavelength of light most efficiently absorbed is due to differences in the protein component, and in the manner in which the retinene is bound to it (75,81).

Relatively little is known about the opsins. Cattle opsin is a lipoprotein with a molecular weight of about 40,000, of which some 45 per cent is phospholipid (73,80). Opsin is reportedly free of any trace of metals in cattle (56), although a more recent report indicates the possible presence of iron in the frog (54). The protein has no free terminal α-amino or α-carboxyl groups (1). Its main attachment to retinene is through a Schiff base linkage formed by condensing the aldehyde group of retinene with an ε-amino group of lysine (73).

The absorption of light by pigment molecules embedded in the visual cell outer segments sets in motion a complex series of metabolic events involving the entire cell, as well as neighboring cells. Most of the available information concerns rhodopsin, the retinene$_1$ rod pigment.

Rhodopsin is a reddish pigment with a maximum absorption (in mammals) near 500 mμ, and consists of opsin combined with a specific, unusually bent and twisted (11-*cis*) isomer of retinene. Although the probability of absorption is enormously greater for wavelengths in the blue-green region, the pigment is capable of absorbing all visible wavelengths (11,117). The visual cell is probably incapable of discriminating between different wavelengths of light absorbed in its outer segment. The pigment molecule manifests the same reaction, as does the cell itself, independently of the energy of each absorbed quantum. Similar considerations presumably apply to the three classes of cone pigments with different absorption maxima—in the red, blue, and green—which appear to underlie the phenomenon of color vision (88,145).

When a quantum of light is absorbed by a rhodopsin molecule, the absorbed energy causes the isomerization of retinene from the bent (11-*cis*) to the straight-chain (all-*trans*) form. Light supplies the activation energy for this exergonic process. This, the only action of light energy in the visual process, apparently destroys the correspondence of the "lock and key" relationship between retinene and opsin. A sequence of molecular rearrangements of the protein follows immediately, manifested by the appearance of two sulfhydryl groups and one acid-binding group (75,94). Excitation of the visual cell occurs at some early stage during these sequential changes. The end result of the molecule modifications initiated by light absorption is the "bleaching" step, in which the all-*trans* retinene is liberated from opsin. To maintain the visual capacity, the cell must be able to resynthesize this pigment. This is done by re-isomerizing retinene to the 11-*cis* form, which is then trapped by an "empty" opsin molecule, thereby recreating the photosensitive rhodopsin.

The basic process in the bleaching and regeneration of visual pigment is therefore (*a*) the absorption of light energy, causing isomerization of retinene to the all-*trans* form, which is subsequently liberated from the opsin, and (*b*) re-isomerization of retinene to the 11-*cis* isomer, which is recaptured by opsin, somehow altering the protein configuration, thereby regenerating the pigment. The formation of the 11-*cis* form requires an expenditure of energy, since this isomer represents a higher energy state than the all-*trans* form (144). This process, which must take place rapidly enough to support the persistence of vision in bright light, would be expected to occur in the outer segments. In fact, an isomerase which mediates the all-*trans* to 11-*cis* conversion has been extracted from cattle retinae (74). The equilibrium of this reversible reaction actually favors formation of the more stable all-*trans* isomer. However, trapping of the 11-*cis* form by binding to opsin would keep the reaction moving in the 11-*cis* direction.

There is abundant evidence to suggest that the *in vivo* situation is more complex. Although all-*trans* retinene is liberated upon rhodopsin bleaching, it never accumulates in the outer segments, even in very bright light (36). Some of the all-*trans* retinene may be immediately re-isomerized and trapped by opsin, although much of it is apparently reduced to vitamin A by alcohol dehydrogenase, at least under conditions of severe bleaching.* This enzyme is strategically located

* Much of the work on rhodopsin bleaching and regeneration has involved non-physiological conditions of extreme light stimulation—e.g., 95 per cent bleaching in 30 minutes (32). Under the conditions of dim light in which the rods normally function, less than 0.02 per cent of the pigment is bleached in an hour (117).

as a constituent of the outer segment disks (57,58,61,147). The retinene-vitamin A interconversion is also a reversible reaction, favoring formation of the vitamin A.* The necessary function of alcohol dehydrogenase is the conversion of vitamin A to retinene, the molecular form required for vision. Nevertheless, when the retina is strongly bleached, there is a net production of vitamin A from the liberated retinene. Furthermore, much of this newly generated vitamin A is subsequently esterified with a long-chain fatty acid (59,79)† and may leave the outer segments, being displaced to the pigment epithelium, where most of the remaining vitamin A is apparently esterified. Displacement of vitamin A in light adaptation has been demonstrated in the rat (32,67) and strongly suggested in the frog (76), but there is apparently no evidence on this topic in other species. To regenerate the bleached rhodopsin, the vitamin A ester must diffuse *back* to the outer segment, and be hydrolyzed by an esterase to liberate the vitamin A (79), which must then be oxidized (by alcohol dehydrogenase) back to its original retinene form. And at some point, of course, it must be converted to the 11-*cis* isomer.

Are any of these "additional" phenomena *obligatory* for regeneration of the visual pigment? Probably not, with one possible exception: the trip to the pigment epithelium may be necessary if the isomerase is confined to that cell type. An isomerase is present in the pigment epithelium of frogs and in the retina of cattle, but it is not necessarily restricted to these areas (74). The variable anatomical distribution of isomerase may account for the fact that bleached retinae of cattle can regenerate rhodopsin in the dark *in vitro* without the pigment epithelium, whereas frog (and rat) retinae cannot (23). So little information is available concerning the isomerase that the question must remain largely academic until further research is conducted. Whether isomerization occurs in the outer segments or in the pigment epithelium, or uses vitamin A ester, alcohol, or retinene as substrate is simply not yet known (77).

Amplification, Conduction, and Transmission of the Signal

When a vertebrate retina is stimulated by a flash of light, an almost instantaneous electrical response is generated by the photoreceptor cells. This response has been termed the early receptor potential (ERP) by Brown & Murakami (12), who first observed it. The latency of the first phase of the ERP (which is biphasic in form) does not exceed 25 microseconds (15), suggesting that it is generated after photo-isomerization of the retinene, but before it leaves the opsin, during the early molecular rearrangements of the protein (112). The latency of the second phase is so short that it could also arise as a result of events occurring in the outer segment, prior to conduction down the visual cell fiber (13,26). Since

* NADH (reduced nicotinamide adenine dinucleotide) is capable of acting as the hydrogen donor or acceptor in this reversible reaction. It seems more likely, however, that the reduction is performed by NADPH, a product of the HMP shunt. The resulting NADP might then activate the HMP shunt, possibly in the outer segment itself (57).

† Cell-free preparations from cattle retinae can perform this esterification (2,58,79). The outer segments themselves may (3) or may not (2) be active in this regard. However, the most potent source of the esterifying enzyme in cattle is the pigment epithelium (79). The function of esterification may simply be to prevent the vitamin A from escaping into the bloodstream, where it occurs only as the free alcohol.

the ERP is not generated as a change of membrane potential resulting from ion movement, it is the result of phenomena fundamentally different from those underlying the electrical responses of nerve cells which have been analyzed (15). The second phase of the ERP (but not the first) is abolished by cooling the eye to freezing temperatures, indicating that the two are generated by different mechanisms (112). Both are resistant to the loss of oxygen.

The amplitude of the ERP is linearly proportional to the number of visual pigment molecules excited by the stimulus (25). This implies that each molecule makes the same contribution to the final response (26).

After stimulation by light energy, the early receptor potential is followed by a potential of greater magnitude, with a latency of some 1.7 milliseconds, which is also generated by the photoreceptors. The latency of this late receptor potential (LRP, the a-wave of the electroretinogram) is probably due to conduction time through the receptor cell (12). The LRP, which is believed to be generated near the synaptic end of the visual cells (14), has the characteristics of a neuronal action potential involving membrane depolarization, accompanied by the flow of ions across the membrane (112). This is consistent with the structure of the rod fiber, which resembles a nerve axon (137,138).

The amplitude of the LRP is enormously larger than that of the ERP. The ERP is probably an unamplified response (26), and a significant process of amplification (long suspected on theoretical grounds) must intervene before the potential associated with conduction down the fiber is generated.

How is excitation transmitted from the altered pigment molecule (which may be embedded in a "free-floating" disk) to the cell membrane, down which transmission to the synaptic body presumably occurs? What is the nature of the amplification process? These critical questions remain unanswered. A variety of suggestions have been offered (100,146), but there is little evidence on which to evaluate any of them.

The ellipsoidal mitochondria, interposed between the sites of the unamplified ERP and the amplified LRP, and known to be a source of energy-yielding substances (ATP), may possibly be involved in the amplification process (22,137). There are some hints of increased enzymatic activity in this zone after light stimulation (42,50). Ubiquinone, which normally functions in mitochondrial electron transport, has been reported to be present in the outer segments (114, 115).* This and other evidence has suggested the possibility that electron transport might be involved in amplification of the signal. The schemes which have been offered involve variously electron transport from one side of the disk membranes to the other (78), from the outer segment to the mitochondria (114,115), or from the mitochondria to the outer segments (22).

Presumably, depolarization of the presynaptic membrane (associated with generation of the LRP) involves the release of a transmitter from the synaptic end of the cell, giving rise to an action potential in the bipolar cell. The nature of the

---

*Cytochrome oxidase, another component of the mitochrondrial electron transport chain, was reported to occur in photoreceptor outer segments (103), but subsequent work has not supported this claim (5,54,55,95).

hypothetical transmitter is not known. It is apparently not acetylcholine, judging by the absence of acetylcholinesterase in the outer plexiform layer (43,44,71). Nor does it appear that the photoreceptors are adrenergic (39), although the evidence is as yet sparse and inconclusive (43,130).

SUMMARY

Vertebrate photoreceptor cells respond to the stimulus of light and transmit this response to adjoining neurons. This functional specialization is achieved through a remarkable segmental organization. Within each segment resides a specialized assemblage of organelles which mediate particular metabolic pathways. This compartmentalization creates a requirement for intracellular supply lines, since regions of synthesis tend to be separated from sites of utilization.

The photoreceptor cells are differentiated during development of the retina and do not thereafter proliferate. The functional integrity of the cell during its prolonged life-span is maintained by the continual renewal of practically all of its constituents. Only the genetic material, DNA, appears to be stable.

DNA is restricted to the cell nucleus, where it controls the synthesis of RNA. RNA is continually displaced from the nucleus to the inner segment, where it regulates the formation of the specific group of photoreceptor proteins. Much of this newly synthesized protein moves through the ellipsoid zone and connecting structure to the base of the outer segment, where it is used in the formation of double-membrane disks. The lipid constituents of the outer segment disks are probably synthesized, displaced, and assembled into the membrane by a similar sequence of events. Continual formation of disks at the base of the outer segment displaces older disks in a scleral direction. A balanced removal of material occurs at the apical end of the cell. The pigment epithelium appears to be an active participant in the disposal phase of this outer segment renewal mechanism.

Glucose metabolism also shows signs of intracellular compartmentalization. Anaerobic glycolysis is largely restricted to the neuronal end of the cell, whereas the oxidative pathway is essentially confined to the ellipsoid zone. Neither of these pathways—the sources of energy-bearing ATP—appear to operate in the outer segment. The HMP shunt is active throughout the myoid and fiber portions of the cell, and possibly in the outer segments as well. Visual cells contain variable amounts of glycogen. Mucopolysaccharide is synthesized in the inner segments, then released into the extracellular region between the outer segments, where it undergoes rapid renewal.

The vertebrate photoreceptor cell not only renews gradually its pigment-containing outer segment, it also rapidly regenerates the pigment molecules *in situ* after they have been bleached by the absorption of light energy. Light absorption causes isomerization of 11-*cis* retinene to the all-*trans* form, which is subsequently liberated from the opsin. Regeneration involves re-isomerization of retinene to the 11-*cis* form, which is then captured by opsin. In some species, under conditions of severe bleaching, the liberated all-*trans* retinene may be reduced to vitamin A, displaced to the pigment epithelium, esterified, and temporarily stored, later to return to the outer segments during dark adaptation.

Stimulation of photoreceptor cells by light results in an almost instantaneous, biphasic, electrical response, apparently generated during the molecular rearrangements of the opsin molecule which result from the photo-isomerization of retinene. A subsequent electrical potential then arises near the synaptic end of the visual cells. This second, highly amplified response has the characteristics of a neuronal action potential and presumably involves depolarization of the plasma membrane.

Discussion

Question from the floor: Dr. Young, I noticed some scattered grain counts over the pigment epithelium in some of your pictures, and wondered if you consider that as background or if they have some significance.

Young: My findings are equivocal at the moment with regard to the question of whether the radioactive material which disappears from the apex of the photoreceptors is actually removed by the pigment epithelium. I have an intuitive feeling that this is what happens, bolstered by micrographs (Figure 89) of Bairati & Orzalesi (3), which seem to show such ingestion. My own material does not yet demonstrate it, however.

Hall: Dr. Young, has anyone looked at the pigment epithelium for the presence of proteolytic or hydrolytic enzymes which might take care of these fragments of outer segments which possibly find their way into the pigment epithelium? It seems that there should be a high concentration of such enzymes.

Young: Acid phosphatase has been demonstrated, as well as lysosome-like bodies, a lipase, and lamellated inclusions. These are generally associated with intracellular digestion. I do not believe that any specific proteolytic enzyme has been directly demonstrated.

REFERENCES

1. Albrecht, G., Terminal amino acids of rhodopsin. *J. Biol. Chem.*, 1957, **229**: 477–487.
2. Andrews, J. S., and Futterman, S., Metabolism of the retina. V. The role of microsomes in vitamin A esterification in the visual cycle. *J. Biol. Chem.*, 1964, **239**: 4073–4076.
3. Bairati, A., Jr., and Orzalesi, N., The ultrastructure of the pigment epithelium and of the photoreceptor-pigment epithelium junction in the human retina. *J. Ultrastruct. Res.*, 1963, **9**: 484–496.
4. Bartley, W., Lipids of intracellular organelles. In: *Metabolism and Physiological Significance of Lipids* (R. M. C. Dawson and D. N. Rhodes, Eds.). Wiley, New York, 1964: 369–381.
5. Berkow, J. W., and Patz, A., Histochemistry of the retina. I. Introduction and methods. *Arch. Ophthal.* (Chicago), 1961, **65**: 820–827.
6. Berman, E. R., The biosynthesis of mucopolysaccharides and glycoproteins in pigment epithelial cells of bovine retina. *Biochim. Biophys. Acta*, 1964, **83**: 371–373.
7. Bernstein, M. H., and Hillenberg, M. J., Fine structure of the choriocapillaris and retinal capillaries. *Invest. Ophthal.*, 1965, **4**: 1016–1025.

8. Bok, D., RNA and DNA metabolism in rat photoreceptors. *Anat. Rec.*, 1966, **154**: 320.

9. Bonavita, V., Guarneri, R., and Ponte, F., Neurochemical studies on the inherited retinal degeneration of the rat. II. NAD- and NADP-linked enzymes in the developing retina. *Vision Res.*, 1965, **5**: 113–121.

10. Bonting, S. L., Caravaggio, L. L., and Canady, M. R., Studies on sodium-potassium-activated adenosine triphosphatase. X. Occurrence in retinal rods and relation to rhodopsin. *Exp. Eye Res.*, 1964, **3**: 47–56.

11. Boynton, R. M., Discussion: Competing theories of receptor excitation. *Psychol. Bull.*, 1964, **61**: 262–267.

12. Brown, K. T., and Murakami, M., A new receptor potential of the monkey retina with no detectable latency. *Nature* (London), 1964, **201**: 626–628.

13. ———, Biphasic form of the early receptor potential of the monkey retina. *Nature* (London), 1964, **204**: 739–740.

14. Brown, K. T., and Watanabe, K., Rod receptor potential from the retina of the night monkey. *Nature* (London), 1962, **196**: 547–550.

15. Brown, K. T., Watanabe, K., and Murakami, M., The early and late receptor potentials of monkey cones and rods. *Sympos. Quant. Biol.*, 1965, **30**: 457–482.

16. Cohen, A. I., The ultrastructure of the rods of the mouse retina. *Am. J. Anat.*, 1960, **107**: 23–48.

17. ———, The fine structure of the extrafoveal receptors of the Rhesus monkey. *Exp. Eye Res.*, 1961, **1**: 128–136.

18. ———, Vertebrate retinal cells and their organization. *Biol. Rev.*, 1963, **38**: 427–459.

19. ———, Some observations on the fine structure of the retinal receptors of the American gray squirrel. *Invest. Ophthal.*, 1964, **3**: 198–216.

20. ———, New details of the ultrastructure of the outer segments and ciliary connectives of the rods of human and macaque retinas. *Anat. Rec.*, 1965, **152**: 63–80.

21. Cohen, L. H., and Noell, W. K., Glucose catabolism of rabbit retina before and after development of visual function. *J. Neurochem.*, 1960, **5**: 253–276.

22. ———, Relationships between visual function and metabolism. In: *Biochemistry of the Retina* (C. N. Graymore, Ed.). Academic Press, New York, 1965: 36–50.

23. Collins, F. D., Green, J. N., and Morton, R. A., Studies in rhodopsin. 7. Regeneration of rhodopsin by comminuted ox retina. *Biochem. J.*, 1954, **56**: 493–498.

24. Collins, F. D., Love, R. M., and Morton, R. A., Studies in rhodopsin. 5. Chemical analysis of retinal material. *Biochem. J.*, 1952, **51**: 669–673.

25. Cone, R. A., Early receptor potential of the vertebrate retina. *Nature* (London), 1964, **204**: 736–739.

26. ———, The early receptor potential of the vertebrate eye. *Sympos. Quant. Biol.*, 1965, **30**: 483–490.

27. Dartnall, H. J. A., and Tansley, K., Physiology of vision: retinal structure and visual pigments. *Ann. Rev. Physiol.*, 1963, **25**: 433–458.

28. Denton, E. J., The contributions of the oriented photosensitive and other molecules to the absorption of whole retina. *Proc. Roy. Soc. London B*, 1959, **150**: 78–94.

29. De Robertis, E., Electron microscope observations on the submicroscopic organization of the retinal rods. *J. Biophys. Biochem. Cytol.*, 1956, **2**: 319–330.

30. De Robertis, E., Some observations on the ultrastructure and morphogenesis of photoreceptors. *J. Gen. Physiol.*, 1960, **43**, Supp. 2: 1–14.

31. De Robertis, E., and Lasansky, A., Ultrastructure and chemical organization of photoreceptors. In: *The Structure of the Eye* (G. K. Smelser, Ed.). Academic Press, New York, 1961: 29–49.

32. Dowling, J. E., Chemistry of visual adaptation in the rat. *Nature* (London), 1960, **188**: 114–118.

33. Dowling, J. E., and Gibbons, I. R., The effect of vitamin A deficiency on the fine structure of the retina. In: *The Structure of the Eye* (G. K. Smelser, Ed.). Academic Press, New York, 1961: 85–99.

34. ———, The fine structure of the pigment epithelium in the albino rat. *J. Cell Biol.*, 1962, **14**: 459–474.

35. Dowling, J. E., and Sidman, R. L., Inherited retinal dystrophy in the rat. *Ibid.*: 73–110.

36. Dowling, J. E., and Wald, G., The biological function of vitamin A acid. *Proc. Nat. Acad. Sci. USA*, 1960, **46**: 587–608.

37. Droz, B., Dynamic condition of proteins in the visual cells of rats and mice as shown by radioautography with labeled amino acids. *Anat. Rec.*, 1963, **145**: 157–168.

38. Droz, B., Rambourg, A., and Olivier, L., Action de la lumière sur l'incorporation de méthionine ^{35}S au niveau de la rétine de la souris. *C. R. Soc. Biol.* (Paris), 1963, **157**: 2136–2140.

39. Ehinger, B., Adrenergic nerves to the eye and to related structures in man and in the cynomolgus monkey (*Macaca irus*). *Invest. Ophthal.*, 1966, **5**: 45–52.

40. Eichner, D., Über Histologie und Topochemie der Sehschicht in der Netzhaut des Menschen. *Zschr. mikr.-anat. Forsch.*, 1957, **63**, 82–93.

41. Eichner, D., and Themann, H., Zur Frage des Netzhautglykogens beim Meerschweinchen. *Zschr. Zellforsch.*, 1962, **56**: 231–246.

42. Enoch, J. M., The use of tetrazolium to distinguish between retinal receptors exposed and not exposed to light. *Invest. Ophthal.*, 1963, **2**: 16–23.

43. Eränko, O., Niemi, M., and Merenmies, E., Histochemical observations on esterases and oxidative enzymes of the retina. In: *The Structure of the Eye* (G. K. Smelser, Ed.). Academic Press, New York, 1961: 159–171.

44. Esilä, R., Histochemical and electrophoretic properties of cholinesterases and non-specific esterases in the retina of some mammals, including man. *Acta Ophthal.*, (Kobenhavn) 1963, Supp. **77**.

45. Feeney, L., Grieshaber, J., and Alvarado, J., New observations on human retinal pigment epithelium. *Invest. Ophthal.*, 1966, **5**: 111.

46. Fernández-Morán, H., Cell membrane ultrastructure: low-temperature electron microscopy and x-ray diffraction studies of lipoprotein components in lamellar systems. *Res. Publ. Ass. Nerv. Ment Dis.*, 1962, **15**: 235–267.

47. Fine, B. S., Limiting membranes of the sensory retina and pigment epithelium. *Arch. Ophthal.* (Chicago), 1961, **66**: 847–860.

48. Fine, B. S., and Zimmerman, L. E., Müller's cells and the "middle limiting membrane" of the human retina; an electron microscopic study. *Invest. Ophthal.*, 1962, **1**: 304–326.

49. ———, Observations on the rod and cone layer of the human retina; a light and electron microscopic study. *Invest. Ophthal.*, 1963, **2**: 446–459.

50. Fowlks, W. L., and Peterson, D. E., Substrate inhibition of tetrazolium salt reduction in dark adapted retinae. *Proc. Soc. Exp. Biol. Med.*, 1965, **118**: 491–494.
51. Francis, C. M., Lipids in the retina. *J. Comp. Neurol.*, 1955, **103**: 355–383.
52. Frank, R. N., and Goldsmith, T. H., Adenosine triphosphatase activity in the rod outer segments of the pig's retina. *Arch. Biochem. Biophys.*, 1965, **110**: 517–525.
53. Freeman, M. I., and Wortman, B., Mucopolysaccharides in beef retina and small cerebral vessels. *Invest. Ophthal.*, 1966, **5**: 88–92.
54. Fujishita, S., The organo-iron compound in the digitonin extract of the rod outersegment. *Jap. J. Physiol.*, 1962, **12**: 460–466.
55. ———, Non-respiratory nature of oxygen uptake by rod outer segments. *Jap. J. Physiol.*, 1964, **14**: 551–559.
56. Fukami, I., Vallee, B. L., and Wald, G., Does rhodopsin contain a trace metal? *Nature* (London), 1959, **183**: 28–30.
57. Futterman, S., Metabolism of the retina. III. The role of reduced triphosphopyridine nucleotide in the visual cycle. *J. Biol. Chem.*, 1963, **238**: 1145–1150.
58. ———, Stoichiometry of retinal vitamin A metabolism during light-adaptation. In: *Biochemistry of the Retina* (C. N. Graymore, Ed.). Academic Press, New York, 1965: 16–21.
59. Futterman, S., and Andrews, J. S., Metabolism of the retina. IV. The composition of vitamin A ester synthesized by the retina. *J. Biol. Chem.*, 1964, **239**: 81–84.
60. Futterman, S., and Kinoshita, J. H., Metabolism of retina. I. Respiration of cattle retina. *J. Biol. Chem.*, 1959, **234**: 723–726.
61. Futterman, S., and Saslaw, L. D., The estimation of vitamin A aldehyde with thiobarbituric acid. *J. Biol. Chem.*, 1961, **236**: 1652–1657.
62. Geeraets, W. J., Williams, R. C., Chan, G., Ham, W. T., Jr., Guerry, D., and Schmidt, F. H., The relative absorption of thermal energy in retina and choroid. *Invest. Ophthal.*, 1962, **1**: 340–347.
63. Graymore, C., Metabolism of the developing retina. III. Respiration in the developing normal rat retina and the effect of an inherited degeneration of the retinal neuro-epithelium. *Brit. J. Ophthal.*, 1960, **44**: 363–369.
64. Graymore, C., and Tansley, K., Iodoacetate poisoning of the rat retina. II. Glycolysis in the poisoned retina. *Brit. J. Ophthal.*, 1959, **43**: 486–493.
65. Graymore, C., and Towlson, M., Levels of soluble NAD-linked α-glycerophosphate dehydrogenase and lactic acid dehydrogenase in rat retina. *Exp. Eye Res.*, 1963, **2**: 48–52.
66. ———, The metabolism of the retina of the normal and alloxan diabetic rat. *Vision Res.*, 1965, **5**: 379–389.
67. Greenberg, R., and Popper, H., Demonstration of vitamin A in the retina by fluorescence microscopy. *Am. J. Physiol.*, 1941, **134**: 114–118.
68. Grignolo, A., Orzalesi, N., and Calabria, G. A., Studies on the fine structure and the rhodopsin cycle of the rabbit retina in experimental degeneration induced by sodium iodate. *Exp. Eye Res.*, 1966, **5**: 86–97.
69. Hall, M. O., Ocumpaugh, D. E., and Young, R. W., The utilization of ^{35}S-sulfate in the synthesis of mucopolysaccharides by the retina. *Invest. Ophthal.*, 1965, **4**: 322–329.

70. Hanawa, I., Kimura, E., and Hosoya, Y., The respiration of the isolated outer-segments of rods. *Jap. J. Physiol.*, 1955, **5**: 322–333.
71. Hebb, C. O., Silver, A., Swan, A. A. B., and Walsh, E. G., A histochemical study of cholinesterases of rabbit retina and optic nerve. *Quart. J. Exp. Physiol.*, 1953, **38**: 185–191.
72. Hubbard, R., The respiration of the isolated rod outer limb of the frog retina. *J. Gen. Physiol.*, 1954, **37**: 373–379.
73. ———, The molecular weight of rhodopsin and the nature of the rhodopsin-digitonin complex. *Ibid.*: 381–399.
74. ———, Retinene isomerase. *J. Gen. Physiol.*, 1956, **39**: 935–962.
75. Hubbard, R., Bownds, D., and Yoshizawa, T., The chemistry of visual photo-reception. *Sympos. Quant. Biol.*, 1965, **30**: 301–315.
76. Hubbard, R., and Colman, A. D., Vitamin-A content of the frog eye during light and dark adaptation. *Science*, 1959, **130**: 977–978.
77. Hubbard, R., and Dowling, J. E., Formation and utilization of 11-*cis* vitamin A by the eye tissues during light and dark adaptation. *Nature* (London), 1962 **193**: 341–343.
78. Jahn, T. L., A possible mechanism for the amplifier effect in the retina. *Vision Res.*, 1963, **3**: 25–28.
79. Krinsky, N. I., The enzymatic esterification of vitamin A. *J. Biol. Chem.*, 1958, **232**: 881–894.
80. ———, The lipoprotein nature of rhodopsin. *Arch. Ophthal.* (Chicago), 1958, **60**: 688–694.
81. Kropf, A., and Hubbard, R., The mechanism of bleaching rhodopsin. *Ann. N. Y. Acad. Sci.*, 1958, **74**: 266–280.
82. Kuwabara, T., and Cogan, D. G., Retinal glycogen. *Arch. Ophthal.* (Chicago), 1961, **66**: 680 688.
83. Lasansky, A., Morphological bases for a nursing role of glia in the toad retina. Electron microscope observations. *J. Biophys. Biochem. Cytol.*, 1961, **11**: 237–243.
84. ———, Functional implications of structural findings in retinal glial cells. *Progr. Brain Res.*, 1965, **15**: 48–72.
85. Lillie, R. D., Histochemical studies on the retina. *Anat. Rec.*, 1952, **112**: 477–495.
86. Lowry, O. H., Roberts, N. R., and Lewis, C., The quantitative histochemistry of the retina. *J. Biol. Chem.*, 1956, **220**: 879–892.
87. Lowry, O. H., Roberts, N. R., Schultz, D. W., Clow, J. E., and Clark, J. R., Quantitative histochemistry of the retina. II. Enzymes of glucose metabolism. *J. Biol. Chem.*, 1961, **236**: 2813–2820.
88. MacNichol, E. F., Jr., Three-pigment color vision. *Sci. Amer.*, 1964, **211**: 48–56.
89. Majima, K., Studien über die Struktur der Sehzellen und der Pigmentepithel-zellen der Froschnetzhaut. *Graefe Arch. klin. exp. Ophthal.*, 1924, **115**: 286–304.
90. Maraini, G., and Franguelli, R., Radioautographic investigations on nucleic acids and protein metabolism of the retina in vitro. *Ophthalmologica*, 1962, **144**: 141–150.
91. Maraini, G., Franguelli, R., Pasino, L., and Diotti, G., Influenze della prolungata mancanza di stimolazione luminosa sul metabolismo proteico della retina e dei neuroni del corpo genicocolato laterale. *Boll. Oculist.*, 1963, **42**: 175–181.

92. Maraini, G., Franguelli, R., and Peralta, S., Studies on the metabolism of the retina and lateral geniculate nucleus. *Invest. Ophthal.*, 1963, **2**: 567–570.

93. Matschinsky, F. M., Passonneau, J. V., and Lowry, O. H., Quantitative histochemistry of metabolites of glycolysis in retina. *J. Histochem. Cytochem.*, 1965, **13**: 707.

94. Matthews, R. G., Hubbard, R., Brown, P. K., and Wald, G., Tautomeric forms of metarhodopsin. *J. Gen. Physiol.*, 1963, **47**: 215–240.

95. McConnell, D. G., The isolation of retinal outer segment fragments. *J. Cell Biol.*, 1965, **27**: 459–473.

96. Missotten, L., L'ultrastructure des cones de la rétine humaine. *Bull. Sọc. Belg. Ophtal.*, 1953, **132**: 472–502.

97. ———, L'ultrastructure des tissus oculaires. *Bull. Soc. Belg. Ophtal.*, 1964, **136**: 1–204.

98. ———, *The Ultrastructure of the Human Retina*. Arscia, Brussels, 1965.

99. Missotten, L., Appelmans, M., and Michiels, J., L'ultra-structure des synapses des cellules visuelles de la rétine humaine. *Bull. Soc. Franc. Ophtal.*, 1963, **76**: 59–82.

100. Moody, M. F., Photoreceptor organelles in animals. *Biol. Rev.*, 1964, **39**: 43–86.

101. Moody, M. F., and Robertson, J. D., The fine structure of some retinal photoreceptors. *J. Biophys. Biochem. Cytol.*, 1960, **7**: 87–92.

102. Niemi, M., and Merenmies, E., Cytochemical localization of the oxidative enzyme systems in the retina. I. Diaphorases and dehydrogenases. *J. Neurochem.*, 1961, **61**: 200–205.

103. ———, Cytochemical localization of the oxidative enzyme systems in the retina. II. Cytochrome oxidase. *Ibid.*: 206–209.

104. Nilsson, S. E. G., An electron microscopic classification of the retinal receptors of the leopard frog (*Rana pipiens*). *J. Ultrastruct. Res.*, 1964, **10**: 390–416.

105. ———, Interreceptor contacts in the retina of the frog (*Rana pipiens*). *J. Ultrastruct. Res.*, 1964, **11**: 147–165.

106. ———, Receptor cell outer segment development and ultrastructure of the disk membranes in the retina of the tadpole (*Rana pipiens*). *Ibid.*: 581–620.

107. ———, The ultrastructure of the receptor outer segments in the retina of the leopard frog (*Rana pipiens*). *J. Ultrastruct. Res.*, 1965, **12**: 207–231.

108. Noell, W. K., Cellular physiology of the retina. *J. Opt. Soc. Amer.*, 1963, **53**: 36–48.

109. ———, Aspects of experimental and hereditary retinal degeneration. In: *Biochemistry of the Retina* (C. N. Graymore, Ed.). Academic Press, New York, 1965: 51–72.

110. Nover, A., and Schultze, B., Autoradiographische Untersuchung über den Eiweissstoffwechsel in den Geweben und Zellen des Auges. (Untersucht mit S^{35}-Thio-Aminosäuren, C^{14}-Aminosäuren, H^3-Leucin an Maus, Ratte und Kaninchen). *Graefe Arch. klin. exp. Ophthal.*, 1960, **161**: 554–578.

111. Ocumpaugh, D. E., and Young, R. W., Distribution and synthesis of sulfated mucopolysaccharides in the retina of the rat. *Invest. Ophthal.*, 1966, **5**: 196–203.

112. Pak, W. L., Some properties of the early electrical response in the vertebrate retina. *Sympos. Quant. Biol.*, 1965, **30**: 493–499.

113. Pearse, A. G. E., Localization of oxidative enzymes in rat and chick retina in various physiological conditions. In: *The Structure of the Eye* (G. K. Smelser, Ed.). Academic Press, New York, 1961: 53–72.

114. PEARSE, A. G. E., Cytochemical localization of ubiquinones in the retina. *Nature* (London), 1965, **205**: 708–709.

115. ———, The localization of ubiquinones in the cornea and retina. In: *Biochemistry of the Retina* (C. N. Graymore, Ed.). Academic Press, New York, 1965: 110–114.

116. PEDLER, C., The fine structure of the radial fibres in the reptile retina. *Exp. Eye Res.*, 1963, **2**: 296–303.

117. PIRENNE, M. H., Light quanta and vision. *Endeavour*, 1961, **20**: 197–209.

118. PORTER, K. R., and YAMADA, E., Studies on the endoplasmic reticulum. V. Its form and differentiation in pigment epithelial cells of the frog retina. *J. Biophys. Biochem. Cytol.*, 1960, **8**: 181–205.

119. RABINOVITCH, M., MOTA, I., and YONEDA, S., Note on the histochemical localization of glycogen and pentosepolynucleotides in the visual cells of the chick (*Gallus gallus*). *Quart. J. Micr. Sci.*, 1954, **95**: 5–9.

120. RASCH, E., SWIFT, H., RIESEN, A. H., and CHOW, K. L., Altered structure and composition of retinal cells in dark-reared mammals. *Exp. Cell Res.*, 1961, **25**: 348–363.

121. RAVIOLA, E., and RAVIOLA, G., Studio istochimico della retina di coniglio adulto e nel corso dello sviluppo postnatale e nell'adulto. *Ann. Histochim.*, 1963, **8**: 263–267.

122. READING. H. W., Activity of the hexose monophosphate shunt in the normal and dystrophic retina. *Nature* (London), 1964, **203**: 491–492.

123. ROBERTSON, J. D., A possible ultrastructural correlate of function in the frog retinal rod. *Proc. Nat. Acad. Sci. USA*, 1965, **53**: 860–866.

124. RODRIGUEZ-PERALTA, L., Experiments on the site of the blood-ocular barrier. *Anat. Rec.*, 1962, **142**: 273.

125. SCHIMKE, R. T., Histochemical determination of glyceraldehyde phosphate and glycerophosphate dehydrogenases in brain. *Fed. Proc.*, 1957, **16**: 334.

126. SCHMIDT, W. J., Polarisationsoptische Analyse der Verknüpfung von Protein- und Lipoidmolekeln, erläutert am Aussenglied der Sehzellen der Wirbeltiere. *Pubbl. Staz. Zool. Napoli*, 1951, Supp. **23**: 158–183.

127. SCHULTZE, B., APPONI, G., and NOVER, A., Autoradiographische Untersuchung mit H^3-Thymidin über die Desoxyribonucleinsäure-Neubildung in den Geweben des Rattenauges. *Graefe Arch. Ophthal.*, 1961, **163**: 130–138.

128. SEKOGUTI, Y., On the ATPase activities in the retina and the rod outer segments. *J. Cell. Comp. Physiol.*, 1960, **56**: 129–136.

129. SHANTHAVEERAPPA, T. R., and BOURNE, G. H., Histochemical studies on the distribution of acid phosphatase in the eye. *Acta Histochem.* (Jena), 1964, **18**: 317–327.

130. ———, Monoamine oxidase distribution in the rabbit eye. *J. Histochem. Cytochem.* 1964, **12**: 281–287.

131. ———, Histochemical demonstration of thiamine phrophosphatase and acid phosphatase in the Golgi region of the cells of the eye. *J. Anat.*, 1965, **99**: 103–117.

132. SHIMIZU, N., and MAEDA, S., Histochemical studies on glycogen of the retina. *Anat. Rec.*, 1953, **116**: 427–438.

133. SIDMAN, R. L., The structure and concentration of solids in photoreceptor cells studied by refractometry and interference microscopy. *J. Biophys. Biochem. Cytol.*, 1957, **3**: 15–30.

134. Sidman, R. L., Histogenesis of mouse retina studied with thymidine-H^3. In: *The Structure of the Eye* (G. K. Smelser, Ed.). Academic Press, New York, 1961: 487–506.

135. Sidman, R. L., and Wislocki, G. B., Histochemical observations on rods and cones in retinas of vertebrates. *J. Histochem. Cytochem.*, 1954, **2**: 413–433.

136. Sjöstrand, F. S., Ultrastructure of retinal rod synapses of the guinea pig eye as revealed by three-dimensional reconstructions from serial sections. *J. Ultrastruct. Res.*, 1958, **2**: 122–170.

137. ———, The ultrastructure of the retinal receptors of the vertebrate eye. *Ergebn. Biol.*, 1959, **21**: 128–160.

138. ———, Electron microscopy of the retina. In: *The Structure of the Eye* (G. K. Smelser, Ed.). Academic Press, New York, 1961: 1–28.

139. ———, The synaptology of the retina. In: *Colour Vision; Physiology and Experimental Psychology* (A. V. S. de Reuck and J. Knight, Eds.). Churchill, London, 1965: 110–151.

140. Sjöstrand, F. S., and Nilsson, S. E., The structure of the rabbit retina as revealed by electron microscopy. In: *The Rabbit in Eye Research* (J. H. Prince, Ed.). Thomas, Springfield, 1964: 449–513.

141. Smelser, G. K., and Ozanics, V., Distribution of radioactive sulfate in the developing eye. *Am. J. Ophthal.*, 1957, **44**(4/II): 102–109.

142. Tokuyasu, K., and Yamada, E., The fine structure of the retina studied with the electron microscope. IV. Morphogenesis of outer segments of retinal rods. *J. Biophys. Biochem. Cytol.*, 1959, **6**: 225–230.

143. Villegas, G. M., Ultrastructure of the human retina. *J. Anat.*, 1964, **98**: 501–513.

144. Wald, G., The visual function of the vitamins A. *Vitamins Hormones* (NY), 1960, **18**: 417–430.

145. Wald, G., and Brown, P. K., Human color vision and color blindness. *Sympos. Quant. Biol.*, 1965, **30**: 345–359.

146. Wald, G., Brown, P. K., and Gibbons, I. R., The problem of visual excitation. *J. Opt. Soc. Amer.*, 1963, **53**: 20–35.

147. Wald, G., and Hubbard, R., The reduction of retinene$_1$ to vitamin A_1 *in vitro*. *J. Gen. Physiol.*, 1949, **32**: 367–389.

148. Walters, P. T., Anaerobic glycolysis in rats affected with retinitis pigmentosa; its significance in relation to various forms of primary degeneration of the retina. *Brit. J. Ophthal.*, 1959, **43**: 686–696.

149. Wislocki, G. B., and Ladman, A. J., The demonstration of a blood-ocular barrier in the albino rat by means of the intravitam deposition of silver. *J. Biophys. Biochem. Cytol.*, 1955, **1**: 501–510.

150. Wislocki, G. B., and Sidman, R. L., The chemical morphology of the retina. *J. Comp. Neurol.*, 1954, **101**: 53–91.

151. Wortman, B., Acid mucopolysaccharides in beef retina. I. Isolation and fractionation. *Am. J. Ophthal.*, 1959, **47**(2): 203–207.

152. Yamada, E., Observations on the fine structure of the photoreceptive elements in the vertebrate eye. *J. Electron Micr.* (Tokyo), 1960, **9**: 1–14.

153. Yoshida, M., Microspectrophotometric studies on desoxyribonucleic acid of an individual nucleus in the ox retina. *Jap. J. Physiol.*, 1958, **8**: 57–66.

154. Young, R. W., The renewal of photoreceptor cell outer segments. *J. Cell Biol.*, 1967, **33**: 61–72.

155. Zimmerman, L. E., Acid mucopolysaccharides in ocular histology and pathology. *Proc. Inst. Med. Chicago*, 1961, **23**: 267–277.

MUCOPOLYSACCHARIDES OF THE RETINA

MICHAEL O. HALL and **JORAM HELLER** *
UCLA School of Medicine
Los Angeles, California

This paper will be concerned with one structural and functional component of the retina †—the interstitial material in which the visual cells are embedded. Histological and biochemical studies have shown that this material is comprised mainly of a complex mixture of mucopolysaccharides (MPS) and proteins. Since the MPS component has been most extensively studied in our own and other laboratories, we will review in some detail present knowledge concerning the chemistry and biosynthesis of retinal MPS, with emphasis on those of the photo-receptor layer.

TABLE 2

COMPONENTS OF CONNECTIVE TISSUE MUCOPOLYSACCHARIDES (MPS)

MPS	Amino sugar	Uronic acid	Sulfate
Hyaluronic acid	Glucosamine	Glucuronic acid	None
Chondroitin	Galactosamine	Glucuronic acid	None
Chondroitin sulfate A	Galactosamine	Glucuronic acid	1
Chondroitin sulfate B	Galactosamine	Iduronic acid	1
Chondroitin sulfate C	Galactosamine	Glucuronic acid	1
Keratosulfate	Glucosamine	Galactose (neutral sugar)	1

MPS are high-molecular-weight heteropolysaccharides isolated from connective tissue and other intercellular material. Their present classification is based on the nature of their sugar monomers and the bond between them; Table 2 shows the monomer units of some common MPS. While most of the MPS are straight-chain

* The authors wish to express their gratitude for permission to include original figures and tables in this review to Dr. E. R. Berman (Hadassah University Hospital, Jerusalem, Israel), Dr. B. S. Fine (Armed Forces Institute of Pathology, Washington, D.C.), and Dr. R. W. Young (UCLA School of Medicine, Los Angeles, California). The technical assistance of Mrs. Anita Beck and Mrs. Joyce Harbison is gratefully acknowledged. One of us (M.O.H.) is supported by a U.S. Public Health Service Grant, NB-5214, and by a Fight for Sight Grant-in-Aid of the National Council to Combat Blindness, Inc., New York, N.Y.

† An overall picture of the morphological and biochemical structure of the retina was presented by Dr. Young (pp. 177–210).

Figure 92. Suggested linkage between mucopolysaccharides and proteins.

polymers, composed of alternating hexosamine and uronic acid monomers, an exception to this is keratosulfate, in which uronic acid is replaced by galactose. An important aspect of the MPS structure is that ester sulfate and/or carboxyl groups are interspaced at regular intervals on the polysaccharide backbone, giving the MPS a strong polyanionic character. Present evidence suggests that most or all MPS are covalently bound to proteins in their native state (17). As shown in Figure 92, the bridge between the protein and the MPS is a glycosydic bond between a galactosyl-xylosyl sequence at the end of the MPS polymer and a serine or threonine hydroxyl group on the protein (8,13,14,15). Other covalent linkages between the MPS and protein have been suggested (21).

Although the chemical structure of most MPS is now fairly well established, the biosynthetic pathways have only recently been partially clarified. The known facts about the biosynthesis of connective tissue MPS are summarized below and in Figure 93.

a. Glucose can serve as the source of the monomer units for all known MPS.

b. The sugar units are incorporated into the polysaccharide chain via their activated forms, namely UDP-GNAc, UDP-Gal NAc and UDPGA* (4,24). The

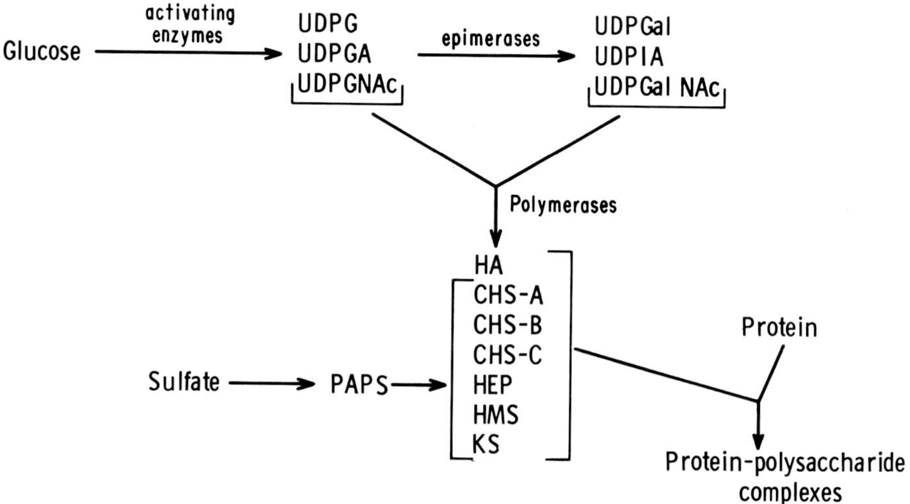

Figure 93. Pathways for the formation of mucopolysaccharides. *CHS:* Chondroitin sulfate; *Gal:* galactose; *Gal NAc:* N-acetylgalactosamine; *G:* glucose; *GNAc:* N-acetylglucosamine; *GA:* glucuronic acid; *HA:* hyaluronic acid; *HEP:* heparin; *HMS:* heparin monosulfate; *IA:* iduronic acid; *KS:* keratosulfate; *PAPS:* 3′-phosphoadenosine 5′-phosphosulfate *UDP:* uridine diphosphate.

* See Figure 93 for abbreviations.

activating enzymes and the epimerases which interconvert the activated sugars have been demonstrated in tissue preparations (20).

c. Once the polysaccharide backbone is synthesized, sulfate is attached to it. Prior to this step, the sulfate has to be activated in the form of PAPS.* Both the activating and transferring enzymes have been demonstrated in tissue preparations (20).

d. The biosynthetic route for the formation of the MPS-protein complex remains unclear. Preliminary evidence (27) suggests a mechanism which involves addition of carbohydrate units to preformed protein to yield a protein-polysaccharide complex.

The presence or absence of a matrix surrounding the visual cells, and the source of the material constituting this matrix, were in dispute for almost a hundred years. As Sidman put it in 1958 (22), "[In 1855] Henle and others suggested that the rods were embedded in a homogeneous matrix. However, little evidence of such a matrix was obtained . . . and Henle's idea lost favor. In 1909, Kolmer presented

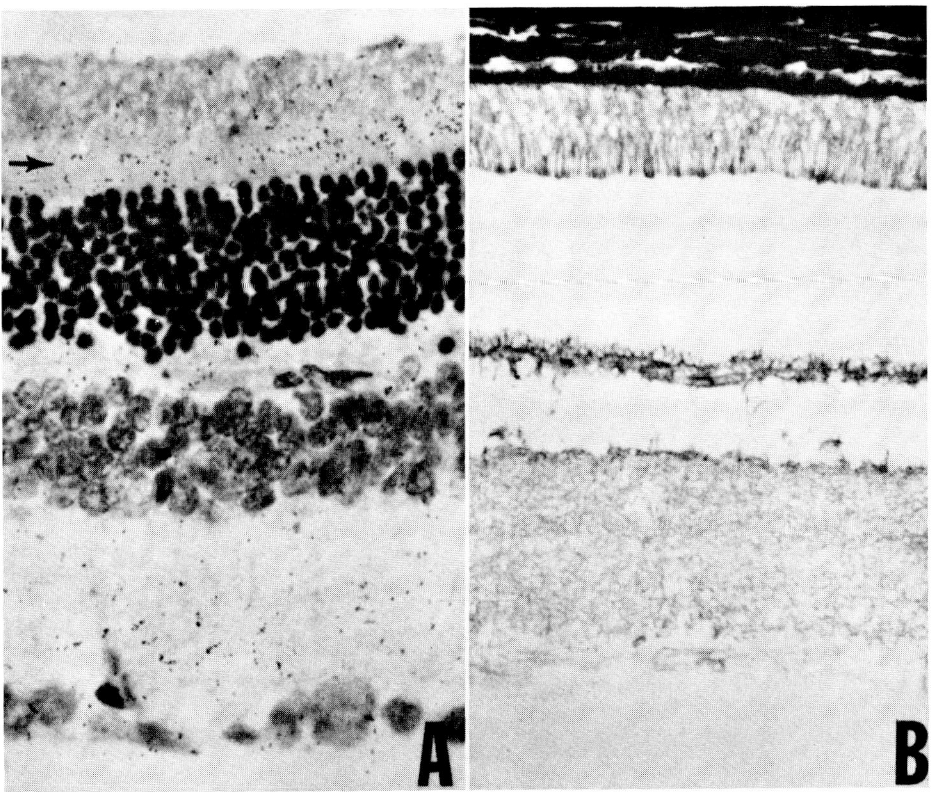

Figure 94. *A:* Retina of an 8-week-old rat killed 24 hours after injection of S^{35}-sulfate; the greatest autoradiographic reaction occurs over the rod inner segments (arrow); there is also a moderate labeling of the inner and outer plexiform layers; (autoradiogram, PAS and hematoxylin; ×370). *B:* A comparable section stained with the colloidal iron technique for mucopolysaccharides; the most intense staining reaction occurs in the photoreceptor layer below the pigmented choroid; there is also a strong reaction over the inner and outer plexiform layers. (From Ocumpaugh & Young, 19.)

some evidence for the secretory function of the pigment epithelium, but he withdrew the claim at a later date. [In 1952] Lillie . . . described metachromasia of rod outer segments. Subsequently the metachromasia was localized to a fibrillar and amorphous material between the outer segments. . . . Later the homogeneous acid mucopolysaccharide component was demonstrated with alcian blue in the human retina. . . . So it is that we have now come full circle and again believe that an interstitial matrix material does exist. Furthermore, the pigment epithelial cells with their granules and fibrils have the appearance of secretory cells, supporting Kolmer's opinion of 1909."

The existence of an MPS matrix in the photoreceptor region of the retina is now an established fact, based on histochemical staining procedures of various types applied in many species of animals (6,11,12,22,23,28,31,32,33). Figure 94B shows a section of the rat retina stained for MPS (19).

Our laboratory studies on the retinal MPS were aimed at elucidating the following problems: isolation and characterization, site and mechanism of biosynthesis, physiological function. Some progress has been made in the past two or three years in a number of laboratories towards answering these questions.

Isolation and Chemical Properties of Retinal Mucopolysaccharides

For quantitative reasons, our initial studies on the isolation of MPS were carried out on cattle retinae, using the classical methods of digestion with proteolytic enzymes (18). The histological studies cited above had shown that the visual cell layer and the pigment epithelium were particularly rich in acid MPS. In order to detect differences between these MPS and those in the inner retinal layers, the retina was carefully removed from the optic cup and laid flat on a glass plate with the visual cell layer facing up. The visual cells were gently brushed off and the pigment epithelial cells remaining in the optic cup were collected in the same manner. These two fractions were then combined and called FS; the remainder of the retina was called FR. After digestion of these fractions with proteolytic enzymes, the MPS were precipitated and purified. A portion of each sample was hydrolyzed and separated by paper chromatography. Table 3 shows the analytical composition of these two fractions and the compounds which could be identified by paper chromatography (9). The visual cell-pigment epithelial MPS contain considerably less neutral sugar and show a higher degree of sulfation than do those of the inner retinal layers. This simple experiment thus indicates a difference between the MPS of the inner layers of the retina and those of the visual cell-pigment epithelial layer.

Berman (3) recently isolated MPS from cattle retinae by saline extraction, without using proteolytic enzymes or base. The MPS obtained after purification by precipitation and column chromatography contained only 8.3 per cent protein. This method is significant not only for its simplicity, but for the fact that it allows the MPS to be extracted without breaking the cells by homogenization, which indicates that most of the MPS extracted was extracellular, a finding that correlates well with histological evidence.

A comparison of the results obtained by this method with those we obtained

TABLE 3

Analysis of Mucopolysaccharides
Isolated from Different Fractions of the Retina

Component	FR		FS	
	μmoles *	Ratio to hexosamine (μmoles)	μmoles *	Ratio to hexosamine (μmoles)
Uronic acid	3.8	0.6	4.7	0.8
Neutral sugar	15.0	2.5	7.1	1.0
Hexosamine	6.1	1.0	6.8	1.0
Ester sulfate	2.9	0.5	4.5	0.7
Sugars identified by chromatography	Glucose Galactose Mannose Fucose Glucosamine Galactosamine Glucuronic acid		Glucose Galactose Glucosamine Galactosamine Glucuronic acid	

* Isolated from 25 cattle eyes.

after proteolytic digestion is interesting. As can be seen from Table 4, Berman's method, in addition to being simple, yields a product in which the ratio of uronic acid to hexosamine is almost unity—as would be expected for a pure MPS or even a mixture of MPS.

Wortman (7,29) isolated MPS from beef retinae after proteolytic digestion and attempted to separate the purified MPS by passage through columns of ECTEOLA-cellulose. By eluting at different pH's it was possible to separate two main uronic acid-containing fractions; analysis of these fractions showed that they were extremely heterogeneous and contained neutral, nonsulfated, and sulfated acid MPS.

Labeled mucopolysaccharides have also been isolated from rat retinae after the animals were injected with S^{35}-sulfate (9). Although the MPS represented less

TABLE 4

Analysis of Retinal Mucopolysaccharides
Isolated by Two Different Methods

Component	Ratio to Hexosamine (μmoles)			
	Crude *	Pure *	FR	FS
Uronic acid	0.7–0.8	1.1–1.3	0.6	0.8
Neutral sugar	1.6	0.9	2.5	1.0
Hexosamine	1.0	1.0	1.0	1.0
Ester sulfate	—	0.7	0.5	0.7

* Calculated from Berman (3).

than 5 per cent of the total retinal dry weight, this fraction contained 70 per cent of the total retinal radioactivity and essentially all of the bound S^{35}. Chromatography of this MPS fraction on DEAE-Sephadex resulted in a separation into two radioactive fractions, both of which were extremely heterogeneous with regard to their MPS components.

The analytical and chromatographic data from the studies cited above indicate that the isolated retinal MPS contain both sulfated and nonsulfated components. Some of the findings are consistent with the hypothesis that the major component is either chondroitin or an undersulfated chondroitin sulfate, whereas the minor component may be a keratosulfate-like substance. However, certain findings are difficult to reconcile with the known chemical composition of MPS isolated from other sources. Of particular interest is the large amount of neutral sugar which appears to be intimately associated with the uronic acid-containing MPS. Similar results have been found in brain tissue by Stary and coworkers (26). It is unlikely that glycogen is the source of the neutral sugar, since the methods of precipitation used in the isolation procedure (e.g., use of quaternary ammonium bases) would result in the removal of this compound. The presence of keratosulfate has been eliminated in both retina and pigment epithelium (2,3,30). Thus, the retinal MPS appear to be more complex chemically and structurally than was previously supposed, and may contain unique components.

Susceptibility of Retinal Mucopolysaccharides to Hyaluronidase

It was initially believed that retinal MPS were nonsulfated and resistant to hyaluronidase (6,25,31). In the rat and the cow, however, at least part of the MPS in the retina are sulfated and contain fractions susceptible to digestion with bovine testicular hyaluronidase (9,19). In studies in which the retinal MPS of the rat were labeled with S^{35}-sulfate, there was some loss of MPS-bound radioactivity from all layers of the retina after extraction of tissue sections with hyaluronidase: about 70 per cent of the labeling was removed from the photoreceptor region,

TABLE 5

Loss of Labeling in Different Layers of the Retina and Corneal Stroma after Hyaluronidase Extraction *

Ocular Tissue	Percentage Loss Compared to Controls
Retina	
Outer segment	70
Inner segment	67
Outer nuclear	23
Outer plexiform	48
Inner nuclear	31
Inner plexiform	34
Ganglion cells	43
Optic nerve	47
Corneal stroma	27

* From Ocumpaugh & Young (19).

and between 20 to 50 per cent from the other retinal layers (Table 5). In the same experiment, only about 27 per cent of the radioactivity was removed from the corneal stroma, which agrees with other studies showing lability of about one-third of the corneal MPS to hyaluronidase (1). Our own and other studies have shown that about 20 per cent of the total retinal MPS from cattle is susceptible to digestion with testicular hyaluronidase (3,7,29). As shown in Table 5, however, different layers of the retina appear to contain MPS which vary in their hyaluronidase lability, those in the photoreceptor region being most susceptible. Thus, studies on the digestion of total retinal MPS produced a figure which was an average of the different species of MPS and lower than that for, say, the photoreceptor layer. It is, however, very probable that a species difference exists, with some animals having a higher percentage of the hyaluronidase-resistant classes of MPS; this would account for the variation found by different workers in different animals, ranging from no digestion of human retinal MPS by hyaluronidase (25,31) to 70 per cent digestion in the photoreceptor layer of the rat retina (19).

Site of Synthesis of Retinal Mucopolysaccharides

Studies *in vivo* (9,19) have shown that, in the rat, S^{35}-sulfate is rapidly incorporated into the retinal MPS, particularly into the photoreceptor zone (Figure 94A). Histological evidence showing that S^{35}-sulfate is first incorporated into the inner segment of the visual cell and subsequently displaced into the extracellular spaces between the outer segments has been briefly reviewed by Dr. Young.* It therefore seems that the inner segment of the visual cell is the most probable site of synthesis of the MPS surrounding the outer segments. Evidence to support this hypothesis is available from both biochemical and electron microscopic investigations.

A number of investigators (20,24), using cell-free preparations from various sources, have shown that the enzymes responsible for the polymerization of the activated monomers into high-molecular-weight MPS reside in the particulate fraction of the cell, that is, the ribosomal or rough membrane fraction. It therefore seems probable that the part of the visual cell containing the ribosomes is responsible for the synthesis of MPS in this tissue.

Fine & Zimmerman (6) have shown that the apical part of the photoreceptor cell (i.e., the rod and cone inner segments) is especially rich in ribosomes and associated membranes (Figure 95). In addition, the Golgi complex, generally considered to play an important role in the secretory activities of the cell, is very prominent in the apical part of the photoreceptors, where a large number of associated vesicles is also found. Many of the larger vesicles contain a finely granular or filamentous material that is electron-lucent and closely resembles that which occupies the intercellular spaces between the outer limiting membrane and the pigment epithelium (Figure 96).

The above observations strongly suggest that the apical cytoplasm is the synthetic site of these mucinous substances. The MPS are then probably concentrated

---

* See pages 197–198.

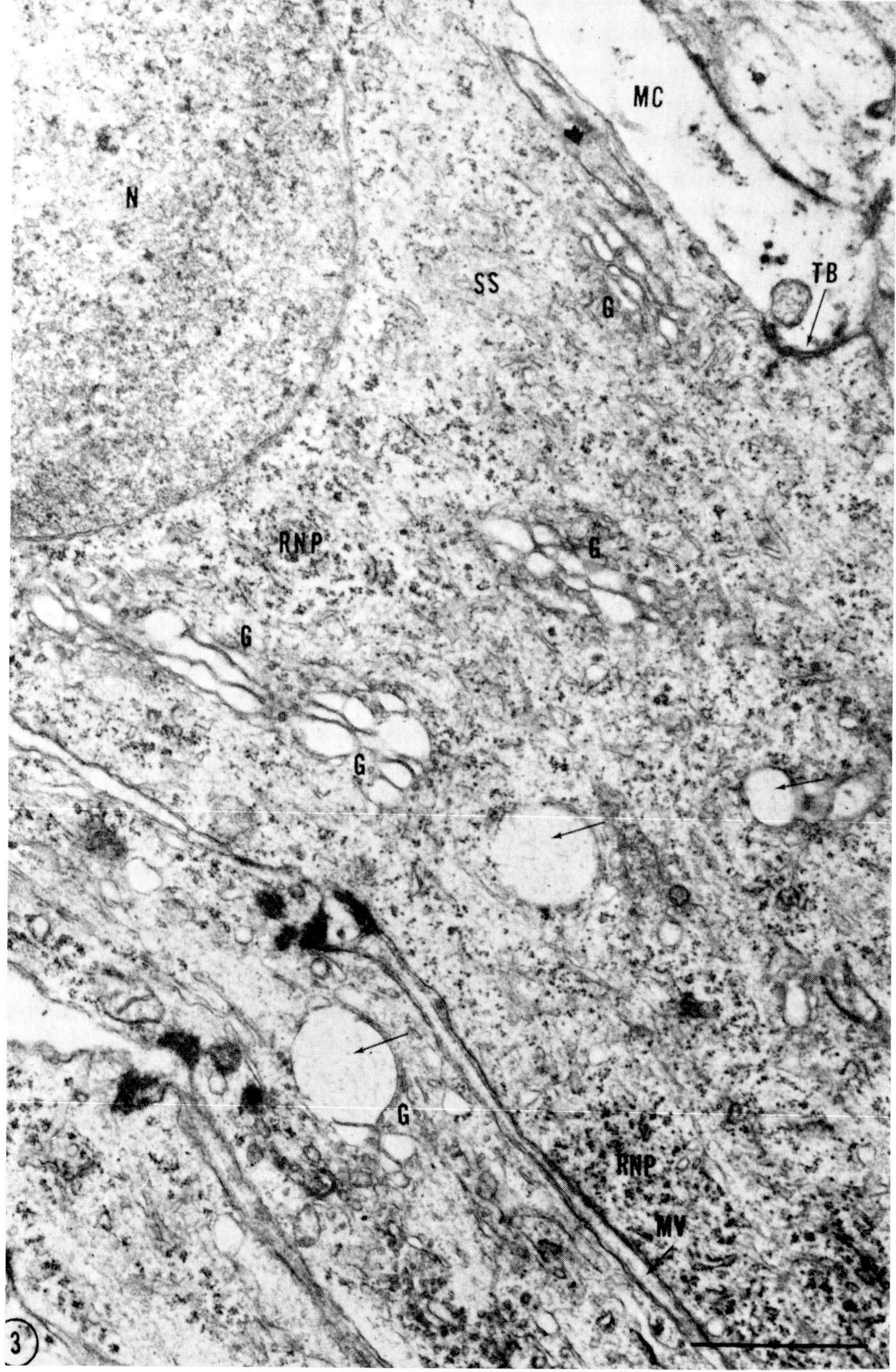

Figure 95 →

in the Golgi complex, from where they are eventually extruded into the intercellular space.

Our recent *in vitro* studies of the synthesis of MPS by the rat retina (10) show that the enzymes responsible for the synthesis of 3′-phosphoadenosine 5′-phosphosulfate (PAPS), a prerequisite for the transfer of sulfate to MPS, were present in this tissue. However, initial attempts to obtain synthesis of MPS *de novo*, using C^{14}-glucose as a precursor, have been unsuccessful. At present it is impossible to tell whether this is a consequence of some unknown requirement of this system in the retina, or of some rate-limiting step in the conversion of glucose to MPS precursors.

Berman (2) has studied the synthesis of MPS *in vitro* by bovine pigment epithelial cells. Incubation of the cells with C^{14}-glucose resulted in the incorporation of a considerable quantity of isotope into newly synthesized MPS, which could be separated from the pigment cells by gentle agitation, indicating that they were extracellular and had possibly been "secreted" by these cells. In addition, the amelanotic "pigment" granules of the albino mouse have been shown to stain very intensely with MPS stains (33). The pigment cells themselves send out delicate fingerlike processes which interdigitate with the developing outer segments of the visual cells; these processes stain positively for acid MPS. This retinal layer cannot therefore be precluded as at least a partial source of the MPS of the visual cell matrix in some animals.

Mucopolysaccharides and Disease

Nothing conclusive is known about the physiological function of the MPS surrounding the visual cells. One obvious possibility is that they merely provide a supporting matrix to maintain the physical orientation of the photoreceptor cells, or that they act as an adhesive which keeps the retina in close apposition to the pigment epithelium.

A class of genetically determined diseases in which there is an abnormal accumulation of MPS in various tissues has been recognized in recent years (16). These diseases—the mucopolysaccharidoses, known by the trivial name of Hurler's syndrome and its varieties (Hunter, Sanfilippio, Morquio, and Scheie syndromes)—are characterized by typical facies ("gargoyle"), bone and joint changes, and other systemic manifestations. In most cases there is slight to severe mental deficiency. The ocular symptoms are a cloudy cornea and a retinal degeneration of the pigmentary type. Gills (cited by McKusick et al., 16) found a diminished or extinguished electroretinogram in many patients suffering from

Figure 95. Apical region of cone photoreceptor (top) and two rod photoreceptors (lower left). The apical part of the visual cell, which is continuous with the myoid portion, contains a very large Golgi complex (*G*) with many associated vesicles varying in size. Some of these larger vesicles contain a lucent, almost filamentous material (unlabeled arrows) that closely resembles the extracellular material observed more distally (Figure 96). The cytoplasm also contains large clusters of ribonucleoprotein (*RNP*) particles, most of which lie "free" or in small clusters. Moderate numbers of these ribosomes are observed to be associated with short fragments of a double membrane system. *MC:* Müller cell; *MV:* Müller cell villi; *N:* nucleus; *SS:* smooth-surfaced endoplasmic reticulum; *TB:* terminal bar. (Nasal macula, uranyl acetate treated; ×31,900.) (From Fine & Zimmerman, 6.)

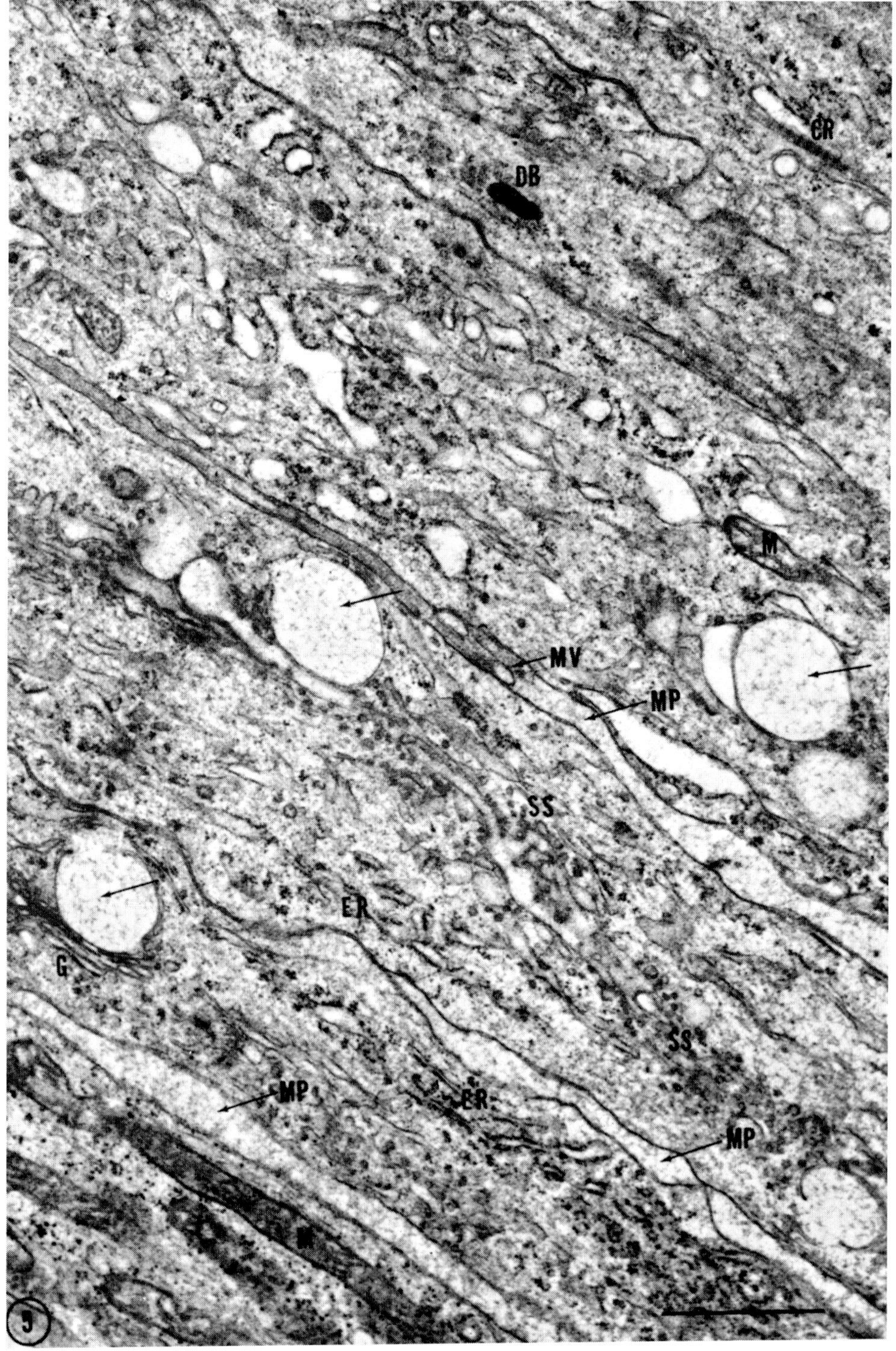

Figure 96 →

mucopolysaccharidoses. The genetic transmission in most cases is X-linked recessive. Various types of MPS can be found in the urine in amounts greater than normal.

McKusick and coworkers (16) have attempted to classify the various mucopolysaccharidoses on the basis of the MPS type excreted. As was pointed out by Dorfman (5), however, the analytical tools are not yet refined enough to offer an unambiguous classification on the basis of urinary MPS. Moreover, no direct correlation could be shown between the MPS excreted in the urine and that found in excess in various tissues. The exact nature of the underlying biochemical defect in the mucopolysaccharidoses is not known. Dorfman suggests a defect in the binding of the polysaccharide to the protein, leading to the accumulation of excessive amounts of the polysaccharide in the tissues and to its excretion in the urine (5).

It is interesting that pigmentary retinal degeneration occurs in a disease that apparently affects mostly the extracellular ground substance. A provocative hypothesis is that an excessive accumulation of polysaccharide in the visual cell-pigment epithelium zone interferes with the normal diffusion mechanisms through which the visual cells derive their nutrients from the choroid. One function of the MPS might thus be that of a normal mediator and regulator in the exchange of metabolites between the retina and choroid and in the exchange of vitamin A between the retina and pigment epithelium.

The above observations provide indirect evidence that these seemingly innocent intercellular substances, the MPS, whose real physiological function is little known, are an integral part of the retina and are essential to its normal functioning and to the integrity of its cytoarchitecture as a whole.

SUMMARY

The visual cells are embedded in a matrix consisting predominantly of a complex mixture of mucopolysaccharides (MPS) and proteins. Several procedures for the isolation of MPS from the retina are available. The major component of this MPS mixture appears to be a chondroitin sulfate-like compound. The components of this matrix vary in different species of animals and show diverse susceptibility towards hyaluronidase.

Available evidence indicates that these MPS are synthesized in the myoid region of the visual cell and extruded into the intercellular spaces, although the pigment epithelium is a possible contributor.

Figure 96. Photoreceptor (rod) inner segments just external to the portions depicted in Figure 95. The villi of Müller cells protrude between these inner segments; one villus can be seen cut obliquely at *MV*. Beyond this villous process, lying in the space between adjacent cells, is a lucent, finely granular to filamentous material (*MP*), which occupies more space as the cells are more widely separated distally (towards lower right). Within these cells is an extensive Golgi complex system (*G*), together with several large vesicles frequently observed to contain finely granular to filamentous lucent material (unlabeled arrows) that resembles the material (*MP*) lying between the cells. *CR:* Portion of a crossbanded ciliary rootlet; *DB:* dense body; *ER:* granular endoplasmic reticulum; *M:* mitochondria; *SS:* smooth-surfaced endoplasmic reticulum. (Nasal macula, uranyl acetate treated; × 29,700.) (From Fine & Zimmerman, 6.)

In the mucopolysaccharidoses, such as Hurler's syndrome, a retinal degeneration of the pigmentary type occurs, indicating that these MPS may have important physiological functions in the eye.

Discussion

Michaelson: It is possible that the retinal mucopolysaccharides tend to keep the pigment and sensory layers adherent to each other, and that a difference in their chemistry may explain the variations in the tendency of the retina to detach in the presence of retinal holes. This variation is very marked among Africans, who show the Caucasian incidence of retinal holes, but in whom retinal detachment is much rarer compared with Caucasians.

Hall: As you know, it is very difficult to detach the retina in some animals. In most mammals one can do so by merely shaking the optical cup in saline solution after removal of the anterior segment, which suggests that, whatever the forces may be, they are not very strong in most cases. However, when a retina is pulled off, one very often finds pigment granules attached to the visual cells, indicating a sticky property for this material, but we do not know how important it is in terms of retinal detachment.

Some of our recent experiments have shown that there is a marked difference between the retinal mucopolysaccharides of the albino versus the pigmented rat, and this includes those mucopolysaccharides surrounding the visual cells. Thus the retinal mucopolysaccharides of the albino rat appear to be largely resistant to digestion by hyaluronidase, while those of the pigmented rat retina are quite labile to the action of this enzyme; this is a case in which the same genus shows a considerable difference in this respect. Although I have no information regarding the differences between the retinal mucopolysaccharides of Africans versus Caucasians, it is quite possible that a variation does exist, and may be important in detachment prevention.

REFERENCES

1. Anseth, A., and Laurent, T. C., Studies on corneal polysaccharides. I. Separation. *Exp. Eye Res.*, 1961, **1**: 25–38.
2. Berman, E. R., The biosynthesis of mucopolysaccharides and glycoproteins in pigment epithelial cells of bovine retina. *Biochim. Biophys. Acta*, 1964, **83**: 371–373.
3. ———, Isolation of neutral sugar-containing mucopolysaccharides from cattle retina. *Biochim. Biophys. Acta*, 1965, **101**: 358–360.
4. Dorfman, A., Biosynthesis and metabolism of acid mucopolysaccharides of connective tissues. *Fed. Proc.*, 1962, **21**: 1070–1074.
5. ———, Heritable diseases of connective tissues: the Hurler syndrome. In: *The Metabolic Basis of Inherited Disease* (J. B. Stanbury, J. B. Wyngaarden, and D. S. Fredrickson, Eds.). McGraw-Hill, New York, 1966: 963–994.
6. Fine, B. S., and Zimmerman, L. E., Observations on the rod and cone layer of the human retina; a light and electron microscopic study. *Invest. Ophthal.*, 1963, **2**: 446–459.
7. Freeman, M. I., and Wortman, B., Mucopolysaccharides in beef retina and small cerebral vessels. *Invest. Ophthal.*, 1966, **5**: 88–92.

8. GREGORY, J. D., LAURENT, T. C., and RODÉN, L., Enzymatic degradation of chondromucoprotein. *J. Biol. Chem.*, 1964, **239**: 3312–3320.

9. HALL, M. O., OCUMPAUGH, D. E., and YOUNG, R. W., The utilization of ^{35}S-sulfate in the synthesis of mucopolysaccharides by the retina. *Invest. Ophthal.*, 1965, **4**: 322–329.

10. HALL, M. O., and STRAATSMA, B. R., The synthesis of 3′-phosphoadenosine 5′-phosphosulfate by retinae and livers of normal and vitamin A-deficient rats. *Biochim. Biophys. Acta*, 1966, **124**: 246–253.

11. LARSEN, G., An autoradiographic study on the uptake of S^{35}-labeled sodium sulfate. *Am. J. Ophthal.*, 1959, **47**: 519–530.

12. LILLIE, R. D., Histochemical studies on the retina. *Anat. Rec.*, 1952, **112**: 477–495.

13. LINDAHL, U., CIFONELLI, J. A., LINDAHL, B., and RODÉN, L., The role of serine in the linkage of heparin to protein. *J. Biol. Chem.*, 1965, **240**: 2817–2820.

14. LINDAHL, U., and RODÉN, L., The role of galactose and xylose in the linkage of heparin to protein. *Ibid.*: 2821–2826.

15. ———, The chondroitin 4-sulfate-protein linkage. *J. Biol. Chem.*, 1966, **241**: 2113–2119.

16. MCKUSICK, V. A., KAPLAN, D., WISE, D., HANLEY, W. B., SUDDARTH, S. B., SEVICK, M. E., and MAUMENEE, A. E., The genetic mucopolysaccharidoses, *Medicine* (Baltimore), 1965, **44**: 445–483.

17. MEYER, K., Introduction: mucopolysaccharides. *Fed. Proc.*, 1966, **25**: 1032–1034.

18. MORETTI, A., and WHITEHOUSE, M. W., Changes in the mucopolysaccharide composition of bovine heart valves with age. *Biochem. J.*, 1963, **87**: 396–402.

19. OCUMPAUGH, D. E., and YOUNG, R. W., Distribution and synthesis of sulfated mucopolysaccharides in the retina of the rat. *Invest. Ophthal.*, 1966, **5**: 196–203.

20. PEARLMAN, R. L., TELSER, A., and DORFMAN, A., The biosynthesis of chondroitin sulfate by a cell-free preparation. *J. Biol. Chem.*, 1964, **239**: 3623–3629.

21. SENO, N., MEYER, K., ANDERSON, B., and HOFFMAN, F., Variations in keratosulfates. *J. Biol. Chem.*, 1965, **240**: 1005–1010.

22. SIDMAN, R. L., Histochemical studies on photoreceptor cells. *Ann. N. Y. Acad. Sci.*. 1958, **74**: 182–195.

23. SIDMAN, R. L., and WISLOCKI, G. B., Histochemical observations on rods and cones in retinas of vertebrates. *J. Histochem. Cytochem.*, 1954, **2**: 413–433.

24. SILBERT, J. E., Incorporation of ^{14}C and ^{3}H from nucleotide sugars into a polysaccharide in the presence of a cell-free preparation from mouse mast cell tumors. *J. Biol. Chem.*, 1963, **238**: 3542–3546.

25. SMELSER, G. K., and OZANICS, V., Distribution of radioactive sulfate in the developing eye. *Am. J. Ophthal.*, 1957, **44**(4/II): 102–109.

26. STARY, Z., WARDI, A. H., TURNER, D. L., and ALLEN, W. S., Arabinose as a mucopolysaccharide component in human and animal brain tissue. *Arch. Biochem.*, 1965, **110**: 388–394.

27. TELSER, A., ROBINSON, H. C., and DORFMAN, A., The biosynthesis of chondroitin-sulfate protein complex. *Proc. Nat. Acad. Sci. USA*, 1965, **54**: 912–919.

28. WISLOCKI, G. B., and SIDMAN, R. L., The chemical morphology of the retina. *J. Comp. Neurol.*, 1954, **101**: 53–91.

29. WORTMAN, B., Acid mucopolysaccharides in beef retina. I. Isolation and fractionation. *Am. J. Ophthal.*, 1959, **47**(2): 203–207.

30. WORTMAN, B., and FREEMAN, M., Resolution of retinal mucopolysaccharides by anion-exchange chromatography. *Fed. Proc.*, 1962, **21**: 170.

31. Zimmerman, L. E., Applications of histochemical methods for the demonstration of acid mucopolysaccharides to ophthalmic pathology. *Trans. Am. Acad. Ophthal. Otolaryng.*, 1958, **62**: 697–703.
32. ———, Acid mucopolysaccharides in ocular histology and pathology. *Proc. Inst. Med. Chicago*, 1961, **23**: 267–277.
33. Zimmerman, L. E., and Eastham, A. B., Acid mucopolysaccharide in the retinal pigment epithelium and visual cell layer of developing mouse eye. *Am. J. Ophthal.*, 1959, **47**: 488–499.

CIRCULAR DICHROISM AND THE CONFORMATIONAL PROPERTIES OF VISUAL PIGMENTS

WILFRIED F. H. M. MOMMAERTS
UCLA School of Medicine
Los Angeles, California

The primary process of excitation in the visual pigments poses an intriguing problem. While it is generally held that cellular mechanisms of excitation are a limited or self-propagated local response in the cell membrane, leading to a differential change in ionic permeabilities, the nature of the transient molecular change in the membrane remains a problem for future elucidation. In the retinal photoreceptor, excitation can be induced by the absorption of a single quantum, too small an energetic magnitude to give rise directly to such a membrane alteration. One is led to assume that something comparable to the latter occurs only after an amplification process, triggered cascade fashion by a much smaller primary change localized in the single rhodopsin or other pigment molecule involved in the absorption of a photon. Of the two problems arising in this connection, the nature of the primary event and the nature of the amplification process, only the former will be discussed here.

The experimental work addressed to this problem (2) can be traced to the views expressed by Wald (17) and Hubbard (6), the essentials of which are schematically presented in Figure 120.* It is assumed that, in the native molecule of rhodopsin, the prosthetic group 11-*cis* retinal—the chromophore responsible for the absorption of visible light—is held in a specific strained configuration. This in turn forces a specific conformation on a part of the protein moiety. Upon the absorption of a photon, the retinal is isomerized to the all-*trans* conformation and is detached from the protein. The Wald-Hubbard hypothesis proposes that both the retinal and the protein lose the forced conformations contingent upon their superimposition, and that this represents the trigger which eventually leads to the excitatory phenomenon.

It was not erewhile obvious which measurements to employ for the detection of these surmised phenomena, nor was it certain that both aspects would express themselves by comparable manifestations. It was thought possible, however, that the strained attachment of the retinal would confer a dissymmetric feature upon its optical transitions, detectable by means of circular dichroism in its absorption

* Page 283, in Dr. Wald's paper on " The Molecular Basis of Human Vision ".

band. It was equally (but independently) possible that the conformational change in the protein would affect a region with a helical or otherwise dissymmetrical character, and would likewise be detectable by a change of circular dichroism in the far ultraviolet. Both hypotheses have been found to be true.

By way of introduction, it may be mentioned that, while the interaction between matter and a photon can be described as the induction of a dipole, and absorption as a transition to a higher energy level in case of sufficient vibrational resonance, the existence of a certain dissymmetry of polarizability gives rise to the complex of phenomena known as optical activity. Its fundamental manifestation is *circular dichroism*, meaning a preferential absorption of left- or right-handed circularly polarized light; its alternate manifestation, evident also in spectral regions of wavelengths other than the absorption bands, is *optical rotation*, meaning a greater refractivity for left- or right-handed circularly polarized light. The set of conjugate properties in a region of absorption, namely circular dichroism and optical rotatory dispersion, is known as a Cotton effect. Our work has dealt with Cotton effects in the visible and ultraviolet, measured by the recording of circular dichroism (CD) which provides the essential information in a simpler and more explicit form than does rotatory dispersion.

Since in most instances circular dichroism is a very small effect, the difference in extinction coefficients for the two oppositely polarized beams being only a few ten-thousandths of the mean extinction, it is very difficult to measure (10,15). This difficulty can now be overcome, for equipment for the continuous recording of circular dichroism over most of the desired wavelength range is now available and quite satisfactory. The results are presented as spectra, of which the band maxima can be positive or negative, depending upon the sign of the quantity $(\varepsilon_L - \varepsilon_R)$.

Let us first consider the phenomena in the visible region of the spectrum and in the proximal ultraviolet. The absorption spectrum of rhodopsin in this region is well known—there is a major band (α) with a maximum at about 500 mμ, and a lesser β-band around 350 mμ. These bands are functions of the prosthetic group, 11-*cis* retinal, the vibrational frequencies of which have shifted bathochromically by the attachment to protein. Both bands are optically active, as evidenced by their circular dichroism, the β-band proportionally more so (Figure 97).

The possible origin of this anisotropy should be examined. Retinal can exist in a number of isomeric forms (Figure 98), based upon the possibility of *cis-trans* isomerism at each of the conjugated double bonds. Of particular importance are the all-*trans* isomer, which results from rhodopsin upon bleaching, and the 11-*cis* isomer, which occurs in rhodopsin in all cases tested. The all-*trans* form (Figure 98A) is capable of variations in its molecular conformation by rotation around the single bonds. *Cis-trans* isomerism as such does not produce optical activity. Unlike the other *cis*-retinals, however, the 11-*cis* isomer (Figure 98C) is not formed freely; indeed, it was excluded in the first survey of predictable possibilities, since the methyl group would interfere sterically with the adjacent part of the polyene chain and its apposite hydrogen atom. The substance does exist, however, and a study of molecular models suggests that it can be formed without strain by a

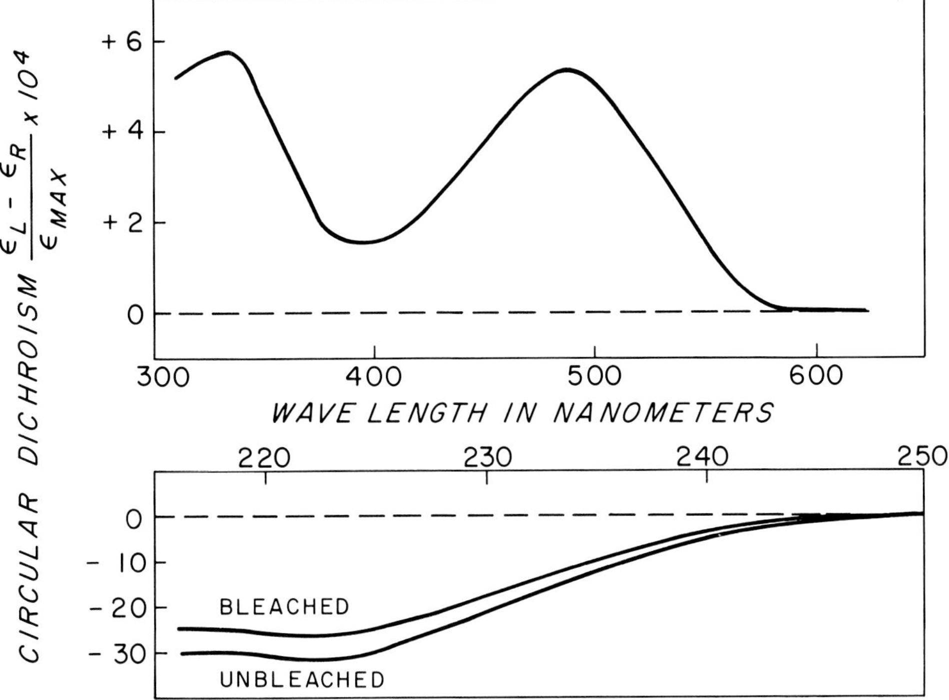

Figure 97. Circular dichroism of frog rhodopsin as a function of wavelength. *Above:* The positive CD associated with the α- and β-absorption bands in the visible and near-ultraviolet region, referred to a solution with an optical density of 1.0 at the maximum of the A-band; the dotted line indicates absence of CD, and the measurements of bleached rhodopsin fall upon this line within their accuracy. *Below:* The negative CD in the far ultraviolet, referred to the same solution upon bleaching; the CD is reduced in magnitude but does not approach the baseline, and a significant amount remains. (Data from Crescitelli, Mommaerts & Shaw, 2.)

special twisting operation which can be carried out in two different ways, leading to short, helix-like conformations of opposite sense (Figure 99). We might note here that the nature of the steric hindrance in retinal has been studied by Jurkowitz et al. (7), and that usually the interconversion of the opposite forms will proceed at room temperature in the case of "soft" hindrance; only in exceptional cases of large hindrance can the enantiomorphs be actually resolved (11). In a random population of 11-*cis* retinal, both forms would occur in equal amounts and an interconversion among them is possible, but if a population of one form were isolated and maintained, it would certainly display circular dichroism. It is therefore proposed that, in the biological formation of an 11-*cis* retinal and its attachment to the opsin, one or the other form is preferentially stabilized.

To be sure, this specific formulation in terms of steric hindrance combined with *cis-trans* isomerism may not be essential: once it is assumed that the attachment to a complementary structure in a protein isolates one of the forms, it can equally be assumed that the protein can induce a certain dissymmetric conformation in the retinal, and this may well be the case. Opsin can also combine with the 9-*cis*

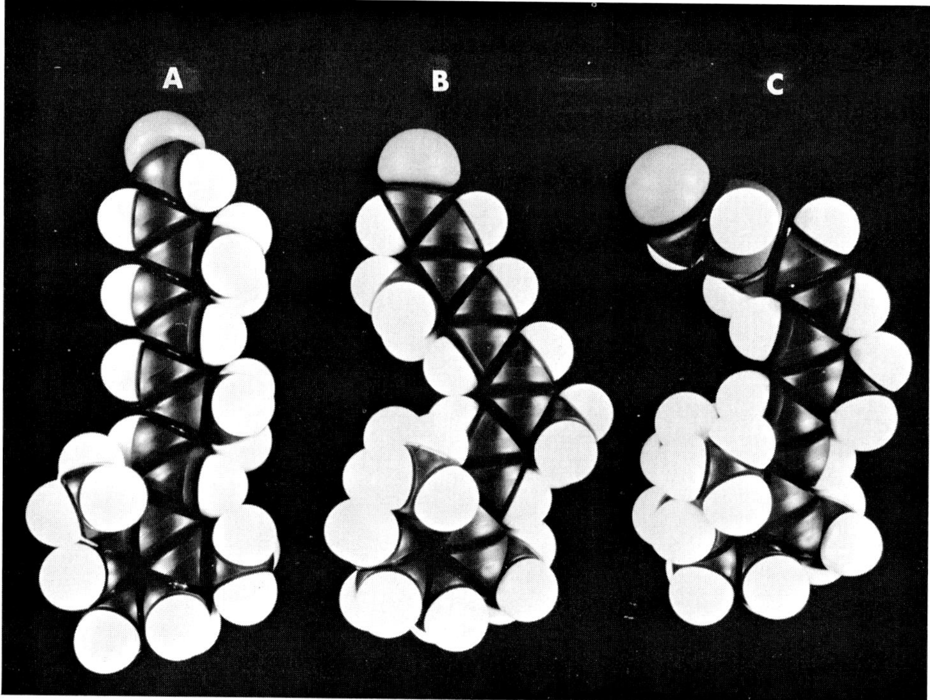

Figure 98. Scale models of three stereoisomers of retinal. *A:* All-*trans*; *B:* 9-*cis*; *C:* 11-*cis*.

isomer, which is not subject to steric limitations (Figure 98B), and it should be established whether this isorhodopsin is circularly dichroic. The special limitations inherent in 11-*cis* retinal are of interest, however, in that they restrict the potential structures imposed by the protein, while themselves specifying the possibility of optical dissymmetry. Without the steric hindrance, some preferred conformation would have to result spontaneously from the interaction of the polyene and part of the protein; in the special instance of the 11-*cis* isomer, two preferred forms are inherent in the polyene, one of which is selected and stabilized by the protein. It is probable that this is the reason for the unlikely evolutionary choice of an isomer that until recently was declared impossible.

In porphyropsin, found in fresh water fish, there is an additional double bond in the ring of the retinal (retinal$_2$) which extends the conjugated system and hence shifts the absorption maxima bathochromically, both in the free and in the protein-bound condition. Again, the α-band is circularly dichroic, to exactly the same degree as in rhodopsin. The β-band, however, is now isotropic. It is not yet known, although the experimental route towards the decision is straightforward, whether this is due to different vibrational modes and dissymmetries within the chromophore itself, retinal$_1$ versus retinal$_2$, or to a different inductive influence of the protein moiety.

The properties described are all contingent upon the presence of unbleached visual pigments. Upon complete bleaching in strong light, the absorption spectra change to those of the yellow bleached pigments because of the isomerization of

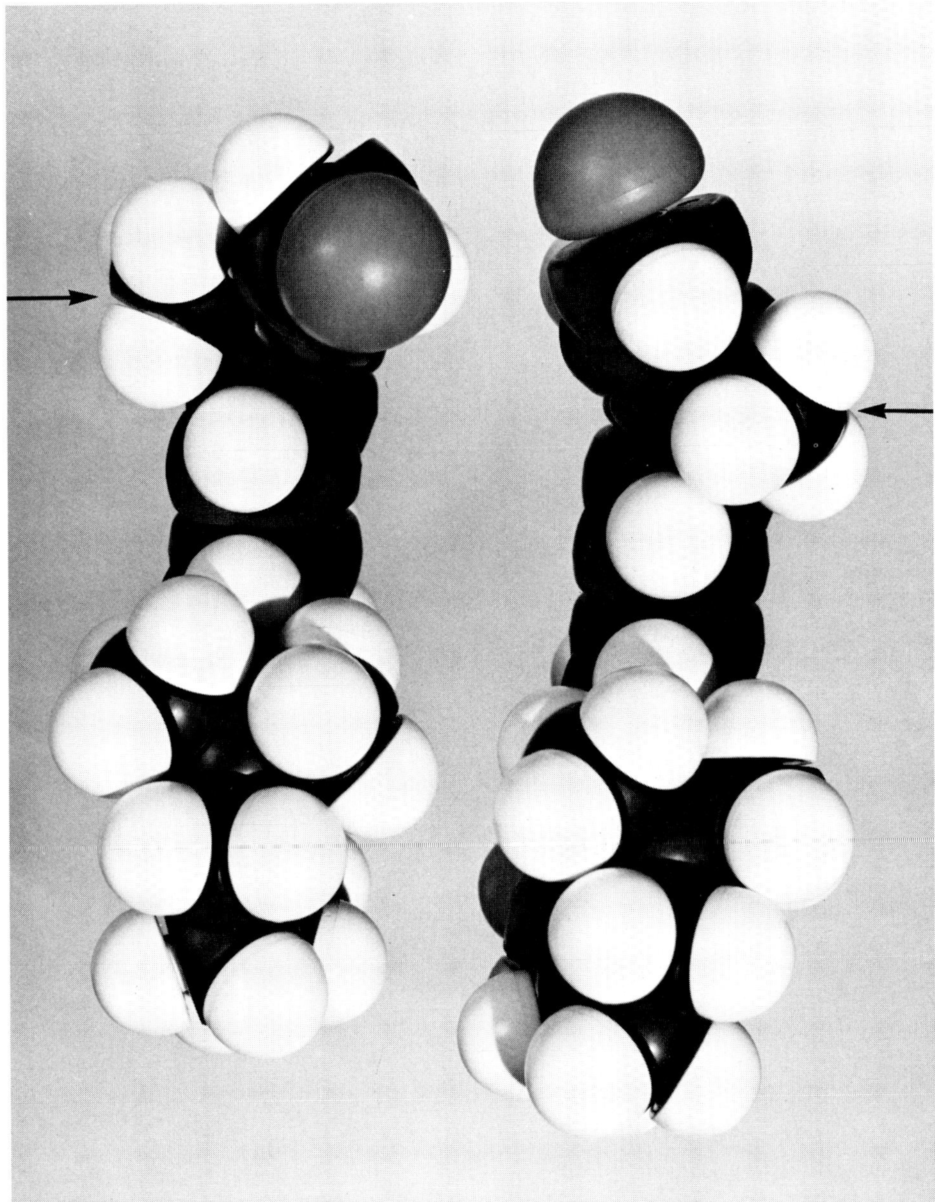

Figure 99. Two selected conformations of 11-*cis* retinal, based upon steric interference with the placing of the methyl group marked by the arrow. The two choices result from placing this group to the left or to the right.

the retinal to the all-*trans* form and its partial, if not complete, detachment from the opsin. The circular dichroism of both α and β absorption bands (where present) vanishes completely (Figure 97). Again, it is not known whether this is because the all-*trans* form does not lend itself to suitable juxtaposition to the relevant protein site, or whether it is primarily the absence of a choice between two sterically hindered conformations that is decisive; the distinction may not be crucial by itself. The circular dichroism also vanishes upon thermal bleaching, which is held to loosen the retinal without isomerization, but this would lead to a randomization between the two steric forms of the 11-*cis* isomer.

A different set of phenomena is encountered in the far ultraviolet, where certain proteins display a set of three circular-dichroic bands, *a* (positive) and *b* and *c* (negative). These were first described for apomyoglobin (4) and myosin (9) and, on the basis of synthetic polypeptide measurements (4), were thought to be the characteristic pattern of the α-helical conformation. Transformation of a helical polypeptide into the β-form gives an entirely different pattern, and proteins in which this or other conformations predominate over the α-helix have circular-dichroic spectra which differ from the described pattern (12). The ultraviolet CD-spectrum of visual pigment is clearly of the α-helical type (Figure 97). Since our pigment preparations were of unspecified purity, it is not possible to derive quantitative conclusions. Assuming, however, that our frog rhodopsin approached the purity of Hubbard's preparations (5), it can be calculated from the absolute extinction coefficient and the molecular weight that a major part (about 75 per cent) of the opsin is in the form of a right-handed α-helix.

Upon bleaching, this circular dichroism diminishes (Figure 97). While the absolute intensities varied in different pigment preparations (due undoubtedly to varying amounts of accompanying protein), the absolute amount of the decrease appeared to be rather constant, indicating that about 10 per cent of the opsin reverts from the α-helical to a different conformation. Whether this means a transformation to a random coil is not explicitly certain; there is some indication that the *b* and *c* bands may not diminish to exactly the same degree, which would leave open the possibility of the occurrence of some β-form or of other structural features. The molecule remains predominantly α-helical, however, and thus the transconformation is localized.

These findings would seem to give a very substantial specification of Hubbard's and Wald's proposals, but some further discussion is still required for full appreciation. The circular dichroism in the region of the α (and β) absorption bands represents a case of an external or induced Cotton effect (cf. Ulmer & Vallee, 14), but this exists in two rather different categories. The classical example is the binding of certain dyes to helical peptides, discovered by Stryer & Blout (13) in terms of anomalous rotatory dispersion in the region of the dye's absorption bands. These are dyes which would, by themselves, have a tendency to polymerize; their polymerization is promoted by the charge pattern on the peptide, and the helical placement of these charges on the peptide matrix induces the dye molecules to form a dissymmetric array. This explanation does not hold here: one retinal molecule is attached to one protein molecule, and in digitonin solution these protein molecules exist singly in the form of protein-detergent micells. Thus, the optical dissymmetry is induced in single retinal chromophores, along the lines already implied in this essay, and in agreement with the views of Hubbard and Wald. Further, the presence of the strained chromophore acts back upon the protein and maintains helical order in a large section of the protein molecule, a

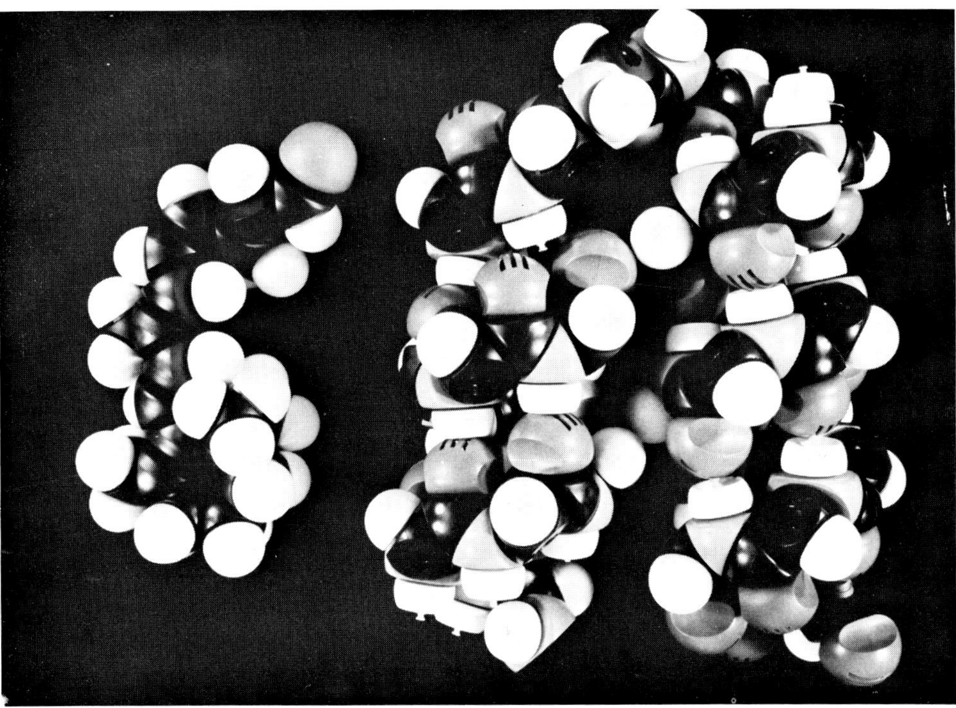

Figure 100. *Left:* An 11-*cis* retinal molecule. *Right:* A largely α-helical section of a protein molecule, stripped of its side chains, of about the relative size of the area imagined to lose its helical structure upon bleaching.

region estimated to measure about 4000 daltons, some 14 times the size of the prosthetic group. This is a very profound organizing influence, one that extends farther than would have been envisaged; whether to call it an *allosteric* effect is a matter of definition, and the point will not be belabored. In addition, it might be a striking illustration of the principle of *induced fit* developed in enzymology (8). The size of the protein region affected by the presence of the prosthetic group (Figure 100) may appear beyond belief, yet it is not altogether out of proportion to existing precedent: in myoglobin, the presence of heme induces helicity in a region about half of the size estimated here (1,3).

As to the direct physiological consequences, we clearly tend toward the view of Wald and Hubbard that the conformational transition of the protein may represent the primary event of excitation. However, some reservation is still needed: the changes in circular dichroism have so far been detected only as the end result of total bleaching. An investigation of the intermediary stages will be required to provide a more specific basis for the discussion of possible physiological mechanisms (cf. Figure 120*).

Assuming, however, that Wald and Hubbard are correct, a reason could be discerned as to why Nature employed the unlikely 11-*cis* isomer instead of one of

---

* Page 283.

the more obvious forms which, without steric hindrance, could accommodate themselves more easily to the contour of the protein molecule. The point might seem to be that such a flexible retinal would be less effective in altering the structure of the protein and might be unable to force upon it a specific conformation to achieve an induced fit; 11-*cis* isomers alone would have the required rigidity. This point is also accessible to experimentation: we would venture to predict that isorhodopsin, in which 9-*cis* retinal is bound to give a pigment with an absorption spectrum similar to that of rhodopsin, might or might not be circularly dichroic in the visible region, but will not change its ultraviolet circular dichroism upon bleaching. This would show that, while more than one retinal can be used to make a pigment of the accustomed spectral characteristics, only the 11-*cis* isomer can do this and at the same time "cock" the protein to a condition from which it can be triggered so as to incite the excitatory event.

SUMMARY

The circular-dichroic spectrum of rhodopsin shows a positive band in the visible region, associated with the major absorption band, and a negative pair of bands in the far ultraviolet characteristic for helical proteins. Upon bleaching, the former disappears and the latter diminish.

These findings have been interpreted in the light of the stereochemistry of retinal. It is concluded that, upon its transformation from a 9-*cis* to an all-*trans* form, a sizable region of the protein loses its helicity. Whether this represents an aspect of the primary excitation process is suggested and discussed.

Discussion

MacNichol: Dr. Mommaerts, I believe that Theodore Williams of Brown University reached exactly the same conclusion by optical rotatory dispersion methods. Would you comment on the use of the two methods for arriving at the same conclusion?

Mommaerts: While Williams' work (18) was restricted to the visible region, the two methods definitely point in the same direction. It had become traditional to study this field by means of rotatory dispersion, but circular dichroism is more directly informative.

I would draw a comparison between the relation of optical rotation and circular dichroism and that of refractivity and absorption. One can derive an absorption spectrum from the study of refractive index dispersion by using a spectrophotometer to measure the spectrum; but, of course, nobody does this. The same concept applies to rotary dispersion versus circular dichroism. Rotatory dispersion has been very uninformative, especially in nucleic acids, and it was not until circular dichroism was applied that this field became penetrable; the same is also true about proteins, although a substantial amount of work had been done previously.

By all means, as far as it goes, the work by Williams is exactly comparable to ours.

Wald: I think it would be most interesting to pursue the information being provided by this new method in the following direction. Not only can free 11-*cis* retinal exist in two screw forms, right- and left-handed, of which the protein opsin almost surely selects one, but the attachment of retinal to opsin probably influences its shape, as well, perhaps, as the degree of screw rotation. The first light product, prelumirhodopsin, should be examined at temperatures close to liquid nitrogen because, although it is the first step leading to bleaching of the molecule, it itself is not less but more of a pigment than rhodopsin. The spectrum of prelumirhodopsin is both higher and shifted far towards the red compared with that of rhodopsin, yet its chromophore is now all-*trans*. That need not mean that the chromophore has taken on the geometry of free all-*trans* retinal; its attachment to opsin may be holding it in a very strained geometry that may even still present some degree of twist. We have wondered whether precisely this strained geometry may account for the striking character of the absorption spectrum (19).

Mommaerts: We are tooling up for work at lower temperatures and also for illumination at low temperatures. There is a choice between two forms or the conformation imposed by the protein; the extent to which this choice predominates would be somewhat hard to decide as long as we work with ordinary rhodopsin only. I think the experiment with isorhodopsin will be very informative, because there is no twofold choice with 9-*cis* retinal. This would perhaps give rise to the possibility of an induced conformation, which would suggest the extent of that effect's contribution.

REFERENCES

1. Breslow, E., Beychok, S., Hardman, K. D., and Gurd, R. N., Relative conformations of sperm whale metmyoglobin and apomyoglobin in solution. *J. Biol. Chem.*, 1965, **240**: 304–309.
2. Crescitelli, F., Mommaerts, W. F. H. M., and Shaw, T. I., Circular dichroism of visual pigments in the visible and ultraviolet spectral regions. *Proc. Nat. Acad. Sci. USA*, 1966, **56**: 1729–1734.
3. Harrison, S. C., and Blout, E. R., Reversible conformational changes of myoglobin and apomyoglobin. *J. Biol. Chem.*, 1965, **240**: 299–303.
4. Holzwarth, G., and Doty, P., The ultraviolet circular dichroism of polypeptides. *J. Am. Chem. Soc.*, 1965, **87**: 218–228.
5. Hubbard, R., The molecular weight of rhodopsin and the nature of the rhodopsin-digitonin complex. *J. Gen. Physiol.*, 1954, **37**: 381–399.
6. Hubbard, R., Bownds, D., and Yoshizawa, T., The chemistry of visual photoreception. *Sympos. Quant. Biol.*, 1965, **30**: 301–315.
7. Jurkowitz, L., Loeb, J. N., Brown, P. K., and Wald, G., Photochemical and stereochemical properties of carotenoids at low temperatures. *Nature* (London), 1959, **184**: 614–624.
8. Koshland, D. E., Jr., The active site and enzyme action. *Advances Enzym.*, 1960, **22**: 45–97.
9. Mommaerts, W. F. H. M., Ultraviolet circular dichroism of myosin. *J. Molec. Biol.*, 1966, **15**: 377–380.
10. ———, Ultraviolet circular dichroism in nucleic acid structural analysis. In: *Methods in Enzymology*, Vol. XIIB (S. P. Colowick and N. O. Kaplan, Eds.). Academic Press, New York, 1968: 302–329.

11. Rieger, M., and Westheimer, F. H., The calculation and determination of the buttressing effect for the racemization of 2,2′,3,3′-tetraiodo-5,5′-dicarboxybiphenyl. *J. Am. Chem. Soc.*, 1950, **72**: 19–28.
12. Sarkar, P. K., and Doty, P., The optical rotatory properties of the beta-configuration in polypeptides and proteins. *Proc. Nat. Acad. Sci. USA*, 1966, **55**: 981–989.
13. Stryer, L., and Blout, E. R., Optical rotatory dispersion of dyes bound to macromolecules; cationic dyes: polyglutamic acid complexes. *J. Am. Chem. Soc.*, 1961, **83**: 1411–1418.
14. Ulmer, D. D., and Vallee, B. L., Extrinsic Cotton effects and the mechanism of enzyme action. *Advances Enzym.*, 1965, **27**: 37–104.
15. Velluz, L., Legrand, M., and Grosjean, M., *Optical Circular Dichroism; Principles, Measurements, and Applications.* Academic Press, New York, 1965.
16. Wald, G., Receptor mechanisms in human vision. In: *XXIII International Congress of Physiological Sciences; Lectures and Symposia.* Excerpta Medica Foundation, Amsterdam, 1965: 69–79.
17. Wald, G., Brown, P. K., and Gibbons, I. R., The problem of visual excitation. *J. Opt. Soc. Amer.*, 1963, **53**: 20–35.
18. Williams, T. P., Induced asymmetry in the prosthetic group of rhodopsin. *Vision Res.*, 1966, **6**: 293–299.
19. Yoshizawa, T., and Wald, G., Pre-lumirhodopsin and the bleaching of visual pigments. *Nature* (London), 1963, **197**: 1279–1286.

THE PHOTOCHEMICAL APPROACH TO VISUAL PROBLEMS

H. J. A. DARTNALL*
Medical Research Council Vision Research Unit
Institute of Ophthalmology
London, England

More than 40 years ago Hecht (14) began the studies on visual adaptation and brightness discrimination that led to his celebrated "stationary"-state equations (16,18). He postulated that the photosensory system of many organisms, including man, is expressed by the reversible reaction

$$S \underset{\text{dark}}{\overset{\text{light}}{\rightleftharpoons}} P + A$$

where S is the photosensitive material (e.g., rhodopsin) and P and A are products of the photochemical change.

The net rate of breakdown of S at time t was represented by the equation

$$\frac{dx}{dt} - k_1 I(a - x)^m - k_2 x^n$$

where x is the concentration of the products P and A at time t; $a - x$ is the concentration of S, a being its original concentration; I is the luminance of the light; k_1 and k_2 are velocity constants for the photolytic and regenerative reactions respectively, and m and n are exponents representing the orders of these reactions.

A sensory system continuously exposed to a steady light flux eventually reaches an equilibrium in which the rate of photochemical decomposition of S is balanced by its rate of formation from P and A. At this stage,

$$KI = \frac{x^n}{(a - x)^m}$$

where K has been written for k_1/k_2.

Hecht supposed that a just-appreciable difference between two adjacent stimuli I_1 and I_2 (to both of which the mechanism was adapted) was possible when the difference in the amounts x equalled a certain constant value c. Thus,

$$x_2 - x_1 = \sqrt[n]{KI_2(a - x_2)^m} - \sqrt[n]{KI_1(a - x_1)^m} = c$$

*My thanks are given to Dr. W. S. Stiles, Dr. R. A. Weale, and Dr. G. B. Arden for helpful discussions, and to Dr. C. D. B. Bridges for providing retinas or extracts of some of the species (Gwyniad, Powan and Smelt) used in the photosensitivity measurements.

Hecht (17) also considered the case where an eye, after being adapted to a luminous field, is presented with a superimposed increment luminance of short duration, i.e., one to which the eye had no time to adapt. Assuming the exponents m and n to have the value 2, he showed that the ratio of increment threshold ΔI to field intensity I is given by

$$\frac{\Delta I}{I} = \frac{c'}{a^2 k_2}\left(1 + \frac{1}{\sqrt{KI}}\right)^2$$

where c' is the value of the rate term dx/dt resulting from the increment stimulus. Hecht assumed that for threshold to be reached this term should have a certain critical value c'.

By inserting in these equations appropriate assumed values for m and n (e.g., $m = 1, n = 2$, or $m = n = 2$), for the velocity constants k_1 and k_2, and for c and c', Hecht had much success in accounting for brightness discrimination and other experimental data; this material has been reviewed by Bartlett (2,3) and Brown & Mueller (4).

Hecht's theory had an immediate effect on visual science and was in vogue for a number of years, but it has steadily lost ground. As experimental data advanced knowledge, the values he assumed for the parameters in the above equations were replaced, revealing an enormous gulf between theory and experiment. Thus Stiles (28), using Rushton's data for the pigment kinetics (23), showed that the theory was incapable of explaining the relation between the increment threshold and field brightness (log ΔI versus log I), since there was a discrepancy of 7 log units of field intensity in the case of the extrafoveal data, and of more than 3 log units in that of the foveal data.

The crux of the issue was well expressed by Rushton (23), who wrote: "According to the photochemical theory, a steady adaptation light I bleaches the pigment to some fraction $1/p$ of the initial concentration. It will now need p times the original flash intensity to photolyse a fixed 'threshold' amount of pigment. It follows that the pigment must be half bleached away by an intensity I which causes ΔI to be twice the absolute threshold. . . . It is a remarkable thing that the chief proponents of the theory that rod function hangs upon the quantitative relations of rhodopsin bleaching appear neither to have themselves measured this rate of bleaching nor paid attention to the results of Dartnall, Goodeve, and Lythgoe, who did. Otherwise it would have been obvious that this goes on so slowly at a background field where ΔI is twice threshold, that even in the absence of any regeneration, the required bleaching of half the total rhodopsin would take 30 years!"

In recent years much has been learned about the reaction kinetics of the visual pigments. Data now exist for the calculation of bleaching rates under any given conditions of irradiation; the regenerative properties of pigments in living eyes, thanks to the work of Rushton (24,25) and of Weale (33,34), can be quantitatively stated; retinal concentrations of pigments are known or can be shrewdly estimated; and the relation between pigment density and molecular concentration can be obtained via the molar extinction coefficient of rhodopsin, as measured by

Wald (30). It therefore seems opportune to redevelop the equilibrium ("stationary")-state equation in modern terms, and to reexamine the power of the photochemical approach to explain certain visual data.

But dressing up an old theory does not absolve us from attempting to find an answer to the criticism presented by Rushton in the above quotation. On examination it seems that his stricture is not necessarily so much against a photochemical approach per se as against the consequence of assuming (as Hecht did) that an increment threshold corresponds to a fixed increment of bleaching. We must therefore seek another and more acceptable chemical equivalent of increment threshold.

Over a limited range of intensity, the increment threshold ΔI for large fields is proportional to the field intensity I, i.e., $\Delta I/I$, the Weber fraction, is constant (22). Since the response of a visual mechanism is a function of the light that the pigment absorbs (6), and not of that which is incident, it is more realistic to replace the Weber fraction by $\Delta A/A$, where A is the light absorbed by pigment, and ΔA the increment of absorption necessary for threshold. Thus we assume that an increment threshold corresponds not to a constant increment of bleaching (or absorption) but to a constant *percentage* increment, say x. On this new basis, if a certain steady adaptation light bleaches 10^{-3} per cent of the pigment, the corresponding increment threshold will be $10^{-3}\,x$. If the intensity of the adaptation light were raised to the level at which twice as much pigment is bleached, viz. 2×10^{-3} per cent, then the increment threshold would become $2 \times 10^{-3}\,x$, or twice what it was before. The bleaching of only a minute amount of pigment could therefore substantially raise the increment threshold.

If we assume (for a given subject) that $\Delta A/A$ is constant for all levels of field intensity, we can then ascertain whether the observed variation of the Weber fraction $\Delta I/I$ can be attributed to variations in the absorbed fractions due to pigment concentration changes.

The effects of various parameters on the equilibrium state will be examined next, and an attempt made to assess the value and limitations of the photochemical approach to certain visual problems.

The Equilibrium-State Equation

The position of equilibrium eventually assumed by a visual mechanism when irradiated by a field of constant intensity is determined by, among others, the photosensitivity, the regeneration kinetics, and the original concentration of the pigment that mediates the mechanism. Before setting up the equilibrium-state equation, the range of variability of these three parameters in different animal species will be briefly reviewed.

The first measurements of visual pigment photosensitivity in absolute units were made by Dartnall, Goodeve & Lythgoe (7,8) who obtained the value $2.3 \times 10^4\,\text{cm}^2$ for the photosensitivity of frog rhodopsin in solution at a wavelength close to the absorbance maximum. Photosensitivity is defined as the product of the decadic molecular extinction coefficient ε_λ, and γ, the quantum efficiency of bleaching, and has its maximum value at the wavelength of maximum absorbance.

In 1958, Dartnall (5) investigated the bleaching rates of four other visual pigments in comparison with frog rhodopsin and found that the relative maximum photosensitivities ($\varepsilon_{max}\gamma$) ranged only downwards from the frog value to about two-thirds of this value. Two of the four pigments studied were retinaldehyde derivatives ("A_1" pigments), and two were 3-dehydroretinaldehyde derivatives ("A_2" pigments).

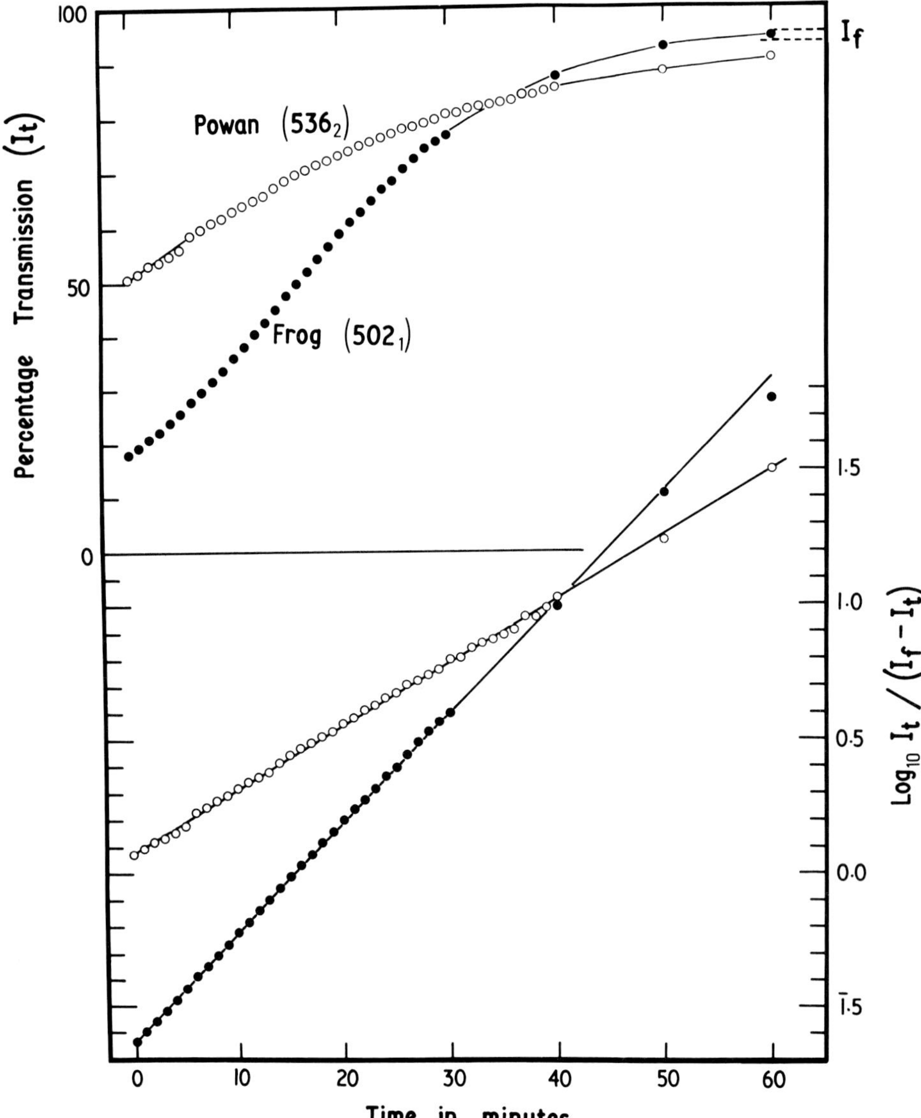

Figure 101. *Above:* Typical curves showing the changes of transmission with time when visual pigment solutions are bleached by a constant-intensity light of wavelength 500 nm; the transmissions of the fully bleached solutions are indicated by I_f. *Below:* Straight lines obtained by plotting $\log_{10} I_t/(I_f - I_t)$ *vs.* time; the gradients of these lines are measures of photosensitivity at 500 nm ($\varepsilon_{500}\lambda$).

The present study has again used this comparative method, measuring the relative rates of bleaching of a number of different visual pigments at one wavelength (500 nm). The apparatus and procedures were as previously described (5), except that 0.10 volume of 2M neutral hydroxylamine solution was added to each pigment solution to inhibit regeneration, which in certain cases would be sufficiently marked to interfere with the measurements. Typical experimental curves are shown in Figure 101, and the results for all experiments are listed in Table 6. The relative maximum photosensitivities for the visual pigments are plotted versus λ_{max} of pigment in Figure 102 and it is clear that they fall into two groups; all the "A_1" pigments have nearly the same values, while the "A_2" pigments, though likewise nearly constant, are only about 70 per cent as photosensitive as the former. Thus, there is little, if any, variation of photosensitivity among different pigments of the same group, and only a modest difference between those of the two groups.

The regenerative process, on the other hand, has a much wider range of rates. Measurements taken *in vivo* indicate that, for both scotopic and photopic pigments, regeneration follows the kinetics of monomolecular reactions, the rate of regeneration being proportional to the concentration of bleached pigment (see, however, Weale, 35). Thus, in the case of rabbit rhodopsin the half-return period is about 25 minutes (26); for human rhodopsin, about 7 minutes (26) or 5 minutes (25); and for the human cone pigments, chlorolabe and erythrolabe, about 1.2 minutes (24). Similarly, Weale (33,34) found that regeneration of the scotopic pigment of the cat and frog was slow (half-return time, about 20 minutes), but a much faster regeneration, maximal at c. 550 nm (half-return time less than 1 minute) was also occasionally observed in these animals. These differences between the scotopic and photopic regeneration rates are possibly related to the observation of Wald, Brown & Smith (32) that the velocity constant for the synthesis of chicken iodopsin *in vitro* is more than 500 times that of chicken rhodopsin.

However, although in general the scotopic pigments are more slowly regenerated *in vivo* than are the photopic ones, this is not an invariable rule, for Wald, Brown & Kennedy (31) found an extremely rapid regeneration of rhodopsin in the Mississippi alligator.

The third parameter, the concentration of pigment in the photoreceptor, is also very variable. The decadic optical density (at λ_{max}) in the axial direction may range from nearly zero, through 0.1 to 0.2—values appropriate for rhodopsins in the rods of rat and man—up to densities in excess of 1.0 in the receptors of certain deep-sea fishes (9).

The rate of photochemical breakdown of visual pigment is given by the product of the quantum efficiency, γ, and the rate of light absorption (7). Thus

$$-\frac{dn}{dt} = \gamma f I$$

where n is the number of visual pigment molecules per square centimeter of retina, I is the light flux in quanta per square centimeter per second, and f is the fraction of this flux that is absorbed.

TABLE 6
RELATIVE PHOTOSENSITIVITIES OF VISUAL PIGMENTS AT 25° C

Species		λ_{max} of pigment in nm	Based on A_1 or A_2	$\varepsilon_{500}\gamma$ *	$\varepsilon_{max}/\varepsilon_{500}$	$\varepsilon_{max}\gamma$ †
Common name	Latin name					
Frog	*Rana temporaria* ‡	502	A_1	0.0421	1.00	0.0421
				0.0421	1.00	0.0421
				0.0423	1.00	0.0423
				0.0426	1.00	0.0426
				0.0427	1.00	0.0427
				0.0424	1.00	0.0424
Crab-eating frog	*Rana cancrivora*	500	A_1	0.0407	1.00	0.0407
				0.0396	1.00	0.0396
Bush baby	*Galago crassicaudatus agisymbanus*	501	A_1	0.0417	1.00	0.0417
Gwyniad	*Coregonus clupeoides pennantii*	520	A_1	0.0388	1.10	0.0427
				0.0380	1.10	0.0418
Conger eel	*Conger conger*	487	A_1	0.0379	1.07	0.0406
				0.0372	1.07	0.0398
Gurnard	*Trigla cuculus*	493	A_1	0.0423	1.01	0.0427
Common carp	*Cyprinus carpio*	523	A_2	0.0265	1.09	0.0289
Crucian carp	*Carassius carassius*	523	A_2	0.0273	1.09	0.0297
Roach	*Rutilus rutilus*	536	A_2	0.0256	1.23	0.0314
Powan	*Coregonus clupeoides*	536	A_2	0.0247	1.23	0.0304
Smelt	*Osmerus eperlanus*	543	A_2	0.0228	1.31	0.0299

* The relative photosensitivities at 500 nm ($\varepsilon_{500}\gamma$) are the slopes ($\min^{-1}$) of the straight lines obtained by plotting $\log_{10} I_t/(I_f - I_t)$ *vs.* time, after correction by the function Φ and for the small variation of bleaching light intensity from experiment to experiment (5).

† Relative maximum photosensitivities, obtained by multiplying the relative photosensitivities at 500nm by the appropriate absorbance ratio, $\varepsilon_{max}/\varepsilon_{500}$.

‡ The six values for *R. temporaria* were obtained at times interdigitating with those of the experiments on other species; the constancy of the values shows that conditions were constant throughout the series.

The rate of regeneration of visual pigment is proportional to the concentration of bleached pigment. If we assume that the stoichiometric relation between pigment and photoproduct is unity, the concentration of photoproduct at any time is given by the loss in concentration of pigment, i.e., by $(n_{max} - n_t)$, where n_{max}

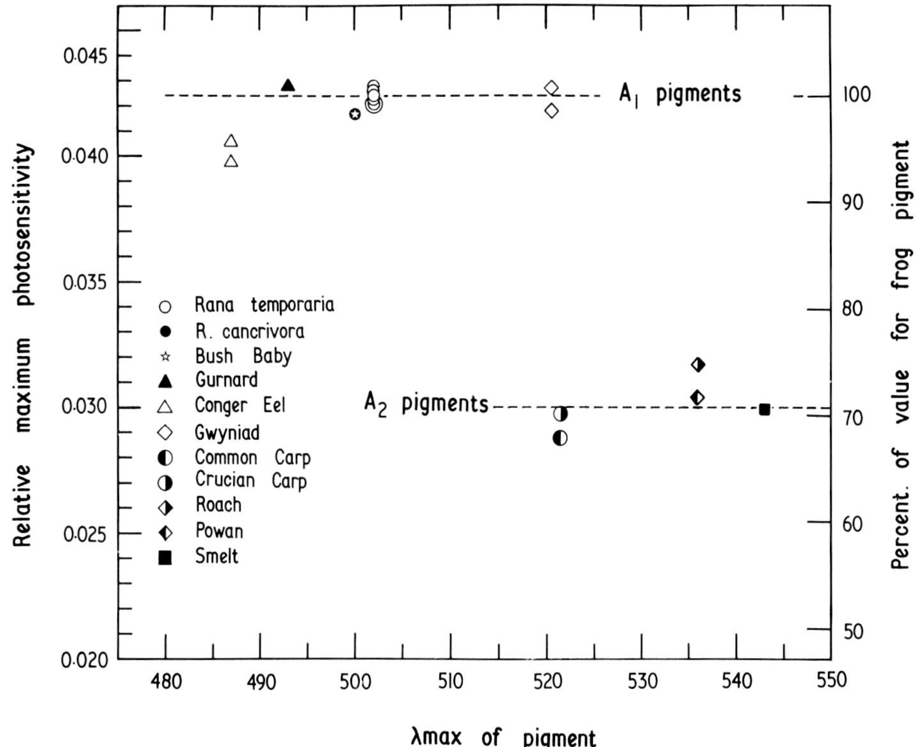

Figure 102. Maximum photosensitivity ($\varepsilon_{max}\gamma$) in relative units (see text) as a function of pigment λ_{max} in nm. Note that the data fall into two groups, depending on whether a pigment is based on retinaldehyde (A_1 pigments) or 3-dehydroretinaldehyde (A_2 pigments), and that within each group the maximum photosensitivity is independent of λ_{max}.

is the original ("dark-adapted") number of visual pigment molecules per cm^2 of retina, and n_t that remaining after t seconds exposure. Thus we may write

$$+\frac{dn}{dt} = k(n_{max} - n_t)$$

where k is a constant that has approximate values as follows: 5×10^{-4} sec^{-1} for rabbit rhodopsin (half-return time = 25 minutes), 2×10^{-3} sec^{-1} for human rhodopsin (half-return time = 5–7 minutes) and 1×10^{-2} sec^{-1} for human chlorolabe and erythrolabe (half-return time = 1.2 minutes).

The net rate of decrease in the number of visual pigment molecules is given by the difference between the opposing processes of bleaching and regeneration, i.e.,

$$-\frac{dn}{dt} = \gamma fI - k(n_{max} - n_t)$$

An exact integration of this differential equation has not been found. Useful information can be obtained, however, from a consideration of the equilibrium state ($dn/dt = 0$), where the rate of regeneration balances the rate of photochemical bleaching. We then have

$$\gamma f_e I = k(n_{max} - n_e)$$

where the subscripts e refer to equilibrium values. This equation may be put in the form

$$\gamma f_e I = \frac{kn_{max} P_e}{100} \qquad [1]$$

where P_e, the percentage of pigment bleached at equilibrium, has been written for $100(1 - n_e/n_{max})$.

Now, f_e, the fraction of light absorbed by the visual pigment at its equilibrium concentration, is strictly given by

$$f_e = \frac{D_e}{D_e + D_e'}(1 - 10^{-(D_e + D_e')})$$

where D_e and D_e' are the optical densities of pigment and product respectively. However, if the density $D_e + D_e'$ does not exceed 0.1 (which is frequently the case), pigment and product absorb light nearly as though each were the only species present, and the fraction obtained by visual pigment is

$$f_e = 1 - 10^{-D_e}$$

This simpler formula clearly also applies for any pigment density whenever D_e' can be neglected in comparison with D_e. For the illustrative purpose of this paper, the simpler formula is used, which on substitution in equation [1] yields the relation

$$P_e = \frac{100\gamma I(1 - 10^{-D_e})}{kn_{max}} \qquad [2]$$

In order to apply equation [2] to some actual problems we need to obtain a value for n_{max}, the original number of pigment molecules per square centimeter of retina. This can be arrived at from D_{max}, the optical density (at dark adaptation) of pigment in the photoreceptors* via the value for the molar extinction coefficient. Thus the molar extinction at λ_{max} of rhodopsin (for example†) is 4.06×10^4 cm² in solution (30). This means that a molar solution of this pigment has an optical density (1 cm path) of 4.06×10^4 at 500 nm. Since any molar solution contains 6.1×10^{23} molecules per liter, i.e., 6.1×10^{20} molecules per cm³, it follows that a rhodopsin solution of density D_{max} contains 1.5×10^{16} D_{max} molecules per cm³. In the photoreceptor, however, the pigment is oriented so that its effective extinction is increased by 50 per cent (10). For this reason a receptor density of D_{max} corresponds to a concentration of 1.0×10^{16} D_{max} molecules per cm² of retina, and this is the appropriate value for n_{max} in equation [2].

---

* Strictly, a correction should be made for the percentage of retinal area covered by the photoreceptors.

† Since the maximum photosensitivities ($\varepsilon_{max}\lambda$) of all "A_1" pigments measured are substantially the same (Figure 102), it seems reasonable to conclude that both γ and ε_{max} are constant. The lower value of $\varepsilon_{max}\gamma$ for "A_2" pigments suggests that ε_{max} for these is about 70 per cent of the "A_1" value of 4.06×10^{-4} cm².

Inserting this value for n_{max} in equation [2] we obtain

$$P_e = \frac{\gamma I(1 - 10^{-D_e})}{10^{14}kD_{max}} \qquad [3]$$

Equation [3] expresses the percentage of pigment bleached at equilibrium (P_e) in terms of the quantum efficiency (γ), the incident light intensity (I), the equilibrium density of pigment (D_e) and the original density of pigment (D_{max}).

With equation [3] we are now in a position to calculate the light intensities required to produce any given percentage bleaching of visual pigment and to examine the effects of the two parameters that show considerable species variation, viz. pigment density (D_{max}) and regeneration constant (k). For example, if we take γ to be unity, and assume values of 0.1 for D_{max} and 1×10^{-3} sec^{-1} for k, equation [3] becomes

$$10^{10} P_e = I(1 - 10^{-D_e})$$

where D_e can have any value between 0.1 and 0 to correspond with bleaching percentages between 0 and 100. Thus, for 30 per cent bleaching the left-hand side of the equation is 3×10^{11} and this, in the units of quanta/sec/cm^2, is the flux of light *absorbed*, i.e., $I(1 - 10^{-D_e})$. For 30 per cent bleaching D_e is 0.07 and $(1 - 10^{-D_e})$, the fraction absorbed, is 0.1489. From this it follows that I, the *incident* flux, is $3 \times 10^{11} \div 0.1489$, i.e., 2.015×10^{12} quanta/sec/cm^2. Table 7 lists the values of I for various bleaching values between 0 and 100 per cent.

TABLE 7

THE INTENSITIES OF INCIDENT LIGHT, I, REQUIRED TO PRODUCE VARIOUS EQUILIBRIUM STATES BETWEEN 0 AND 100% BLEACHING OF PIGMENT ($D_{max} = 0.1$; $k = 10^{-3}$ sec^{-1})

Percentage of Rhodopsin Bleached at Equilibrium P_e	Density at Equilibrium D_e	Fraction of Incident Light Absorbed $1 - 10^{-D_e}$	Flux Absorbed at Equilibrium $I(1 - 10^{-D_e})$	Flux Incident I	Log I
0	0.1	0.2057	0	0	$-\infty$
1	0.099	0.2038	1×10^{10}	4.91×10^{10}	10.691
5	0.095	0.1965	5×10^{10}	2.54×10^{11}	11.406
10	0.09	0.1872	1×10^{11}	5.34×10^{11}	11.728
20	0.08	0.1682	2×10^{11}	1.19×10^{12}	12.075
30	0.07	0.1489	3×10^{11}	2.01×10^{12}	12.304
40	0.06	0.1290	4×10^{11}	3.10×10^{12}	12.491
50	0.05	0.1087	5×10^{11}	4.60×10^{12}	12.663
60	0.04	0.0880	6×10^{11}	6.82×10^{12}	12.834
70	0.03	0.0667	7×10^{11}	1.05×10^{13}	13.021
80	0.02	0.0450	8×10^{11}	1.78×10^{13}	13.250
90	0.01	0.0228	9×10^{11}	3.95×10^{13}	13.596
95	0.005	0.01145	9.5×10^{11}	8.30×10^{13}	13.919
99	0.001	0.00230	9.9×10^{11}	4.31×10^{14}	14.635
100	0	0	1×10^{12}	∞	$+\infty$

In Figure 103 the percentage of rhodopsin bleached, P_e, is plotted as a function of the logarithm of the incident light flux, I, for various values of the parameters k and D_{max}. The curves are S-shaped, the values of log I ranging from $-\infty$ (for zero bleaching) to $+\infty$ (for 100 per cent bleaching).

The effect of varying k, the regeneration constant, while keeping D_{max} constant at 0.1, is shown by the four curves through the circles. It is clear from equation [3] that a tenfold increase (for example) in k would require a compensating tenfold increase in the incident flux if the percentage of pigment bleached is to remain constant. Thus a change in the value of k merely results in a displacement of the curve along the log I axis. The curves through the circles in Figure 103 give the positions for values of k equal to 10^{-4}, 10^{-3}, 10^{-2}, and 10^{-1} sec^{-1}. These curves are located at 1 log unit intervals on the intensity axis, in correspondence with the tenfold changes in k. A teleological explanation is thus provided for the fact that the regeneration constants for photopic pigments are generally greater than those for scotopic pigments. As already noted, the value of k for chlorolabe and erythrolabe is five times that of human rhodopsin, thus shifting their operative range to proportionately higher intensities.

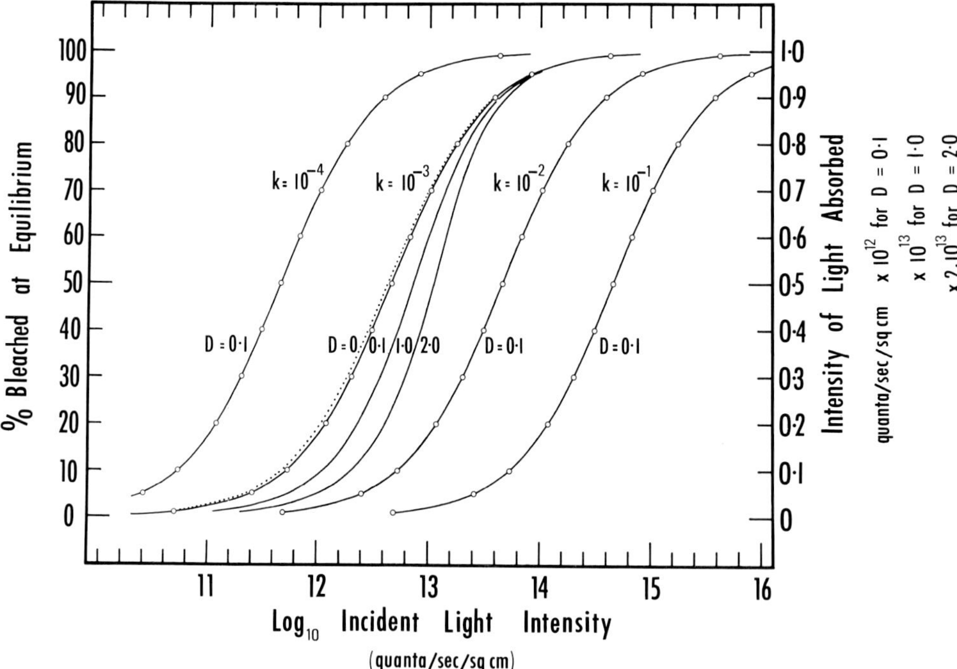

Figure 103. Relation between the percentage of pigment bleached and the logarithm of the field intensity (of wavelength $= \lambda_{max}$) when equilibrium conditions have been reached. The curves were calculated from the equilibrium-state equation (see text) for retinaldehyde-based (A_1) pigments for various values of the regeneration constant k ranging from 10^{-4} to 10^{-1} sec^{-1}, and for various retinal concentrations (density) of pigment between 2.0 and the limit as D tends to zero. Note that the effect of increasing or decreasing k tenfold is to displace the function by 1 log unit along the horizontal axis. Note also that the percentage of pigment bleached at equilibrium, and the intensity of light absorbed by unbleached pigment at equilibrium (scales on right) are proportionate quantities.

The influence of D_{max}, the retinal density of pigment, on the P_e/log I function is shown in Figure 103 for values of D_{max} equal to 2.0, 1.0, 0.1, and for the limit as D_{max} tends to zero. The value of 2.0 is extremely high (99 per cent absorption) and, with the possible exception of some deep-sea fishes, it is doubtful whether such a value is reached in retinas. The great majority of species have D_{max} in the range 0.1 to 1.0. Figure 103 shows that raising D_{max} increases the slope of the P_e/ og I function, but with otherwise comparatively little effect on the position of the curve relative to the intensity axis. In one respect, however, the effect of D_{max} is direct, as in determining the quantity of light absorption (and hence the intensity of visual response). Thus in equation [3] the quantity $I(1 - 10^{-D_e})$, i.e., the intensity of absorbed light, occurs in the numerator of the left-hand side, while D_{max} occurs in the denominator. Hence a tenfold increase (for example) in D_{max} entails a tenfold increase in the absorbed light for a given value of P_e.

The ordinate scale in Figure 103 (left) is the percentage of pigment bleached at equilibrium, or alternatively (right), the intensity of light flux absorbed at equilibrium, these two quantities being proportional to each other (equation [3]). Since the response of a visual mechanism is a function of the light it absorbs (6), we can regard the ordinates as a function of response. More specifically, if we assume for the present that visual response is *directly* proportional to the absorbed light, the right-hand side ordinates in Figure 103 provide a scale of response.

With this assumption, the curves in Figure 103 become the plots of response versus log intensity; according to the Weber-Fechner law, they should be straight lines. In fact, the central parts of these plots are nearly linear, and the Weber-Fechner law can be regarded as valid over these ranges.

Adaptational State and Incremental Threshold

Over a fair range of intensity (brightness) the just noticeable increment of brightness, ΔI, is proportional to the brightness I (22). Thus

$$\frac{\Delta I}{I} = \text{constant, the Weber fraction}$$

Fechner (13) assumed that the sensation increment ΔQ corresponding to the brightness increment ΔI was constant, and hence

$$\Delta Q = \frac{c\,\Delta I}{I}$$

whence by "integration"

$$Q = k \log_e I + c'$$

where c and c' are constants.

This relation, the Weber-Fechner law, states that visual sensation varies linearly with the logarithm of the light intensity. While the above derivation of this law is sometimes regarded as mathematically unsound because finite quantities instead of infinitesimal ones are "integrated", Wright (36) has shown how this difficulty can be avoided and how an identical relation can be obtained by impeccable mathematics.

But since it is only absorbed light that can be visually effective, it is not realistic to consider such terms as I and ΔI, which are incident intensities. Only a fraction of these quantities—a fraction that depends on the pigment concentration—is absorbed. As already mentioned, the innovation proposed here is the replacement of the Weber fraction by

$$\frac{\Delta A}{A} = \text{constant}$$

where A is the light absorbed by visual pigment, and ΔA the increment of absorption. Since the absorbed flux is proportional to the percentage of pigment bleached at equilibrium (see equation [3] and Figure 103), this is also equivalent to the ratio of increment bleached to total amount bleached.

Intensity discrimination measurements can be made either by comparing two adjacent fields to both of which the eye is adapted, or by adapting the eye to a single field and then superimposing a brief test flash on it. In the former case equilibrium conditions are assumed to be reached, and if the two fields compared have intensities I_1 and I_2, the corresponding absorbed fluxes A_1 and A_2 are given by

$$A_1 = f_1 I_1 \quad \text{and} \quad A_2 = f_2 I_2$$

where f_1 and f_2 are the fractions absorbed by the pigment at the corresponding equilibrium concentrations. We may then write,

$$\frac{\Delta A}{A} = \frac{A_2 - A_1}{A_1} = \frac{\Delta I}{I_1} - \frac{I_2}{I_1} \cdot \frac{(f_1 - f_2)}{f_1} \qquad [4]$$

where ΔI has been written for $I_2 - I_1$. This equation shows the relation between $\Delta A/A$ and the classic Weber fraction $\Delta I/I$. Since f_1, the fraction absorbed at the lower intensity, is greater than f_2, it follows that $\Delta I/I$ is always greater than $\Delta A/A$. However, at very low intensities, i.e., when the degree of bleaching is small, the fractions absorbed will not differ greatly from f_{max}, the value corresponding to D_{max}, the density at full dark adaptation. In this low intensity range (say, up to 10 per cent bleaching) $\Delta I/I$ will have practically the same value as $\Delta A/A$. Thus, on the basis of the present hypothesis, one would expect the Weber fraction $\Delta I/I$ to have a constant minimum value ($\Delta A/A$) in the low intensity range, and to increase at higher intensities. Again, it is obvious that f_1 and f_2 will be more nearly equal (and hence that $\Delta I/I$ will approximate more nearly to $\Delta A/A$) when $\Delta A/A$ is small than when it is large. The minimum values of the contrast sensitivity ($\Delta I/I$) are about 0.2 and 0.02 for the scotopic and photopic mechanisms respectively (27). One would therefore expect the intensity range over which $\Delta I/I$ remains constant (and equal to $\Delta A/A$) to be greater in the photopic mechanism, and this in fact is the case (27).

In the other kind of intensity-discrimination measurement, such as when a brief test flash is superimposed on a steady field, the eye does not have time to come into equilibrium with the flash. We may assume that the eye is adapted to the steady field and that, as before, the absorbed flux A_1 is given by

$$A_1 = f_1 I_1$$

If the intensity of the flash is I_2 (quanta per second) and its duration is Δt (sec.) then, assuming that Δt is shorter than the visual summation time, we have to consider the effect of a "dose" of $I_2 \, \Delta t = \Delta I$ quanta superimposed on the adapting field. If, for the present, we assume that the entire dose of quanta is delivered to the eye instantaneously, then the fraction absorbed will be that appropriate to the equilibrium set up by the adapting field, namely f_1. In this case

$$A = f_1 \, \Delta I$$

and hence

$$\frac{\Delta A}{A_1} = \frac{\Delta I}{I_1} \qquad [5]$$

Thus, under these conditions the Weber fraction should be constant, and equal to $\Delta A/A$ at all intensities. It is not permissible, however, to assume that the entire dose of quanta is delivered instantaneously to the eye—it is, on the contrary, spread evenly over the period Δt. Consequently, we may not always assume that the fraction absorbed remains sensibly constant at the value f_1. As bleaching proceeds during the flash period, the value of f_1 tends to diminish towards a value, f_2, that would obtain if the eye were to come into equilibrium with a continuous light flux of the same intensity, I_2, as that of the flash. For this reason one would expect the values of $\Delta I/I$ obtained in the "superimposed flash" type of experiment to lie between $\Delta A/A$ and the higher value defined in equation [4] for the equilibrium case.

Some exemplary calculations of the increment thresholds (ΔI) at various equilibrium states of a visual mechanism are listed in Table 8. In these calculations it has been assumed that D_{max}, the density of pigment in the fully dark-adapted state, is 0.1; that the value of k, the regeneration constant, is 10^{-3} sec^{-1}, and that a 20 per cent increase in the light absorbed by pigment ($\Delta A/A = 0.2$) is required to reach increment threshold. In other words, the calculations apply approximately to the human scotopic mechanism based on rhodopsin. In section B of Figure 104 (curves through black circles), these data are plotted as log increment threshold (ΔI) versus log field intensity (I). At the lower intensities the relation is strictly linear but at higher intensities there is progressive divergence from linearity, as expected from equation [4] and previous discussion. The strictly linear portion of the plot and its dashed-line extension give the relation one would expect between log ΔI and log I when the incremental threshold is measured for an instantaneous flash. For a brief (i.e., not instantaneous) flash, the expected relation would lie between the dashed line and the curve appropriate to measurements at equilibrium (black circles).

There are three parameters that affect the relationship between the increment threshold and the field intensity: the increment ratio required for threshold ($\Delta A/A$), the value of D_{max}, and the value of k. The various curves in Figure 104 show the effects of varying these parameters.

In section A of the figure, the relationship when $\Delta A/A$ is 0.02 and k is 10^{-3} sec^{-1} is shown for $D_{max} = 0.1$ (white circles) and for $D_{max} = 1.0$ (black circles).

TABLE 8

EXEMPLARY CALCULATIONS OF THE INCREMENT THRESHOLDS FOR VARIOUS EQUILIBRIUM STATES ON THE SUPPOSITION THAT A 20% INCREASE IN THE LIGHT ABSORBED BY VISUAL PIGMENT ($\Delta A/A = 0.2$) IS REQUIRED FOR THRESHOLD ($D_{max} = 0.1$; $k = 10^{-3}$ sec^{-1})

Percentage of Rhodopsin Bleached at Equilibrium P_e	Density at Equilibrium D_e	Fraction of Incident Light Absorbed $1 - 10^{-D_e}$	Flux Absorbed at Equilibrium $I(1 - 10^{-D_e})$	Flux Incident I	Log Field Intensity $\log I$	Log Increment Threshold $\log \Delta I$
0.1	0.0999	0.2055	1.0×10^9	4.866×10^9	9.687	
0.12	0.09988	0.2054	1.2×10^9	5.841×10^9		
				0.975×10^9		8.989
1.0	0.099	0.2038	1.0×10^{10}	4.906×10^{10}	10.691	
1.2	0.0988	0.2035	1.2×10^{10}	5.898×10^{10}		
				0.992×10^{10}		9.997
40	0.06	0.1290	4.0×10^{11}	3.100×10^{12}	12.491	
48	0.052	0.1128	4.8×10^{11}	4.254×10^{12}		
				1.154×10^{12}		12.062
80	0.02	0.0450	8.0×10^{11}	1.777×10^{13}	13.250	
96	0.004	0.00917	9.6×10^{11}	10.468×10^{13}		
				8.691×10^{13}		13.939
83.3	0.01667	0.0376	8.3×10^{11}	2.213×10^{13}	13.345	
100.0	0	0	10.0×10^{11}	∞		
				∞		∞

It is clear from these curves that D_{max} has only a minor effect and that an increase in density increases slightly the intensity range over which the relation is linear.

Section B of Figure 104 shows the effect of changing $\Delta A/A$ from 0.02 (white circles) to 0.2 (black circles). The linear portions of these plots are separated by 1 log unit. This follows from the fact that, over the linear portions, $\Delta A/A = \Delta I/I$, and that if ΔA is increased x-fold the line is displaced by $\log x$.

Finally, in section C of Figure 104 curves are shown ($\Delta A/A = 0.02$ and $D_{max} = 0.1$) for $k = 10^{-3}$ sec^{-1} (white circles) and for $k = 10^{-2}$ sec^{-1}(black circles). From these it is clear that a higher regeneration rate (such as applies in photopic vision) extends the range of intensities over which the relationship is linear.

Attempted Interpretation of Experimental Data

Aguilar & Stiles (1) measured the incremental threshold response of the human scotopic mechanism using the two-color threshold method, with a red-adapting field of 20° diameter and a green test stimulus of 9°. The subjects were adapted

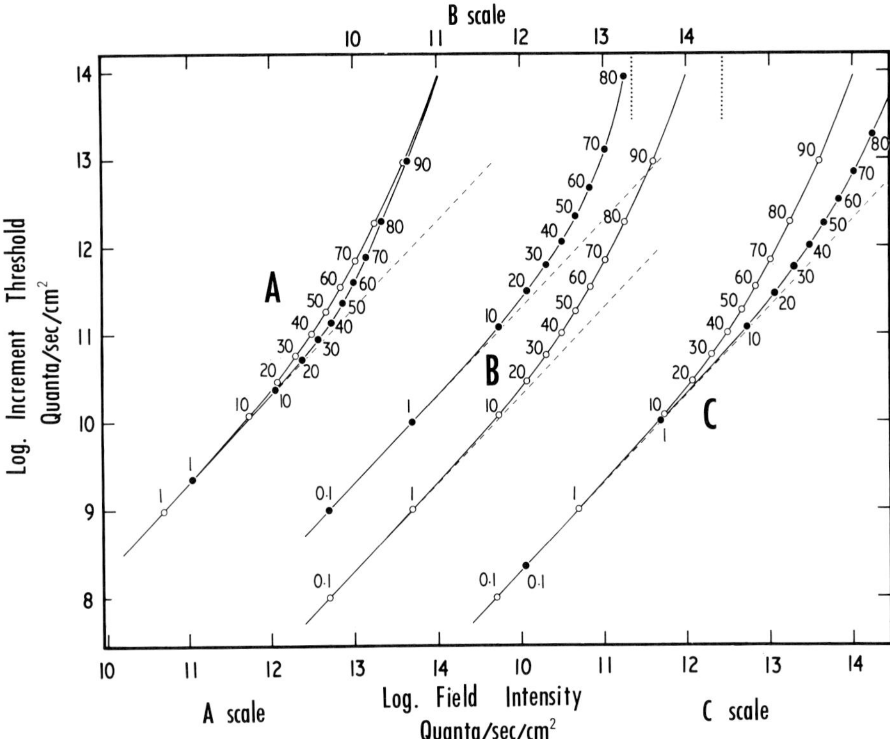

Figure 104. Relations between log field intensity and log increment threshold according to present hypothesis, and the effects of changing the values of various parameters, viz. pigment concentration (density) D (curves **A**), increment ratio $\Delta A/A$ (curves **B**), and regeneration constant k (curves **C**). The solid-line curves through the symbols give the relations when the increment stimulus is determined under equilibrium conditions; the straight dashed lines show them when the stimulus is presented as a flash (see text). The curves through the black circles are identical and relate to $D = 0.1$, $\Delta A/A = 0.02$, and $k = 10^{-3}$ sec^{-1}. The curves through the white circles are as those for the black circles, with the following variations: **A**, for $D = 1.0$; **B**, for $\Delta A/A = 0.2$; **C**, for $k = 10^{-2}$ sec^{-1}. The figures against the symbols are the percentages of pigment bleached. The short vertical dotted lines at the top of the figure show the asymptotic values for the B curves.

first to darkness for three minutes, and then to the red field. The green test stimulus was subsequently superimposed on the field for 0.2 sec. once every second, and the intensity of the stimulus adjusted to threshold. After each increment threshold had been determined the field intensity was raised, and the subject was then exposed to the new field for two to three minutes before the next series of stimulus presentations.

By this technique and other ingenious details of experimentation, Aguilar & Stiles were able to explore the relation between field intensity and increment threshold for the scotopic mechanism alone, up to relatively high field intensities.

The results obtained for one of their four observers (subject B) are given by the circles in Figure 105. These data give the relation between log (field intensity) and log (increment threshold) in units of scotopic trolands; the absolute threshold (i.e., field intensity = zero) is indicated by the cross. All other observers gave generally similar results.

Following Aguilar & Stiles (1), we can regard the experimental data as lying on a curve with four characteristics: (*a*) An initial horizontal section corresponding

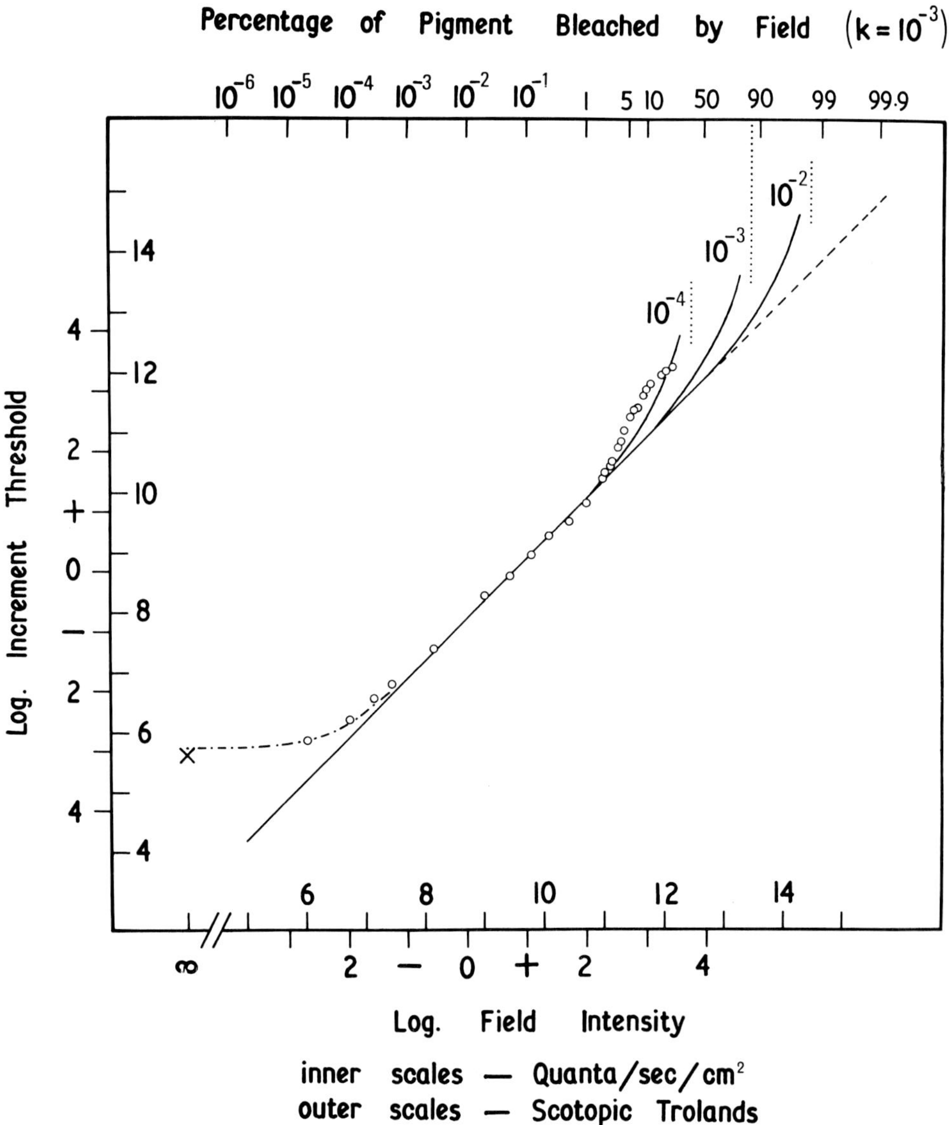

Figure 105. Attempted interpretation of Aguilar & Stiles' (1) measurements (circles) of increment threshold as a function of field intensity. Solid-line curves give the expected relationship on the present hypothesis when equilibrium conditions apply, and for various values of the regeneration constant between 10^{-4} and 10^{-2} sec^{-1} as indicated. The straight portion of these curves and its dashed extension give the expected relationship when the increment stimulus is presented as a flash. The dash-and-dot curve gives the expected relationship when the hypothesis is modified to include the concept of an absolute threshold (X) (see text). Vertical dotted lines at top indicate asymptotic values (86.3 per cent pigment bleached) for the solid-line curves.

to absolute threshold; (*b*) an ascending linear section of unit gradient extending over about 4 log units of intensity; (*c*) a section of much higher gradient; and (*d*) a final section of low gradient. Sections *a*, *b*, and *c* are attributed by Aguilar & Stiles to rod vision, section *d* to cone vision. These conclusions were based on the fact that, in section *d* but not in the other sections, a directional (Stiles-Crawford) effect was found for the test stimulus; the observers also reported that over most of the range the test flash was perceived as a white or colorless patch, but at high intensities—corresponding approximately to section *d*—it appeared green.

In order to test the present hypothesis against these data, we must determine the value of $\Delta A/A$ for observer B and convert the intensities of field and stimulus into absolute units. With regard to the value of $\Delta A/A$, it has already been shown that this is given by the value of $\Delta I/I$ over the linear portion (section *b*) of the plot. From Figure 105, log $(\Delta I/I)$ has the value of $\bar{1}.2$ in section *b*, i.e., $\Delta I/I$ $(= \Delta A/A)$ is 0.16.

According to the present hypothesis, the relation in absolute units between log ΔI and log I for a $\Delta A/A$ of 0.16 is given in Figure 105 (for the equilibrium condition) by the solid-line curve, which trifurcates at the higher field intensities, and (for the "instantaneous flash" condition) by the linear portion of this curve and its linear dashed extension. The trifurcation of the solid-line curve relates to three different assumed values for the regeneration constant *k*, viz. 10^{-4}, 10^{-3}, and 10^{-2} sec^{-1} as indicated in the figure (cf. curves C in Figure 104).

Aguilar & Stiles' experimental data are expressed in scotopic trolands, the hypothetical data in quanta/sec/cm^2. Since both coordinate axes in Figure 105 are scaled logarithmically, the size of the intensity unit is immaterial, but for a comparision of hypothesis with experiment it is necessary to equate the two sets of data at one point. For calculation purposes, one can suppose that in Aguilar & Stiles' experiments both test and field stimuli had been provided by monochromatic light of 507 nm (the maximum of the scotopic visibility curve, and close to the maximum absorbance of human rhodopsin). As these authors point out, "this will not alter our conclusions as far as rod vision is concerned because whatever the energy distribution of a stimulus it will produce the same number of absorbed quanta in the rods as a stimulus of wavelength 507 mμ provided the scotopic intensities of the two stimuli are the same" (1). Aguilar & Stiles calculated that, at an intensity of one scotopic troland, one square degree of field delivered 4.46×10^5 quanta per second into the eye. This being equivalent to an illumination of 5×10^8 quanta/sec./cm^2 of retina, the hypothetical and experimental data have been registered in Figure 105 by making 1 scotopic troland (log $= 0$) equal to 5×10^8 quanta/sec/cm^2 (log $= 8.7$).

This having been done, it is at once apparent from Figure 105 that the present hypothesis does not provide an explanation for the departure of the experimental data (circles) from linearity at high field intensities: the hypothesis would lead one to expect this departure to take place somewhere *between* the solid-line curve (equilibrium condition) and the dashed line (instantaneous-flash condition). As Figure 105 shows, however, the experimental data diverge before the "equilibrium" curve whatever value, within reason, is assumed for *k*, the regeneration constant. Thus, for $k = 10^{-3}\,\text{sec}^{-1}$ the deviation from linearity should commence at the point where about 20 per cent of pigment is bleached (scale at top of Figure 105), whereas the experimental data begin to deviate at about 3 per cent bleached (on this assumed value for k). For higher values of k, the disparity is greater. Moreover, lower values do not help the interpretation, for, if regeneration is very slow, the data should adhere more closely to the instantaneous-flash condition and be linear throughout. In fact, as mentioned earlier, the value of k calculated from Rushton's (25) *in vivo* measurements for human rhodopsin is about $2 \times 10^{-3}\,\text{sec}^{-1}$.

A further divergence of hypothesis from experiment relates to section a, that part of the data in Figure 105 corresponding approximately to the range 0 to 10^{-3} per cent of pigment bleached. This divergence arises because the present hypothesis takes no account of the existence of an absolute threshold: on the contrary, it predicts that the linear portion of unit slope—section b—should extend indefinitely downwards to zero field intensity ($\log = -\infty$).

The hypothesis was developed on the basis that the fraction $\Delta A/A$ is constant, A being the flux absorbed by visual pigment and ΔA the increment of absorption necessary for the perception of a change. The size of ΔA is thus proportional to A (16 per cent of it for observer B), and hence approaches zero as A itself approaches zero, i.e., at very low field intensities. The existence of an absolute threshold implies, however, that the signal ΔA must be of a certain minimum size, and that this requirement overrides at low intensities the requirement that it must be 16 per cent of A.

For the quantitative development of this argument we may start from the first point in Figure 105 for Aguilar & Stiles' observer. This point shows that for a log (field intensity) of 6.02 in absolute units (quanta/sec/cm^2) the log (increment threshold) is 5.88 instead of 5.22, as would be expected on hypothesis (solid line in the figure). Very little pigment is bleached in these regions of low intensity, and the pigment density may be assumed, without appreciable error, to remain at D_{max} ($= 0.1$), at which a fraction around 0.2 of incident light is absorbed. Bearing this in mind, plus the fact that the stimulus light was presented for a period of 0.2 seconds, the increment threshold flux of $10^{5.88}$ quanta incident per sec. per cm^2 corresponds to $4 \times 10^{3.88}$, i.e., 3.0×10^4 quanta absorbed per cm^2. Similarly, the increment threshold flux expected on hypothesis, viz. $10^{5.22}$, corresponds to 0.7×10^4 quanta absorbed per cm^2. The difference between these figures, i.e., 2.3×10^4 quanta absorbed per cm^2, thus represents the difference between hypothesis and experiment. When similar calculations are made for other experimental points near threshold, substantially the same values for the differences from hypothesis are obtained.

The "extra" number of absorbed quanta per cm^2 required for this observer, that is, about 2.3×10^4, corresponds to an *incident* flux of 5.75×10^5 quanta/sec/cm^2 ($\log = 5.76$), and this is close to the experimental value for his log (absolute threshold), namely 5.62 (X in Figure 105). Values for increment thresholds calculated on the assumption that 2.3×10^4 absorbed quanta per cm^2 are required *in addition* to those predicted by hypothesis are shown in Figure 105 by the dashed and dotted curve. This curve merges into the 45° line at about one log unit above absolute threshold, and interprets reasonably the experimental data in this region. The deviation from hypothesis of the data for Aguilar & Stiles' other observers in the near absolute-threshold region can be similarly interpreted. The effect of this amendment on the original hypothesis is to replace the simple concept $\Delta A/A$ = constant by $(\Delta A - T)/A$ = constant, where T, the absolute threshold, is expressed in the same units as ΔA and A.

SUMMARY

When the retina is irradiated by a field of constant intensity and wavelength composition, a state of equilibrium is eventually reached in which the rate of photolysis of visual pigment in the photoreceptors is just balanced by the rate of regeneration. The position of this equilibrium is determined, among other things, by the photosensitivity, the kinetics of regeneration, and the original concentration of the visual pigment. This paper is concerned with the effects of variation in the values of these three parameters on the equilibrium states corresponding to any field.

Experimental data are presented showing that there is little or no variation in the photosensitivities at λ_{max} of different visual pigments, those based on 3-dehydroretinaldehyde ("A_2" pigments) having maximum photosensitivities about 70 per cent of those based on retinaldehyde ("A_1" pigments). On the other hand, the regeneration rates and concentrations (densities in photoreceptors) of pigments, as reported in the literature, are subject to fairly wide variation in different species and different kinds of receptors.

An attempt is then made to interpret Aguilar & Stiles' (1) experimental data for the variation of increment threshold with field intensity for the human scotopic mechanism, and hence to re-assess the value and limitations of the photochemical approach initiated by Hecht (14) more than 40 years ago. For this purpose it is tentatively assumed that an increment threshold corresponds, not to a constant amount of pigment bleached (as Hecht assumed), but to a constant percentage increment of the equilibrium value.

Discussion

Wald: By frequent repetition some things become established in people's minds and in the literature, and I should like to try to clarify Hecht's views concerning the relation between visual thresholds and the concentration of visual pigment. As far as I know, Hecht never assumed that the absolute sensitivity of human vision, i.e., 1/threshold, is proportional to the concentration of visual pigment. There was a period in which he attempted to fit the data of human dark adaptation, cone and rod, on the assumption that the concentration of visual pigment parallels 1/*log* threshold (cf. Hecht, 15). He did not succeed in rationalizing this relationship to his satisfaction, however, and eventually gave it up. After 1934 he never again attempted to fit a theoretical curve to dark-adaptation data. In 1942 he stated his position as follows: "In general, ... human visual dark-adaptation runs roughly parallel with the accumulation of visual purple in the dark-adapting animal retina. Efforts to study this parallelism experimentally have not been successful. ... In fact, even the sensitivity data of human dark-adaptation, though very precise, are still without adequate theoretical treatment in terms of visual purple concentration changes" (21).

As for the human intensity discrimination, beginning in 1934 and thereafter, Hecht went no further than to point out, with great restraint and circumspection, that most of the available data on both rods and cones could be fitted to a photostationary state equation of the form $KI = x^n/(a - x)^m$, in which I is intensity, $(a - x)$ concentration of visual pigment, x the concentration of visual pigment precursors, and K, n, and m are constants.

It was necessary to assume some specific relation between increment threshold, ΔI, and visual pigment concentration; among a variety of possibilities discussed in a long footnote, Hecht decided upon $\Delta I = \text{constant}/(a - x)^m$, on the main basis that this fitted the data best (17).

From the beginning, Hecht found that for cones the best value for the exponents was $m = n = 2$. Lacking adequate data for rods, at first he used the values $m = 1$, $n = 2$ but, as soon as better measurements became available, he set $m = n = 2$ for both rods and cones (19,20).

According to this formulation, therefore, the increment threshold, ΔI, was taken to be inversely proportional to the *square* of the visual pigment concentration, and the Fechner fraction, $\Delta I/I$, was taken to be inversely proportional to x^2, the *square* of the concentration of visual pigment precursors. It should be added that, while Hecht spoke, for mathematical simplicity, as though the precursors of the visual pigments were also the direct products of their bleaching, he pointed out repeatedly that this was not literally true and, indeed, by that time it was known to be untrue.

Some years ago, on the basis of parallelisms with the kinetics of visual pigmen tsynthesis *in vitro* and Rushton's beautiful measurements of the regeneration of human visual pigments *in vivo*, I proposed that in the slow, "photochemical" phase of dark adaptation, the concentration of visual pigment rises as log 1/threshold, or log sensitivity (29,32); this relationship was later established directly with measurements on the rat (11). Over all but the extremes of rhodopsin concentration it is expressed, for the rat, in the equation,

$$1 - (R_t/R_0) = 0.28 \log (I_t/I_0)$$

in which I_0 and R_0 are respectively the threshold and rhodopsin concentration in dark-adapted animals, and I_t and R_t are respectively the thresholds and rhodopsin concentrations during dark adaptation (12).

Dartnall: I can only echo your hopes that this will be cleared up. I thought I was conducting a rescue operation for Hecht.

Wald: Quite right. That is just the point.

Rushton: Dr. Wald had previously made this same protest to me and I sent him a copy of Hecht's 1935 paper (17) in which his theory is clearly set down. What

Dr. Dartnall said Hecht believed is precisely what he said in mathematical terms in that paper, and Dr. Wald had to admit it when he returned my reprint.*

REFERENCES

1. Aguilar, M., and Stiles, W. S., Saturation of the rod mechanism of the retina at high levels of stimulation. *Opt. Acta* (London), 1954, **1**: 59–65.
2. Bartlett, N. R., Thresholds as dependent on some energy relations and characteristics of the subject. In: *Vision and Visual Perception* (C. H. Graham, Ed.). Wiley, New York, 1965: 154–184.
3. ———, Dark adaptation and light adaptation. *Ibid.*: 185–207.
4. Brown, J. L., and Mueller, C. G., Brightness discrimination and brightness contrast. *Ibid.*: 208–250.
5. Dartnall, H. J. A., The spectral variation of the relative photosensitivities of some visual pigments. In: *Visual Problems of Colour*, Vol. 1 (National Physical Laboratory Symposium No. 8). H.M. Stationery Office, London, 1958: 121–146.
6. Dartnall, H. J. A., and Goodeve, C. F., Scotopic luminosity curve and the absorption spectrum of visual purple. *Nature* (London), 1937, **139**: 409–411.
7. Dartnall, H. J. A., Goodeve, C. F., and Lythgoe, R. J., The quantitative analysis of the photochemical bleaching of visual purple solutions in monochromatic light. *Proc. Roy. Soc. London A*, 1936, **156**: 158–170.
8. ———, The effect of temperature on the photochemical bleaching of visual purple solutions. *Proc. Roy. Soc. London A*, 1938, **164**: 216–230.
9. Denton, E. J., and Warren, F. J., The photosensitive pigments in the retinae of deep-sea fish. *J. Mar. Biol. Ass. UK*, 1957, **36**: 651–662.
10. Denton, E. J., and Wyllie, J. H., Study of the photosensitive pigments in the pink and green rods of the frog. *J. Physiol.* (London), 1955, **127**: 81–89.
11. Dowling, J. E., and Wald, G., Vitamin A deficiency and night blindness. *Proc. Nat. Acad. Sci. USA*, 1958, **44**: 648–661.
12. ———, The biological function of vitamin A acid. *Proc. Nat. Acad. Sci. USA*, 1960, **46**: 587–608.
13. Fechner, G. T., Ueber ein wichtiges psychophysische Grundgesetz zur Schätzung der Sterngrössen. *Abhandl. sächs. Ges. Wissensch. Math.-Phys. Klasse*, 1858, **4**: 457.
14. Hecht, S., Intensity discrimination and the stationary state. *J. Gen. Physiol.*, 1924, **6**: 355–373.

* *Dr. Wald's note after the Conference:* I did have a letter from Dr. Rushton on March 18, 1964, explaining that, when he said Hecht claimed that when the background had raised the increment threshold ΔI to twice the absolute (threshold) value of ΔI_0, then the bleaching x was 50 per cent, he based that statement on Hecht's equation discussed above, $\Delta I = \text{constant}/(a - x)^m$ (17). It is true that, lacking adequate data for rods, Hecht tried $m = 1$ for them in that paper, although he set $m = 2$ for cones. Shortly afterward, on the basis of better data for rods, he set $m = 2$ for them also (19,20).

Dr. Rushton's note after the Conference: After the meeting Dr. Wald spoke to me, and it immediately became clear that our disagreement was due to a misunderstanding. The eye adapts in two different ways: (*a*) to the presence of a background, and (*b*) to the effects of recent pigment bleaching—as I have set out at length in my formal contribution to this symposium (see pages 257–280). Dr. Dartnall was referring exclusively to *a*, and Hecht's views on *a* are exactly as he quoted; on the other hand, Dr. Wald was referring to *b* and what he said about *b* was correct, but it did not apply to Dr. Dartnall's communication.

15. Hecht, S., Zur Photochemie des Sehens *Naturwissenschaften*, 1925, **13**: 66–72.
16. ———, Vision II. The nature of the photoreceptor process. In: *Handbook of General Experimental Psychology* (C. Murchison, Ed.). Clark Univ. Press, Worcester, 1934: 704–828.
17. ———, A theory of visual intensity discrimination. *J. Gen. Physiol.*, 1935, **18**: 767–789.
18. ———, The instantaneous visual threshold after light adaptation. *Proc. Nat. Acad. Sci. USA*, 1937, **23**: 227–233.
19. ———, Rods, cones, and the chemical basis of vision. *Physiol. Rev.*, 1937, **17**: 239–290.
20. ———, The nature of the visual process. *Harvey Lect.*, 1937–38, **33**: 35–64.
21. ———, The chemistry of visual substances. *Ann. Rev. Biochem.*, 1942, **11**: 465–496.
22. Koenig, A., and Brodhun, E., Experimentelle Untersuchungen über die psychophysische Fundamentalformel in Bezug auf den Gesichtssinn. *Sitzungber. Akad. Wissensch.*, 1889, **27**: 641–644.
23. Rushton, W. A. H., The intensity factor in vision. In: *Light and Life* (W. D. McElroy and B. Glass, Eds.). Johns Hopkins Press, Baltimore, 1961: 706–723.
24. ———, Colour blindness and cone pigments. *Am. J. Optom.*, 1964, **41**: 265–282.
25. ———, Visual adaptation. *Proc. Roy. Soc. London B*, 1965, **162**: 20–46.
26. Rushton, W. A. H., Campbell, P. W., Hagins, W. A., and Brindley, G. S., The bleaching and regeneration of rhodopsin in the living eye of the albino rabbit and of man. *Opt. Acta* (London), 1955, **1**: 183–190.
27. Stiles, W. S., Visual factors in lighting. *Illum. Engr.*, 1954, **49**: 77–92.
28. ———, Adaptation, chromatic adaptation, colour transformation. *An. Real Soc. Esp. Fis. Quím.*, 1961, **57**: 149–175.
29. Wald, G., Retinal chemistry and the physiology of vision. In: *Visual Problems of Colour*, Vol. I (National Physical Laboratory Symp. No. 8). H.M. Stationery Office, London, 1958: 7–61.
30. Wald, G., and Brown, P. K., The molar extinction of rhodopsin. *J. Gen. Physiol.*, 1953, **37**: 189–200.
31. Wald, G., Brown, P. K., and Kennedy, D., The visual system of the alligator. *J. Gen. Physiol.*, 1957, **40**: 703–713.
32. Wald, G., Brown, P. K., and Smith, P. H., Iodopsin. *J. Gen. Physiol.*, 1955, **38**: 623–681.
33. Weale, R. A., Photochemical reactions in the living cat's retina. *J. Physiol.* (London), 1953, **122**: 322–331.
34. ———, Observations on photochemical reactions in living eyes. *Brit. J. Ophthal.*, 1957, **41**: 461–474.
35. ———, Photo-chemical changes in the dark-adapting human retina. *Vision Res.*, 1962, **2**: 25–33.
36. Wright, W. D., *Researches on Normal and Defective Colour Vision*. Kimpton, London, 1946.

LIGHT AND DARK ADAPTATION OF THE RETINA

WILLIAM A. H. RUSHTON
Cambridge University
Cambridge, England

Everyone is familiar with visual adaptation in two different aspects, one very convenient and one very inconvenient. The convenient aspect is the eye's automatic adjustment to the general level of illumination so as to keep contrast and, indeed, nearly all aspects of appearance unchanged though the actual light energies may alter some thousandfold. This allows an enormous range of input energies (some billionfold, 10^9) to be automatically scaled down to a range that the neural processing mechanisms can handle. And since the input to the brain is nearly identical, appearance learned at one level of illumination can immediately be recognized at another level.

The inconvenient aspect is experienced when, after adaptation to strong light, we go into very dim surroundings, e.g., from sunlight into a darkened theatre. At first we are nearly blind and we only recover full sensitivity after 15–30 minutes.

It is obvious that these two kinds of adaptation are very different. The first, which may be called "adaptation to backgrounds", since it depends upon the general background illumination, follows rapidly the change in illumination. When the sun pops in and out of clouds or extra lights are switched on or off in a room, the eye adapts to the change of illumination in a second or so. The other kind, which may be called "adaptation to bleaching", since it depends upon the fraction of visual pigment in the bleached state, changes very much more slowly, for it is tied to the tedious regeneration of bleached pigments in the rods and cones. We shall now try to form some idea of what is going on in the retina when the eye adapts, and we start with background adaptation in rod vision.

Background Adaptation in Rod Vision

According to the well-known photochemical theory of Hecht (17), a steady background produces some degree of steady bleaching, and thus by removing rhodopsin from the rods it lowers their capacity to catch light and be excited. This view was already discredited when in 1956 (22), by measuring the actual rate of bleaching of rhodopsin in man, I was able to show Hecht's theory in error by a factor of a million. Today no one believes that a weak background that raises the rod threshold threefold has bleached away two-thirds of the pigment—nor indeed any detectable fraction. But the fact remains that this background has raised the threshold three times, and the question is, how does it do it?

What the background does is to rain quanta upon the rod population, and we may well suppose that after some exposure all the rods are sufficiently "quantum sodden" to be substantially changed in sensitivity. It is easy to find how sodden the rods are when the threshold is raised threefold. In an experiment (31) designed to measure this, the background was presented for two seconds and a flash was added to it at the end of the first second and was extinguished with the background one second later. The background luminance was adjusted to raise the rod threshold three times and was measured by ordinary photometry. Knowing the size of the subject's pupil (in the dark) and taking the usual figure (23) that 10 per cent of quanta ($\lambda = 500$ nm) entering the pupil are absorbed by the rods, we easily calculate the total number of quanta caught by the average rod during the two-second exposure. It was less than one per cent. The rods, then, were not very quantum-sodden, for only one in a hundred caught a single quantum. The other 99 could not have "seen" that there was a background there at all, for they did not absorb a single quantum from it. But it was the threshold of those 99 that was raised by the background. If only the one per cent were changed, then, even if their threshold was raised to infinity, the background would remove no more than one per cent from the population and hence change the general threshold by one per cent. But the general threshold was in fact raised not by 1 but by 300 per cent, hence the threshold of the 99 must have been raised threefold. How did those 99 who did not "see" the background know that it was there? They must have been told by the one per cent who saw it.

What is this language of the rods? It seems to be the simplest kind of telegraphic communication. We know from the famous experiments of Hecht, Shlaer & Pirenne (18) that in the fully dark-adapted state a rod can be excited by the catch of a single quantum, and can send a signal to the summation pool (which is probably the ganglion cell) where similar signals from other rods are collected. We know also that a near coincidence of some five to ten signals is required for the light to be *seen*—as though five to ten signals must summate at the ganglion in order to excite it to the point of firing an impulse up the optic nerve.

Now, in the experiment where the background raised the threshold threefold, we have seen that 99 per cent of the rods did not catch a single quantum. Hence those rods themselves must have remained completely dark-adapted, and thus in a state to respond by a signal to each quantum caught from the test flash. But this flash had to be raised threefold to be seen. We thus learn that the effect of background adaptation is to raise the signal requirement of the ganglion from 5 to 15. This might be because the ganglion was desensitized or because the signals were reduced in size by adaptation. Since the electroretinogram (ERG) in the rat is similarly reduced by backgrounds in conditions where ganglia have undergone degeneration,* it is fairly plain that adaptation reduces the size of signal. We thus conclude that there is a special retinal organization, the *adaptation pools*, with the

* Dowling, Easter and Dubin, unpublished data.

following properties: they collect signals from those rods which catch quanta from the background and in some way modify the conducting paths from *all* rods to ganglia in their domain so that the unit signal is reduced in size. In the foregoing experiment, all the rod signals were reduced to one-third, so that three times as many were needed to excite the ganglion, and the threshold was raised threefold. If this idea is correct a remarkable prediction follows.

If, instead of being uniform, the background were made up of alternate bright and dark stripes—a grating of period 1/2° (see inset, Figure 106), and if the test flash presented upon this background were also striped in the same way, then the test might fall upon the background *in-phase* as at (*a*), where bright stripes fall on bright and dark on dark, or the arrangement might be out-of-phase as at (*b*) (Figure 106). If the effect of the background were to desensitize the *rods* exposed to it, it would be chiefly the rods under the bright bars that would be desensitized, and hence the threshold would be far higher for arrangement (*a*) than for (*b*). But, if the adaptation pools collected signals from a region 1/2° in extent and reduced the signals equally over all this region, then phase would not affect the result. The coincidence of black and white circles in the experimental results of Figure 106 shows that over a thousandfold range of background luminances the

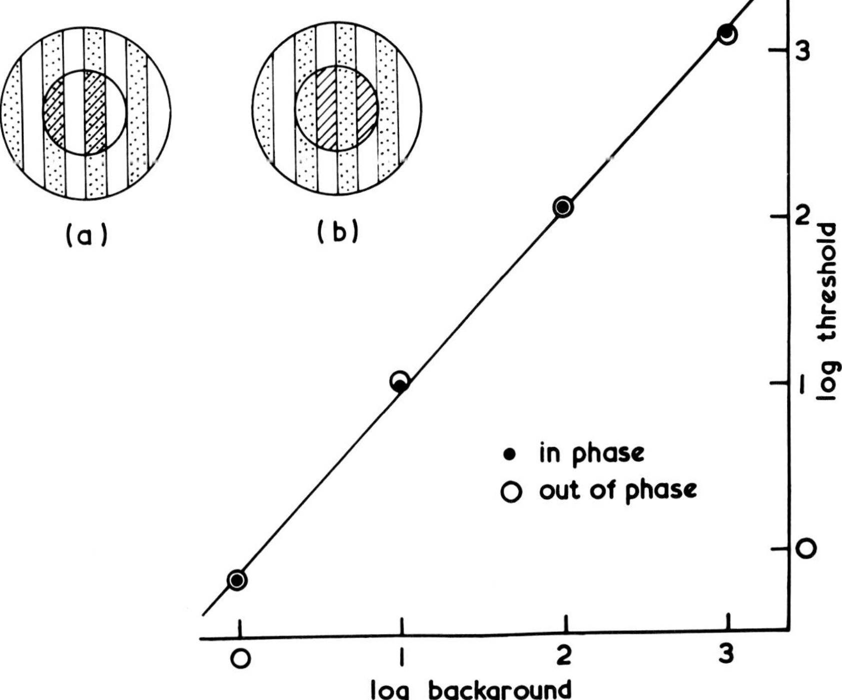

Figure 106. Inset striped background, $\frac{1}{4}$° bright bar, $\frac{1}{4}$° dark bar (dotted). Test flash is similarly striped (dark brown shaded); (*a*) in-phase, (*b*) out-of-phase. Graph plots log increment threshold for rods against log background luminance for a 1000-fold range, well above the absolute threshold. In-phase thresholds (black circles) coincide with out-of-phase thresholds (white circles).

log threshold for in-phase and out-of-phase flashes is the same. The experimental details are given in the original paper (31), but it may be remarked that measurements were made with the stripes stabilized upon the retina so that involuntary eye movements should not smudge the crispness of the grating.

Experiments by Barlow and Martin on man and Easter* on ganglion cells in the retina of goldfish indicate that the exact coincidence of white and black circles in Figure 106 is too perfect. Probably, adaptation is slightly stronger for in-phase than for out-of-phase tests. Thus the influence of adaptation pools in reducing signal size, which certainly does not spread with equal force right across the retina, is slightly stronger at the center of the pool than at 1/2° away.

Conclusion. Every quantum caught by a rod generates a signal, and the ganglion is excited by a quantity proportional to the sum total of these signals within certain space-time limits. But the proportional factor is not constant: it is regulated by adaptation pools. These receive the whole flux of signals and regulate their size so as to constitute more or less of an automatic gain control (A.G.C.). Such a mechanism keeps the output at a fairly constant level and yet preserves the contrast of neighboring regions.

Bleaching Adaptation in Rod Vision

The usual way to measure bleaching adaptation is to plot the dark-adaptation curve. One such curve is shown in Figure 107, taken from Craik & Vernon (10). It is obtained as follows. After a strong illumination, where some visual pigment is bleached, the threshold is measured at various times in the dark. The dark-adaptation curve plots the log threshold against the time in the dark, and in general consists of two branches. The upper, earlier branch is due to cones, for it is present when text flashes fall entirely upon the fovea; this branch shows the spectral sensitivity of photopic vision (= mixed cones). The later and lower branch is due to rods, for it is absent from the fovea, and has the spectral sensitivity of scotopic vision and of rhodopsin.

As is well known, the actual value of the threshold depends on the parameters of the test light used—its wavelength, duration and area, for instance. It might have been hoped that changes in these parameters would simply change the unit of test energy, that is to say, on the logarithmic plot of Figure 107 each branch of the upper curve (10′) should coincide with that of the lower (17°) after a suitable vertical shift. It is obvious, however, that no such coincidence is possible, for the curves are entirely different in shape. Now, a change in the shape of the curve as a result of different *areas* of test cannot represent any effect upon individual rods; it must be an effect upon the rod community. So, we see that one very important aspect of dark adaptation is a change in the organization of the rod population.

It is a striking fact that in the 20 years that followed Craik & Vernon's publication (Figure 107), nearly all the interpretations of dark adaptation followed the dogma of the photochemical theory, according to which the course of the curve

---

* Unpublished data.

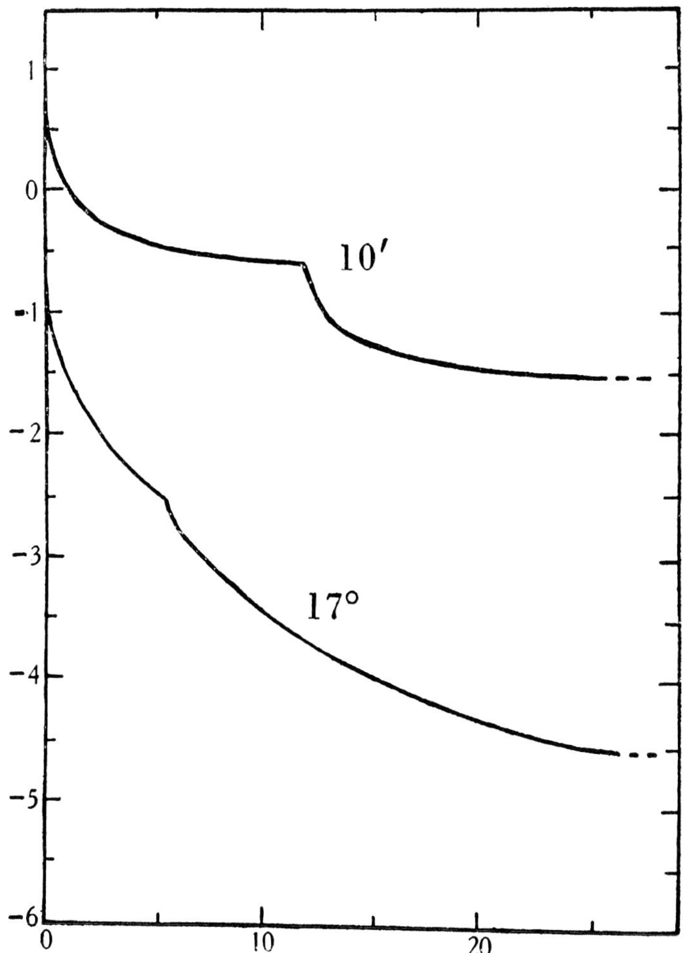

Figure 107. Dark-adaptation-curves taken with 10′ and 17° test fields. (From Craik & Vernon, 10.)

depended simply upon the course of rhodopsin regeneration. The fact that the curve following the same regeneration is so very different with different kinds of tests was seldom referred to. If considered at all, it was pushed aside as a minor parasitic phenomenon. This was a remarkable attitude, for not only is the easily verifiable fact of Figure 107 no minor matter, but there was no evidence whatever in favor of the dogma that dark adaptation was tied to the regeneration of visual pigments. Nor was there any settled view as to what the relation of pigment to threshold was supposed to be. Wald, for instance, in one paper (40) claims that threshold is inversely as the amount of pigment present, and in another (41) that it is an exponential function of the amount absent; in neither case is any objective evidence given to support his conjecture.

The realization that adaptation to bleaching operates through a change in retinal organization reminds us that adaptation to backgrounds operates in this way also, and prompts the questions, "What would be the result of repeating the grating experiment using striped bleachings and tests? Is the in-phase threshold the same as the out-of-phase threshold?" Exactly this experiment has not been done, but Westheimer and I (32) carried out a modification from which the answer can be obtained.

The bleaching was produced by a powerful electronic flash focused upon the dilated pupil. Interposed in the beam was a grating whose image was formed sharply on the retina. Consequently, the result of the flash was to bleach the retina in stripes separated by regions nearly unbleached, the afterimage of the grating being seen crisp. A second retinal region was bleached by the same total amount of light, but spread evenly over the bleached area. The two bleaching fields are shown by the larger circles of the inset in Figure 108. To make the tests comparable, a grating was interposed in the test flash that fell upon the uniformly bleached retina and a uniform flash was presented upon the stripe-bleached region.

On the photochemical theory, the nearly unbleached strips should contain rods of nearly full sensitivity, thus the test flash falling on the stripe-bleached area

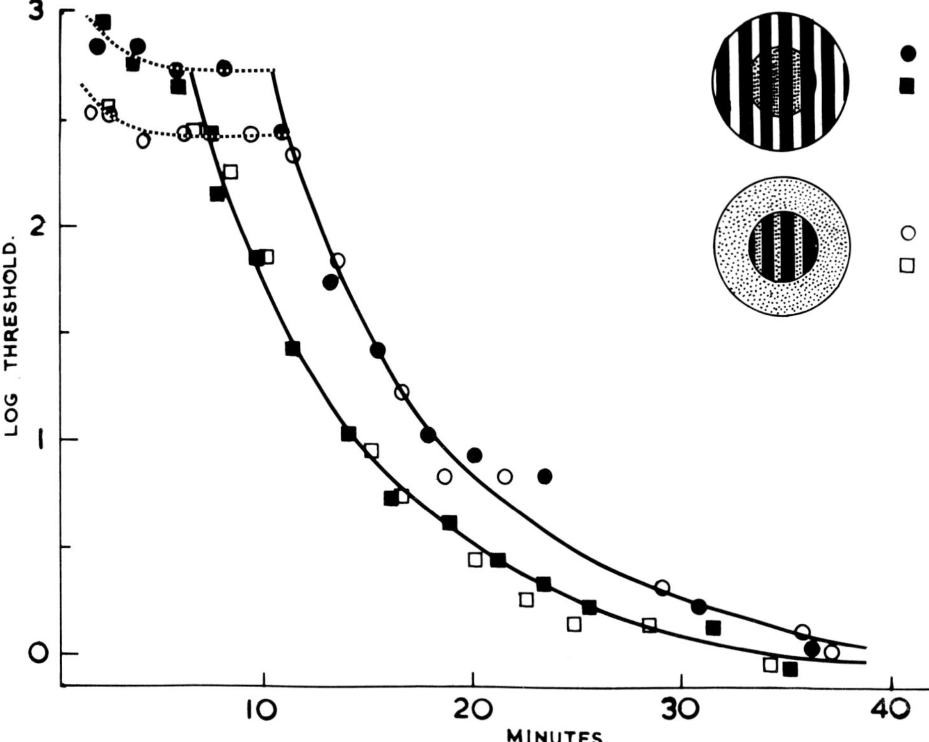

Figure 108. Large circles (inset) show retinal regions bleached by stripes (above) or by a uniform field receiving the same total light (below). Small circles indicate test flash, striped (below) and uniform (above). Black symbols plot dark adaptation with striped bleach, white symbols with uniform bleach. The bleaching light was three times as strong with circles as with squares. Since squares coincide with squares, and circles with circles, but not squares with circles, the threshold depends upon the extent of the total bleach, but not on its retinal distribution (within about 1°).

would be detected by these spared rods at low threshold. But the uniformly bleached area spares no rods, and the thresholds of every one must be raised substantially. Thus the photochemical theory of Hecht and Wald leads to the expectation that the threshold will be raised much less after stripe-bleaching than after bleaching with the same light energy evenly spread over the retina. Consider now an alternative possibility: that the threshold is simply raised for all channels by the total flux of "bleaching signals" that reach the adaptation pools. Then, since the total bleaching light was the same in the two cases, the flux of "bleaching signals" to the adaptation pools would be nearly the same, and hence the threshold would be expected to be raised about equally in the two cases. Consequently, we can distinguish between (*a*) the desensitization of rods by quanta that fall on them, and (*b*) a change in effectiveness organized by the *adaptation pools*, by seeing whether in the experiments of Figure 108 the threshold with striped background is the same as with uniform background, or much lower. Black and white squares show the two comparable thresholds from one experiment, and black and white circles from another where the bleaching light was three times as strong. It is plain that the two comparable thresholds are nearly equal, thus bleaching adaptation depends only upon the total bleach in the area, and not upon the particular rods bleached or tested. This is precisely what was found in background adaptation and it is natural to ask, "Are the adaptation pools the same in the two cases and do they act in the same way?"

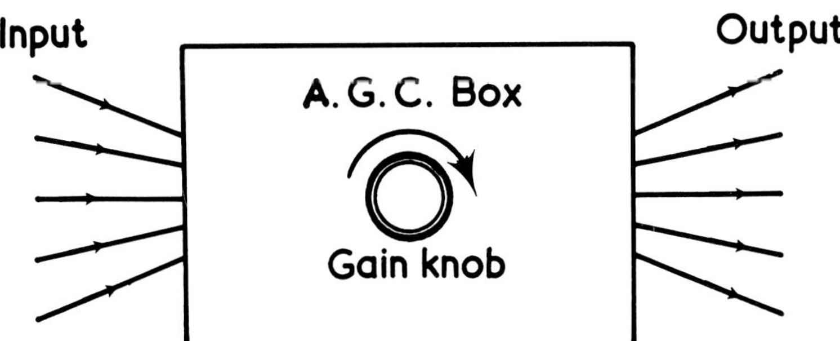

Figure 109. Adaptation pools represented as an Automatic Gain Control (A.G.C.) Box with only one knob to control the entire set of input-output relations, illustrating the *monoparametric* nature of adaptation.

As early as 1932, Stiles & Crawford (38), in a paper of remarkable penetration, tested and substantiated a very important property of adaptation that I shall describe in terms of the model of Figure 109. In this, the adaptation pools are represented by an automatic gain control box with various kinds of input and various kinds of output, but only *one* gain knob. The knob is operated automatically by the action of the inputs, which may be supposed to affect it some more, some less powerfully. For any one position of the knob there is a fixed array of input-output relations and a change in knob position results in a characteristic change in them all.

Now, the adaptation produced by some uniform background may readily be changed over a large range by changing the steady background luminance I. For each I-value, the gain knob of the model will assume some appropriate setting, and all the input-output relations will be modified correspondingly. Thus a very convenient way to specify the "position" of the gain knob in any condition of adaptation is by the value of the background luminance I where the adaptation is the same. Since *all* input-output relations will then be the same, it is necessary to use only one test (for instance, the threshold for the detection of some given flash) in order to find the corresponding I-value. In this way we calibrate the gain knob by affixing a scale of I-values—the *equivalent background* luminances. So, if we wish to specify what is the knob setting corresponding to some stage of dark adaptation at time t after a certain bleaching procedure, all that we have to do is find the threshold at this moment and then (after full recovery) find the background I against which the threshold is the same, using similar test flashes in both cases. The important principle of "*equivalent background of bleaching*" is thus a particular consequence of the more general *monoparametic* nature of adaptation, and is the one that Stiles & Crawford (38) were principally concerned to establish. A well known and very striking example of equivalent background of bleaching is Crawford's (11) demonstration that, no matter what area of test flash was used, the equivalent background in a given state of dark adaptation was always the same. Figure 110 (6) shows the same thing measured on a rod-monochromat in whom cones do not enter to complicate the picture, and where (unlike Crawford's example) the bleaching was substantial.

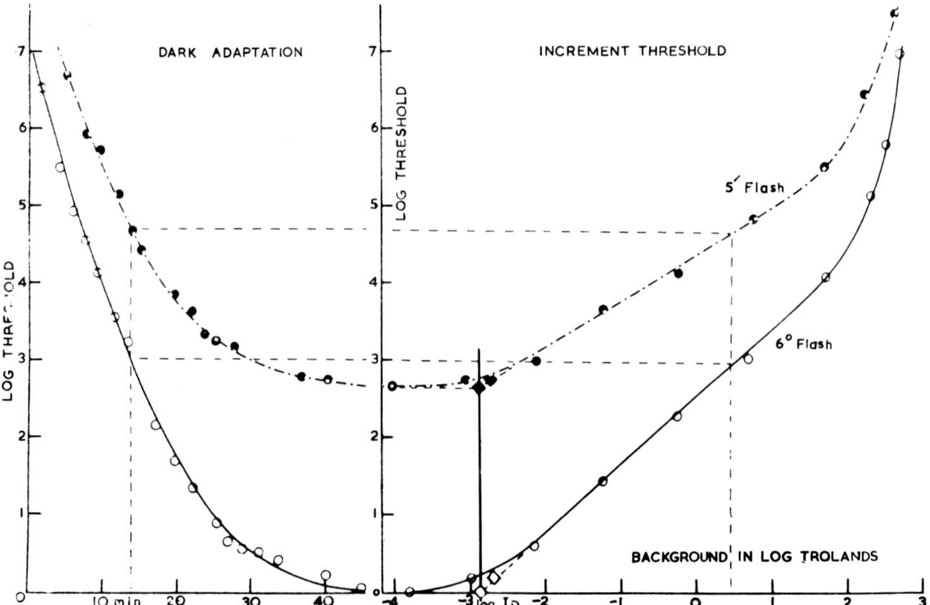

Figure 110. *Left:* Dark-adaptation curves. *Right:* Increment threshold curves. Black circles indicate when the test flash subtended 5′, white circles when it subtended 6°.

The left side of Figure 110 shows dark-adaptation curves taken following the same bleaching exposure when the test flash was either a large "moon" subtending 6° (white circles) or a "star" (black circles) subtending 5′. In confirmation of Figure 107, the white circles give a much larger range of dark adaptation. The principle of equivalent background is shown by the increment threshold curves on the right, obtained with the same test flashes. As the horizontal dotted lines emphasize, the threshold at 14 minutes of recovery is the same as when a background of 0.5 log trolands is present, no matter what the size of test flash. We may therefore say that, in this experiment, 0.5 is the equivalent log background of the bleaching that was still present after 14 minutes of regeneration.

CONCLUSION. Bleaching does not affect the capacity of rods to convert caught quanta into signals but, through the adaptation pools, it reduces the size of those conducted signals. Thus we may say, "In all conditions (up to rod saturation) each quantum caught generates a signal." The adaptation pools reduce the signals after bleaching, just as they do in the presence of a luminous background (the equivalent background of bleaching). But there remains this problem: With backgrounds it is plain that the input to the adaptation pools is the flux of light signals; what is the input that continues so long after the bleaching light has been extinguished?

THE REGENERATION OF RHODOPSIN

At a time when it was fashionable to "explain" biological behavior in terms of mass-action-kinetics in chain reactions of unspecified chemicals, it was a clear, bold step of Hecht's to name rhodopsin as the chemical to whose fate he would tie adaptation. That made his theory alive, because vulnerable, and of its wounds it died. He saw that background adaptation and bleaching adaptation could not *both* depend simply on the rhodopsin level, and he chose background adaptation as the kind directly linked. The guess was unfortunate, for it was a millionfold wrong; bleaching adaptation would have turned out better.

If we are to leave guesswork and actually observe whether rhodopsin regeneration does or does not proceed hand in hand with dark adaptation, we naturally need measurements of two kinds—of the rhodopsin level in the adapting eye and of its visual sensitivity. In 1931, Tansley (39) measured the regeneration of rhodopsin in living rats under standard conditions. But it was 30 years later that Dowling (13) combined this with simultaneous determinations of their ERG threshold and showed for the first time that log threshold (ERG) was proportional to the fraction of rhodopsin still in the bleached state. The following year I (25) was able to demonstrate that the same relation applies to the visual threshold in man. Measurement of the level of rhodopsin in man needs a special equipment that Campbell and I (9) had designed and built five years earlier. It uses the principle of the ophthalmoscope, but the light reflected from the eye goes to a photocell instead of to an ophthalmologist. Since this light has been twice through the retina, it must suffer absorption in the visual pigments there, and the more the pigment present, the greater the absorption. By analyzing the output from the photocell it is possible to measure the amount of rhodopsin in the rods at any stage of bleaching and adaptation.

Our measurements showed that rhodopsin was not bleached away nearly as completely by daylight as had been generally supposed. For instance, when the dilated pupil was exposed indefinitely to the (English) summer sky, only about 50 per cent was bleached. Though we were surprised at this result, it turns out to be about what is to be expected if rhodopsin in the rods is as photosensitive as Dartnall, Goodeve & Lythgoe (12) found it to be in solution, taking into account the observed rate of regeneration. When in the course of dark adaptation the rod branch first appears below the level of the cones, rhodopsin has regenerated some 92 per cent; so, if the ordinary rod dark-adaptation curve is related to the regeneration of rhodopsin, it must relate to this final 8 per cent.

Thus, though in 1955 we showed that the exponential regeneration of rhodopsin had about the same time-course as the exponential dark-adaptation curve, we could not then go so far as to say that log threshold was proportional to the fraction of pigment still bleached. For in the range where the pigment was well measured,

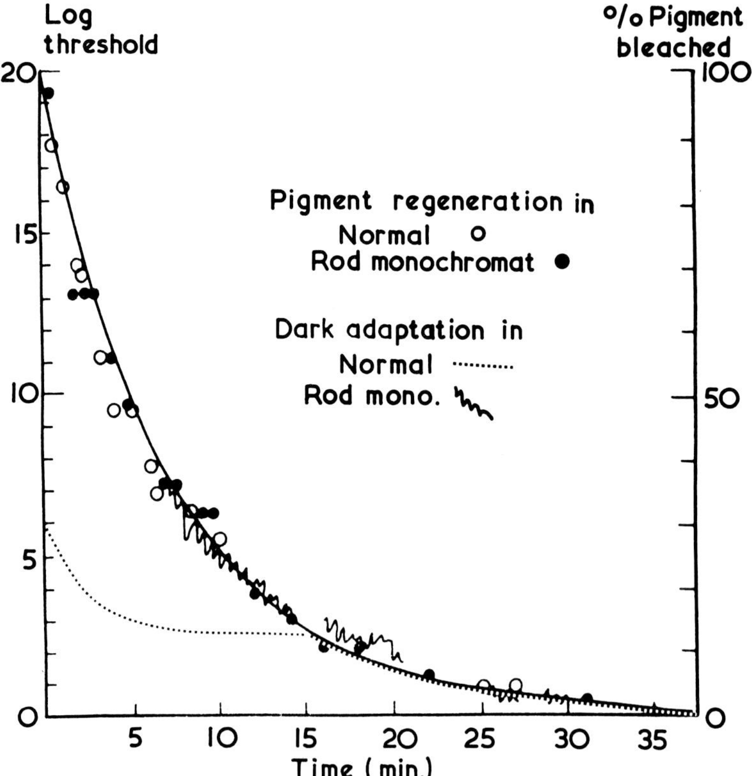

Figure 111. Dark-adaptation curves (scale on left) and regeneration of rhodopsin (percentage still bleached on right) following a full bleaching exposure. White circles: pigment in normal; black circles: in rod monochromat. Irregular tracing, self-recording of dark adaptation (over 6 log units) in rod monochromat. Dotted curve indicates the normal cone and rod branches.

the rod threshold was inaccessible—far above the level of the cones, and where the threshold was well measured there was less than 8 per cent of bleaching left for all comparisons. This difficulty was overcome by making observations upon a rod-monochromat, a subject who had in fact a few foveal cones with which she could fixate adequately, but none outside the fovea to screen the early rod threshold (25). Figure 111 shows the irregular line by which she traced out her dark-adaptation curve (with some short rests). The rod dark-adaptation curve is seen to run a course over six log units of threshold, and coincides throughout with the black circles that plot the regeneration of rhodopsin in her eye. White circles plot the regeneration in the (normal) eye of a subject whose dark-adaptation curve is indicated by the dotted curve that represents cones until, at 16 minutes, it joins the other and thereafter runs with it. It is plain that this result confirms for the visual threshold in man what Dowling found with the ERG threshold in rats. Namely that the log threshold is proportional to the amount of free opsin, that is, rhodopsin still in the bleached state.

The Free Opsin Signal

Though this result is a highly eligible bride, she is not very easy to marry to the Lord of the Adaptation Pools. He sits in the nerve center that we have called the adaptation pool and controls the signal size; she sits in the rods and controls him. How does she do it? Her influence spreads far beyond the pools, it reaches to the pupil of the other eye and also to the sensorium which I suppose is in the brain.

Alpern & Campbell (1) bleached the right eye and measured the size of the left pupil during the next half hour. Over this time the pupil dilated very gradually, keeping pace apparently with the equivalent background of bleaching in the contralateral eye. They proved that the signals which kept the left pupil constricted came from the right eye that had been bleached, for when the circulation to that eye was arrested by pressure on the eyeball which temporarily blinded it, the other pupil suddenly dilated to its full dark value. Removal of pressure allowed nerve messages to flow again from the bleached eye, and with their passage the other pupil constricted again. Clearly, messages from the bleached rods go to the other eye to tell it about the equivalent background brightness. What brightness is that? It appears to be the afterimage!

The afterimage is stabilized upon the retina, and like all stabilized images tends to fade away, so we underestimate its true equivalent luminance. Barlow & Sparrock (5) matched the afterimage against an external luminance whose image was stabilized contiguously upon the retina. The striking result they found can easiest be expressed by saying that the threshold during dark adaptation is raised by exactly the amount that the increment threshold is raised by a background equal in brightness to the afterimage. So, we are tempted to say that it is the brightness of the afterimage which raises the threshold during the course of dark adaptation, for the threshold is raised by just the amount that fits that brightness. Unfortunately this pretty explanation is not correct. Though it fits this particular example it fails in others. There is a more satisfactory alternative.

The Feedback Entry

In my Ferrier Lecture to the Royal Society (29) I presented a mathematical treatment of the input-output relations of the A.G.C. box in equilibrium conditions. I will now give a simplified approximation that will suffice to distinguish between the proposals of H. B. Barlow and of A. L. Hodgkin. We shall consider only backgrounds sufficiently strong for the Weber-Fechner relation $\Delta I = kI$ to hold, and bleachings where the equivalent background lies in this range. Figure 112 indicates an A.G.C. box where the feedback mechanism is such that, when the input is proportional to I the output V is proportional to its logarithm. Then, as Fechner (16) pointed out a century ago, if

$$V = \ln I$$
$$\Delta V = \Delta I/I$$

Thus, if the condition for threshold is that some fixed increment of output ΔV_0 must be generated, the ΔI that does this will be $(\Delta V_0)I$, the observed Weber Law.

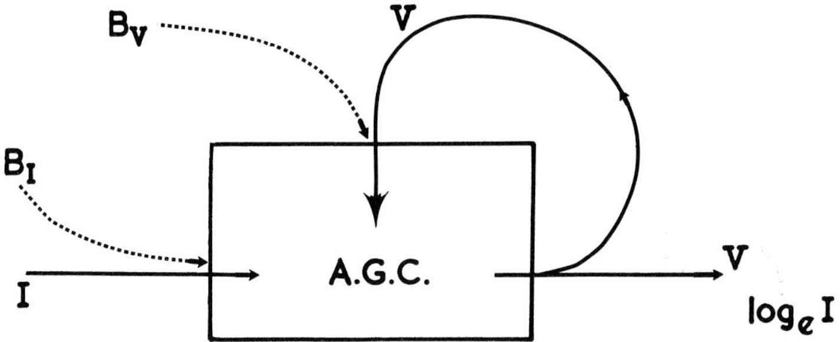

Figure 112. Scheme of Automatic Gain Control Box where input I is transformed into an output V that is $\ln I$, which constitutes a parametric feedback. The bleaching signal might enter as B_I with I (according to Barlow) or as B_V with V (according to Hodgkin).

So much for background adaptation. Bleaching adaptation might occur by the "free opsin" signal B entering with I at input as Barlow has proposed (4), or entering with V by the feedback, as Hodgkin has suggested to me. Now, the experimental fact is that the bleached fraction B is related to threshold, or rather to the "equivalent background" I that is proportional to it, approximately by

$$aB = \ln I \qquad [1]$$

However, as shown in Figure 112, $\ln I$ is the output V, so we see that a signal proportional to B, the fraction of rhodopsin bleached, gets to the feedback and changes the gain. According to Hodgkin's suggestion, the B_V signal goes there directly and B_V is proportional to B. According to Barlow, the B_I signal enters with I and hence must suffer a logarithmic transform before entering the feedback as a signal proportional to B. The input that will do this is of course the antilog of B, and Barlow has to postulate that the signal generated by bleaching is proportional to antilog B, so that by the time it enters the feedback the log of the antilog will be B again. Obviously, it is more direct to suggest with Hodgkin that the B signal enters the feedback direct with no such self-neutralizing transformations. However, what seems the obvious and direct mechanism in biology is not always what actually occurs. An experiment (28) that combines the results of the two grating experiments considered in Figures 106 and 108 goes a long way to decide between the two suggestions.

Figure 106 shows that whether the background stripes were in-phase or out-of-phase with the test made no difference to the threshold. Only the total signal flux from the background signified, not the distribution. And, in fact, that experiment was extended to include the case where the background was uniform but of half the luminance, so again the total signal flux was the same; the threshold in that case was found also to be the same. Turning now to the experiment of Figure 108, it was found (to close approximation) that the log threshold was raised by bleaching in proportion to the total amount of rhodopsin bleached (in the area exposed), independent of its distribution. In other words, the feedback input receives a signal that is the same whether uniform or from an array of stripes with zero bleaching and double bleaching. This is what would be expected on Hodgkin's view, where B_V (Figure 112) is proportional to bleaching. For, if with a uniform bleach the feedback signal is B_V, with the equivalent striped bleach it will be $\frac{1}{2}(0 + 2B_V)$, which is also B_V—as observed.

This, however, would not follow from Barlow's view, in which the uniform bleach generates an input signal according to the anti-logarithmic relation $B_I = e^{aB}$, and the equivalent striped bleach generates $B_I = \frac{1}{2}(0 + e^{2aB})$. These two expressions are far from identical and predict non-equivalence of bleachings where experimentally equivalence is found. Consequently, the experiments of Figures 106 and 108 show that Hodgkin's view fits the facts, but Barlow's does not.

Figure 113 shows the results of an experiment (28) that combines the two procedures just described. Instead of a 1:1 grating, a perforated plate was interposed in the background or the bleaching. As a result, the background appeared formed of a regular array of bright stars that occupied one-third the area, two-thirds being dark. Similarly, such a starry array was seen in the after-image when the plate was interposed in the electronic bleaching flash. From the stabilized image experiments it would be expected that the interposition of the perforated plate, which reduced the flux of signals to one-third, would act like a one-third reduction in the background luminance, a reduction by about 0.5 log unit (log 3 = 0.48). In Figure 113 the results on the right confirm this expectation, for when the plate was interposed the results changed from black circles to white, a drop of 0.5 in the whole of the Fechner line. In this experiment, the background was not stabilized but, if (as we have seen) the effect depends upon the total quantum catch and not (much) upon who catches it, stabilization should make no difference. We may now turn to the left of Figure 113 and, granted C, the dark-adaptation curve with no plate interposed, we may predict the results of interposition upon the expectations of Barlow (D) and Hodgkin (E).

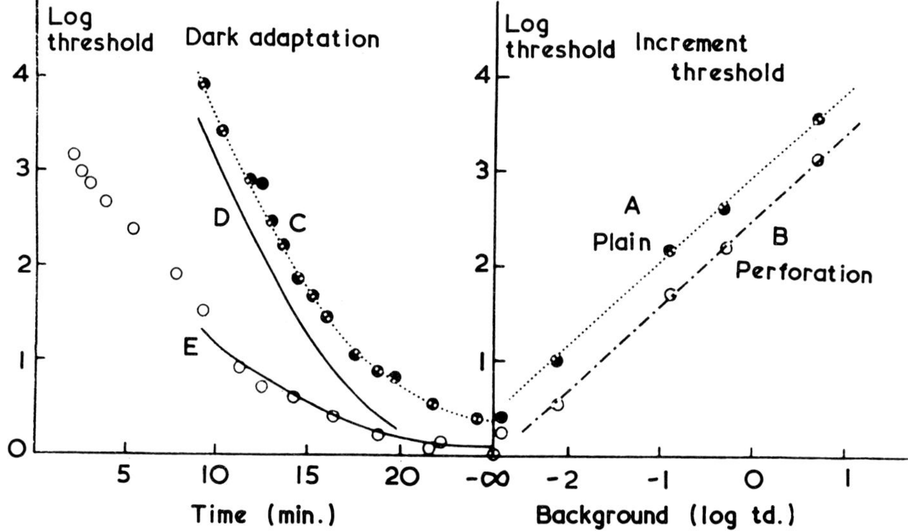

Figure 113. Curve A: Log increment threshold obtained by usual methods. B: Same as A, except that the background was reduced by interposing a perforated plate that blocked $\frac{2}{3}$ of the total background area. C: An ordinary dark-adaptation curve. D: C displaced downwards 0.5 unit (Barlow's prediction). E: C scaled down to $\frac{1}{3}$ ordinate (Hodgkin's prediction). White circles show the experimental results.

On Barlow's view the dark-adapted threshold is the increment threshold with afterimage as background, and hence the starry afterimage background from bleaching through the plate will act like the starry background from viewing through the plate. The latter we have seen changes log threshold from curve A to B, i.e., by dropping 0.5, hence the former must change from curve C to D, also by dropping 0.5.

On Hodgkin's view the perforated plate reduces to one-third the number of "bleaching signals" reaching the feedback. Hence from equation [1] it will reduce ln I to one-third at each stage of recovery. Consequently, we expect on this view that the dark adaptation should follow curve E, which is C scaled down to one-third the ordinate.

It is plain that the experimental results (white circles) fit the expectation of Hodgkin but not that of Barlow. Thus the effect of bleaching is to send to the feedback a signal proportional to the total amount of free opsin in the area at the moment.

In order to make the exceedingly complex question of adaptation as clear as possible, I have somewhat oversimplified the issues. In truth, the picture is not so black-and-white; the lines are blurred and curious possibilities beckon from the half-shadows. Moreover, the story of adaptation that I have given cannot rest firmly unless and until two vital pieces of knowledge are added and found to fit: *a*. What are the anatomical structures referred to as "the adaptation pools", and how do they control signal size? *b*. What are the two kinds of path or two modes of signal referred to as "light signals" and "free opsin signals"? At present I can only guess at these answers; it is essential to establish them.

Adaptation in Cone Vision

Cones are the aristocrats of the receptor population. Whereas rods are herded together for team labor and receive quanta at starvation level, cones are rich in their quantum dividends and the quality of their activity is individual and discriminating. Their superior discrimination is shown in judgments of brightness-difference, color, space (acuity) and time (flicker). Cones also adapt more rapidly than rods and with sharper margins. In spite of these differences in quality, it is natural to suppose that the mechanism of adaptation both to backgrounds and to bleachings is on the same lines as with rods, but the question naturally arises about independence or interdependence of the three color mechanisms of trichromatic vision.

Ever since Young's famous proposal (42), trichromacy has been a likely basis for color vision, and a hundred years ago Clerk Maxwell (21) proved it a fact. The last step in this long analysis is the recent demonstration by Marks, Dobelle & MacNichol (20) that the human (and monkey) retina contains three different kinds of cone maximally sensitive at 445, 535, and 570 nm respectively (Figure 114).

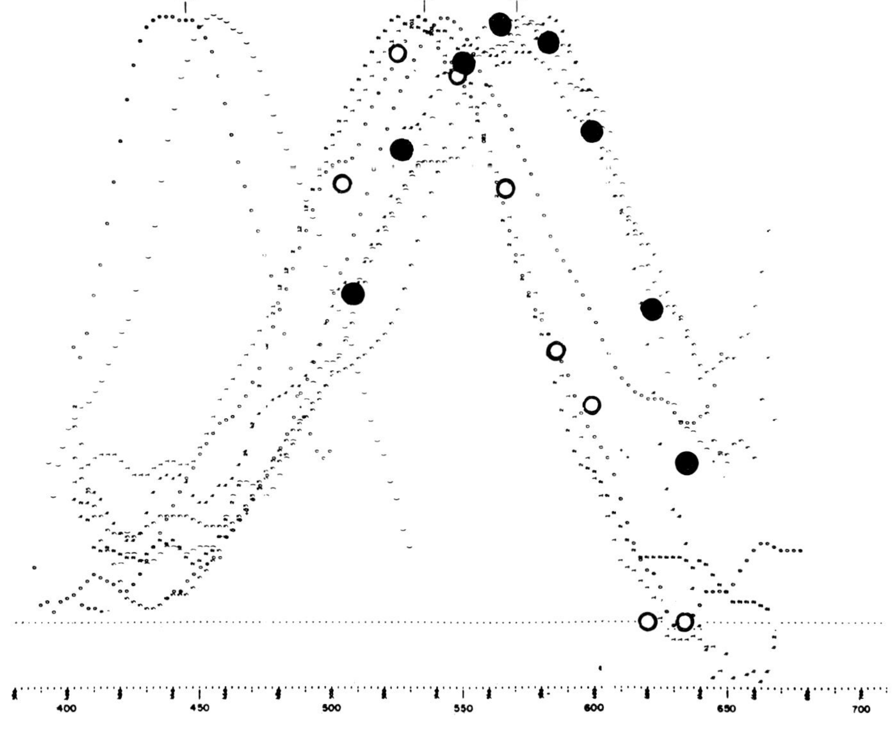

Figure 114. Difference spectra of pigments in single cones. Each point was plotted by a computer after performing certain built-in corrections. Pigments are of three kinds, with maxima at 570, 535, and 445 nm. Black and white circles show difference spectra of erythrolabe and chlorolabe, the cone pigments measured (previously) in the living eye (3). (From Marks, Dobelle & MacNichol, 20.)

It needed a beautifully designed microdensitometer coupled with a computer to obtain these results from single cones, for even such experienced pigment investigators as Brown & Wald (8), using a modification of conventional equipment, found it hard to raise their signal above the noise without bleaching away much of the pigment they wished to measure.

Now, the analysis of cone adaptation actually treats of the three color mechanisms of Stiles (37), independent of whether the pigments are separated in different cones or mixed. But since we now have rather good evidence from Marks, Dobelle & MacNichol that each cone-type contains but one pigment, and that Stiles' π_1, π_4, π_5, and π_0 correspond to the activities of the blue, green, and red cones, and to the rods respectively, it makes our story crisper if we talk of cones than of the less well defined π mechanisms.

Cone Adaptation to Backgrounds

The work of Stiles is rather well known (33–37). Over the space of 20 years he investigated with exceptional accuracy and thoroughness the relation between the energy ΔI of a test flash of wavelength λ_1 when it was presented upon a background of energy I and wavelength λ_2. To a first approximation, the whole array of results can now be expressed in terms of the univariance in output of the three kinds of cone. Simplifying somewhat we may say, "Each cone generates a pattern of signals that depends upon the time pattern of quanta caught, but not upon the wavelength of those quanta." The wavelength, of course, will affect the chance of the quantum being caught by the visual pigment in question and, indeed, the absorption spectrum of the pigment defines this chance. But once any quantum is absorbed, its effect on the receptor is the same as the effect of any other quantum. In the case of rods, then, the effect of λ_1 for flash and λ_2 for background is plain. Wavelength simply alters the units of the two scales and gives appropriate vertical and horizontal shifts to the log plot on the right of Figure 110.

If the three kinds of cones and the rods all had adaptation pools independent one of another, and if threshold was reached whenever the most sensitive of the four mechanisms was excited, then a simply predictable structure of phenomena would be found. As is well known, the work of Stiles has shown that, to a first approximation, this is the structure actually observed.

Cone Adaptation to Bleaching

If cone vision adapts to bleaching as rod vision does, the dark-adaptation curve will depend upon the course of regeneration of the various cone pigments. Naturally, the relevant result cannot be found from isolated cones or excised human eyes. But it can be found by human retinal densitometry, just as in the case of rods (Figure 111). It is as easy to measure the regeneration of cone pigments on the fovea as of rhodopsin in the periphery, and much easier to correlate the result with dark adaptation, since nothing interferes with early measurements of cone thresholds in the way that cones interfere with early measurements of rod thresholds in dark adaptation.

Figure 115 shows two cone pigment regeneration curves measured upon a normal eye and presented to the N.P.L. Symposium in 1957 (24). The upper curve *A* shows that the rate of regeneration is the same when measured by light of 605 or 545 nm, thus the red pigment *erythrolabe* regenerates about as fast as the green pigment *chlorolabe*. The subsequent ten years work on these cone pigments has not revealed any difference in their regeneration rates. Moreover, protanopes and deuteranopes which have been shown to have one pigment each (26,27,28) regenerate at the same rate as each other. Curve B in Figure 115 shows that measurements near the pigment maximum (585 nm) and where the density is much less (625 nm) follow the same curve, which would not be so if erythrolabe were so dense that much self-screening occurred (cf. Brindley, 7).

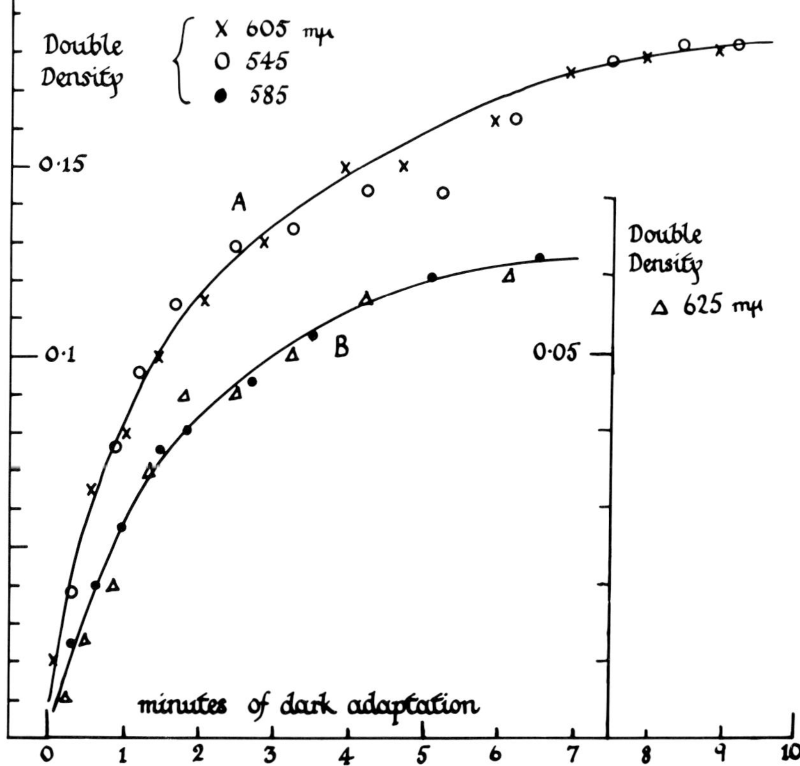

Figure 115. Regeneration of cone pigments on normal fovea. In curve *A* measurements are at 605 and 545 nm to show that red and green pigments return equally fast; in curve *B* they are at 585 and 625 nm to show that self-screening is small.

Figure 116 shows the relation between dark adaptation of red cones in the normal eye and the regeneration of erythrolabe (3). Black and white triangles show two runs of dark adaptation with a red test flash on the fovea of a subject who had normal vision but was rich in red cones. Black and white circles show two runs wherein the rate of regeneration of erythrolabe was plotted (scale on right) as a function of time following the same bleaching exposure. The dashed curve is taken without any change from a similar experiment on a deuteranope who had only erythrolabe present in the red-green range (30).

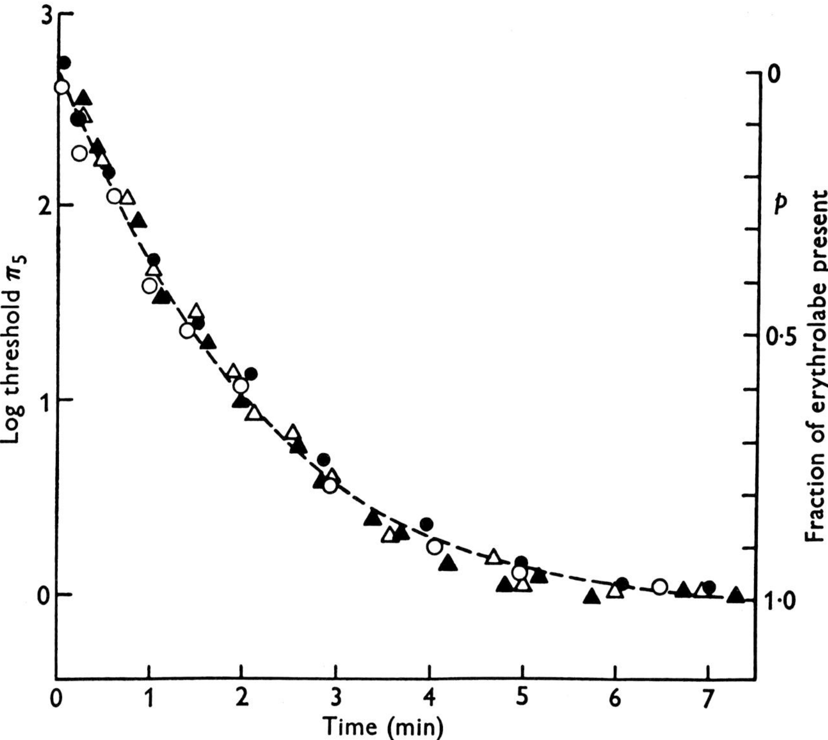

Figure 116. Dark adaptation and regeneration of cone pigment erythrolabe in normal eye. Triangles show two runs of dark adaptation (scale on left) when a deep red test flash was used. Circles show two time-courses of regeneration of erythrolabe (scale on right). Full bleaching exposure given in all cases.

Are Cones Independent in Bleaching Adaptation?

If cones were independent in their adaptation to bleaching, as they are with backgrounds, we might expect, in suitable conditions, breaks in the cone adaptation curves similar (if not so pronounced) to the well-known cone-rod break. I suppose that countless investigators must have looked for this, failed to find it, and left their disappointment unrecorded. The most thorough attempt in the literature appears to be that of Mandelbaum & Mintz (19), who used many colors for bleaching and many colors for test, and never found kinks or much difference in the resulting cone dark-adaptation curves. Their results were recorded in detail, for they were not disappointed; all was as expected from Hecht's theory that the three cone pigments were nearly identical, thus no marked distinctions would be detectable.

We know now that Hecht's view was wrong and, as seen in Figure 114, the three pigments are far from identical. One may ask if Mandelbaum & Mintz' results are to be explained by the view that one type of cone is not as independent of another in its bleaching adaptation as it is in its background adaptation. We know from the photopic spectral-sensitivity curve that various cone types add to the sense of brightness. Perhaps they also add their free-opsin signals to define the adaptation to bleaching.

The results of Auerbach & Wald (2) showed that a complete pooling of signals was unlikely, for after bleaching with a strong orange light the cone adaptation curve measured with a violet test flash showed a small but distinct kink. They correctly supposed that the early cone branch represented Stiles' blue mechanism, but did not make the measurements necessary to prove it. This was done by Du Croz and me (14,15). Figure 117 (like Figure 110) shows on the left dark-adaptation curves, plotted as usual—log threshold against time. On the right are increment thresholds plotted as Stiles did—log threshold against log background intensity of yellow-green light. When the test flash was also yellow-green, only the green chlorolabe cones were excited at threshold and Stiles' π_4 curve (white circles) was obtained. When the test flash was blue, the results are shown as squares. In confirmation of Stiles (34), with very weak backgrounds the *green* cones are still excited at threshold. But a yellow-green background affects green cones much more than blue cones, so that with increasing background the green threshold rises to a point where it lies above the still quiescent blue threshold. At

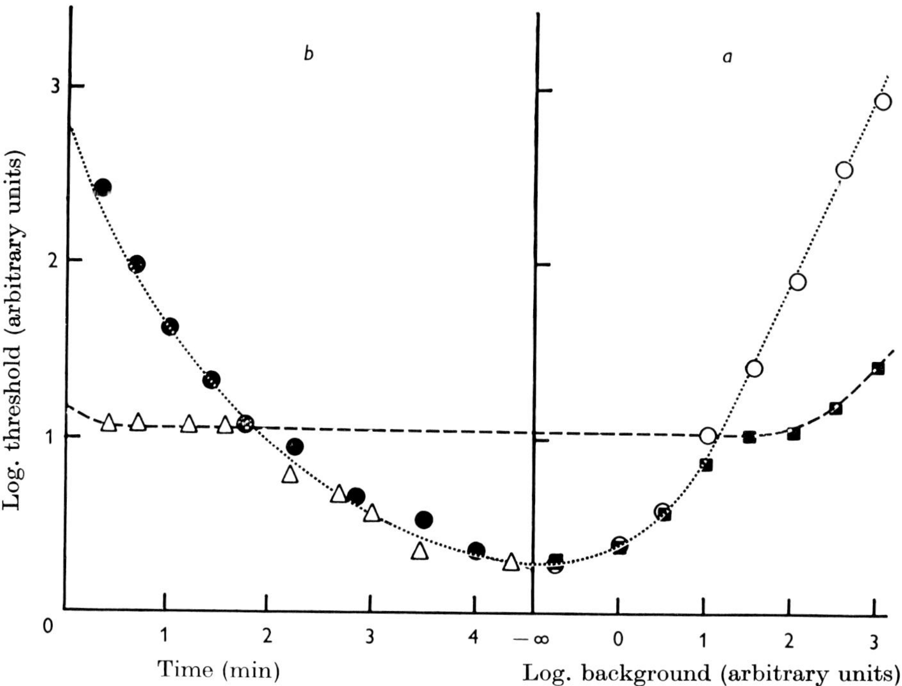

Figure 117. On the left are foveal dark-adaptation curves; on the right, log increment threshold curves on a yellow-green background. White circles indicate yellow-green test flash, which excited only green cones at threshold; squares represent blue test that also excited green cones at absolute threshold but excited blue cones when background was greater than 1 log unit. Triangles show dark adaptation with blue test after an orange bleach; black circles show the same after a white bleach equal to the orange in its excitation of green cones.

this point the curve of squares suddenly reveals the still horizontal increment threshold curve of the blue cones.

So far we have been observing background adaptation and doing no more than confirm what Stiles published 20 years ago. But it enables us to interpret with confidence the new results of bleaching adaptation. On the left of Figure 116 the test flash was always blue, and black circles show the dark adaptation following a white bleach. The curve shows simply the recovery of green cones, which we have seen are most sensitive at full recovery and which we were able to show were the most sensitive throughout recovery from the white bleach. But that was not the case after an orange bleach (triangles), as Auerbach & Wald (2) had already seen. The orange bleach we used was adjusted to be equal to the white in its absorption by chlorolabe, thus green cones would be equally affected by the two bleachings. But the blue cones absorbed hardly any of this orange light and were so little light-adapted by it that they had recovered entirely by 30 seconds of dark adaptation, as may be seen from the horizontal course of the triangles. What is particularly significant about this initial horizontal branch of triangles is that its level is precisely that of the dark threshold for blue cones, as shown on the right by squares. The second branch (triangles) obviously represents the recovery of green cones, for these were bleached as much by orange as by white, and are seen to return along the same dark-adaptation curve as soon as the green cone threshold falls below the dark threshold for blue cones.

The curves of Figure 117 thus give a clear answer to our question, "Are the different kinds of cone as independent in their adaptation to bleaching as Stiles has shown them to be in their adaptation to backgrounds?" It is "Yes." For the recovery of green cones is the same when green bleaching was the same, no matter whether blue cones were not affected at all (triangles) or so much affected (circles) as never to appear at all at threshold even with a blue test flash. And, again, blue cones do not have their threshold raised by an orange bleach that raises greatly the thresholds of green (and red) cones, and these in fact constitute by far the majority of the entire cone population.

It is more difficult to demonstrate a similar break between red and green cone thresholds in the dark-adaptation curve; Figure 118 shows the first recorded example. When a kink is to be demonstrated in a row of experimental points, it is important not to be deceived by some chance irregularity in their alignment. The critical reader will not be favorably impressed by the common practice of drawing the kinks much more exaggerated than is needed to accommodate the points. In Figure 118, as in Figure 117, no curves with kinks are drawn. Two continuous curves are obtained, each representing one color mechanism alone. The triangles are seen in each case to lie partly on one and partly on the other, falling always on the branch where threshold is lowest. In Figure 118 we obtain in comparable conditions the dark-adaptation curve for red cones only (circles), for green cones only (squares), and for the transitional adaptation (triangles) that certainly starts with squares and certainly ends with circles. The comparable conditions to obtain these curves were as follows. Circles and triangles were both measured with a red flash after bleachings that affected the red cones equally. But the bleachings did

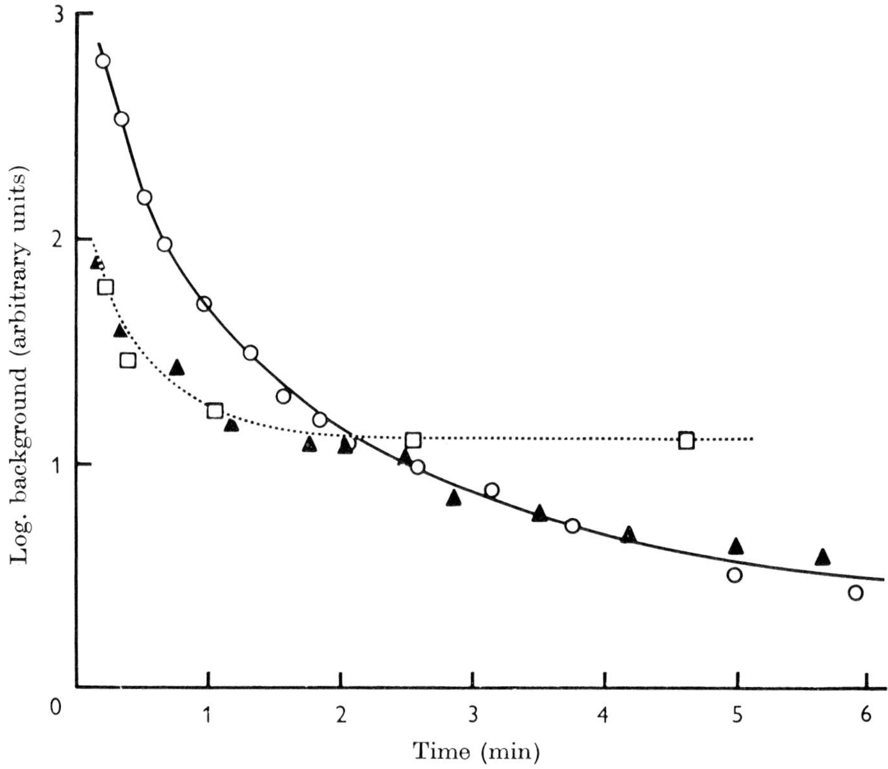

Figure 118. Foveal dark-adaptation curves following bleaches that were equivalent for the red cones. Circles indicate when bleaching light was green and test red, hence red cones were excited throughout; squares, when the bleach was red and the test green, hence green cones were excited throughout; triangles, when the bleach was red and the test was red. First branch runs with squares, since red cone threshold is far above green, but later it runs with circles, since recovered red cones are more sensitive to the red test.

not affect the green cones equally; circles followed a very strong blue-green bleach which made it certain that the red test flash would excite red cones only, so circles show pure red dark adaptation. With triangles, the bleach was a deep red light that affected green cones so much less than red that, in the early stages following, they were more excitable than red cones even in response to the red test flash. When after this same red bleach a green test flash was used (squares), naturally the green cones alone appeared at threshold and recovered as they did with triangles, since the course of dark adaptation of any receptor species is independent of the color of the *test* flash, when (as here) the energy unit is expressed in terms of equal quantum catch.

Conclusion. The adaptation of the cones is therefore to a first approximation very similar to that of the rods. In the same way that rods adapt to backgrounds and to bleachings independent of what is happening to the cones, so each species of cone adapts independently of what is happening to the others. Whichever is most sensitive in any condition defines the threshold.

The organization of the eye is immensely complex, and accurate measurements and special limited conditions reveal some departures from this simple scheme. Stiles has pointed out several aspects in his great and detailed analysis of background adaptations, and Du Croz and I have seen some with bleaching.

We know that the three cone species are not always independent, for the logarithms of their quantum catches seem to add in the appreciation of brightness and to subtract in the appreciation of color, so it would not be surprising if in some conditions a little interaction spilled over and muddied the clear independence of thresholds. But I think we shall better appreciate the nature of these interactions if first we conceive of the simplicity of the isolation into which they burst as intruders.

SUMMARY

The retina may exhibit very great changes in sensitivity, involving a mechanism called "adaptation". It is of two distinct kinds: (*a*) the effect of luminous backgrounds, and (*b*) the effect of pigment bleaching.

A background from which only one per cent of the rods have caught a single quantum may raise the threshold of *all* the rods threefold. Thus, all the signals from an area are controlled by an attenuator that is operated by the average quantum catch in that area.

Similarly, in dark adaptation after the bleaching of rhodopsin, the rise in threshold of rods depends, not on the bleaching in that rod, but upon the average bleach in the area.

The automatic gain or "G-box" is controlled by feedback from its own output signal in the case of background adaptation. But, after bleaching, a signal proportional to the amount of pigment bleached (at each moment) is sent directly into the feedback.

Cone adaptation appears to act in the same manner. The rise in log threshold of red cones in dark adaptation corresponds to the amount of red pigment erythrolabe still remaining bleached. And the various cone mechanisms are as independent in their adaptation to bleaching as Stiles has shown them to be in their adaptation to backgrounds.

REFERENCES

1. Alpern, M., and Campbell, F. W., The behaviour of the pupil during dark adaptation. *J. Physiol.* (London), 1963, **165**: 5–7*P*.
2. Auerbach, E., and Wald, G., Identification of a violet receptor in human color vision. *Science*, 1954, **120**: 401–405.
3. Baker, H. D., and Rushton, W. A. H., The red-sensitive pigment in normal cones. *J. Physiol.* (London), 1965, **176**: 56–72.
4. Barlow, H. B., Dark-adaptation: a new hypothesis. *Vision Res.*, 1964, **4**: 47–58.
5. Barlow, H. B., and Sparrock, J. M. B., The role of afterimages in dark adaptation. *Science*, 1964, **144**: 1309–1314.
6. Blakemore, C. B., and Rushton, W. A. H., Dark adaptation and increment threshold in a rod monochromat. *J. Physiol.* (London), 1965, **181**: 612–628.

7. Brindley, G. S., A photochemical reaction in the human retina. *Proc. Phys. Soc.*, 1955, **68**: 869–870.

8. Brown, P. K., and Wald, G., Visual pigments in single rods and cones of the human retina; direct measurements reveal mechanisms of human night and color vision. *Science*, 1964, **144**: 45–52.

9. Campbell, F. W., and Rushton, W. A. H., Measurement of the scotopic pigment in the living human eye. *J. Physiol.* (London), 1955, **130**: 131–147.

10. Craik, K. J. W., and Vernon, M. D., The nature of dark adaptation. *Brit. J. Psychol.*, 1941, **32**: 62–81.

11. Crawford, B. H., Visual adaptation in relation to brief conditioning stimuli. *Proc. Roy. Soc. London B*, 1947, **134**: 283–302.

12. Dartnall, H. J. A., Goodeve, C. F., and Lythgoe, R. J., The quantitative analysis of the photochemical bleaching of visual purple solutions in monochromatic light. *Proc. Roy. Soc. London A*, 1936, **156**: 158–170.

13. Dowling, J. E., The chemistry of visual adaptation in the rat. *Nature* (London), 1960, **188**: 114–118.

14. Du Croz, J. J., and Rushton, W. A. H., Cone dark-adaptation curves. *J. Physiol.* (London), 1963, **168**: 52–54*P*.

15. ———, The separation of cone mechanisms in dark adaptation. *J. Physiol.* (London), 1966, **183**: 481–496.

16. Fechner, G. T., *Elemente der Psychophysik*. Breitkopf und Härtel, Leipzig, 1860.

17. Hecht, S., Rods, cones, and the chemical basis of vision. *Physiol. Rev.*, 1937, **17**: 239–290.

18. Hecht, S., Shlaer, S., and Pirenne, M. H., Energy, quanta and vision. *J. Gen. Physiol.*, 1942, **25**: 819–840.

19. Mandelbaum, J., and Mintz, E. U., The sensitivities of the color receptors as measured by dark adaptation. *Am. J. Ophthal.*, 1941, **24**. 1241–1254.

20. Marks, W. B., Dobelle, W. H., and MacNichol, E. F., Jr., Visual pigments of single primate cones. *Science*, 1964, **143**: 1181–1183.

21. Maxwell, J. C., Experiments on colour, as perceived by the eye, with remarks on colour blindness. *Trans. Roy. Soc. Edinburgh*, 1857, **21**: 275–298.

22. Rushton, W. A. H., The difference spectrum and the photosensitivity of rhodopsin in the living human eye. *J. Physiol.* (London), 1956, **134**: 11–29.

23. ———, The rhodopsin density in human rods. *Ibid.*: 30–46.

24. ———, The cone pigments of the human fovea in colour blind and normal. In: *Visual Problems of Colour*, Vol. I (National Physical Laboratory Symp. 8). H.M. Stationery Office, London, 1958: 71–105.

25. ———, Rhodopsin measurement and dark-adaptation in a subject deficient in cone vision. *J. Physiol.* (London), 1961, **156**: 193–205.

26. ———, A cone pigment in the protanope. *J. Physiol.* (London), 1963, **168**: 345–359.

27. ———, A visual pigment in the deuteranope. *J. Physiol.* (London), 1963, **169**: 31–32*P*.

28. ———, A foveal pigment in the deuteranope. *J. Physiol.* (London), 1965, **176**: 24–37.

29. ———, The sensitivity of rods under illumination. *J. Physiol.* (London), 1965, **178**: 141–160.

30. ———, Bleached rhodopsin and visual adaptation. *J. Physiol.* (London), 1965, **181**: 645–655.

31. RUSHTON, W. A. H., Visual adaptation. *Proc. Roy. Soc. London B*, 1965, **162**: 20–46.
32. RUSHTON, W. A. H., and WESTHEIMER, G., The effect upon the rod threshold of bleaching neighbouring rods. *J. Physiol.* (London), 1962, **164**: 318–329.
33. STILES, W. S., The directional sensitivity of the retina and the spectral sensitivities of the rods and cones. *Proc. Roy. Soc. London B*, 1939, **127**: 64–105.
34. ———, Separation of the 'blue' and 'green' mechanisms of foveal vision by measurements of increment thresholds. *Proc. Roy. Soc. London B*, 1946, **133**: 418–434.
35. ———, Increment thresholds and the mechanisms of colour vision. *Docum. Ophthal.*, 1949, **3**: 138–163.
36. ———, Further studies of visual mechanisms by the two-colour threshold technique. In: *Coloquio Sobre Problemas Opticos de la Visión*. Madrid, 1953: 65–103.
37. ———, Colour vision: the approach through increment-threshold sensitivity. *Proc. Nat. Acad. Sci. USA*, 1959, **45**: 100–114.
38. STILES, W. S., and CRAWFORD, B. H., Equivalent adaptation levels in localized retinal areas. In: *Report of Discussion on Vision*. Physical Society, London, 1932: 194–211.
39. TANSLEY, K., The regeneration of visual purple: its relation to dark adaptation and night blindness. *J. Physiol.* (London), 1931, **71**: 442–458.
40. WALD, G., Vision: photochemistry. In: *Medical Physics* (O. Glasser, Ed.). Year Book Publishers, Chicago, 1944: 1658–1667.
41. WALD, G., BROWN, P. K., and SMITH, P. H., Iodopsin. *J. Gen. Physiol.*, 1955, **38**: 623–681.
42. YOUNG, T., On the theory of light and colours. *Phil. Trans. Roy. Soc.*, 1802: 12–48.

THE MOLECULAR BASIS OF HUMAN VISION*

GEORGE WALD
Harvard University
Cambridge, Massachusetts

The work of the past few years has begun to yield a surprisingly complete view of the retinal basis of human vision. Until recently, almost all that was known of visual mechanisms had been learned from tissues of other animals and could be applied to man by inference only. We are now beginning to derive much of this essential information directly from human material. There is now an amazingly complete record of the embryological development of the human eye (10,13), and to an already classic microanatomy can now be added the intricate electron microscopical investigations of Yamada and his coworkers (39), Cohen (6), and Bairati & Orzalesi (1). There are also the beginnings of a special biochemistry of human retinas, particularly through the recent microspectrophotometry of the human visual pigments, including those of color vision.

Hardly to be distinguished from these human studies are parallel developments with other primates; in these animals the electrophysiology, which can probably never be pursued very far in man, has reached an exemplary level. For the analysis of retinal mechanisms, man has become one of the principal experimental subjects, with the unique advantage that, while a biophysics can be developed with other animals, with man alone can a psychophysics evolve. The psychophysics of human vision has a long history, but only now can it be developed parallel to the other modes of investigation, thus providing it a firm foundation in the physics, chemistry, and physiology of the retina and visual pathways.

The rods and cones of the vertebrate retina are derived embryonically from ciliated cells, such as those which typically line the ventricles of the brain. The swollen and otherwise modified shaft of a presumptive cilium forms the rod or cone outer segment (7,9,22). The latter has a layered structure, the lamellae taking the form of a pile of flattened sacs enclosed within the plasma membrane (16,17,18). In primate cones these lamellae are arranged similarly to those in rods, except that in the latter the flattened sacs have a differentiated rim (5,6,8). In both rods and cones the lamellar membranes are about 50 Å thick, or approximately the diameter of a molecule of cattle rhodopsin if it is spherical in shape.

* Investigations from our laboratory were supported in part by the U.S. National Science Foundation and the Office of Naval Research. More detailed reviews and references to earlier developments may be found in *Life and Light* (28) and in "The Problem of Visual Excitation" (35).

The visual pigments of vertebrates share a common chemistry (25–28). Each consists of a specific type of protein—an opsin bearing as chromophore a particular configuration of retinaldehyde (vitamin A aldehyde, formerly retinene), the 11-*cis* isomer (Figure 119). *The only action of light in vision is to isomerize this chromophore* from the 11-*cis* to the all-*trans* configuration (11). All other changes—chemical, physiological, indeed psychological—are "dark" consequences of this single light reaction.

The first light product—all-*trans* retinaldehyde bound to as yet unmodified opsin, called pre-lumirhodopsin in the case of rhodopsin—is highly unstable at ordinary temperatures (40). In the dark it is transformed rapidly over a series of intermediates—lumirhodopsin, metarhodopsin I, and metarhodopsin II (15)—hydrolyzing finally to a mixture of opsin and free all-*trans* retinaldehyde (Figure 120). This last reaction is too slow to play a part in visual excitation, which must therefore depend upon one of the earlier intermediates. The latter represent progressive stages in the unfolding of the opsin structure, in the course of which

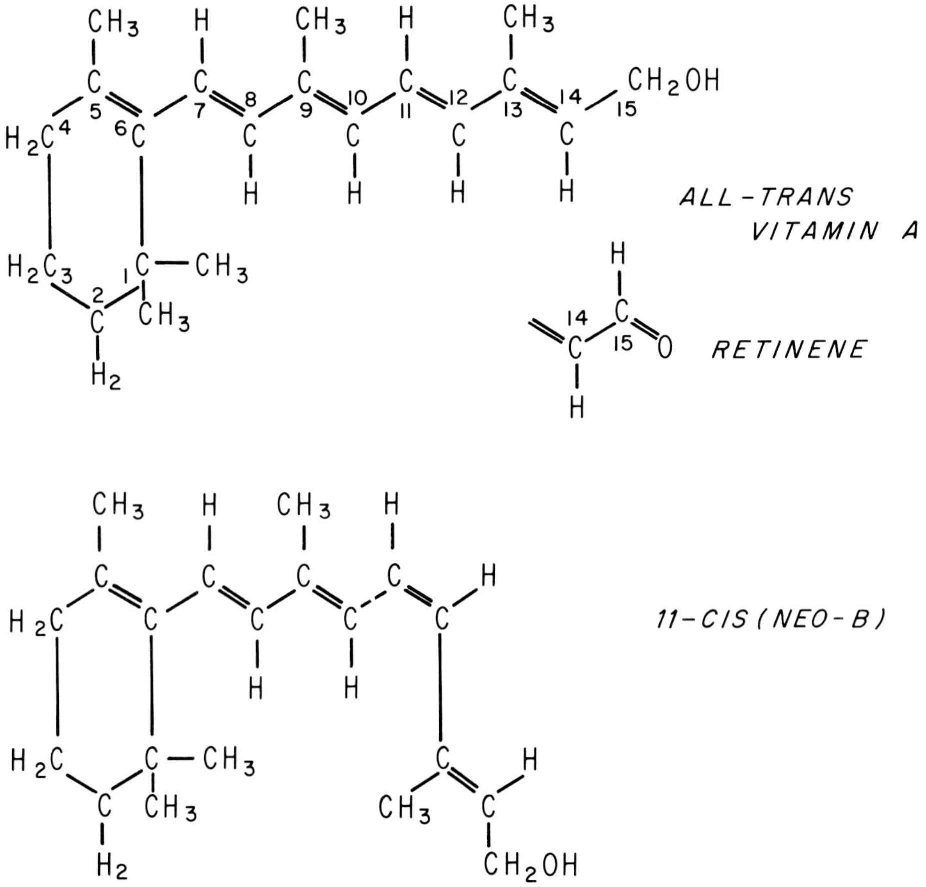

Figure 119. Structures of all-*trans* and 11-*cis* retinol (vitamin A) and retinaldehyde (retinene).

new groups are exposed, including two sulfhydryl (—SH) groups and one H^+-binding group with pK about 6.6 (histidine?).

In vertebrate retinas, the presence of the enzyme, alcohol dehydrogenase, causes the retinaldehyde released by the bleaching of visual pigments to be reduced to retinol (vitamin A). To regenerate a visual pigment, retinol must be reoxidized to retinaldehyde, and either molecule or both must be exchanged for, or isomerized to, the active 11-*cis* configuration.

To these general arrangements, which are shared by other vertebrates, primates add two special features: the presence of a central yellow patch, the *macula lutea*, and color vision, which, though distributed widely among vertebrates and arthropods, is peculiarly accessible in primates and particularly in man.

Human rods contain a typical rhodopsin (33). Its absorption spectrum, measured in suspensions of rod outer segments or by the microspectrophotometry of human retinas (3), has λ_{max} about 500 mμ, and accounts precisely for the spectral sensitivity of human rod vision, whether measured in normal subjects and corrected for ocular transmission, or without correction in lensless eyes. Human rhodopsin extracted into aqueous solution bleaches in the usual way to opsin and all-*trans* retinaldehyde, and can be regenerated in solution from opsin and 11-*cis* retinaldehyde (33). Rhesus monkey rhodopsin exhibits very similar properties. In both man and monkey the rhodopsin molecules are oriented in the rod outer segments in much the same way as in frogs and cattle (3,34), or porphyrhodopsin in the rods of the mudpuppy (2).

After a century of speculation, reliable data on the spectra of the human cone pigments concerned with color vision are becoming available. Difference spectra on the red- and green-sensitive pigments of the cones have been measured by direct microspectrophotometry of human and monkey foveas (3). The spectra of

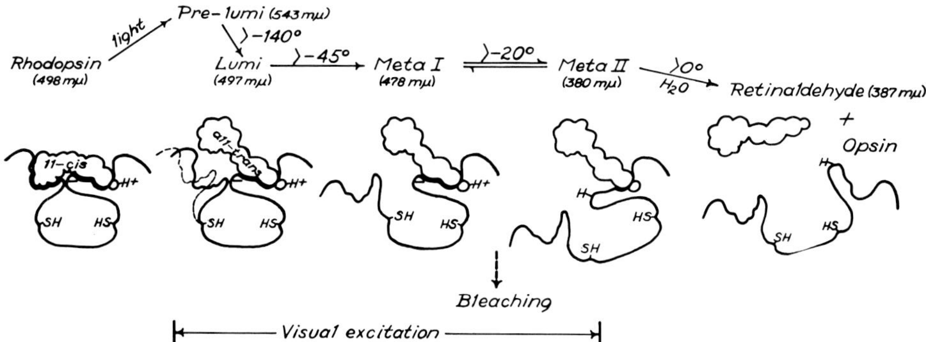

Figure 120. Stages in the bleaching of rhodopsin. Rhodopsin has as chromophore retinaldehyde, which fits closely a section of the opsin structure. The only action of light is to isomerize retinaldehyde from the 11-*cis* to the all-*trans* configuration (pre-lumirhodopsin). Then the structure of opsin opens in stages (lumirhodopsin, metarhodopsin I and II), until finally the retinaldehyde is hydrolyzed away from opsin. Bleaching occurs in the transition from metarhodopsin I to II; by this stage visual excitation must also have occurred. The opening of the opsin structure exposes new groups, including two –SH groups and one H^+–binding group. The absorption maxima shown are for pre-lumirhodopsin at −190° C, lumirhodopsin at −65° C, and the other pigments at room temperature. (From Wald, 30.)

patches of fovea 0.2 mm wide were initially measured in the dark, then after exhaustive bleaching with deep red light, and finally after complete bleaching at shorter wavelengths. The red-sensitive pigment was found to have λ_{max} 565–570 mμ, the green-sensitive pigment λ_{max} about 535 mμ (Figure 121). Both pigments are regenerated on adding 11-*cis* retinaldehyde to the medium, showing this to be their common chromophore, joined to different opsins.

It has recently proved possible to make such measurements in single parafoveal rods and cones of man and monkey (4,14). Recording spectra in such exceedingly small fields inevitably involves some bleaching of the visual pigments. Marks and coworkers (14) incorporate a monitored correction for this factor in their measurements. In our experiments (4) the pigments sometimes bleached as much

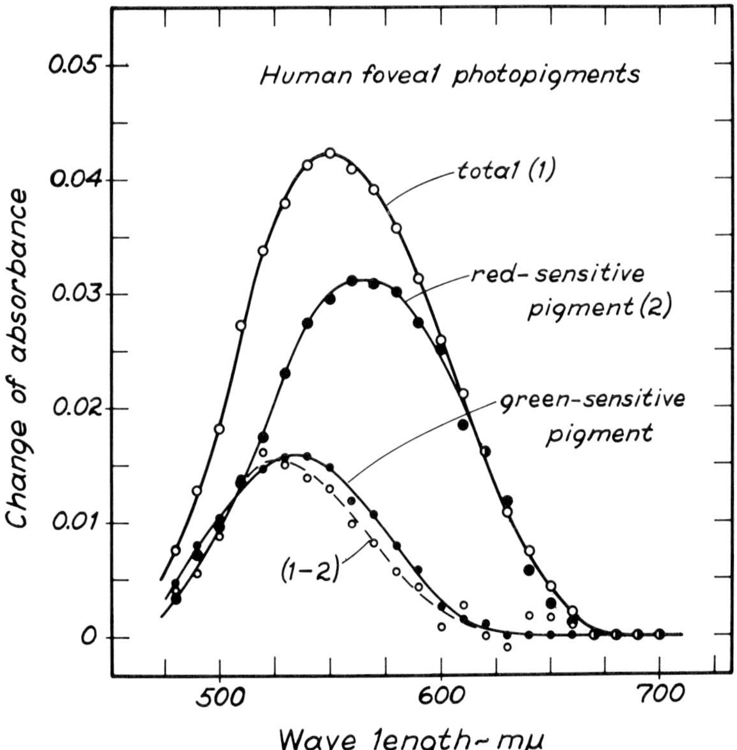

Figure 121. Difference spectra of visual pigments of the human fovea. The foveal spectrum was first recorded in darkness, then after exhaustive bleaching in deep red light, finally after complete bleaching at shorter wavelengths. The difference between the first two spectra measures the red-sensitive pigment (λ_{max} 565–570 mμ); that between the second and third spectra measures the green-sensitive pigment (λ_{max} 535–540 mμ); and that between the first and last spectra, the total foveal pigment (λ_{max} ca. 550 mμ). At wavelengths longer than about 630 mμ, the red-sensitive pigment accounts almost wholly for the total absorption. Subtracting the spectrum of the red-sensitive pigment from the total should yield an estimate of the spectrum of the green-sensitive pigment; this difference (broken line) approximates the directly measured spectrum of the green-sensitive pigment. (From Brown & Wald, 3.)

as 20–30 per cent in the course of a single scan. Nevertheless, by recording the spectrum in both directions—from red to violet and back from violet to red—and averaging the results, spectra that are not greatly distorted in shape or position can be obtained.

Such measurements of the difference spectra of the visual pigments in single human cones reveal the presence of (at least) three groups of cones, red-, green-, and blue-sensitive (Figure 122). These data provide the first direct evidence of the existence of such groups of cones, reasonably consistent in their properties with the hypothetical components of trichromatic theory. Too few cones have as yet been measured in this way to define the absorption maxima reliably. A central problem awaiting such measurements is whether each type of cone contains a single visual pigment, or whether some of them contain mixtures of pigments.

We have recently determined the absorption spectra of human and monkey maculas by direct microspectrophotometry (3). Some years ago, the human macular pigment was shown to be a carotenoid, apparently lutein or leaf

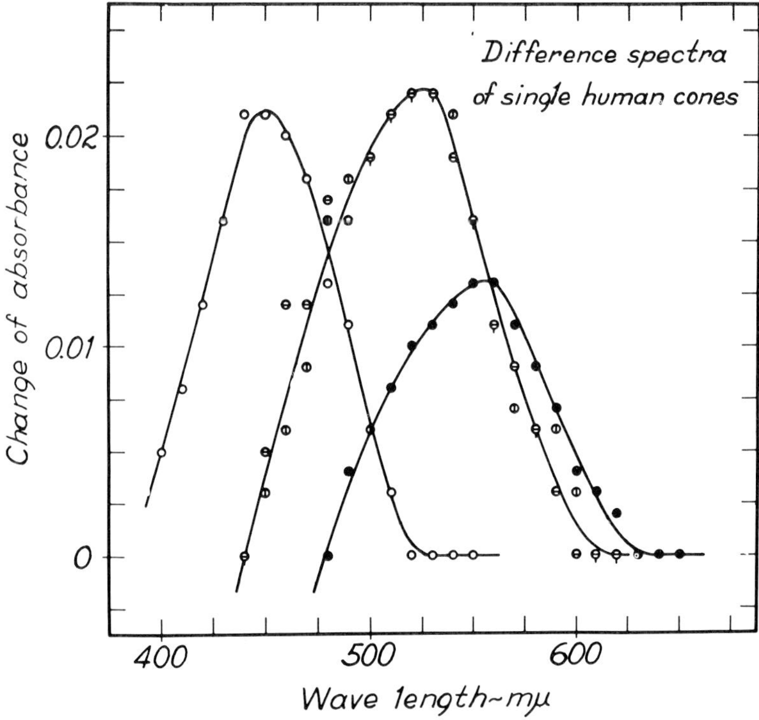

Figure 122. Difference spectra of the visual pigments in single cones of the human parafovea. In each case the absorption spectrum was recorded in the dark, then again after bleaching with a flash of yellow light. The differences between these spectra involve one blue-sensitive cone, two green-sensitive cones, and one red-sensitive cone. In making these measurements, light passed through the cones axially, in the direction of incidence normal in the living eye. (From Brown & Wald, 4.)

xanthophyll, $C_{40}H_{54}(OH)_2$ (23,24). Monkey maculas appear to possess the same pigment. In the microspectrophotometer a patch of human or monkey macula yields a typical carotenoid spectrum, with absorption maxima at about 430, 455, and 484 mμ (Figure 123). The average absorbance at 455 mμ in eight series of measurements of human maculas was 0.49, representing an average absorption at this wavelength of 68 per cent. When allowance is made for ocular and macular absorptions, the absorption spectrum of the total pigments of the human fovea accounts exactly for the foveal spectral sensitivity (3).

A simple psychophysical procedure was recently devised for measuring the spectral sensitivities of the human color vision pigments (29). The spectral sensitivity of the dark-adapted fovea represents the composite action spectrum of all the foveal photopigments. By remeasuring the spectral sensitivity on intense colored backgrounds, one can isolate the action spectra of the individual pigments.

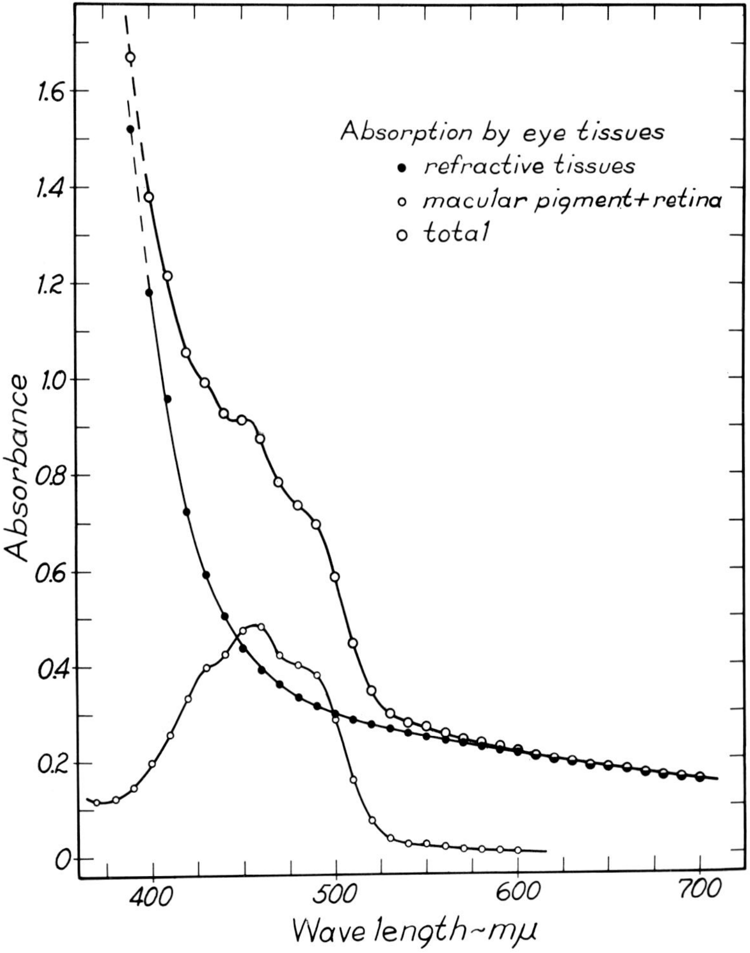

Figure 123. Average absorption by the dioptric tissues of the human eye (cornea to retinal surface) and of the macula lutea in the foveal region (average of eight eyes). (From Brown & Wald, 3; Wald, 29.)

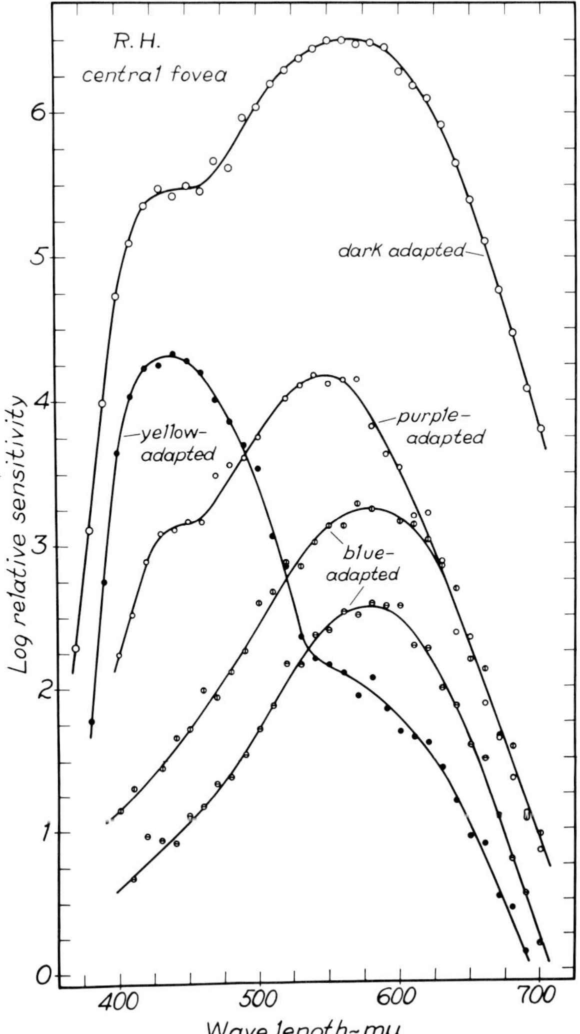

Figure 124. Spectral sensitivity of the dark-adapted fovea and action spectra of the single color-vision pigments, measured in terms of light incident on the cornea of the eye of subject R.H. The dark-adapted fovea is most sensitive at about 562 mμ. Adaptation to yellow light virtually isolates the action spectrum of the blue-sensitive pigment (λ_{max} 438 mμ); adaptation to a mixture of violet and red (purple light) exposes the green-sensitive pigment (λ_{max} 548 mμ), and adaptation to blue light isolates the red-sensitive pigment (λ_{max} 580 mμ). The results of two different blue adaptations demonstrate the invariance of such action spectra with the conditions of adaptation. Ordinates are log relative sensitivity (log 1/threshold), expressed as relative numbers of photons per flash incident upon the cornea of the eye. Absolute sensitivities can be judged from the fact that the threshold of the dark-adapted fovea at about 560 mμ is about 10^4 photons in this observer. (From Wald, 29.)

Thus, for example, determining visual thresholds throughout the spectrum superimposed on a steady background illumination of intense blue light reveals the action spectrum of the red-sensitive pigment. In effect, the blue background selectively adapts the blue- and green-sensitive mechanisms to such levels that the foveal thresholds are due to the red-sensitive pigment alone. Similarly, exposure to bright yellow light isolates the action spectrum of the blue-sensitive pigment, and exposure to a mixture of red and blue (purple light) isolates the spectrum of the green-sensitive pigment (Figure 124).

Measured at the level of the cornea such action spectra vary from one person to another, owing to differences in ocular and macular transmission. The uncorrected spectral sensitivity curves for the blue-, green-, and red-sensitive pigments are maximal at 440–450 mμ, 540–550 mμ, and 575–580 mμ, respectively.

The procedures used in obtaining these curves are closely related to those introduced some years ago by Stiles for the analysis of human color vision (19,20,21). The present spectra of the blue- and green-sensitive pigments agree reasonably well with the sensitivity curves of Stiles's blue-mechanisms ($\pi_1 - \pi_3$) and his green-mechanism (π_4). His red-mechanism (π_5), however, forms an

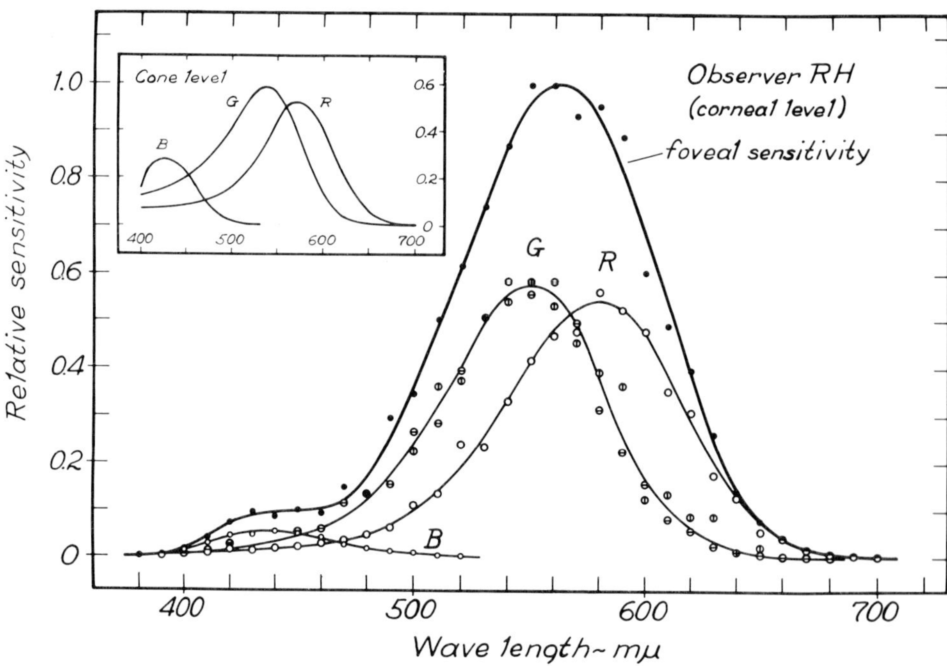

Figure 125. Contributions of the individual color receptor mechanisms to the total foveal sensitivity of observer R.H. The main graph shows measurements at the corneal level; the inset, corresponding curves corrected for ocular and macular transmission, hence as though measured at the level of the cones. In R.H., who is particularly blue-sensitive, when the foveal sensitivity is given a maximal height of 1.0, the heights of the blue-, green-, and red-sensitive components are as B:G:R = 0.053:0.575:0.542 at the corneal level, and 0.28:0.59:0.52 at the level of the cones. In the average observer the blue-component is only about one-third as high. (From Wald, 29.)

almost exact envelope of the action spectra of the red- and green-sensitive pigments shown in Figure 124. The criteria by which Stiles measured these functions were directed more toward isolating physiological mechanisms than individual pigments; this characteristic of the π_5 function may mean that one of the physiological unit mechanisms in color vision may involve the operation of both the red- and green-sensitive pigments.

After correction for ocular and macular transmission, these action spectra become invariant, and acquire the force of absorption spectra of the color-vision pigments. Their maxima lie at about 430, 540, and 570 mμ.

The spectral sensitivities of the three color-vision pigments, measured at the corneal level, add up to yield the average photopic luminosity curve when the maxima are in the proportions, B:G:R: = 0.018:0.58:0.54. Corrected for ocular and macular transmissions, hence as though at the level of the cones, these ratios become about 0.09:0.59:0.52 (Figure 125) (29).

The spectra of these pigments also account for the spectral sensitivities associated with all the major forms of human colorblindness (the dichromias). In a first attempt (29) to explain colorblindness on the basis of information already in the literature, I assumed two kinds of mechanism at work: a "loss" mechanism, in which one of the three color-vision pigments is lacking, and a "fusion" mechanism, in which, despite the presence of the three pigments in normal proportions (and thus of a normal photopic luminosity), two of the pigments excite only one sensation. Such a fusion mechanism would have as principal result the existence of two types of deuteranope, as proposed earlier by Willmer (37).

Using a standardized procedure based on selective adaptation as described above, measurements were recently made of the spectral sensitivities of the dark-adapted fovea and of each of the color-vision pigments in normal and dichromic subjects (31). Typical results are shown in Figure 126. Each of nine normal subjects reveals unequivocally the operation of the three color-vision pigments. Among 20 deutans (13 deuteranopes, 7 deuteranomalous), however, I did not find a single instance of the fusion mechanism. On the contrary, in all 20 deutans this procedure revealed the operation of only two of the three color receptors—the blue- and red-sensitive mechanisms. The deuteranomalous subjects must also possess some diminished representation of the green-receptor but the procedure in current use does not identify it. Nor did these data provide any other basis for dividing the deuteranopes into two groups; on the contrary, they seemed to form a homogeneous distribution.

Similarly, eight protans (five protanopes, three protanomalous) revealed the operation of the blue- and green-sensitive pigments only, and three tritanopes that of the green- and red-sensitive pigments only.

Therefore, despite my expectations, I have not succeeded in finding a "fusion" type of colorblindness and two classes of deuteranope. Each of the colorblind subjects tested lacked one of the three color-vision pigments to some degree. In other words, these measurements have found only one mechanism of colorblindness, the "loss" mechanism first proposed by Thomas Young in 1807 (41) to explain John Dalton's red-blindness.

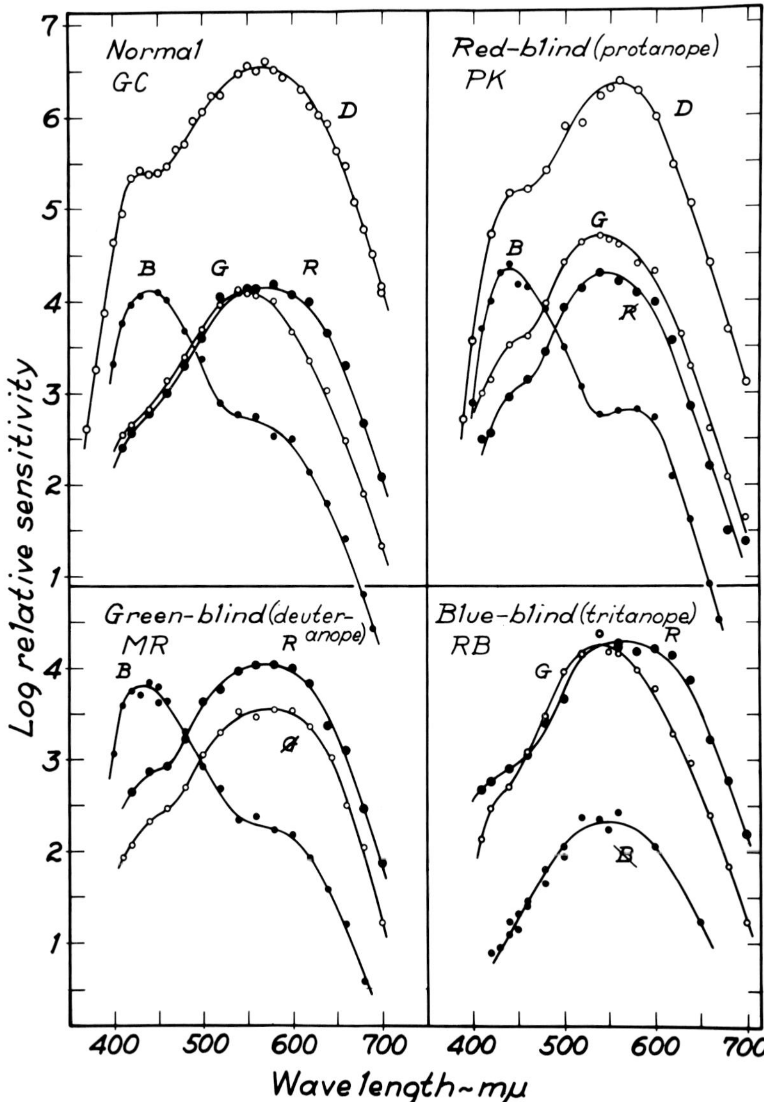

Figure 126. Measurements of spectral sensitivity with a standardized procedure in a normal subject, a red-blind (protanope), a green-blind (deuteranope), and a blue-blind (tritanope). Each of the colorblinds reveals the operation of only two of the three color-vision pigments; in each case the attempt to measure the third pigment reveals only one of the former pigments at a lower level of sensitivity. *D*: Dark-adapted fovea. *B*, *G*, *R*: Blue-, green-, and red-sensitive pigments, measured on bright yellow, purple, or blue backgrounds. The crossed-out letters represent unsuccessful attempts to measure the corresponding pigments in colorblind eyes.

That leaves few distinctions to make, and little terminology needed to make them. Only one syndrome must be dealt with, i.e., dichromia, in its three forms, red-, green-, and blue-blindness, or *anerythropia*, *achloropia*, and *acyanopia*.

Using this same selective adaptation procedure, I also studied (32) the so-called blue-blindness of the fovea, described originally by König & Köttgen (12), and later rediscovered by Willmer (36,38). In both those instances a central region of the normal fovea that was clearly intended to encompass the rod-free area was alleged to behave as though tritanopic. In all seven subjects I have examined in this situation, the contribution of the blue-receptor declined precipitously as centrally fixated foveal fields were reduced in visual angle from 1° to 8′ (Figure 127). In the 8′ field a trace of blue-receptor response could be found in two of the subjects, none at all in the other five. It is clear from these measurements that, though the rod-free area of the fovea—about 1.5°–1.7° in subtense—is well supplied with blue-receptors, its central zone almost or entirely lacks them. This behavior is an aspect of the special topography of the fovea. Thus, an 8′ field centered $\frac{1}{2}$° from the fixation point, i.e., at the border of the 1° zone, reveals a high blue-receptor sensitivity. Similarly, peripheral areas of the retina, 5°–8° from the fixation point, do not develop tritanopia as the test field is decreased in subtense from 1° to 8′.

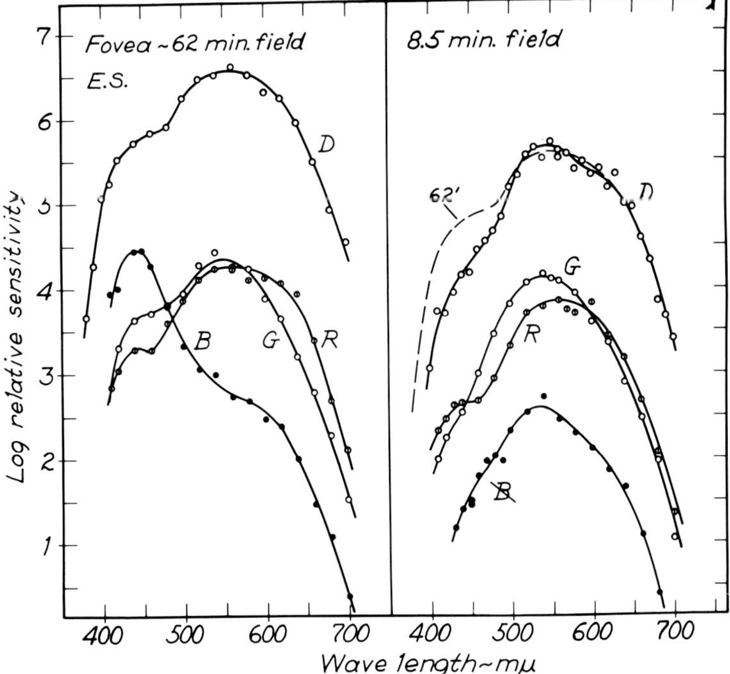

Figure 127. Blue-blindness of the center of the fovea. A centrally fixated 1° field, examined by the standardized procedure, displays the usual spectral sensitivities in the dark-adapted eye (*D*) and the blue-, green-, and red-receptors (*B*, *G*, *R*). When the field is reduced to 8.5′, the dark-adapted sensitivity falls selectively in the blue region, and though the red- and green-receptors are represented normally, no trace is found of the blue-receptor.

SUMMARY

The visual pigments of the human retina share the basic structure common to all known visual pigments, being composed of vitamin A aldehyde (retinal, retinaldehyde; formerly retinene), bound as chromophore to a specific type of protein, an opsin, found in the outer segments of the rods and cones. In all known visual pigments the chromophore is in the distinctive, sterically hindered 11-*cis* configuration. The only action of light in vision is to isomerize such chromophores of visual pigments from 11-*cis* to all-*trans*. All other reactions are "dark" consequences of this one light process. It is followed by a stepwise opening-up of opsin structure that exposes new chemical groups. Some step in this sequence of reactions is responsible for visual excitation.

The human retina contains four such visual pigments: rhodopsin in the rods, and three cone pigments that serve as the basis of color discrimination. All possess 11-*cis* retinal as chromophore, united with four different opsins. The difference spectra of the three cone pigments have been measured by direct microspectrophotometry in human and monkey foveas, and in single parafoveal cones. Their spectral sensitivities can also be measured by selective adaptation of the eye to intense colored lights. All these measurements agree reasonably well in showing the normal retina to possess three pigments, segregated mainly in three classes of cone, with maximum absorptions and sensitivities at about 435, 540, and 565 mμ. In each of the three major classes of colorblind (dichromats), one of these pigments is lacking, the other two apparently remaining normal. Anomalous trichromats yield in this procedure the same results as dichromats; in them, however, a third pigment is present, though reduced in amount (or effectiveness), and displaced in spectrum. In one instance—a deuteranomalous tritanope—this mechanism could be analyzed. This procedure also reveals that a small central area of the fovea, the fixation area, about 8 minutes in diameter, is usually totally blue-blind in the sense of lacking the blue-sensitive mechanism.

Discussion

Question from the floor: Dr. Wald, does your sensitivity curve for protanopes show a reduction in the green-sensitive pigment?

Wald: No. On the contrary, since the protanope has the blue- and green-sensitive pigments, but not the red, the green-sensitive pigment is not depressed, it rather rises slightly. That is, the sensitivity of the green-mechanism is a little higher than normal, probably because a protanope still has the normal number of cones in his retina but, lacking the red-cones, has perhaps almost twice as many green-cones. In any case, it seems that there is a significant increase in sensitivity in the green-receptor in protanopes, and a similar increase in sensitivity in the red-receptor in deuteranopes.

Question from the floor: To avoid bias, why not refer to the red, green, and blue pigments as 1, 2, and 3, as proposed by von Kries? No. 1 pigment has its maximum at 560 mμ, and that is certainly not a red color. In fact, spectrally there is no pure red color, hence calling it pigment No. 1 would be very much fairer.

Wald: It should be noted that the red-sensitive pigment, if it had its peak in the red, should look blue. Actually it does not have its peak in the red, but in the yellow, or even greenish yellow, and it probably looks violet. I therefore disagree with that point of view. I think that the terminology should remain neutral only when one has nothing to say that is not neutral. With our knowledge of a few realities concerning the color-vision pigments and the associated sensitivity curves, we should begin to talk in their terms. The only serious danger in a term such as "blue-blind" is that it might be interpreted to imply that a blue-blind person cannot see blue light, which of course he can, just as a green-blind sees green light, and a red-blind sees red light. These terms are merely meant to imply the lack of one or another of the color-vision pigments and the type of cone in which it occurs.

Brown: Since all the human cone and rod pigments have the same chromophore, and since the chromophore presumably absorbs the light which leads to excitation of retinal receptors, why do the various cone pigments have different absorption spectra, and why does the absorption spectrum of rhodopsin differ from that of the cone pigments?

Wald: On a very simple level, an answer is that in each of the visual pigments the identical chromophore, 11-*cis* retinal, is attached to a different opsin; the different spectra go with the different opsins. On the other hand, we cannot yet specify the intramolecular mechanisms that determine the spectrum in each of these instances. The association of absorption spectra with chemical constitution represents very uncertain territory, involving the nature of the interaction between the side-chain of retinal and neighboring regions of opsin. Despite intense research efforts, there is as yet no clear view of what is going on, even in rhodopsin.

REFERENCES

1. Bairati, A., Jr., and Orzalesi, N., The ultrastructure of the pigment epithelium and of the photoreceptor-pigment epithelium junction in the human retina. *J. Ultrastruct. Res.*, 1963, **9**: 484–496.
2. Brown, P. K., Gibbons, I. R., and Wald, G., The visual cells and visual pigment of the mudpuppy, *Necturus. J. Cell Biol.*, 1963, **19**: 79–106.
3. Brown, P. K., and Wald, G., Visual pigments in human and monkey retinas. *Nature* (London), 1963, **200**: 37–43.
4. ———, Visual pigments in single rods and cones of the human retina. *Science*, 1964, **144**: 45–52.
5. Cohen, A. I., The fine structure of the extrafoveal receptors of the Rhesus monkey. *Exp. Eye Res.*, 1961, **1**: 128–136.
6. ———, New details of the ultrastructure of the outer segments and ciliary connectives of the rods of human and macaque retinas. *Anat. Rec.*, 1965, **152**: 63–80.
7. De Robertis, E., Some observations on the ultrastructure and morphogenesis of photoreceptors. *J. Gen. Physiol.*, 1960, **43**, Supp. 2: 1–14.
8. Dowling, J. E., Foveal receptors of the monkey retina: fine structure. *Science*, 1965, **147**: 57–59.

9. Dowling, J. E., and Gibbons, I. R., The effect of vitamin A deficiency on the fine structure of the retina. In: *The Structure of the Eye* (G. K. Smelser, Ed.). Academic Press, New York, 1961. 85–99.
10. Duke-Elder, S., *System of Ophthalmology* (S. Duke-Elder, Ed.). *Vol. III. Normal and Abnormal Development; Part 2. Congenital Deformities.* Kimpton, London, 1964.
11. Hubbard, R., and Kropf, A., The action of light on rhodopsin. *Proc. Nat. Acad. Sci. USA*, 1958, **44**: 130–139.
12. König, A., and Köttgen, E., Über den menschlichen Sehpurpur und seine Bedeutung für das Sehen. *Sitzber. Akad. Wiss. Berlin*, 1894: 577.
13. Mann, I. C., *The Development of the Human Eye.* Grune & Stratton, New York, 1950.
14. Marks, W. B., Dobelle, W. H., and MacNichol, E. F., Jr., Visual pigments of single primate cones. *Science*, 1964, **143**: 1181–1183.
15. Matthews, R. G., Hubbard, R., Brown, P. K., and Wald, G., Tautomeric forms of metarhodopsin. *J. Gen. Physiol.*, 1963, **47**: 215–240.
16. Sjöstrand, F. S., The ultrastructure of the retinal receptors of the vertebrate eye. *Ergebn. Biol.*, 1959, **21**: 128–160.
17. ———, Fine structure of cytoplasm: the organization of membranous layers. *Rev. Mod. Physics*, 1959, **31**: 301–318.
18. ———, Electron microscopy of the retina. In: *The Structure of the Eye* (G. K. Smelser, Ed.). Academic Press, New York, 1961: 1–28.
19. Stiles, W. S., The determination of the spectral sensitivities of the retinal mechanisms by sensory methods. *Nederl. Tijdschr. Natuurk.*, 1949, **15**: 125–146.
20. ———, Color vision: the approach through increment-threshold sensitivity. *Proc. Nat. Acad. Sci. USA*, 1959, **45**: 100–114.
21. ———, Foveal threshold sensitivity on fields of different colors. *Science*, 1964, **145**: 1016–1017.
22. Tokuyasu, K., and Yamada, E., The fine structure of the retina studied with the electron microscope. IV. Morphogenesis of outer segments of retinal rods. *J. Biophys. Biochem. Cytol.*, 1959, **6**: 225–230.
23. Wald, G., Human vision and the spectrum. *Science*, 1945, **101**: 653–658.
24. ———, The photochemistry of vision. *Docum. Ophthal.*, 1949, **3**: 94–134.
25. ———, The distribution and evolution of visual systems. In: *Comparative Bio-Chemistry. Vol. I: Sources of Free Energy* (M. Florkin and H. S. Mason, Eds.). Academic Press, New York, 1960: 311–345.
26. ———, The significance of vertebrate metamorphosis. *Circulation*, 1960, **21**: 916–938.
27. ———, The visual function of the vitamins A. *Vitamins Hormones* (New York), 1961, **18**: 417–430.
28. ———, The molecular organization of visual systems. In: *Light and Life* (W. D. McElroy and B. Glass, Eds.). Johns Hopkins Press, Baltimore, 1961: 724–753.
29. ———, The receptors of human color vision; action spectra of three visual pigments in human cones account for normal color vision and color-blindness. *Science*, 1964, **145**: 1007–1016.
30. ———, Receptor mechanisms in human vision. In: *XXIII International Congress of Physiological Sciences; Lectures and Symposia.* Excerpta Medica Foundation, Amsterdam, 1965: 69–79.
31. ———, Defective color vision and its inheritance. *Proc. Nat. Acad. Sci. USA*, 1966, **55**: 1347–1363.
32. ———, Blue-blindness in the normal fovea. *J. Opt. Soc. Amer.*, 1967, **57**: 1289–1301.

33. WALD, G., and BROWN, P. K., Human rhodopsin. *Science*, 1958, **127**: 222–226.
34. WALD, G., BROWN, P. K., and GIBBONS, I. R., Visual excitation: a chemoanatomical study. *Symp. Soc. Exp. Biol.*, 1962, **16**: 32–57.
35. ———, The problem of visual excitation. *J. Opt. Soc. Amer.*, 1963, **53**: 20–35.
36. WILLMER, E. N., Colour of small objects. *Nature* (London), 1944, **153**: 774–775.
37. ———, A physiological basis for human colour vision in the central fovea. *Docum. Ophthal.*, 1955, **9**: 235–251.
38. WILLMER, E. N., and WRIGHT, W. D., Colour sensitivity of the fovea centralis. *Nature* (London), 1945, **156**: 119–121.
39. YAMADA, E., TOKUYASU, K., and IWAKI, S., The fine structure of retina studied with electron microscope. III. Human retina. *J. Kurume Med. Ass.*, 1958, **21**: 1979.
40. YOSHIZAWA, T., and WALD, G., Transformations of squid rhodopsin at low temperatures. *Nature* (London), 1964, **201**: 340–345.
41. YOUNG, T., *Lectures on Natural Philosophy*, Vol. II. London, 1807: 345.

INHIBITORY INTERACTION IN THE RETINA

H. KEFFER HARTLINE
The Rockefeller University
New York, New York

The processing of visual information begins in the retina. To be sure, the placement of the eyes, their movements, their cooperation with other sensory systems, all affect the acquisition of information from the animal's lighted surroundings. The nature of the optical system of the eyes also determines the extent to which the properties of the physical stimulus are exploited. But the interpretation of the pattern of light and shade and color, moving and changing, is a nervous function, and the retina, since Ramón y Cajal, has been recognized as a nervous center—the first of a great, complex hierarchy of processing centers in the nervous system.

Properties of the visual receptors, deployed in a mosaic to receive the retinal image of the lighted world, introduce the first step in the interpretation. Their sensitivities, their ranges of transducer action in intensity and wavelength, and their dynamic responses determine the raw data presented to the higher nervous levels. We know much about visual receptors, but we are still ignorant of much. We have no sure knowledge about the steps intermediate between the first photochemical action of light on the visual pigment of the receptor and the generation of a nervous signal. Indeed, with only a few exceptions in the animal kingdom, we do not even know what that nervous signal is. We can, perhaps, feel fairly confident that its ultimate effect is to release a transmitter substance at the synapses between receptors and the next neurons in the visual pathway. But it is not my purpose here to deal with the processing of visual data at the level of the receptors; I will move a little further along, to integrative processes in the retina that are more recognizably neural in character.

A large patch of light is visible at a lower intensity than a small one. More exactly, we know that, while the absorption of one quantum of light can excite a single rod, it takes the cooperation of several excited rods to produce a sensation of light. Moreover, these cooperating rods must be in the same eye and, indeed, within a circumscribed retinal area; there is summation of excitatory influences within neural networks of the retina. The first objective neurophysiological evidence of spatial summation in the retina was Adrian & Matthews' (1) demonstration that the latency of optic nerve discharge in the eel's eye was shorter for four spots of light acting together than for any one of them acting alone. And in the first analysis of single optic nerve fiber discharges in the frog's retina, it became immediately evident that convergent excitatory influences from a sizable receptive field comprising many retinal receptors converge on each retinal ganglion cell (12). The summation of excitatory influences from its entire field determines the response of a ganglion cell (13).

But excitation is only half of the picture of neural integration. Inhibition, whose presence in retinal function was so convincingly demonstrated by Granit's early work (6), forms the other half. And, indeed, the interplay of these two antagonistic influences, according to classical Sherringtonian principles, provides a richness and diversity of retinal action that modern work continues to reveal.

It was a surprise—to me at least—when the first observations of activity of single optic nerve fibers in the frog's retina (11) revealed a remarkable diversity of response, some of the fibers responding only during illumination, some only when light was turned off, others giving brief bursts of impulses only at the onset and cessation of retinal illumination that fell within their receptive fields, but showing exquisite sensitivity to moving spots and shadows (Figure 128).

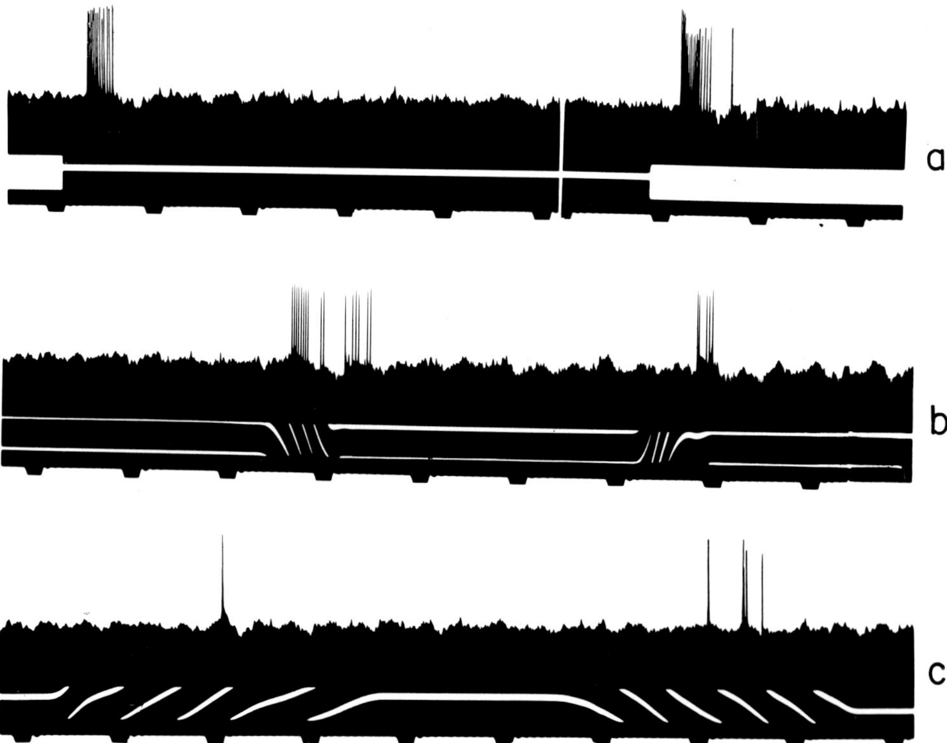

Figure 128. Oscillograms of action potentials of a single optic nerve fiber of the frog, showing responses to onset and cessation of illumination, and to slight movements of a small spot of light (50 μ in diameter) on the retina. The signal marking a period of illumination blackens the white strip above the one-fifth-sec. time marks. There was no discharge during steady illumination if the stimulus spot was stationary, as in *a*. Slight movements of the stimulus spot elicited short bursts of impulses, as in *b* and *c*. Movements of the spot on the retina are signalled by narrow white lines appearing above the time marker; each line corresponds to 7 μ on the retina. (From Hartline, 12.)

We now know, from the work of Lettvin and his associates (25) and of others who are following them (8), that the frog's retina has an even greater variety of sophisticated response types. And in the mammalian retina, Barlow & Levick (2) find some elements which respond only to movements in a particular direction.

It is appropriate to ask to what extent we can understand the diversity of patterns of activity of retinal neurons in terms of an interplay of excitation and inhibition. To the basic excitation furnished by light, inhibition adds a "molding" influence, increasing—as we shall see—temporal and spatial resolution, and supplying a mechanism for increased versatility of response. It was Kuffler's elegant work on the mammalian retina that brought out this versatility with special clarity; receptive fields of ganglion cells in the cat's retina are organized

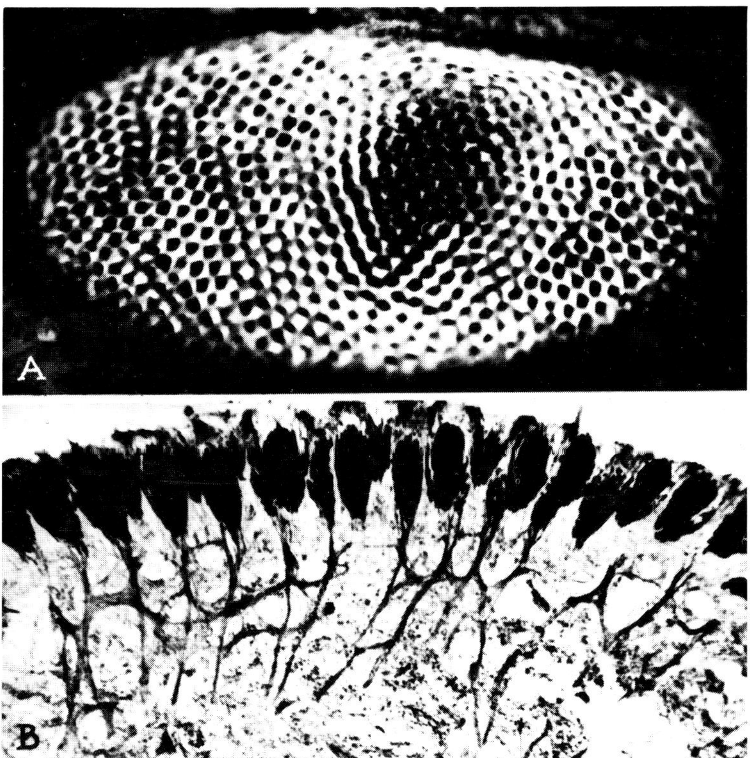

Figure 129. Lateral (compound) eye of *Limulus*. *A*: External view of corneal surface showing faceted structure; ommatidia in the center of the eye point directly toward the camera from a dark "pseudopupil" because they reflect less light than the marginal ones, which point in all directions to cover the hemispherical field of vision of the eye; the long axis of this eye was about 15 mm (from an adult animal, about 30 cm broad). *B*: Light micrograph of a 2 mm portion of a *Limulus* eye, sectioned perpendicularly to the cornea; the heavily pigmented sensory parts of the ommatidia are at the top of the figure; the chitinous cornea has been stripped away; bundles of optic nerve fibers from the ommatidia and interconnecting fiber bundles comprising the lateral plexus have been rendered visible by Samuel's silver stain. (From Hartline, Wagner & Ratliff, 19; Ratliff, 33; preparation *B* by W. H. Miller.)

into antagonistic center versus surround, the final response in an optic nerve fiber depending on the distribution of light over its entire receptive field (21). This holds as well in some coldblooded vertebrate retinas, where the antagonistic areas may in addition have different spectral sensitivities, as in the "color coded" fields of the goldfish retina reported by Wagner, MacNichol & Wolbarsht (44).

There are simpler retinas than the vertebrate; one such is in the compound eye of the horseshoe crab, *Limulus*. In this review I shall confine myself largely to the studies made by my colleagues and myself, over a number of years, on the integrative processes in this relatively simple retina.

In the compound eye of *Limulus* (Figure 129A), each ommatidium is comprised of a cluster of photoreceptor cells (retinula cells) and a bipolar neuron (eccentric cell) which discharges trains of impulses in response to light. The axons of both of these, in passing back to become the optic nerve, give off numerous fine lateral branches to form a network—a retina, indeed—interconnecting the ommatidial units (Figure 129B; cf. Miller, 28). Over these lateral pathways pass inhibitory neural influences, mediated by synapses in clumps of neuropil interspersed liberally throughout the plexus. The ommatidial photoreceptor units thus interact, and the interaction is one of simple mutual inhibition. This offers an opportunity to study, in relatively uncomplicated form, an important integrative process common to visual systems in general, at many levels, from retina to higher centers.

The *Limulus* eye, then, is more than just a mosaic of receptors, deployed to receive light from various directions, each making its own report independently of the others. Rather, the report of each receptor unit is modified by the activity of its neighbors, and the sensory information transmitted over the optic nerve is thus partially processed in the retina.

If an optic nerve fiber from the *Limulus* eye is isolated and its trains of impulses recorded in response to a spot of light focused on the corneal facet of the ommatidium from which it arises, the inhibition exerted by its neighboring ommatidia can be demonstrated readily (19). Steady illumination of the facet of the ommatidia chosen as a "test" receptor results in a steady discharge of impulses from it; illumination of neighboring facets results in a decrease in the impulse frequency of this discharge (Figure 130). The brighter the light on these neighboring elements, the more of them illuminated, and the closer they are to the test receptor, the greater is the decrease in its impulse frequency. This is true for any ommatidium chosen; each, being a neighbor of its neighbors, inhibits them and is inhibited by them. This mutual action can be seen directly by recording from two optic nerve fibers simultaneously; the frequency of firing in each is lower when both are illuminated together than when each is illuminated by itself (Figure 131), and the amount by which the activity of each is lowered is greater the higher the level of activity of the other (16).

A simple mutual inhibitory interaction of retinal elements has significant consequences in the integration of visual information. It is clear that elements in the brightly lighted regions of the retinal image will exert a stronger inhibitory action on their dimly lighted neighbors than will the latter on the former. Thus, the disparity in their responses will be increased, and contrast between unequally lighted regions will be enhanced. Since mutual inhibition is stronger between near neighbors than between widely separated ones, contrast enhancement will be greatest across the steepest gradients of intensity, and edges and contours in the retinal image will be accentuated. This is of course a distortion of sensory

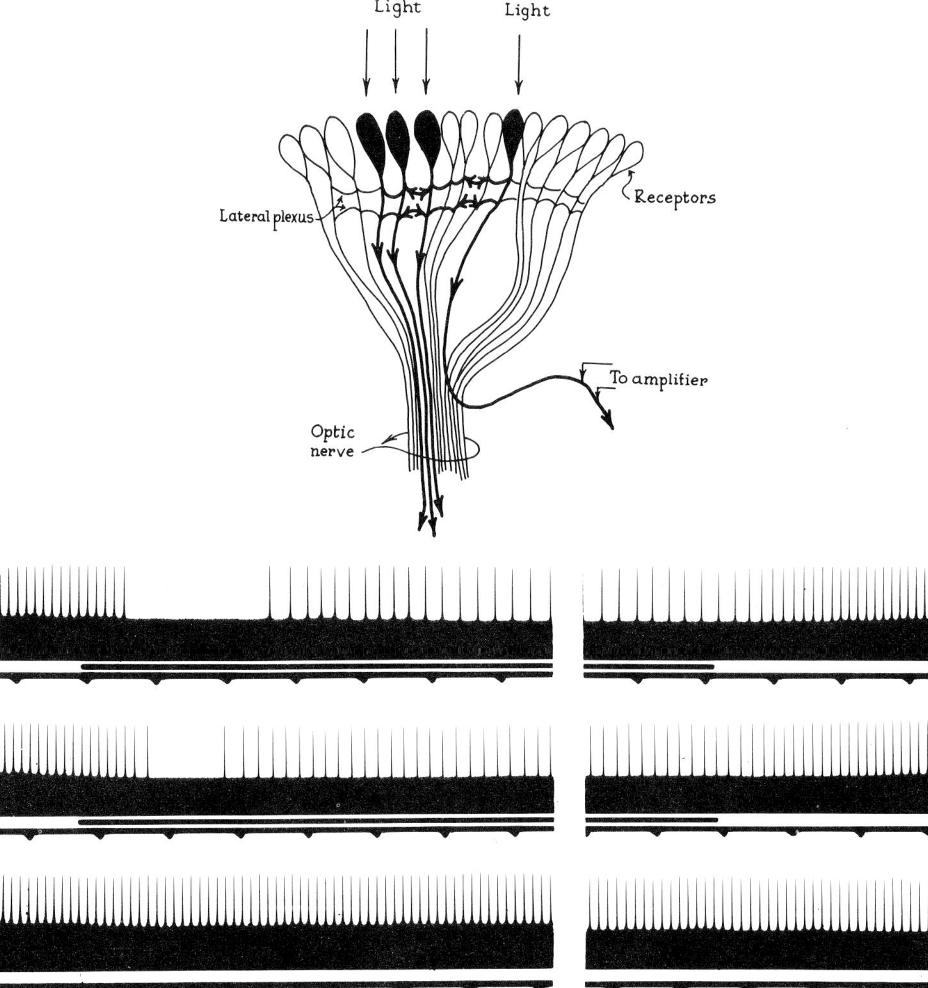

Figure 130. Inhibition of the discharge of impulses in a single optic nerve fiber in the eye of *Limulus*. Sketch (above) shows schematically the eye (see Figure 129B) as used in the experimental arrangement to obtain the three oscillographic records (below). A "test" receptor on the right, whose axon had been isolated by dissection from the optic nerve, was illuminated steadily by a spot of light confined to its facet, starting three seconds before the beginning of each record. The oscillogram shows the trains of impulses thus elicited. For the top and middle records, a small group of neighboring receptors (represented on the left in the sketch) were illuminated during the several seconds marked on the record by the black line in the white strip just above the $\frac{1}{5}$ sec. time marks. For the top record, the intensity of illumination on the neighbors was ten times that used for the middle record. The bottom record is a control, showing the steady discharge in the absence of inhibiting influences. (From Hartline, 15.)

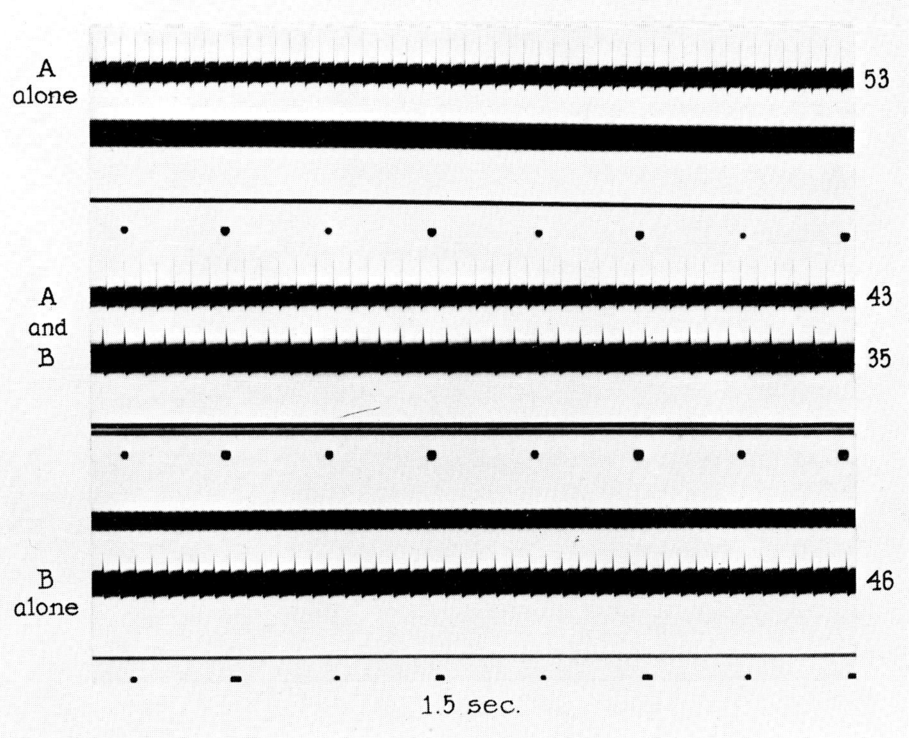

Figure 131. Oscillograms of action potentials recorded simultaneously from two optic nerve fibers, showing the discharge of nerve impulses when the respective ommatidia in which these fibers arose were illuminated separately and together. The numbers on the right give the total number of impulses discharged in the period of 1.5 sec. for the respective cases. The inhibitory effect on *A*, 53–43, is to be associated with the concurrent frequency of *B*, 35; likewise, the effect on *B*, 46–35, is to be associated with the concurrent frequency of *A*, 43 (see text). Time in $\frac{1}{5}$ sec. (From Hartline & Ratliff, 16.)

information, but evidently a useful one, considering the importance of outlines and borders in the recognition of features of the visual scene. Here, then, is a step in the processing of visual information that takes place in the retina, at or close to the level of the receptors themselves.

The role of inhibitory interaction in sensory systems has been recognized for a long time, and interest in it continues to widen. Over a hundred years ago, Ernst Mach invoked it to explain the bright and dark bands bordering steep gradients in intensity. Such "Mach bands" have been demonstrated by direct measurement of the patterns of response of the optic nerve fiber in *Limulus* (34). In the auditory system, von Békésy pointed out many years ago the significance of lateral inhibition in sharpening pitch discrimination (42); he also showed inhibitory interaction within the cutaneous sensory system (43).

An extensive and thorough review of studies concerning the role of inhibitory interaction in sensory systems, with special reference to vision, is to be found in

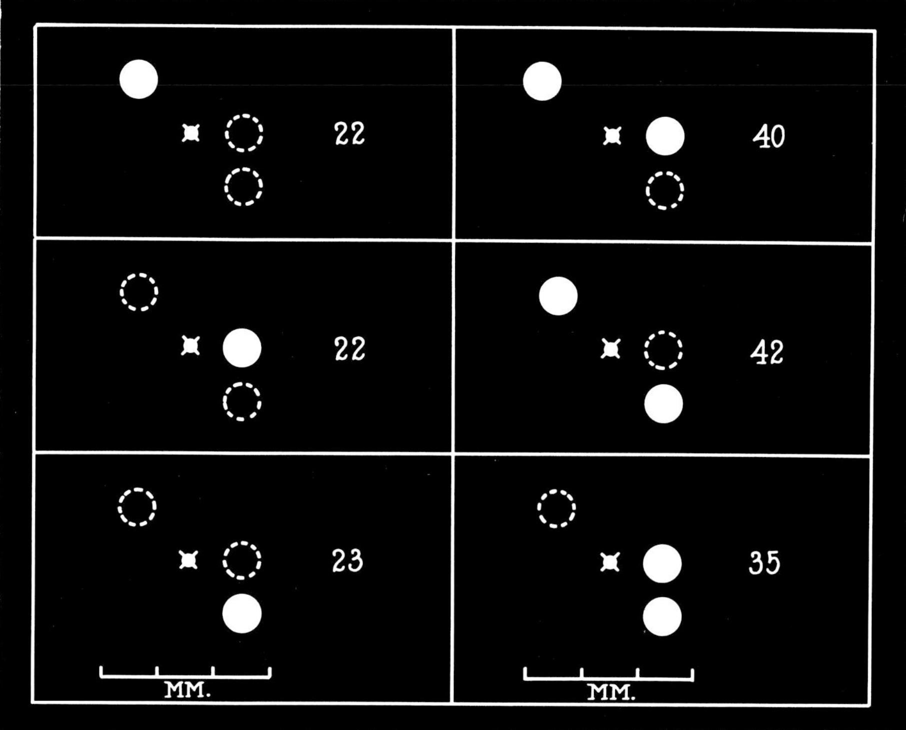

Figure 132. The summation of inhibitory influences exerted by two widely separated receptor groups, and by two groups close together. Each panel maps the same small portion of the eye. A test receptor (X) was illuminated steadily by a small spot of light confined to its facet. Larger spots of light could be placed singly in any of three locations, as shown in the three panels on the left side, or in pairs, as shown on the right. The white circles indicate the spots actually illuminated in each case; the other locations (not illuminated) are indicated in dotted outline merely for purposes of orientation. The number of impulses discharged from the test receptor in a period of 8 seconds was decreased upon illumination of the neighboring spot or spots by the amount shown at the right in each panel. For the widely separated pairs (upper and middle panels), the combined effect of the two was almost equal to the sum of their separate effects, but for the more closely spaced pairs (lower panels), the combined effect fell far short of this sum, as a result of their own mutual inhibition. (From Hartline & Ratliff, 17.)

Ratliff's recent book (33). Beginning with a review of the psychophysical observations made by Mach, and the relation they bore to the development of Mach's wide-reaching philosophical ideas, Ratliff goes on to summarize and document the modern experimental and theoretical work on contrast phenomena in sensory systems, and their physiological foundation in neural interaction. Most of the work he and I have done in collaboration is described and discussed there, in greater completeness than I can attain in this review (see also earlier reviews, 18,32).

The analysis of the interacting system of receptor units in the *Limulus* retina has revealed principles that are of general interest. As has been noted, the inhibition of a particular ommatidium is greater the greater the number of neighboring ommatidia illuminated; spatial summation of inhibitory influences does take place. The first attempt to determine the quantitative laws of this spatial summation led to puzzling, seemingly discordant results. It became evident, however, that the summed inhibitory effects of two separate regions neighboring a "test" receptor depended on how closely they themselves were neighbors to each other. If close together, their combined effects were less than if they were separated (Figure 132). Ommatidia in each region are, of course, inhibited by those in the other, and evidently the net contribution each can make to the summed effect depends on its output as affected by that inhibition (17).

The close reciprocity of the inhibitory interaction of receptor units in the eye of *Limulus* is demonstrated by quantitative measurements from a series of experiments similar to the one shown in Figure 131. Two neighboring receptor units are illuminated independently at various intensities in various combinations, first

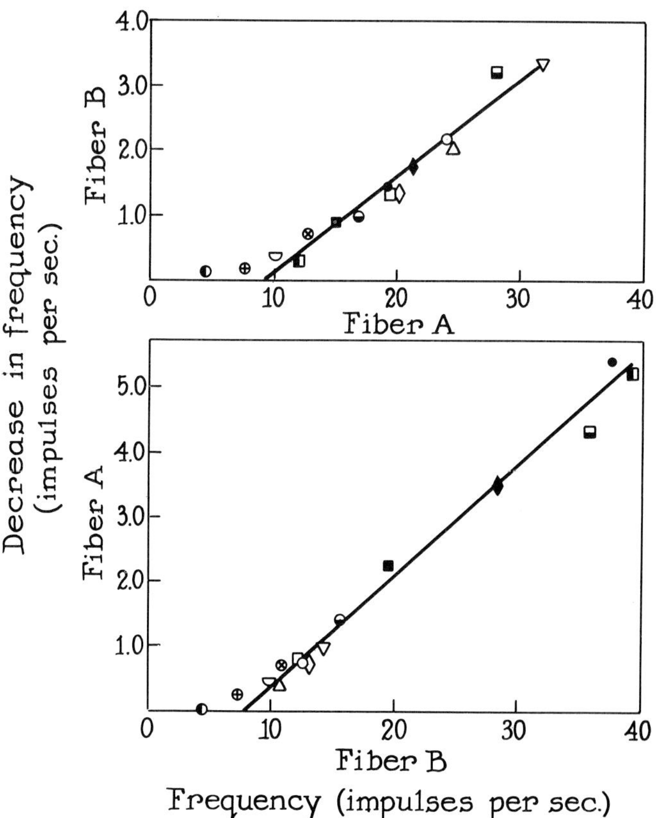

Figure 133. Mutual inhibition of two receptor units. The magnitude of the inhibitory action (decrease in frequency of impulse discharge) exerted on one of the ommatidia is plotted (ordinate) as a function of the degree of concurrent activity (frequency) of the other (abcissa). (See legend, Figure 131.) The different points were obtained by using various intensities of illumination on ommatidia *A* and *B* in several combinations. The data for points designated by the same symbol were obtained simultaneously. (From Hartline & Ratliff, 16.)

separately and then together. The reduction in firing rate of each that results when the other is brought in is taken as a measure of the amount of inhibition exerted on it, and a consistent representation of the measurements results only when the amount of inhibition of one is related to the rate of firing of the other while both are active (Figure 133). Thus, after a steady state is reached the activity of each is affected by the activity of the other; only by stating a pair of simultaneous relationships can the simultaneous responses of both be described without ambiguity. In the case of Figure 133, this means a pair of simultaneous equations, which, as the graphs show clearly, are linear in the range of frequencies above a distinct threshold (16). The closeness of this mutual action, in which the response of each affects and is reciprocally affected by the response of the other, lends a "recurrent" character to the interaction. The inhibition, caused by the streams of impulses passing down the axons of the receptor neurons, acts back on the neurons that generate them, and influences the very stream that causes it.

A digression at this point to consider the cellular mechanisms of the inhibitory action will provide some insight into how this "recurrent" feature arises. By means of a micropipette electrode penetrating an eccentric cell in an ommatidium, electrical changes are observed, such as are usually associated with excitation and inhibition of a neuron. If the electrode has entered the neuron close to the site of impulse generation in the initial segment of its axon, hyperpolarizing potential changes and concomitant conductance changes are observed to accompany inhibition of the neural discharge (Figure 134). These inhibitory postsynaptic potentials (IPSPs) cause inhibition in the well-known manner, by opposing the depolarization induced by the receptor's "generator potential" at the site of origin of the neural discharge. The IPSPs, in turn, are caused by trains of impulses in axons from neighboring receptor elements whose influences pass laterally along branches in the plexus. It is a fact (30,39) that optic nerve impulses are equally effective in causing IPSPs and concomitant inhibition whether they arise naturally as a result of illumination of the receptors neighboring the penetrated eccentric cell, or are generated artificially by electrical shocks applied to the optic

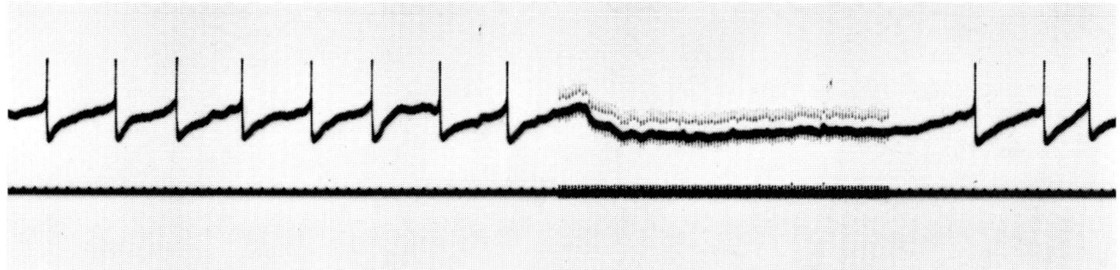

Figure 134. Decrease in magnitude of "generator potential" and concomitant cessation of impulse discharge resulting from inhibitory influences. The inhibition was produced by antidromic stimulation of the axons of neighboring ommatidia (39,40). Antidromic stimuli (66/sec. for 1.5 sec.) are signaled by thickening of lower trace and by shock artifacts on upper trace. Downward movement of the trace indicates increasing negativity of the recording microelectrode in the interior of the cell. Amplitude of spikes, approximately 10 mV. (From Ratliff, Hartline & Miller, 36.)

nerve and travel antidromically into the eye along the same axons. Thus, the inhibitory action is exerted on the pacemaker region, where the frequency of the neural discharge is determined. This inhibitory action itself is a consequence of neural discharges in parallel axons from neighboring receptors, which in the case of natural stimulation are similarly affected at their sites of origin.

Let us return to a consideration of the network properties resulting from the inhibitory interaction. When more than two receptor units in proximity to one another are illuminated, each inhibits and is inhibited by the others; the response of each is affected by the combined inhibition from all the others, which in turn depends on their own inhibited responses. A set of n simultaneous equations must now be used to describe the responses of the systems of n interacting receptor units; each equation must contain a set of terms, each one linear above a specific threshold, expressing the inhibition from all the receptor units. These inhibitory terms must be combined, experimental analysis dictates, by simple addition. The resulting set of "piecewise" linear simultaneous equations provides a satisfactory,

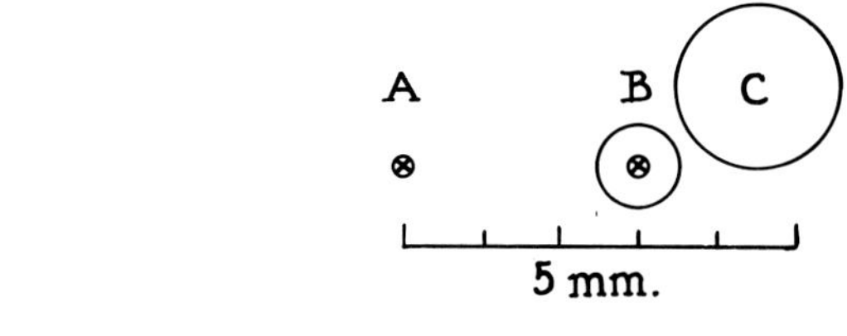

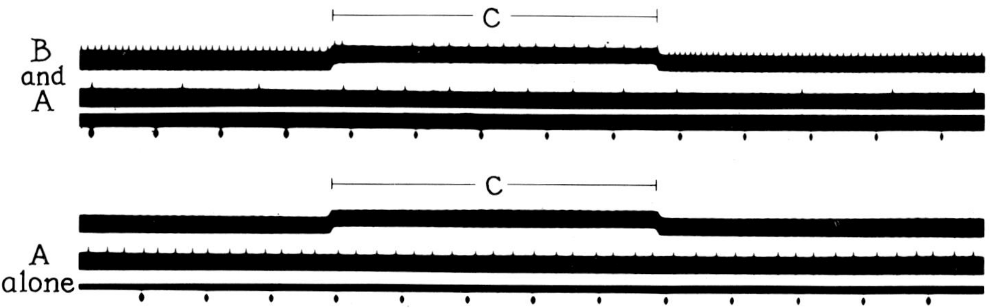

Figure 135. Oscillograms of the electrical activity of two optic nerve fibers, showing disinhibition. In each record the lower oscillographic trace records the discharge of impulses from ommatidium A, stimulated by a spot of light confined to its facet, and the upper trace records the activity of ommatidium B, stimulated by a spot of light centered on its facet, but which also illuminated approximately eight or ten ommatidia in addition to B. A third spot of light (C) was directed to a region of the eye more distant from A than was B (the geometrical configuration of the illumination pattern is sketched above). Exposure of C was signaled by the upward offset of the upper trace. *Lower record:* Activity of ommatidium A in the absence of illumination on B, showing that illumination of C had no perceptible effect under this condition. *Upper record:* Activity of ommatidia A and B together, showing the lower frequency of discharge of A (as compared with lower record) resulting from activity of B, and the effect of illumination of C, causing a drop in frequency of discharge of B and concomitantly an increase in the frequency of discharge of A, as A was partially released from the inhibition exerted by B. Time in $\frac{1}{5}$ sec. The black band above the time marks is the signal of the illumination of A and B, thin when A was shining alone, thick when A and B were shining together. (From Hartline & Ratliff, 16.)

though not absolutely perfect, formal description of the properties of the interacting system, and expresses succinctly the "recurrent" nature of the inhibitory interaction (17,18).

An interesting consequence of the "recurrent" nature of the inhibitory interaction in the *Limulus* retina appears in a special case, when a "test" receptor is acted upon by two groups of receptors at different distances from it. Let one group be chosen which is too far from the test receptor to affect it directly; let a patch of light fall on a second group which is near enough to the test receptor to inhibit it, yet near enough to the first group to be inhibited in turn by it. Then illumination of the first group will cause a release of the test receptor from some of the inhibition acting on it from the second group, and the firing frequency of the test receptor will actually rise (Figure 135). Such "disinhibition" could be mistaken for a spread of excitation from a remote region of the eye, were its dependence on the activity of the nearer receptor group not recognized (16). "Disinhibition" has been detected by psychophysical methods in the human visual system (26); it is commonly discussed in neurophysiology, and has been demonstrated experimentally in a non-visual part of the nervous system, the recurrent Renshaw system in the spinal cord (47,48)—Granit (7) also comments on other parallels between the properties of this system, especially its linearity, with those described in the *Limulus* retina.

As a result of the recurrent mode of inhibitory action, the spatial summation of mutual effects among very near neighbors in the receptor mosaic can affect their activity markedly, depending on the distribution of light upon them. Under steady illumination each receptor unit in a compact group discharges impulses at a much lower rate when the entire group is uniformly illuminated than when only one receives the same intensity of light. The relation between firing frequency of a unit and intensity of stimulating light is consequently much less steep when it is one of a group than when it acts alone (Figure 136). A significant extension of the functional range of visual receptors under steady light is a consequence that may be valuable in the physiology of vision. The effects of such mutual inhibition among members of a group will be termed "group self-inhibition".

Consequences of self-inhibition within a group of receptors are seen in the interactions of several groups of various sizes. A large group exerts a stronger inhibition on its neighbors, as has been said, but the increase does not vary linearly with number of elements in the group, due to the self-inhibition within the group (18). Also, a test receptor is less strongly inhibited by a nearby retinal area if it is illuminated along with a local group of its close neighbors than if it alone is illuminated. In the former case, reduction of the activity of the members of the local group diminishes their group self-inhibition; this opposes the suppressing tendency exerted by the external inhibition.

In addition to the very real process of "group self-inhibition", a comparable "self-inhibition" of the individual receptor units in the *Limulus* eye now seems a reasonable likelihood. Stevens (38), analyzing the transient increase in firing frequency with subsequent exponential decline (time-constant approximately

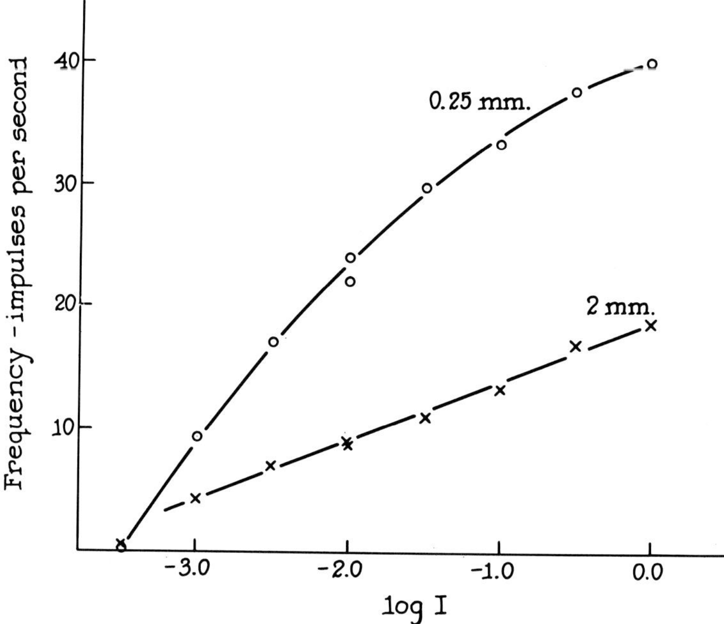

Figure 136. Relations between intensity of light (log *I*, abscissae) and frequency of discharge (ordinates) of a single ommatidium when illuminated alone (upper curve; 0.25 mm spot of light centered on its facet), and when illuminated together with a large number (approx. 40) of neighboring ommatidia surrounding it (lower curve; 2.0 mm spot of light centered on its facet). (From Hartline, Ratliff & Miller, 18.)

0.5 to 1 second) in response to square steps of current injected into an eccentric cell of an ommatidium, concluded that a self-inhibitory action accompanied the discharge of each impulse. Purple (30), by intracellular recording, demonstrated hyperpolarizing potential changes following the discharge of each impulse, with bridge measurements showing concomitant conductance increases; the equilibrium potential he calculated from his measurements led him to conclude that each nerve impulse discharged by an eccentric cell is followed by an IPSP—a true self-inhibitory process—with rapid onset and exponential decay (time constant approximately 1 second).

Whether such self-inhibition arises from actual loops of axon branches returning and synapsing on their cells of origin, whether interneurons as yet unknown are involved, or whether "group self-inhibition" takes place among cells comprising the sensory structure of the ommatidial unit, are questions that cannot yet be answered. Perhaps entirely different mechanisms are involved.

Self-inhibition of the individual receptor units cannot be detected by steady state experiments alone, for it acts whether a test receptor is illuminated alone or together with other receptors (18). Self-inhibition reveals itself, however, as an important factor in the analysis of responses of the interacting system to changing patterns of light on the receptor mosaic. It is to a consideration of the dynamics of the interaction that I will now turn.

An unchanging retinal image is indeed a rarity in nature. All the studies of the *Limulus* retina I have just reviewed concerned responses of receptor cells under steady patterns of illumination, after their mutual inhibitory interactions had established themselves and the system was in a steady state. When a change takes place in the distribution of light on the receptor mosaic, new patterns of interaction must establish themselves, and the transients in neural activity that occur during this rearrangement of mutual influences may well provide the most significant contribution of the intereacting system to visual function.

The study of the dynamics of retinal interaction is hampered by technical difficulties. Mutual actions of individual elements, when they can be isolated for analysis, may be small, yet the interactions of groups of elements, though more easily measured, may be complicated or may have significant details blurred by unresolved diversity of individual actions. Transient responses of the receptors to changes in illumination are complex and difficult to control; artificial stimuli, more easily controlled in some ways, may be less exact in others, or introduce uncertainties of physiological significance. The use of the *Limulus* eye, favorable in many respects, does not resolve all these difficulties. Employment of fiber optics permits very effective isolation of the optical stimulus to single ommatidia at high intensity with a minimum of light scatter into adjacent receptors, but with some loss of control over directional effects that may be important in the natural functioning of each ommatidium. Computer acquisition and processing of data, on line, permit the immediate monitoring during each "run" in an experiment, and allow the prompt averaging of large numbers of repeated runs. Thus, small effects, such as are often all that are seen when only a few cells interact, can be studied quantitatively. Averaging, however, carries a risk of statistical blurring of significant details that may vary slightly in timing from run to run. "Artificial" inhibition induced by antidromic volleys of impulses initiated by electrical shocks to small bundles of optic nerve fibers can be very precisely timed, but at some sacrifice of control of spatial factors, and with some uncertainty as to whether the influences produced are exactly those elicited naturally when receptors are stimulated by light.

Difficulties in dealing with the complexity of dynamic neural interactions are not only technical, but conceptual as well. It is hard enough to grasp the complexity of the interaction of more than just a few retinal elements under steady patterns of illumination. To understand the intricately interdependent transients in response to changes in patterns of light is much more difficult. For the steady state, analytic solutions of the system of simultaneous equations can be achieved in limited cases, as in the treatment of Mach bands (20). For more general cases, analog models (3,18) and computer solutions* have been devised to solve the simultaneous equations, or their integral equation counterpart. If it could be found, a corresponding mathematical formulation which would describe the dynamic responses in detail and reduce to the succinct expressions for the steady state would be highly useful. The disadvantage exists, however, that any empirical

---

* D. Quarles, personal communication.

theory rich enough to encompass the variety of observations might itself be almost as difficult to comprehend as the system it purported to describe. An alternative is to construct somewhat more mechanistic models, based on underlying physiological processes as far as they are known. Workable models are necessarily oversimplified approximations and must supply assumptions where knowledge is imperfect. The appeal of such models to the mechanistically minded physiologist lies perhaps in their realistic pretentions—a trap for the unwary, however—but they can have solid worth if, in addition to predictive value, they are fruitful in suggesting new experiments.

An electronic analog devised by Dodge (31) has been useful in visualizing the effects of self-inhibition in the *Limulus* ommatidium. Harmon (9,10) has devised an electronic analog consisting of circuit units that can be interconnected so as to simulate with great diversity systems of interacting neurons. A model designed by Lange (22,23) specifically for the study of the dynamics of the inhibitory interaction in the *Limulus* retina uses a computer program to simulate the processes of excitation by light and inhibition by synaptic action; suitable scaling permits the introduction of realistic parameter values, and the outputs of the program can be displayed so as to be directly comparable to the computer outputs resulting from actual experiments. I will refer to some of Lange's results below.

In the remainder of this survey I would like to describe a few features of the dynamics of the inhibitory action in the retina of *Limulus*; our studies are still in a preliminary phase.

Inhibitory influences take time to build up, and take time to decay. A brief burst of impulses from a receptor in response to short flashes of light induces a transient dip in frequency of firing of a steady-lighted neighbor, but only after a delay of about two-tenths of a second (Figure 137). The inhibition requires time to build up to its threshold before it takes effect; if a background of steady inhibition is provided—even if sub-threshold—the time delay is reduced (35). A time delay

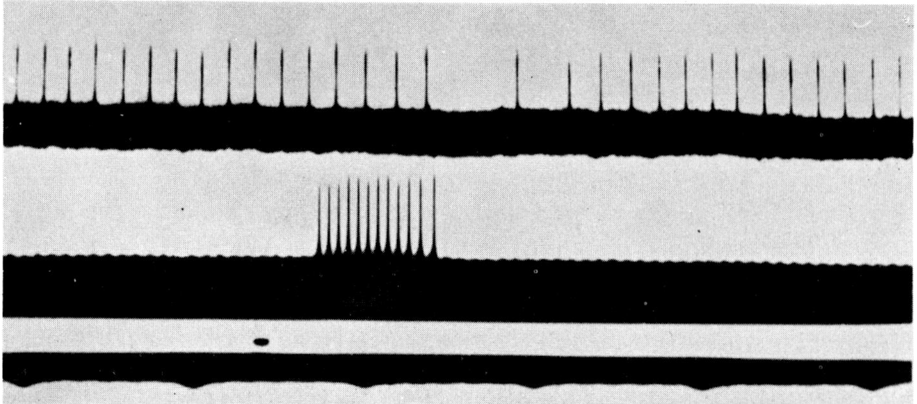

Figure 137. Transient inhibition of the discharge from a steadily illuminated ommatidium (upper trace) caused by a burst of impulses discharged from a second ommatidium nearby (bottom trace) in response to a 0.1 sec. flash of light (signaled by the black dot in the white band above the time marks). Time in $\frac{1}{5}$ sec. (From Hartline, Ratliff & Miller, 18.)

for inhibition to take effect also appears when a small group of receptors is suddenly illuminated. The response of a single receptor shows the familiar initial high frequency "on" transient, with subsequent decline—sensory adaptation—to a steady level (Figure 138, upper curve). The response of the same receptor to an exposure of the same intensity but which includes a number of the receptor's near neighbors shows a much more precipitous drop in frequency; the mutual inhibition of all the receptors in the small group takes effect quickly, but not quickly enough to prevent the first part of the "on" transient to appear undiminished. A steady level of discharge is reached eventually, but not without oscillations, as the mutual effects come into balance (Figure 138, lower curve). Of

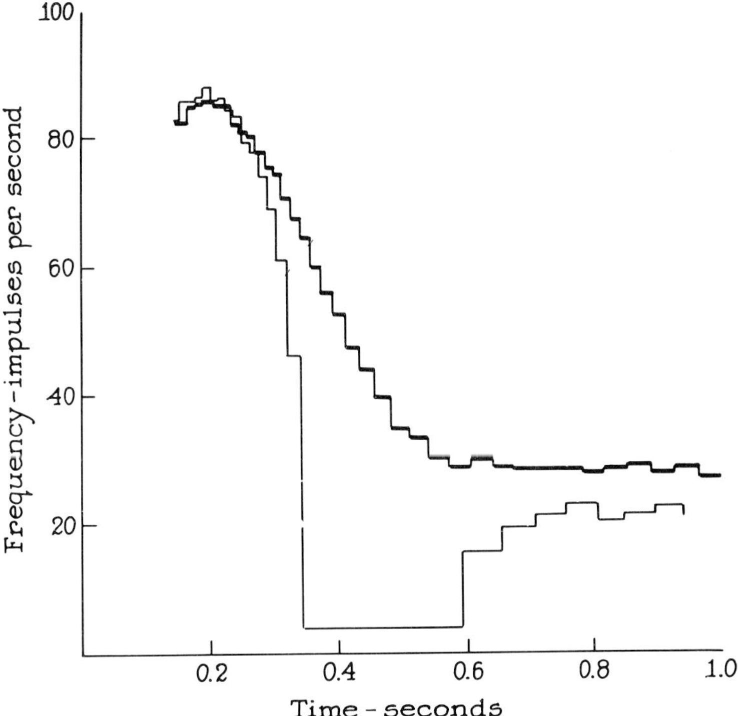

Figure 138. Inhibitory action of a group of receptors on one of its members. The upper, heavy trace shows the frequency of impulses from an ommatidium illuminated alone ("test" receptor). The lower, light trace shows the frequency of discharge from the same receptor when the area of illumination (same intensity as before) was enlarged so that neighboring ommatidia were also illuminated. The time delay of their inhibitory action on the test receptor was long enough for the initial peak of the discharge to be unaffected; this peak was reached before the inhibitory influences affected the test receptor. Soon after, however, the inhibitory influences affected the test receptor and its response dropped abruptly. Since the inhibition is mutual, similar effects were produced on the neighboring receptors themselves, the inhibition they exerted became smaller, and the response of the test receptor increased slightly to a steady level that remained below that reached when the test receptor alone was illuminated (cf. Figure 136). (From Hartline, Ratliff & Miller, 18.)

course, when the group is illuminated, the final steady discharge is at a lower frequency than that achieved by any one receptor illuminated alone; this has already been described as "group self-inhibition". Physiologically, this delay in inhibitory action permits receptors to act at their full sensitivity, without inhibitory restraints, in the first part of their transient responses to sudden increases in light intensity. They thus are enabled to detect small sudden increments in spite of the inhibitory feedback that serves to extend their range of action over a wide range of intensity of steady illumination.

We must note, of course, that the familiar sensory adaptation of the individual receptor has this same function of emphasizing sudden changes, and the inhibitory influences in group action only accentuate this. The dominant factor in receptor adaptation surely resides in the excitatory mechanism, as evidenced by the large initial transient and low plateau of the generator potentials observed by intracellular recording (4,5,27,41). In addition, however, self-inhibition of the individual receptor must be a substantial component of receptor adaptation, in the same manner described for group inhibition.

A feature of inhibitory dynamics that is perhaps of more general interest is the transient that follows the cessation of inhibition. As may be seen from the spacing of impulses in the records of Figures 130, 134, 135, and 137, and in the plots of

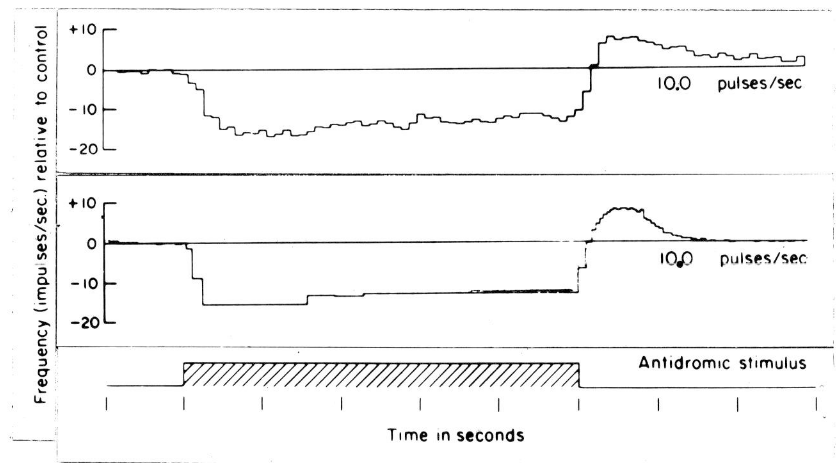

Figure 139. *Upper trace:* record of the activity of a steadily illuminated receptor subjected to a 5-second period of inhibition by antidromic excitation of a bundle of optic nerve fibers from neighboring receptors; as ordinate is plotted the difference in the frequency of impulse discharge during "inhibited" *vs.* "control" (no antidromic stimulation) runs; note the slight "undershoot" at the onset of the inhibition, and the pronounced, slowly subsiding "overshoot" at its cessation. *Lower trace:* simulation by Lange's computer "model" of the inhibition shown in the upper trace; parameters, including values of the inhibitory coefficients and thresholds, were chosen to match those directly measured in the actual experiment, except for the time-constant of decay of the lateral and self-inhibitory processes (set at 0.67 and 1.00 sec. respectively), not measured directly for this preparation but in the range found in other experiments. (From Lange, 22.)

"instantaneous" frequency in Figure 139, the firing of a test receptor overshoots in returning to its uninhibited rate after a period of inhibition. Such "post-inhibitory rebound" is familiar in neurophysiology; in the visual system, "off" responses are its direct manifestations (29,41,45). In general, a number of factors no doubt contribute to postinhibitory rebound. In the present case, we seek its explanation in a discrepancy between the relative rate of decay of lateral inhibition, on the one hand, and the rate of build-up of self-inhibition as the test receptor resumes discharging impulses at its uninhibited frequency, on the other. If the two processes proceeded at the same rate, recovery would be simultaneous; evidently, however, the lateral inhibition disappears more rapidly than the self-inhibition is restored, and an "overshoot" results. This discrepancy in rates reflects perhaps inherent differences between self-inhibition and lateral inhibition; alternatively, as the lateral inhibition falls below the threshold, its last subsiding remnant will be hidden, so that only the rapid early limb of the exponential decays is manifest. Thus, the lateral inhibition acts as though it had a rapid decay which is over before the self-inhibition is fully restored. This interpretation is not at all evident from simple inspection of responses; it was suggested by examination of the changes in those numbers in Lange's computer program model that represented the values of self- and lateral inhibitory influences, as the model simulated the transient at the end of a period of inhibition (Figure 139) (24).

Both of these dynamic features, i.e., the crispening of the "on" transient and the generation of an "off" overshoot, seem feeble details of the firing pattern to compare with the vigorous "on" and "off" responses seen in, for example, the

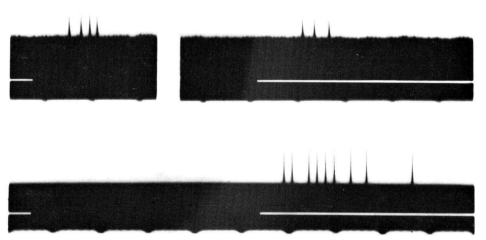

Figure 140. Oscillograms of diverse "types" of impulse discharge patterns in single fibers of *Limulus* optic nerve. *Upper record:* a synthetic "on-off" response (approximately 1 sec. was cut from the middle of this record). *Lower record:* a synthetic "off" response. Time is marked in $\frac{1}{5}$-sec. periods. Signal of exposure of eye to light blackens the white line above the time marker. Fibers whose activity is shown in the two records gave a sustained discharge when the ommatidia from which they arose were illuminated alone. Only by adjusting conditions of adaptation, and the distribution of light over the neighboring receptors, could these somewhat anomalous patterns of response be contrived. (From Ratliff & Mueller, 37.)

vertebrate retina. It is intended here only to demonstrate concretely how transients of an interacting system of receptor units can lead in the direction of more highly developed response patterns. The analogy can go a little farther. By the judicious choice of conditions, Ratliff & Mueller (37) were able to "synthesize" actual "on-off" and "off" response patterns in the *Limulus* eye (Figure 140). In each case there was nothing anomalous about the receptors they chose; only the patterns of light on the chosen receptor and its neighbors and, to some extent, conditions of adaptation, were adjusted in a manner that could scarcely occur in nature so as to accentuate the weaker transients we have just described and suppress the steady component of the discharge from the receptor under observation. What was contrived was indeed an "interplay of excitation and inhibition" that exploited the dynamics of interaction in this simple retina to produce an anomalous result in imitation of functional properties that are inherent in more highly organized visual centers. To this we should add that *Limulus* itself does have, in its own higher visual centers, neural elements that generate quite typical "off" discharges in response to reduction of illumination on the eye (Figure 141) or to cessation of trains of artificially generated volleys of impulses in the optic nerve (46).

It would be unwarranted at the present time to insist that the diverse and complex types of responses exhibited by neurons of highly organized retinas and visual centers are to be explained solely by simple algebraic combination of excitatory and inhibitory influences exerted upon them, even given diverse rates of rise and fall of these influences. Other mechanisms may well be equally significant: various membrane properties of individual neurons, special effects of strategically placed synapses, influence of glial elements, and others yet to be discovered. It is mainly the purpose of this review to show how, in a comparatively simple retina,

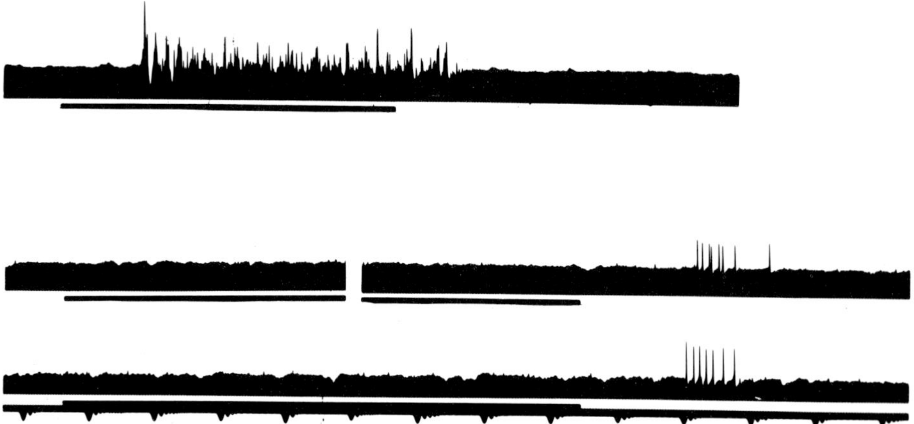

Figure 141. Action potentials recorded by microelectrodes in the optic ganglion of *Limulus*. *Upper record:* responses to illumination of the eye recorded by a large electrode inserted in the ganglion at the point of entrance of the optic nerve. *Lower records:* responses to illumination of the eye recorded by a small electrode inserted in the same ganglion approximately 2 mm posterior to the point of entrance of the optic nerve. Signal of illumination above time marker; time in $\frac{1}{5}$ sec. (From Hartline, 14.)

an interplay of excitatory and inhibitory influences can contribute to the integration of visual information by modifying the sensory message transmitted to the higher centers. But it is also to be hoped that the analysis of these relatively uncomplicated processes may point the way to an understanding of the sophisticated mechanisms of data processing that take place in intricately organized neural centers.

SUMMARY

The processing of visual information begins at the level of the receptors. Their spectral sensitivities fix the range of wavelengths that are visible, their thresholds set the lower limits of vision, and their static and dynamic characteristics determine the basic properties of the excitatory events that initiate vision. Spatial and temporal summation of excitation takes place in the retinal pathways. Inhibition is also a basic process in retinal action; the interplay between excitatory and inhibitory influences early in the retinal process generates the diverse patterns of neural activity that are passed on to the higher visual centers.

Inhibitory interaction was studied in the comparatively simple retina of *Limulus*: its basic properties are described and its mechanism analyzed. Its role in accentuating contrast at edges and in steep intensity gradients in the retinal image is examined, and the dynamics of this lateral inhibitory interaction is studied in detail. A number of the features of the impulse discharges in optic nerve fibers can be understood on the basis of the rise and fall of inhibitory influences exerted by neighboring receptor units on one another. The inhibitory component of retinal interaction is essential in the generation of the highly complex patterns of neural activity observed in the vertebrate retina, and in the higher visual centers of vertebrates and invertebrates—patterns that underlie the visual perception of form and motion.

REFERENCES

1. Adrian, E. D., and Matthews, R., The action of light on the eye. III. The interaction of retinal neurones. *J. Physiol.* (London), 1928, **65**: 273–298.
2. Barlow, H. B., and Levick, W. R., The mechanism of directionally selective units in the rabbit's retina. *J. Physiol.* (London), 1965, **178**: 477–504.
3. Beddoes, M. P., Conner, D. J., and Melzak, Z. A., Simulation of a visual receptor network. *IEEE Trans. Biomed. Engin.*, 1965, BME**12**: 136–138.
4. Fuortes, M. G. F., Initiation of impulses in visual cells of *Limulus. J. Physiol.* (London), 1959, **148**: 14–28.
5. Fuortes, M. G. F., and Hodgkin, A. L., Changes in the time scale and sensitivity in the ommatidia of *Limulus. J. Physiol.* (London), 1964, **172**: 239–263.
6. Granit, R., *Sensory Mechanisms of the Retina*. Hafner, New York, 1947.
7. Granit, R., Pascoe, J. E., and Steg, G., The behavior of tonic α and γ motoneurones during stimulation of recurrent collaterals. *J. Physiol.* (London), 1957, **138**: 381–400.
8. Grüsser-Cornehls, U., Grüsser, O.-J., and Bullock, T. H., Unit responses in the frog's tectum to moving and nonmoving visual stimuli. *Science*, 1963, **141**: 820–822.

9. Harmon, L. D., Neural analogs. *Spring Joint Comp. Conf.*, 1962, **21**: 153–158.

10. ———, Neuromimes: action of a reciprocally inhibitory pair. *Science*, 1964, **146**: 1323–1325.

11. Hartline, H. K., The response of single optic nerve fibers of the vertebrate eye to illumination of the retina. *Am. J. Physiol.*, 1938, **121**: 400–415.

12. ———, The receptive fields of the optic nerve fibers. *Am. J. Physiol.*, 1940, **130**: 690–699.

13. ———, The effects of spatial summation in the retina on the excitation of the fibers of the optic nerve. *Ibid.*: 700–711.

14. ———, The neural mechanisms in vision. *Harvey Lect.*, 1941, **37**: 39–68.

15. ———, Receptor mechanisms and the integration of sensory information in the eye. *Rev. Mod. Physics*, 1959, **31**: 515–523.

16. Hartline, H. K., and Ratliff, F., Inhibitory interaction of receptor units in the eye of *Limulus*. *J. Gen. Physiol.*, 1957, **40**: 357–376.

17. ———, Spatial summation of inhibitory influences in the eye of *Limulus*, and the mutual interaction of receptor units. *J. Gen. Physiol.*, 1958, **41**: 1049–1066.

18. Hartline, H. K., Ratliff, F., and Miller, W. H., Inhibitory interaction in the retina and its significance in vision. In: *Nervous Inhibition* (E. Florey, Ed.). Pergamon Press, New York, 1961: 241–284.

19. Hartline, H. K., Wagner, H. G., and Ratliff, F., Inhibition in the eye of *Limulus*. *J. Gen. Physiol.*, 1956, **39**: 651–673.

20. Kirschfeld, K., and Reichardt, W., Die Verarbeitung stationärer optischer Nachrichten im Komplexauge von *Limulus* (Ommatidien-Sehfeld und räumliche Verteilung der Inhibition). *Kybernetik*, 1964, **2**: 43–61.

21. Kuffler, S. W., Discharge patterns and functional organization of mammalian retina. *J. Neurophysiol.*, 1953, **16**: 37–68.

22. Lange, D., *Dynamics of Inhibitory Interaction in the Eye of* Limulus; *Experimental and Theoretical Studies.* Thesis, The Rockefeller University, New York, 1965.

23. Lange, D., Hartline, H. K., and Ratliff, F., Inhibitory interaction in the retina: techniques of experimental and theoretical analysis. *Ann. N.Y. Acad. Sci.*, 1966, **128**: 955–971.

24. ———, The dynamics of lateral inhibition in the compound eye of *Limulus*. II. In: *The Functional Organization of the Compound Eye* (C. G. Bernhard, Ed.). Pergamon, Oxford, 1966: 425–449.

25. Lettvin, J. Y., Maturana, H. R., McCulloch, W. S., and Pitts, W. H., What the frog's eye tells the frog's brain. *Proc. Inst. Radio Engrs.*, 1959, **47**: 1940–1951.

26. Mackavey, W. R., Bartley, S. H., and Casella, C., Disinhibition in the human visual system. *J. Opt. Soc. Amer.*, 1962, **52**: 85–88.

27. MacNichol, E. F., Jr., Visual receptors as biological transducers. In: *Molecular Structure and Functional Activity of Nerve Cells* (R. G. Grenell and L. J. Mullins, Eds.). American Institute of Biological Sciences, Washington, D.C., 1956: 34–62.

28. Miller, W. H., Fine structure of some invertebrate photoreceptors. *Ann. N.Y. Acad. Sci.*, 1958, **74**: 204–209.

29. Naka, K., Inoma, S., Kosugi, Y., and Tong, C., Recording of action potentials from the single cells in the frog retina. *Jap. J. Physiol.*, 1960, **10**: 436–442.

30. Purple, R. L., *The Integration of Excitatory and Inhibitory Influences in the Eccentric Cell in the Eye of* Limulus. Thesis, The Rockefeller University, New York, 1964.

31. Purple, R. L., and Dodge, F. A., Interaction of excitation and inhibition in the eccentric cell in the eye of *Limulus*. *Sympos. Quant. Biol.*, 1965, **30**: 529–537.
32. Ratliff, F., Inhibitory interaction and the detection and enhancement of contours. In: *Sensory Communication* (W. A. Rosenblith, Ed.). Wiley, New York, 1961: 183–203.
33. ———, *Mach Bands: Quantitative Studies on Neural Networks in the Retina*. Holden Day, San Francisco, 1965.
34. Ratliff, F., and Hartline, H. K., The responses of *Limulus* optic nerve fibers to patterns of illumination on the receptor mosaic. *J. Gen. Physiol.*, 1959, **42**: 1241–1255.
35. Ratliff, F., Hartline, H. K., and Lange, D., The dynamics of lateral inhibition in the compound eye of *Limulus*. I. In: *The Functional Organization of the Compound Eye* (C. G. Bernhard, Ed.). Pergamon, Oxford, 1966: 399–424.
36. Ratliff, F., Hartline, H. K., and Miller, W. H., Spatial and temporal aspects of retinal inhibitory interaction. *J. Opt. Soc. Amer.*, 1963, **53**: 110–120.
37. Ratliff, F., and Mueller, C. G., Synthesis of "on-off" and "off" responses in a visual-neural system. *Science*, 1957, **126**: 840–841.
38. Stevens, C. F., *A Quantitative Theory of Neural Interactions: Theoretical and Experimental Investigations*. Thesis, The Rockefeller Institute, New York, 1964.
39. Tomita, T., Mechanism of lateral inhibition in the eye of *Limulus*. *J. Neurophysiol.*, 1958, **21**: 419–429.
40. Tomita, T., Kikuchi, R., and Tanaka, I., Excitation and inhibition in lateral eye of horseshoe crab. In: *Electrical Activity of Single Cells* (Y. Katsuki, Ed.). Igaku Shoin, Tokyo, 1960: 11–23.
41. Tomita, T., Murakami, M., Hashimoto, Y., and Sasaki, Y., Electrical activity of single neurons in the frog's retina. In: *The Visual System: Neurophysiology and Psychophysics* (R. Jung and H. Kornhuber, Ed.). Springer, Berlin, 1961: 24–31.
42. von Békésy, G., Zur Theorie des Hörens: Die Schwingungsform der Basilarmembrane. *Physik. Zschr.*, 1928, **29**: 793–810.
43. ———, Neural inhibitory units of the eye and skin; quantitative description of contrast phenomena. *J. Opt. Soc. Amer.*, 1960, **50**: 1060–1070.
44. Wagner, H. G., MacNichol, E. F., Jr., and Wolbarsht, M. L., The response properties of single ganglion cells in the goldfish retina. *J. Gen. Physiol.*, 1960, **43**(6), Supp. 2: 45–62.
45. Wiesel, T. N., Recording inhibition and excitation in the cat's retinal ganglion cells with intracellular electrodes. *Nature* (London), 1959, **183**: 264–265.
46. Wilska, A., and Hartline, H. K., The origin of "off-responses" in the optic pathway. *Am. J. Physiol.*, 1941, **133**: 491–492.
47. Wilson, V. J., and Burgess, P. R., Changes in the membrane during recurrent disinhibition of spinal motoneurons. *Nature* (London), 1961, **191**: 918–919.
48. Wilson, V. J., Diecke, F. P. J., and Talbot, W. H., Action of tetanus toxin on conditioning of spinal motoneurons. *J. Neurophysiol.*, 1960, **23**: 659–666.

THE ELECTRORETINOGRAM: ITS COMPONENTS AND THEIR ORIGINS*

KENNETH T. BROWN
University of California Medical Center
San Francisco, California

Discovery of the electroretinogram (ERG) in 1865 by Holmgren (55) was an important event in visual physiology, which initiated the use of electrophysiological methods for studying visual systems. This type of response has now been recorded from the retinas of all of the many vertebrate species which have been studied, and responses which are generally simpler have been found from the visual organs of invertebrates. The complexity of the vertebrate ERG indicates that it is not unitary, but consists of a number of separate components. Since it may be recorded across the whole retina by gross electrodes, which cannot detect single cell activity, each component must consist of the summed activity of many cells of a given class which are responding in synchrony to the light stimulus. Thus the ERG offers the unique advantages of a readily recorded response which reveals electrical activity from certain classes of retinal cells.

The primary problems of the ERG have always been to analyze this complex response into its components, and to identify the type of retinal cell which generates each component. These problems are important for retinal physiology, and are also of clinical interest, since the normal ERG must be understood before the ERG of a human patient can attain its maximum value in the diagnosis of retinal disorders. The purpose of this paper is to examine the present status of our knowledge concerning components of the ERG and their origins. This will be done primarily by reviewing work in which the author has been engaged during the last ten years, including recent results not published previously. No attempt will be made to cover all studies in this field, but other lines of work will be included which seem particularly relevant to the central problems. The emphasis will be upon results obtained or confirmed in mammals, and many of the critical findings have been obtained in primates, so these results should apply to

* This paper has been published in *Vision Research*, Vol. 8, 1968 (pp. 633–677), and is republished in this volume by permission of that journal.

The author is indebted to Mrs. Kay M. Howell for preparing histological sections, and to Kosuke Watanabe and Motohiko Murakami, each of whom assisted in some of the recent experiments. This work was supported by grant No. B-1903 from the National Institute of Neurological Diseases and Blindness, U.S. Public Health Service.

interpretation of the human ERG. A brief summary of this work has been published previously (17) and earlier work on these problems has been reviewed by Granit (46–49).

ERGs from Rod and Cone Retinas, and the Analyses of Granit

In early work the active electrode was usually placed upon the cornea, while the reference electrode was at a remote location which was effectively behind the eye. If the active electrode is placed in the vitreous humor, it is closer to the retina and the responses are considerably larger (33). Also, if the reference electrode is in the orbit, directly behind the eye, there is less recording of extraneous bioelectric signals, and the noise level is reduced. Hence these electrode locations were used for Figure 142, while the usual more remote locations were used for Figure 143. In early ERG work the convention became established that positivity of the active electrode was recorded as an upward deflection, and that convention is used for all records of this paper. The cat ERG of Figure 142 seems typical of ERGs recorded from predominantly rod retinas under light-adapted conditions, except that the cat's c-wave is unusually large. Following the rapid a- and b-waves, there is a period of negativity which continues during the remainder of the stimulus. When the stimulus terminates there is a simple negative deflection which constitutes the off-response. This is followed by the rising phase and peak of the c-wave, but the c-wave is not an off-response. Granit (45) showed that if the stimulus is sufficiently long the peak of the c-wave occurs during the stimulus, as

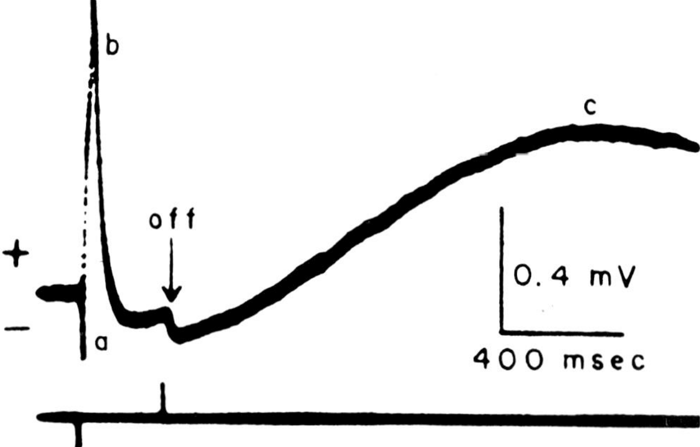

Figure 142. The ERG of the cat, recorded between a chlorided silver wire in the vitreous humor and a chlorided silver reference electrode in the orbit behind the eye. Positivity of the active electrode is recorded as an upward deflection in this and all other records of this paper, in accordance with the convention for ERG work. Direct-coupled amplification. The retina was stimulated by a 2.18 mm light spot delivered in the area of the tapetum, and the retinal illumination in the focused spot was 4.6 log lumen/m^2. The lower record shows when the stimulus began and terminated. The stimulus duration was 320 msec., and it was repeated every 10 sec.

illustrated in Figure 144, and Figure 146 shows that the c-wave begins to rise soon after onset of the stimulus. Thus the c-wave is elicited by turning the stimulus on, but its time-course is quite slow, so in Figure 142 its peak is not reached until after the stimulus has terminated. Figure 143 shows an ERG from the pure cone retina of a squirrel, which illustrates that the main differences between ERGs from predominantly rod and pure cone retinas occur after the stimulus has terminated. In the cone ERG the off-response is a d-wave, consisting of a rapid positive deflection followed by a slower negative fall to the baseline, and there is no detectable c-wave.

Because of these differences, Granit recognized the necessity for separate analyses of ERGs from predominantly rod and pure cone retinas. These analyses form the best starting point for the present work, and are shown in Figure 144. At the top is the cat ERG, analyzed into three major components, which were designated PI, PII, and PIII. In this terminology the term "P" stands for process, since at that time the cellular origin was not known for any of the potentials. The components were then numbered in the order in which they disappeared following the administration of ether anesthesia. After this procedure Granit found that the deflections of the cat ERG disappeared in three major steps. The c-wave disappeared first, then the b-wave and off-response disappeared at about the same time, while the a-wave disappeared last (45). Thus in Figure 144 the analysis at high stimulus intensity shows that the c-wave results from PI. The b-wave is due to a peak of PII, which includes a very slow positive phase, the decay of which gives the negative off-response. The a-wave is then accounted for by the onset of PIII, a negative potential which is well maintained during the stimulus. After the negative off-response of this cat ERG there is a small positive deflection, which is labeled the d-wave and which is accounted for by the decay of PIII. At lower stimulus intensity the cat ERG is shown to consist almost entirely of PII.

At the bottom of Figure 144 is the analysis by Granit & Riddell (51) of the light-adapted ERG from the frog retina, which contains numerous cones. In this case there is a prominent d-wave, which is shown to result from the decay of PIII, followed by the decay of PII. In this animal the light-adapted ERG showed no distinct c-wave, but a relatively small c-wave was found in the frog's

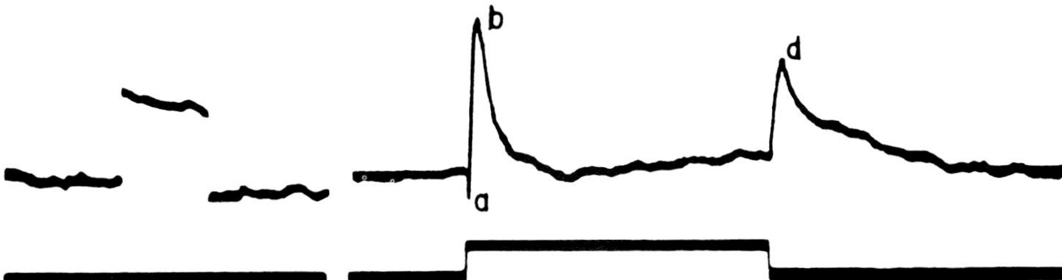

Figure 143. Electroretinogram from the pure cone retina of the squirrel, as recorded under light-adapted conditions by a contact lens electrode on the cornea and a reference electrode on the skin of the forehead. Preceding the response is a 0.5 mV calibration signal, and the stimulus duration was 1 sec. After Arden & Tansley (7), with labels added.

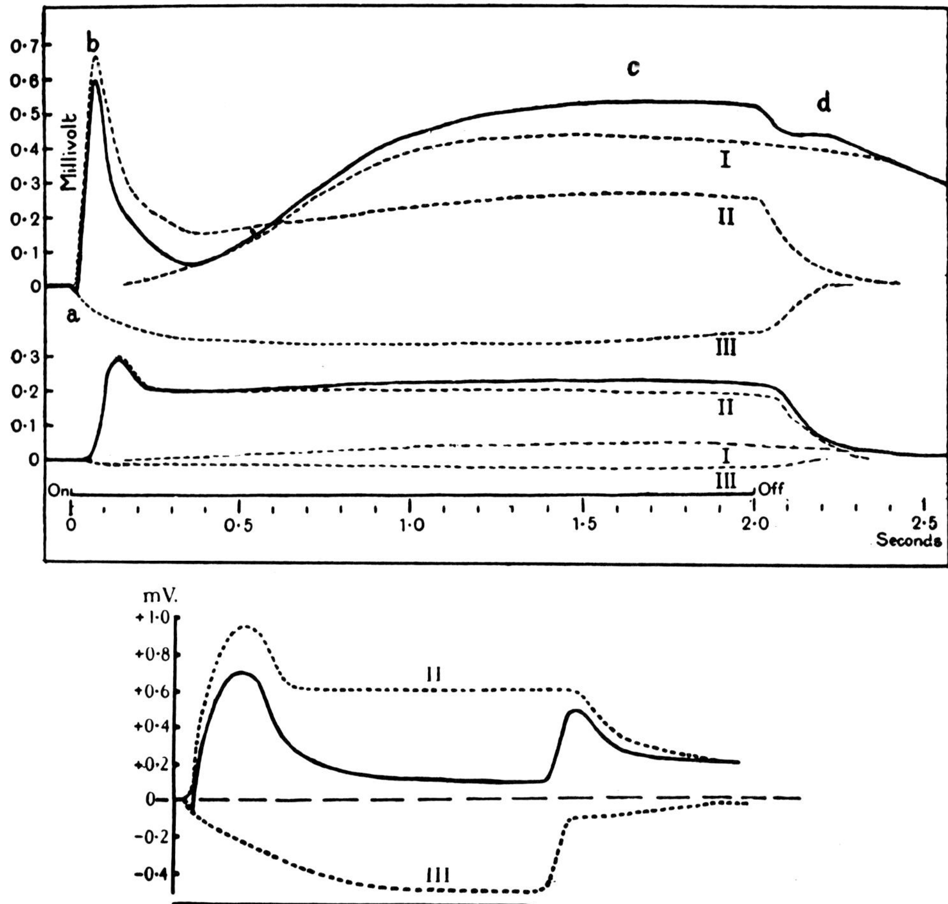

Figure 144. The enclosed top portion shows analyses of the predominantly rod ERG of the cat, when evoked at stimulus intensities of 14 ml (upper analysis) and 0.14 ml (lower analysis); (from Granit, 45). The bottom portion shows an analysis of the cone-type ERG of the light-adapted frog retina. Stimulus duration, 2 sec. (From Granit & Riddell, 51.)

dark-adapted ERG. Hence these analyses of rod and cone ERGs were based upon evidence for three components, which were found capable of explaining major features of ERGs from both rod and cone retinas.

Microelectrode Methods in Intact Mammalian Eyes

The use of microelectrodes for intraretinal recording of the ERG was first reported in isolated eyes and retinas of cold-blooded vertebrates by Tomita (76) and by Ottoson & Svaetichin (66). Since each component should have maximum amplitude as an electrode passes the cells which generate it, microelectrodes offered promising new techniques for analyzing the ERG and determining the origins of its components. But the early studies gave conflicting results, probably because of technical problems (34,49). Methods were then developed by Brown & Wiesel (32) for using microelectrodes in the intact mammalian eye (58), a preparation which yielded some helpful technical advantages. Following further development, including necessary special equipment, the methods now used have been described and have proved satisfactory for a variety of problems (15). They are best suited to relatively large eyes, and experimental animals have included the cat, cynomolgus monkey (*Macaca irus*), and night monkey (*Aotus trivirgatus*).

The animal is anesthetized by barbiturate anesthetic, and skeletal muscle movements are abolished by a continuous intravenous infusion of succinylcholine. The animal is then artificially respirated, and body temperature is automatically controlled at normal levels. A special device is attached to the eye which incorporates channels for three needles which are inserted into the vitreous humor. Each needle then serves as a channel for introducing an electrode or other device into the eye. When recording the ERG of the entire retina, a chlorided silver wire is placed in the vitreous humor and the reference electrode is a coil of chlorided silver wire which is wrapped with saline-soaked cotton and placed in the orbit behind the eye. For microelectrode work, one needle channel is used for either a micropipette filled with 3M KCl, or for a tungsten microelectrode which is insulated except for the very tip. In either case the diameter of the electrode tip is less than 0.5 μ. The microelectrode may be directed toward a wide variety of retinal areas, and is advanced through the retina by a hydraulic electrode advancer. In this type of work the reference electrode is usually a chlorided silver wire in the vitreous humor. The third needle channel may be used for any of several special devices, such as a rod for applying pressure upon the optic disk to clamp selectively the retinal circulation. Since the normal optics of the eye are maintained and well protected by a glass contact lens, a hand ophthalmoscope may be used for positioning intraocular devices under visual control. The retina is also viewed directly for focusing and positioning the stimulus spot. Light stimuli from a tungsten source are provided by a special optical stimulator, which permits the control of all relevant parameters of the stimulus (15).

In using intraretinal microelectrodes to study the ERG, two technical difficulties were encountered in early studies which were especially troublesome. One was the problem of knowing the actual depth of the microelectrode. The other was the difficulty of relating intraretinal responses to the ERG recorded across the entire retina. These problems were solved in the cat eye by Brown & Wiesel (32,33). It was discovered that micropipette electrodes are extremely sensitive mechanoelectric transducers, which can record the pulse beat of blood vessels in the tissue through which the electrode passes (32). Thus a pulse beat first appeared in the record when the retina was contacted, remained strong throughout the surface layers of the retina, and disappeared or was sharply reduced when the electrode passed the outer margin of the inner nuclear layer. The retinal circulation of the cat extends only to that level (60); deeper layers of the retina are avascular, and little or no pulse beat was recorded in the avascular layers. But as the electrode contacted the pigment epithelium, back by Bruch's membrane, a strong pulse beat reappeared which was due to the choroidal circulation. A slight additional advance resulted in penetration of the R-membrane, an entity with especially high electrical resistance, which was first described in the frog by

Brindley (12). In the cat the structure which constitutes this R-membrane was found to be in the complex of Bruch's membrane and pigment epithelium (26,31,32), and results in the frog are now in agreement with this finding (14,79). After penetrating the R-membrane, a strong pulse beat was recorded throughout the choroid. Thus recording the pulse beat provided a means for identifying three major electrode locations, including the retinal surface, the outer margin of the inner nuclear layer, and the retinal side of the pigment epithelium. Certain intermediate retinal levels were also identified by correlating other types of responses with retinal anatomy. These physiological methods of electrode location were later validated with electrode marking work by Brown & Tasaki (26). The physiological methods have proved especially useful, since they permit identification of electrode location during any given penetration and at the time when recordings are being made.

The intraretinal responses of the cat were next analyzed (33). In accord with previous work, the ERG recorded across the entire retina in the usual manner proved to be a summated response from essentially the entire retina. When evoked by a relatively small stimulus spot, this gross ERG is recorded primarily from the large retinal area stimulated by low-intensity stray light. An intraretinal electrode can likewise record this gross ERG, provided that the reference electrode is effectively behind the eye at a remote location. But the intraretinal electrode will also record a *local* response, which is only from a small retinal area surrounding the electrode, and having a diameter of about 0.75–1.5 mm. The local response has the same general form as the ERG, and was found to be composed of the same components. Minor differences in time-course between the gross ERG and the local response were found to be explained from the different recording conditions, which cause the *effective stimuli* for the two responses to be different. If the stimulus is a focused spot which is centered upon the electrode, the gross ERG is elicited primarily from distant retinal areas by low-intensity stray light, while the local response is elicited by the high-intensity light in the focused spot.

Since the minor differences in time-course are readily explained, the local response is simply an ERG from a small area of retina surrounding the electrode. But the distinction between gross and local responses is of great importance from the standpoint of experimental methods, so the local ERG was designated the LERG. Since the LERG is generated by the cells in the retinal area penetrated by the microelectrode, the amplitude of a given component of this response should be maximum as the electrode passes the cells which generate the component. The gross ERG, on the other hand, is generated primarily from retinal areas remote from the electrode; thus changes in amplitude of this response, which occur during a retinal penetration, are due only to passive electrical resistance of the tissue and have no significance for the origins of components. Since the gross ERG sums with the LERG, it must be eliminated to record the LERG in pure form. It was found that when the reference electrode was placed in the vitreous humor, the gross ERG was not recorded. This is probably because the electrical resistance of the retina itself is small compared to that of the R-membrane, so that most of the gross ERG appears only as a voltage drop across the R-membrane. Thus, if the reference electrode is in the vitreous humor, the LERG may be recorded without interference from the gross ERG, and this method has been used in most further studies of the LERG.

The Splitting of PII into Two Separate Components

Granit's analysis of the cat ERG shows that at lowered stimulus intensity PII tends to become isolated, and the b-wave portion of PII becomes less prominent. With the new recording methods, which gave larger responses, it was found that stimulus intensity could be reduced sufficiently to abolish the b-wave of the cat without abolishing the steady portion of PII (33). This was demonstrated both by intraretinal recording of the LERG, and by recording the gross ERG with an active electrode in the vitreous humor. Since the remaining response had a time-course similar to that of a D.C. current pulse, it was designated the D.C. component (33). The effects of reduced stimulus intensity upon the cat ERG are better illustrated by recent experiments, one of which is shown in Figure 145. As stimulus intensity is reduced, all portions of the response are attenuated, but at different rates. The a-wave disappears first, and is not seen at 1.5 log units below the maximum stimulus intensity. As the c-wave is diminished, its peak occurs at progressively earlier times, and the c-wave disappears at about minus 2.0 log units. Beyond this point the b-wave declines more rapidly than the D.C. component. At minus 3.4 log units the b-wave has disappeared, and the D.C. component appears to be isolated. Beyond this point the amplitude of the D.C. component decreases steadily until it disappears. Constant conditions of light adaptation were maintained for all records, as described in the legend, and the final control record shows that during this experiment there was no appreciable change in the preparation or recording conditions.

Lowered stimulus intensity is the only method known thus far which can reveal the approximate time-course of the D.C. component by showing it under conditions where the recorded amplitudes of all other components have been reduced to negligible levels. Experiments like that of Figure 145 have also been performed in the night monkey and cynomolgus, where lowered stimulus intensity likewise reveals the D.C. component. The results of this procedure indicate that the b-wave and D.C. component are separately generated, but other methods are required to demonstrate this convincingly. Such evidence seems provided by Figure 146, which shows that the b-wave may be selectively blocked by local anesthetic. In this work it is necessary for the anesthetic to produce its effects over the entire retinal area from which the records are obtained. Hence the LERG of the cat was recorded intraretinally by a microelectrode near the retinal side of the pigment epithelium. In such responses all components, except for the c-wave, are inverted in polarity with respect to components recorded in the gross ERG by conventional methods. The reasons for this will become evident from results given later in this paper. Thus in Figure 146 the control response at zero time shows a small positive a-wave and a negative b-wave; the D.C. component is also negative, as shown by a rapid positive deflection after termination of the stimulus. Xylocaine was then injected from a pipette located directly over the site where the microelectrode

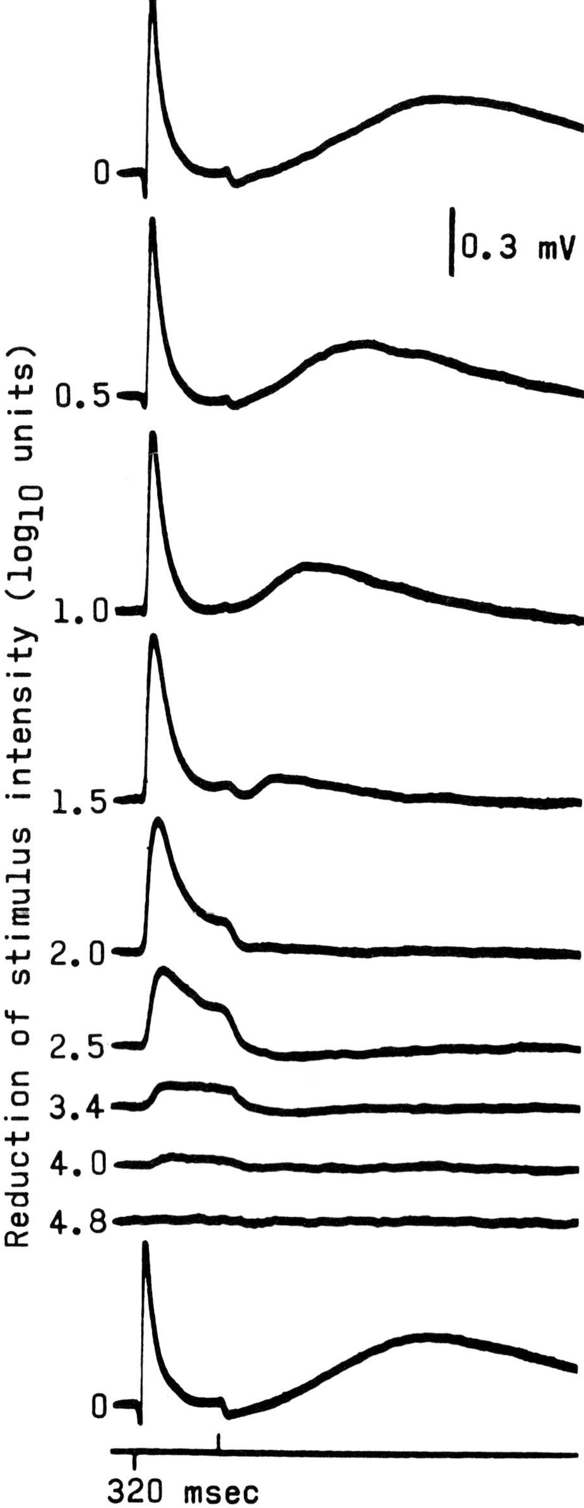

Figure 145. The ERG of the cat as a function of stimulus intensity. Responses recorded between a chlorided silver wire in the vitreous humor and a chlorided silver reference electrode in the orbit behind the eye, using direct-coupled amplification. The retina was stimulated by a 2.18 mm light spot delivered in the area of the tapetum, and at maximum intensity the retinal illumination in the focused spot was 4.6 log lumen/m^2. Constant conditions of light adaptation were obtained by stimulating every 10 sec. at maximum intensity until the response stabilized; then a given filter was inserted and the first response after inserting the filter was recorded. Intensities are specified in $\log_{10}$ units below the maximum intensity by specifying the optical densities of the neutral filters. Responses were recorded in sequence from top to bottom, and the lowest record is a final control response. The rapidly rising phase of the b-wave has been made more distinct in some records by retouching, as has also been done for the rapidly rising phases of certain responses in later figures of this paper.

entered the retina. Following this procedure the b-wave was diminished, and after 2.5 minutes appears to be abolished. At this time the response consists of an a-wave which is enlarged, due to abolition of the b-wave, and the c-wave appears unaffected. After the a-wave there is a negative deflection, of similar amplitude to the positive deflection after termination of the stimulus, and these deflections appear to represent the onset and decay of the D.C. component. Since the magnitude of the off-deflection is no less than that of the original control record, the D.C. component has not been reduced. Thus xylocaine appears to abolish

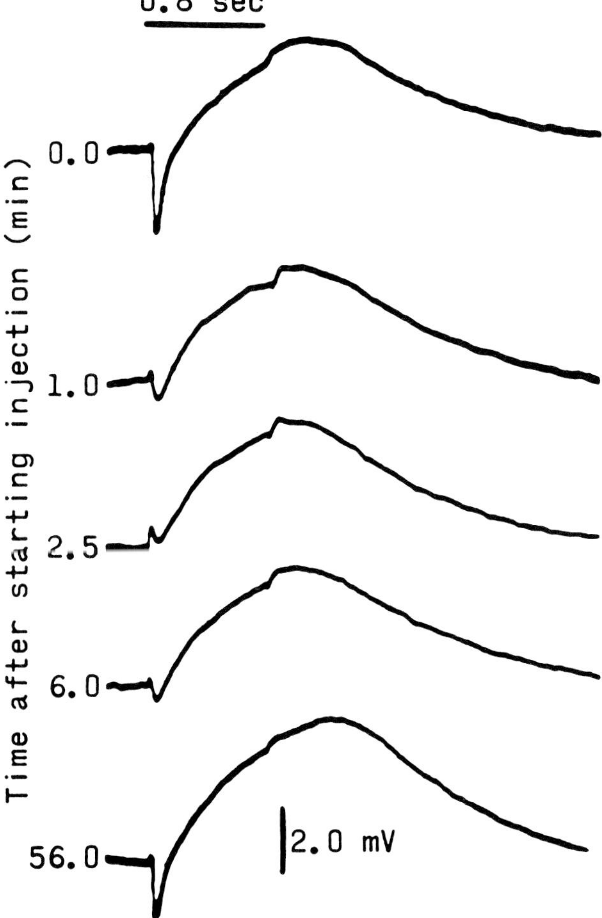

Figure 146. Selective and reversible block of the locally recorded b-wave of the cat by local anesthetic. The micro-pipette electrode was near the retinal side of the pigment epithelium and the reference electrode was placed on the back of the head. Then 0.01 ml of a 2 per cent xylocaine solution was injected slowly, over a period of 1 min., into the vitreous humor close to where the microelectrode entered the retina. The stimulus was a 0.5 mm spot which was centered on the electrode; it gave a retinal illumination of 71 lumen/m^2, and was repeated every 5 sec. Amplification direct-coupled. (After Brown & Wiesel, 34.)

the b-wave, without affecting the D.C. component or c-wave, and the a-wave is secondarily enlarged. This interpretation has now been confirmed by clamping the retinal circulation while maintaining the choroidal circulation. This procedure abolishes both the b-wave and D.C. component, as shown later in the present paper, and it abolishes the deflections in the 2.5-minute record of Figure 146 which appear to represent the onset and decay of the D.C. component, as illustrated previously (30: Fig. 7). In Figure 146 some recovery of the b-wave may be seen after 6 minutes, and after 56 minutes the amplitude of the b-wave is almost normal. Thus the effects of xylocaine upon the b-wave are highly selective and reversible. This means that the b-wave and D.C. component must be generated by different mechanisms, so Granit's PII consists of these two components. Figure 146 also shows that if there is a causal relation between these two components, the D.C. component must be generated at an earlier level of the retinal pathway than the b-wave. Although the mechanism whereby xylocaine blocks the b-wave is not known, the initial effect of a local anesthetic in low concentration is to block nerve impulses. Since xylocaine affected *only* the b-wave, the results of Figure 146 suggest that the b-wave occurs after an impulse stage in the retinal pathway (34).

Amplitudes of Components of the Cat LERG as a Function of Electrode Depth

The amplitudes of all four major components were next studied in the cat retina as a function of electrode depth, as shown in Figures 147 and 148. Figure 147

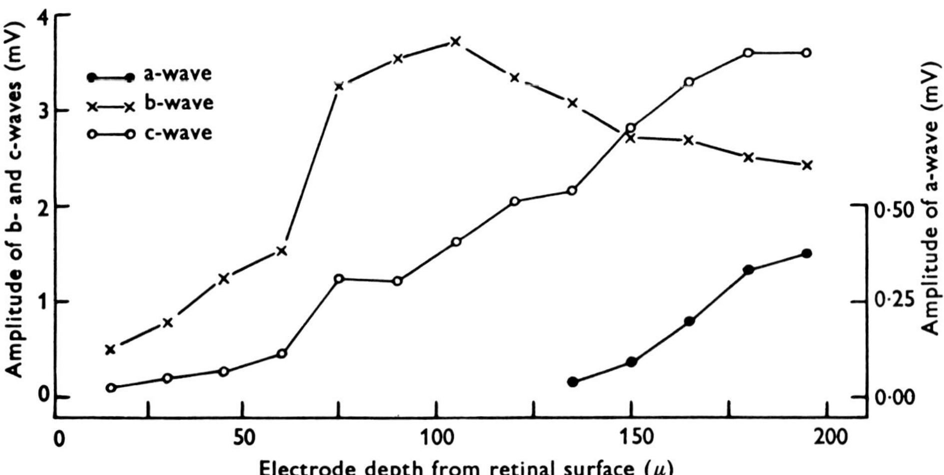

Figure 147. Amplitudes of a-, b-, and c-waves plotted as a function of depth of a micropipette electrode during a single penetration of the cat's peripheral retina. The penetration was approximately perpendicular, and at a measured depth of 195 μ the electrode was against the retinal side of the pigment epithelium. Reference electrode in the vitreous humor. The stimulus spot was 3.0 mm in diameter, centered upon the electrode, and provided a retinal illumination of 71 lumen/m². The stimulus had a duration of 50 msec. and was repeated every 5 sec. (From Brown & Wiesel, 34.)

shows the a-, b-, and c-waves plotted from a single penetration. The deepest electrode position for which results are shown was adjacent to the retinal side of the pigment epithelium, and when the R-membrane was penetrated all responses were sharply reduced in amplitude. Thus the amplitude maxima for both the a- and c-waves were found close to the retinal side of the pigment epithelium, while the amplitude maximum for the b-wave was about halfway through the retina, in the region of the inner nuclear layer. The results of Figure 148 were obtained after reducing stimulus intensity just sufficiently to abolish the a- and c-waves, leaving only the b-wave and D.C. component. The amplitudes of these components were then plotted during a single penetration, the amplitude of the D.C. component being measured from the amplitude of the off-deflection. Figure 148 shows that the amplitude maxima of the b-wave and D.C. component are at about the same retinal level, which is in or near the inner nuclear layer. The locations of all these amplitude maxima have been confirmed by electrode marking (26). Similar results have also been obtained now in the cynomolgus monkey and night monkey, so the results of Figures 147 and 148 seem typical of mammalian retinas. From the standpoint of component analysis, these results divide the ERG into responses generated at two distinctly different retinal levels.

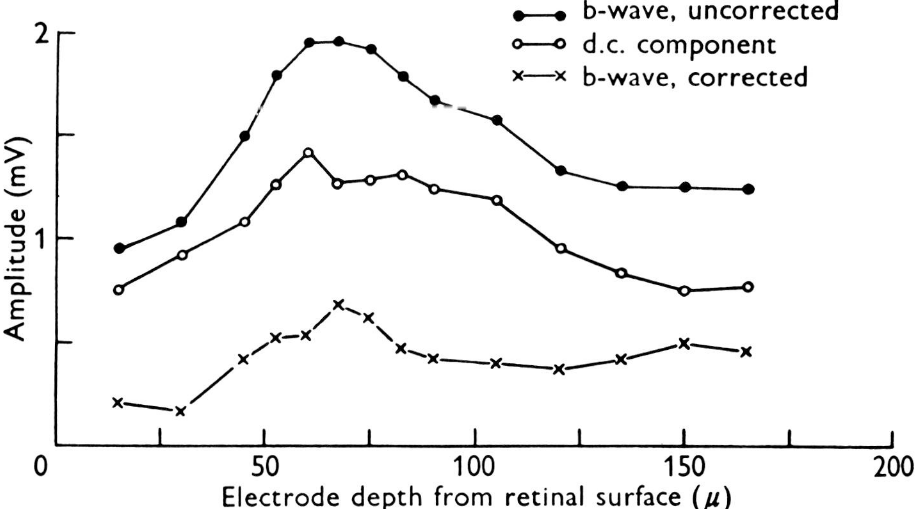

Figure 148. Amplitudes of the b-wave and D.C. component as a function of depth of a micropipette electrode during a single penetration of the cat's peripheral retina. At a depth of 165 μ the electrode was against the retinal side of the pigment epithelium. Reference electrode in vitreous humor. The stimulus intensity was sufficiently low to eliminate both the a- and c-waves. The uncorrected b-wave was measured from the baseline to the peak, while the D.C. component was measured from the magnitude of the deflection at termination of the stimulus. The corrected b-wave was then plotted by subtracting the D.C. component curve from that for the uncorrected b-wave. The stimulus was a 1.0 mm spot, centered upon the electrode and giving a retinal illumination of 0.022 lumen/m^2. Stimulus was 0.8 sec. in duration, repeated every 5 sec. (From Brown & Wiesel, 34.)

Evidence for Separate Origins of the a- and c-Waves

There is strong evidence that the a- and c-waves are not only generated by separate mechanisms, but arise from two different cell types. Noell (64) showed that sodium iodate selectively reduces the c-wave, correlated with selective destruction of the pigment epithelium, and was the first to conclude that the c-wave is generated by cells of the pigment epithelium. Also, Yamashita (84) and others have not recorded the c-wave from isolated retinas of cold-blooded animals which give all of the other major components. Hence the c-wave appears to be generated by cells which are not present in the isolated retina. Sickel (71) recently reported from the isolated frog retina a potential which has a time-course similar to that of the c-wave, but an interpretation of this finding was not offered and its significance is not clear.

In the cat, intracellular responses have been obtained by Brown & Wiesel (34) which show a time-course similar to that of the c-wave. These responses were found only on rare occasions during the process of penetrating the complex of pigment epithelium and Bruch's membrane, and appeared only in conjunction with a large negative D.C. shift, presumably representing the membrane potential of a cell. The intracellular response was of opposite polarity to the extracellular c-wave, and considerably larger in amplitude, as may be expected. Since the c-wave has a time-course which is rather distinctive among retinal potentials, and since the intracellular response had a similar time-course, it seems assured that the response recorded intracellularly was the c-wave. Both the membrane potential and the response declined rapidly, as is typical of intracellular recordings from small cells. Hence high quality records were not obtained, but the observations were made repeatedly, usually when using micropipette electrodes with especially high electrical resistance and therefore having especially small tips. The pigment epithelium cells are the only ones from which it seems possible that these intracellular responses could have been obtained. The a-wave also has maximum amplitude near the retinal side of the pigment epithelium, but is readily recorded from isolated retinas of cold-blooded animals. Thus it was concluded that the a-wave must be a response of the retinal photoreceptors (34).

Methods of Determining the Origins of Components in the Cynomolgus Monkey Retina

Since there are subtle difficulties in interpreting curves which show the amplitude of a given component as a function of electrode depth (30,34), it was next desired to find methods of localizing the origins of components which are entirely independent of electrode depth studies. Two such methods seemed feasible in macaque monkeys and were applied by Brown & Watanabe (27). Figure 149 shows the peripheral retina of a macaque monkey with all of the major layers and structures labeled. For comparison, Figure 150 is a section through the center of the fovea. In the central fovea the ganglion cell layer is entirely absent, and the inner nuclear layer is reduced to a few scattered cells, while the receptor layer is especially well developed. Hence if local responses are compared between

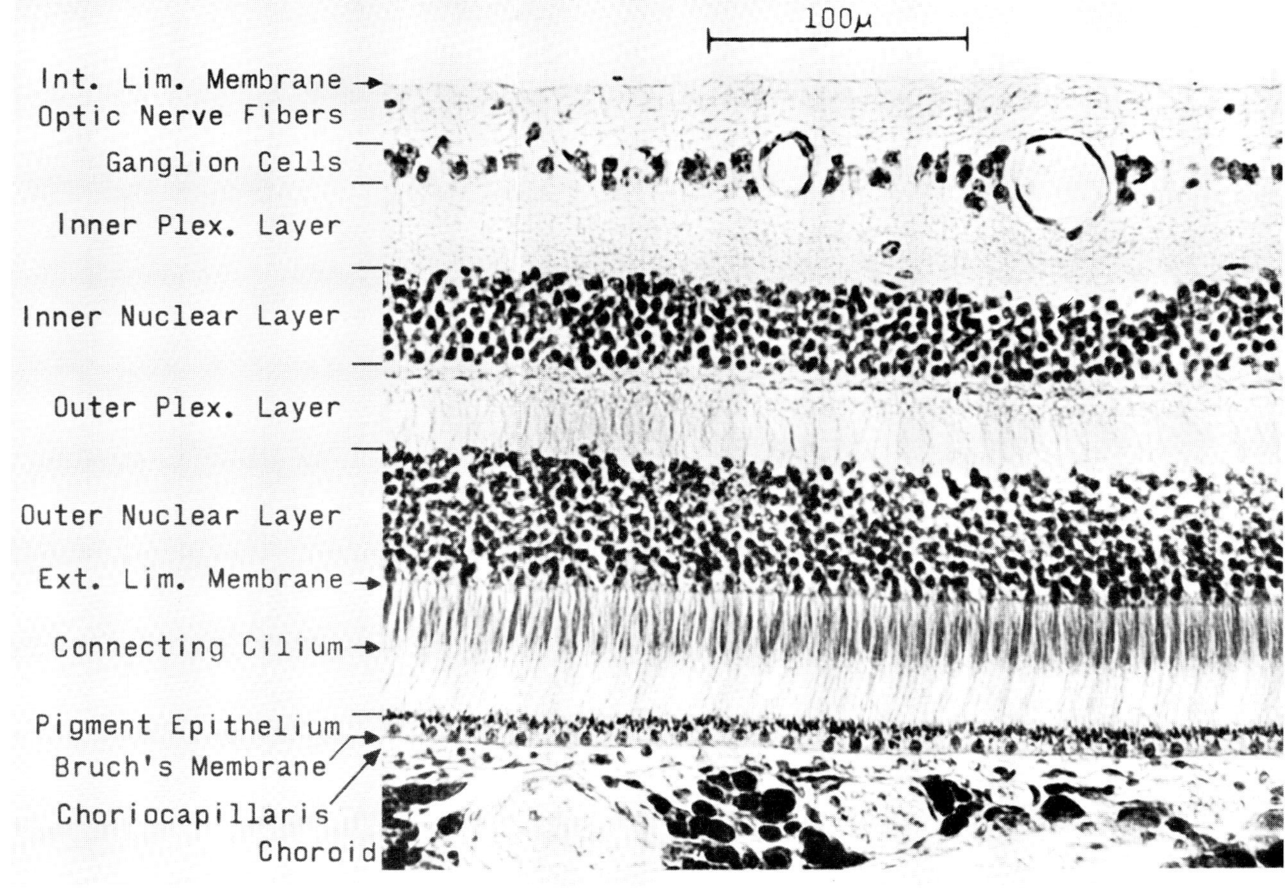

Figure 149. The peripheral retina on the nasal side of a rhesus macaque eye, with all major layers and structures labeled. This retina is quite comparable to that of the cynomolgus macaque, which is only a different race of the same species (43). Techniques of fixation and embedding were as described by Brown & Tasaki (26). The section was cut perpendicular to the retinal surface, as assured by alignment of the inner segments of receptors in the plane of the section. The thickness of the section was 10 μ, and the stain was hematoxylin and eosin.

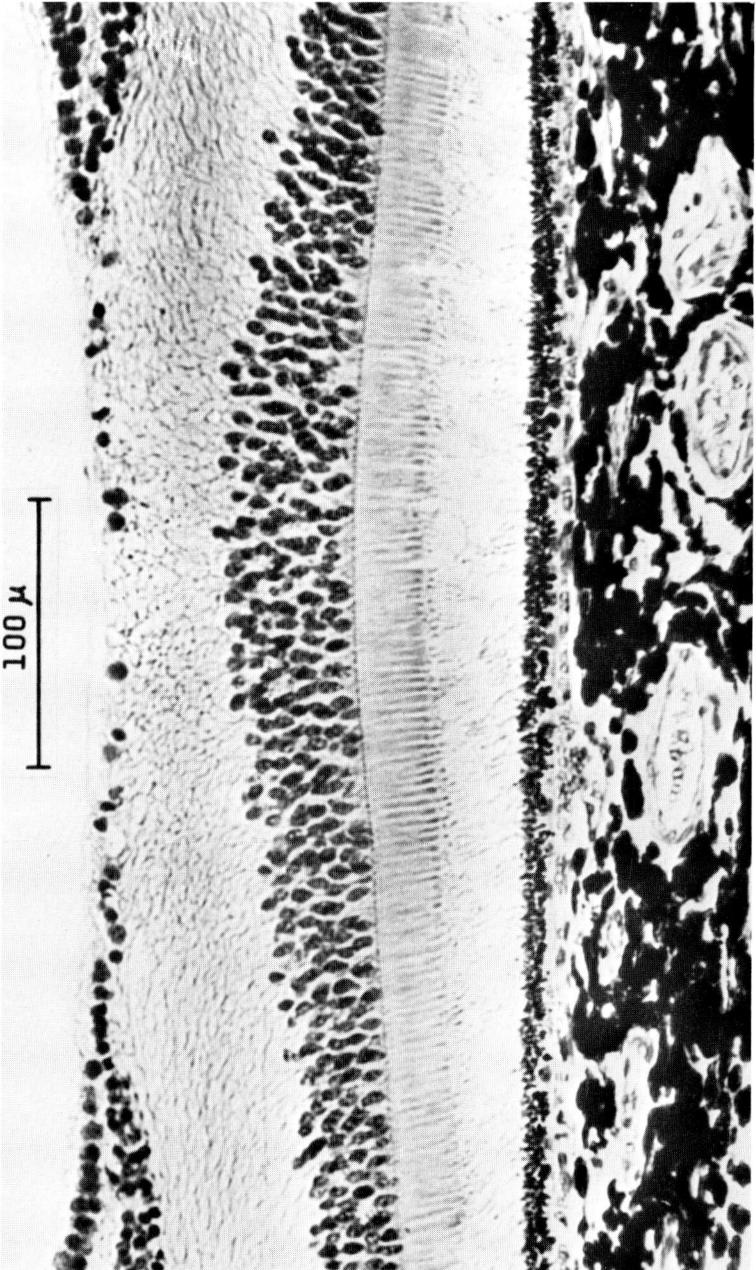

Figure 150. A histological section through the center of the cynomolgus fovea, as indicated by the maximum size of this area in serial sections. Histological technique as in Figure 149. (From Brown, Watanabe & Murakami, 30.)

the peripheral retina and fovea of this animal, any components generated by cells proximal to the receptors should be greatly reduced or absent in the fovea, while responses generated by the receptors should be unaffected or larger. It proved possible to manipulate a tungsten microelectrode for penetration of the fovea under visual control. An intraretinal electrode records from a larger area than that of the central fovea, but the stimulus spot could be made smaller than this area. Thus small stimulus spots were accurately focused and directed to the central fovea, so that the receptors stimulated were primarily those in this pure cone area. Foveal responses were then compared with responses which were similarly evoked and recorded from the peripheral retina.

The other method was selective clamping of the retinal circulation without affecting the choroidal circulation. This was done by using the third needle channel to insert a stainless steel rod with a rounded end into the eye. This rod was then manipulated under visual control to apply pressure upon the optic disk, thus mechanically clamping the entire retinal circulation whenever desired during an experiment. The cessation of blood flow in the retinal vessels was visually verified, and the choroidal circulation was unaffected, since the major choroidal vessels penetrate the sclera at a distance from the optic disk (70). Because the retinal circulation extends only to the outer margin of the inner nuclear layer, and terminates sharply at that level (70: p. 600), it has long been thought that in the monkey retina the ganglion cells and the cells of the inner nuclear layer are supported primarily by the retinal circulation. Since there is no retinal circulation in the fovea, it has also been thought that the receptors satisfy their metabolic requirements primarily from the choroidal circulation (70: p. 600). These views have been supported by the histological effects of clamping the retinal circulation, which causes severe degeneration of the ganglionic and inner nuclear layers (64,75). Hence selective clamping of the retinal circulation was expected to abolish quickly those components generated by cells of the inner nuclear layer, while components generated by the receptors or pigment epithelium cells were expected to be maintained by the choroidal circulation.

It is evident that this method requires an accurate assessment of which cells are strongly dependent upon the retinal circulation. Thus photocoagulation was used to close permanently the major retinal vessels serving certain areas of the cynomolgus retina, and histological studies were performed to determine which cells degenerated following this procedure. Figure 151 shows portions of a single section from the retina of a cynomolgus monkey, proceeding from the normal parafovea on the left to an area of the peripheral retina on the right where the retinal circulation had been permanently clamped by photocoagulation twenty days before sacrificing the animal. The ganglion cell layer is completely absent in the experimental area, and the inner nuclear layer has been thinned to a single row of cells, while the receptor layer is intact. The pigment epithelium of this area was also intact. Similar histological effects were seen by Noell (64) after a transient surgical interruption of the retinal circulation of a rhesus monkey, but Figure 151 shows that after permanent clamping of the retinal circulation the degeneration of the inner nuclear layer is somewhat more severe.

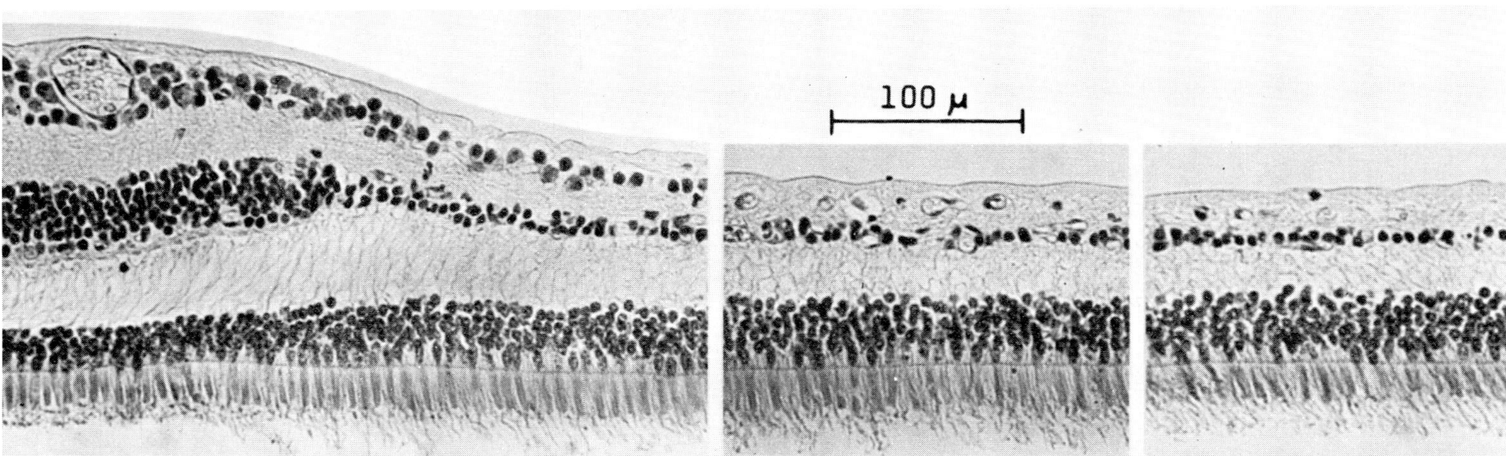

Figure 151. The degeneration of surface layers of the cynomolgus retina following permanent closure by photocoagulation of the retinal blood vessels serving the superior-temporal part of the retina. The animal was sacrificed 20 days later. All three pictures were taken from a single section; reading from left to right, this section passes from the inferior to the superior portion of the temporal retina. The left view shows rapid transition from the normal parafovea, containing a large patent retinal blood vessel, to the ischemic part of the retina. Following a 340 μ gap, the middle picture shows only a few ganglion cells, which appear abnormal, and the inner nuclear layer is severely thinned. Following a gap of 220 μ, the right picture shows no distinct ganglion cells, and the inner nuclear layer is thinned to a single row of cells. Histological technique as in Figure 149, except that this section was 6 μ thick. (From Brown, Watanabe & Murakami, 30.)

Results of Recording from the Fovea of the Cynomolgus Monkey and of Clamping the Retinal Circulation

The results of both these procedures are shown in Figure 152. Note that all responses were obtained from the same animal by using four separate penetrations. Also, all responses were recorded from adjacent to the retinal side of the pigment epithelium, and the stimulus was a 0.25 mm spot which was well-focused and centered upon the electrode. In the peripheral retina, with the retinal circulation normal, the normal LERG was obtained. This response consists of a positive a-wave and negative b-wave, followed after termination of the stimulus by a negative d-wave. The c-wave of cynomolgus is relatively small and readily abolished by light adaptation. In Figure 152 the retina was light-adapted by repetitive stimulation, and no c-wave has been detected under these conditions (30). In the normal foveal response the b-wave is greatly reduced, but is not abolished. The remaining b-wave is probably due partly to foveal receptors activating parafoveal cells of the inner nuclear layer, and partly to stimulation of the parafovea by low-intensity stray light. The falling phase of the d-wave is sufficiently reduced not to be seen in the foveal record; this deflection is small even in the peripheral record, and results from decay of the D.C. component of the inner nuclear layer, as shown by later results of this paper. On the other hand, both the a-wave and the rising phase of the d-wave are recorded at larger amplitude in the fovea, as expected if these deflections result from the onset and decay of a receptor response, which is more clearly revealed by reducing the contributions of components of opposite polarity which are generated by cells of the inner nuclear layer.

When recording from the peripheral retina, clamping the retinal circulation completely abolished both the b-wave and the falling phase of the d-wave. Thus

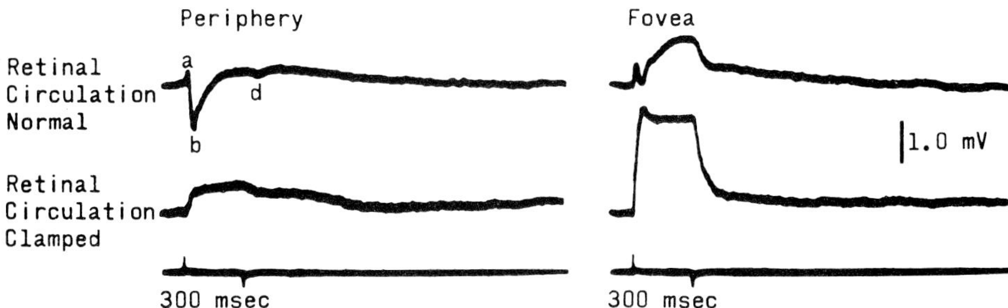

Figure 152. Comparison of responses from the periphery and fovea of the cynomolgus monkey, with the retinal circulation both normal and clamped. All responses were recorded from the same retina by making four separate penetrations with a tungsten microelectrode, and all records were obtained from adjacent to the retinal side of the pigment epithelium. The reference electrode was in the vitreous humor, and amplification was direct-coupled. In each case the stimulus spot was carefully focused and centered upon the electrode. The size of the retinal stimulus spot was about 0.25 mm, and the retinal illumination in the focused spot was 3.29 log lumen/m^2. The stimulus was repeated every 10 sec. (After Brown & Watanabe, 27.)

both the b-wave and D.C. component are generated by cells which are supported by the retinal circulation. The remaining response rises quickly to a level which is well maintained during the stimulus, and which decays in two phases after the stimulus terminates. There is first a rapid decay phase, followed by a much slower decay to the baseline. The onset of this response corresponds to the a-wave of the normal LERG, as shown more clearly by records at high sweep speed (30). Also, the rapid decay phase corresponds to the rising phase of the d-wave, as shown more clearly by Figure 162. Hence this isolated response is the one which Granit designated PIII. This component had been isolated previously, in the case of cold-blooded animals, by treating the retinas with KCl, cooling, or massage (46). When isolated by these earlier methods, PIII was not stably maintained but showed a progressive decline in amplitude. With the new method in mammals the isolation can be complete, the response is in near-normal condition, and the response may be stably maintained for many hours by the choroidal circulation (30). Thus, systematic experiments may be performed upon the isolated response. Such work has identified PIII as generated by the receptors, as will be shown in this paper. When an even earlier receptor potential was found (22), Granit's PIII was designated the late receptor potential (late RP), and that terminology will be used in the remainder of this paper.

Figure 152 shows that, when recording from the fovea, clamping the retinal circulation completed the abolition of responses from the inner nuclear layer and isolated the foveal late RP. Since the fovea is a pure cone area, this foveal response must closely approximate the time-course of the cone late RP. The response shows a rapid rise, followed by a slight fall to a plateau which is well maintained during the remainder of the stimulus. When the stimulus terminates there is a rapid decay almost all the way to the baseline. Thus the results of Figure 152 indicate that the cone late RP decays rapidly, and suggest that the rod late RP decays slowly, thus accounting for the peripheral late RP as a simple summation of a rapidly decaying cone response superimposed upon a slowly decaying rod response.

Effects of Clamping the Retinal Circulation in the Cat and Night Monkey

It was next necessary to determine the time-course of the rod late RP. The predominantly rod retina of the cat gave preliminary results on this point, and showed further effects of clamping the retinal circulation. The cat retina has no fovea, but only an area centralis, where the ganglion cell layer is thicker than in the remainder of the retina (73). In the absence of a fovea, local recording offers little advantage for demonstrating the effects of clamping the retinal circulation, so Figure 153 shows the effects of this procedure upon the gross ERG. An advantage of this method of recording is that the late RP and c-wave are opposite in polarity, and hence may be readily distinguished. In the left column a stimulus of maximum intensity evoked a typical normal cat ERG. After clamping the retinal circulation, the rapidly rising phase of the negative late RP is followed by a small positive notch. This notch is not fully understood (30), but is especially prominent

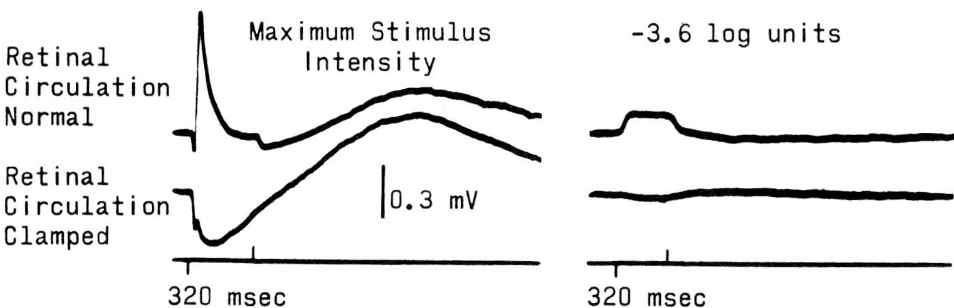

Figure 153. The effects of clamping the retinal circulation upon the ERG of the cat. Responses recorded between a chlorided silver wire in the vitreous humor and a chlorided silver reference electrode in the orbit behind the eye, using direct-coupled amplification. The retina was stimulated by a 2.18 mm light spot delivered in the area of the tapetum, and at maximum intensity the retinal illumination in the focused spot was 4.6 log lumen/m^2. The responses at maximum intensity were obtained from one preparation, and the responses at 3.6 log units lower intensity were recorded from a separate preparation at somewhat slower sweep speed. All records were obtained with a repetition rate of one every 10 sec. In the case of responses to low intensities, the retina was stimulated at maximum intensity until the response stabilized, and then the first response was photographed after inserting the neutral filters. This assured a constant level of light adaptation for all responses.

in the cat, so in this animal a small portion of the b-wave may be supported by the choroidal circulation. After termination of the stimulus there is no rapid off-deflection, indicating abolition of the D.C. component, and the c-wave survives at large amplitude. In the right column the stimulus intensity was reduced sufficiently to isolate the D.C. component when the retinal circulation was normal, and this D.C. component was abolished by clamping the retinal circulation. Hence these results in the cat supplement those from cynomolgus in several ways. First, since there is no true d-wave in the cat, the D.C. component is more readily identified in normal records and the abolition of this component by clamping the retinal circulation may be more clearly demonstrated. Second, the large c-wave of the cat makes it possible to show that this component, like the late RP, is well supported by the choroidal circulation alone. Third, although the rapid rise of the negative late RP has considerable amplitude, there is no indication of a rapid positive deflection after termination of the stimulus. Thus the entire decay of the predominantly rod late RP in this record must be quite slow, and must be masked by the c-wave. Although a small rapid decay phase of the late RP is sometimes seen in the cat, especially with intraretinal recording (30), it is quite small in relation to the amplitude of this response at its onset. Hence the cat provides further evidence that the decay of the rod late RP is much slower than that of cones.

Although retinas containing exclusively rods are difficult or impossible to find (82: pp. 215–216), this condition is closely approached in nocturnal animals. Thus studies were undertaken in the strictly nocturnal night monkey, which has a large enough eye to permit intraocular recording techniques. Although Polyak (70: p. 922) reports a fovea in this animal, Walls (81: p. 62) considers this a vestigial characteristic occurring only in certain members of the species, since it

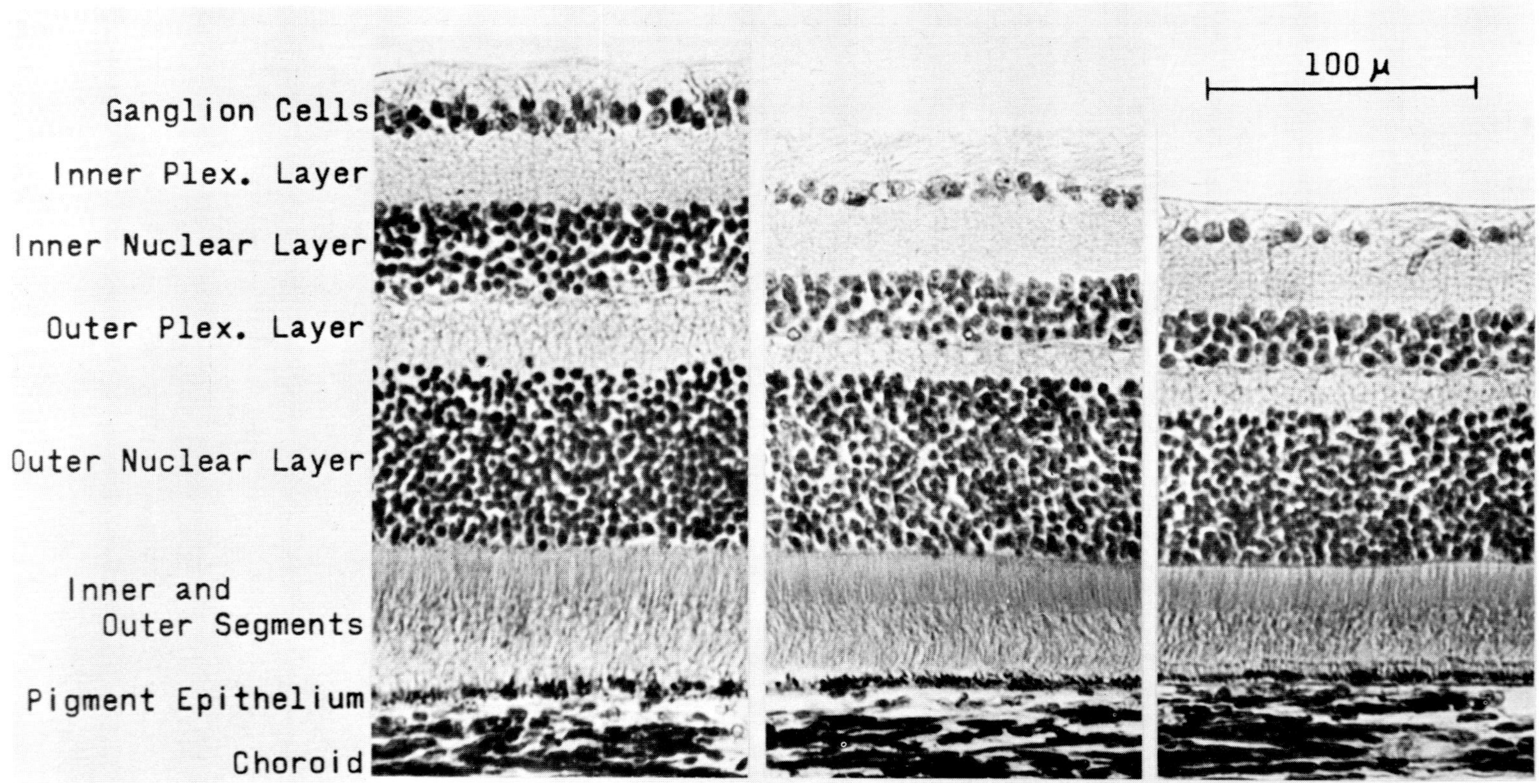

Figure 154. Histological sections from three representative areas of the night monkey retina. The left section is from the center of the area centralis, where the ganglion cell layer is thickest. The middle section is from near the area centralis, and the right section is from the peripheral retina about halfway to the ora serrata. Histological technique as in Figure 149.

has not been found by other investigators. Kolmer (57) found only an area centralis, similar to that of the cat, where the ganglion cell layer and the inner nuclear layer are thicker than in the remainder of the retina. This is also the only specialized area which I have found in serial sections; Figure 154 shows this area centralis, compared with an intermediate retinal area and the peripheral retina. Further details of the night monkey retina are shown by Figure 155. The inner segments of all receptors are very slender and give no sign of cones, in marked contrast to the peripheral retina of cynomolgus. A few cones are present, however, as revealed by the demonstration of cone pedicles in the outer plexiform layer (57). Polyak (70: p. 601) states that the retinal circulation of the night monkey is similar to that of other primates. In agreement with this, the deepest blood vessels I have found are on the outer margin of the inner nuclear layer, and one of these is shown in Figure 155.

Since the night monkey also has no fovea, gross recording is used in Figure 156 to show the effects of clamping the retinal circulation. The normal response is similar to that of the cat, but this retina offers two advantages over the cat's. In addition to having an almost exclusive rod population of receptors, the c-wave is much smaller and permits more accurate recording of the time-course of the rod late RP. After clamping the retinal circulation, both the b-wave and the off-deflection are abolished. The remaining late RP shows an initial rapid rise, followed by a slower rise during the stimulus, so the rod late RP is quite large during the later part of the stimulus. But termination of the stimulus is not followed by any indication of rapid decay, and the recorded decay is quite slow, although any c-wave which may be present in this record would make the decay of the rod late RP appear more rapid than the true decay rate. Thus the results of Figure 156 show that decay of the pure rod late RP is very slow, especially by comparison with that of cones.

The Different Decay Rates of Cone and Rod Late RPs

If a high-intensity stimulus evokes a late RP from a retinal area containing strong proportions of both cones and rods, the response appears to consist of a rapidly decaying cone response superimposed upon a slowly decaying rod response, as shown by the late RP from the peripheral retina of cynomolgus in Figure 152. When large stimulus spots are used under light-adapted conditions, the rapid and slow decay phases of this response are typically about equal in amplitude (30). One wonders why this is the case, since there are so many more rods than cones in the peripheral retina of cynomolgus. This is probably because the extracellularly recorded response of a single cone is larger than that of a single rod under light-adapted conditions, since there is evidence for this principle (30). There is also evidence that this is at least partly a consequence of interacting pathways between receptors, which mediate a suppression of the rod late RP by cone activity under light-adapted conditions; this work has been reported in preliminary form (24), and a full report is in press (25a). These findings also appear to explain why the late RP from the fovea of cynomolgus is so much larger than the late RP of the peripheral retina under light-adapted conditions.

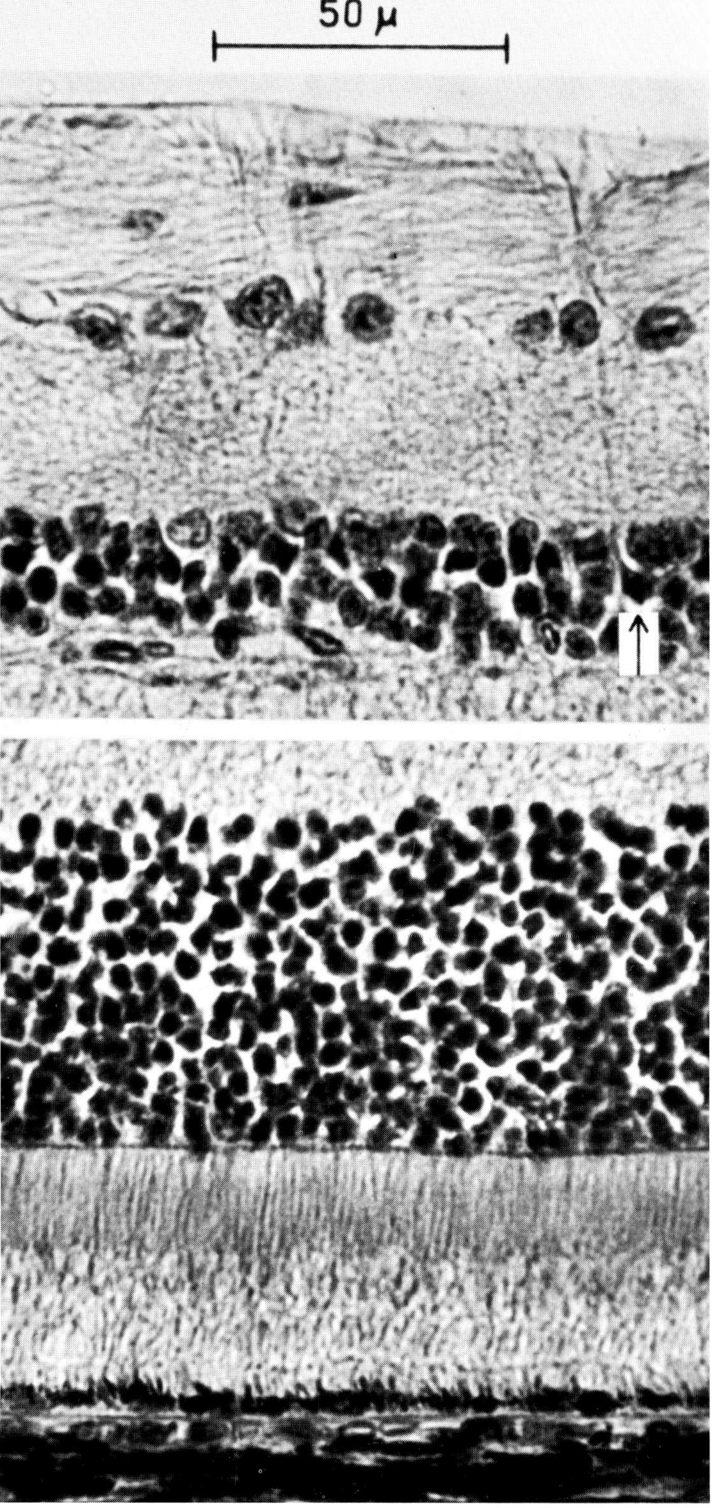

Figure 155 →

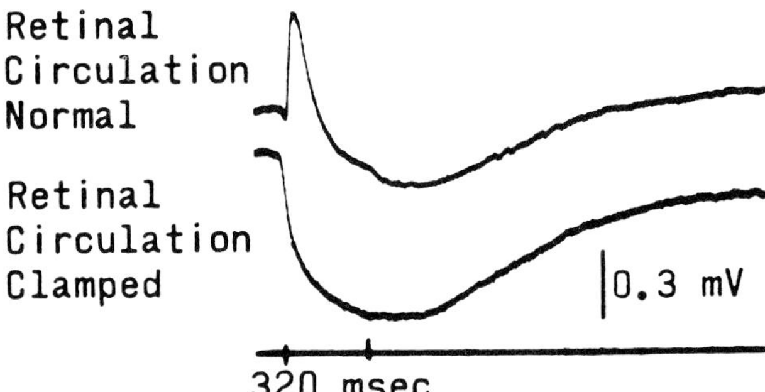

Figure 156. The ERG of the night monkey before and after clamping the retinal circulation. The active electrode was a chlorided silver wire in the vitreous humor, and a chlorided silver reference electrode was in the mouth. Amplification direct-coupled. The stimulus was an approximately 4.0 mm light spot delivered to the nasal side of the retina, and the retinal illumination within the focused spot was 3.74 log lumen/m^2. This stimulus was repeated every 30 sec. (From Brown & Watanabe, 28.)

The different decay rates of cone and rod late RPs permit both cone and rod potentials to be measured separately in a response from a mixed population of receptors. Thus a variety of tests may be applied to see if the different decay rates constitute a general principle for cone and rod responses. When the relative amounts of cone and rod activity which contribute to the response are deliberately varied, the expected effects occur in the relative amplitudes of the rapid and slow decay phases of the late RP. This has been shown by comparing responses of different species, recording from different areas of the cynomolgus retina, varying the size of the stimulus spot while recording from the cynomolgus fovea, and varying stimulus intensity (30). Thus the different decay rates of cone and rod late RPs seem to constitute a general principle. This means that cones and rods differ not only in their anatomy and in their contained photopigments, but also in the rates of decay of their electrical responses. Hence the different decay rates constitute another aspect of the duplicity theory, and appear to account for some of the well-known functional differences between cones and rods (30).

Since the cone and rod responses have been identified, perhaps the best demonstration of the relative decay rates of cone and rod late RPs has been obtained in cynomolgus. Here the decays of both responses may be seen in the same records without any detectable distortion from the c-wave. In Figure 157

Figure 155. More detailed photomicrographs of the peripheral retina of the night monkey, showing levels both superficial to, and deeper than, the outer plexiform layer. Note that this animal has no tapetum lucidum in the choroid, such as that which occurs over a large portion of the peripheral cat retina, and which is shown in Figure 165. Also, the pigment epithelium cells are heavily pigmented, as found only in the non-tapetal areas of the cat retina. An especially distinctive soma of a Müller cell is present which is marked by an arrow, and a fiber of this cell may be seen ascending toward the internal limiting membrane. A horizontally oriented blood vessel may also be seen at the outer margin of the inner nuclear layer. Histological technique as in Figure 149.

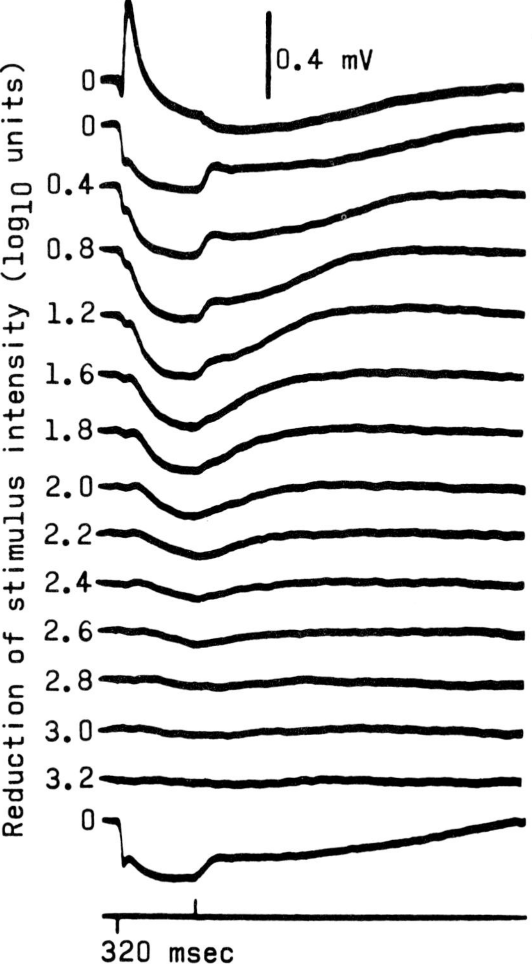

Figure 157. Effects of clamping the retinal circulation upon the ERG of cynomolgus, and the effects of stimulus intensity upon the response after clamping. Responses were recorded between a chlorided silver wire in the vitreous humor and a chlorided silver reference electrode in the orbit behind the eye, using direct-coupled amplification. The top record shows the normal ERG, and all other records were obtained after clamping the retinal circulation. The stimulus spot was delivered to the nasal side of the retina and had a diameter of 2.72 mm; at maximum intensity the retinal illumination within this focused spot was 3.69 log lumen/m^2. Constant conditions of light adaptation were obtained by stimulating every 10 sec. at maximum intensity until the response stabilized; then the first response after inserting a given filter was recorded. Intensities are specified in $\log_{10}$ units below the maximum intensity by specifying the optical densities of the neutral filters. Responses were recorded in sequence from top to bottom; the final control record shows that there was no appreciable change in the preparation or recording conditions during the intensity series. (From Brown, Watanabe & Murakami, 30.)

the top record shows the gross ERG of cynomolgus under normal conditions. Then the retinal circulation was clamped, and at maximum stimulus intensity the late RP shows both rapid and slow decay phases of large amplitude. As stimulus intensity was reduced, the rapid decay phase declined and disappeared, and at minus 2.0 log units only the slowly decaying rod late RP remained. With further reduction of stimulus intensity, the rod late RP also declined and disappeared. Hence Figure 157 shows another method of varying the relative amounts of cone and rod activity which contribute to the response, and the results are in accord with the well-known principle that the rod receptor system is capable of mediating lower thresholds than the cone receptor system. Note that the time-course of decay of the rod late RP is not fixed, but varies with stimulus intensity. At maximum stimulus intensity the decay requires about 1.5 seconds, but the decay becomes increasingly rapid as stimulus intensity is reduced. Experiments like that of Figure 157 have also been performed in the night monkey and cat, where the rod late RP likewise decays more rapidly as stimulus intensity is reduced. This principle has also been demonstrated in cynomolgus with intraretinal recording (25), which permits accurate control of stimulus intensity over the retinal area from which the response is recorded. Hence the more rapid decay of the rod late RP with lowered stimulus intensity appears to be a general principle, which probably accounts for the fact that rods can mediate off-responses of higher-order neurons under scotopic conditions (30).

The Isolated Late RP of Cynomolgus as a Function of Electrode Depth

If the retinal circulation of cynomolgus is clamped, the isolated late RP may then be studied as a function of electrode depth. This type of experiment has provided further evidence identifying the late RP with the receptors, as well as information concerning the nature of this response. The results of Figure 158 were obtained in the peripheral retina, and electrode depth is given on a percentage scale, in which the 100 per cent value is against the retinal side of the pigment epithelium. This percentage scale eliminates the factor of the angle at which the electrode passes through the retina, and with tungsten microelectrodes it has proved both accurate and reliable (30). The responses were evoked by an intense brief flash from a condenser-discharge lamp, which has advantages for stimulation. The high intensity elicits large and rapidly rising responses, while light adaptation resulting from the flash is minimized by its short duration, permitting responses to be elicited at convenient repetition rates. The stimulus flash for Figure 158 had a duration of only about 20 μsec., and the time of its delivery is shown in the bottom record. At the 92 per cent electrode depth, where the response amplitude was maximum, the response shows a rapidly rising phase followed by a notch. There is then a rather long plateau before the response decays. When the decay does occur, it is about half rapid and half slow, as in response to longer stimuli of lower intensity. Thus when the stimulus flash is sufficiently intense, the rapid decay of the cone late RP occurs only after a rather long delay, on the order of 150 msec. in this case. When the intensity of the flash is reduced, the delay in decay of the cone late RP decreases and disappears (25). For

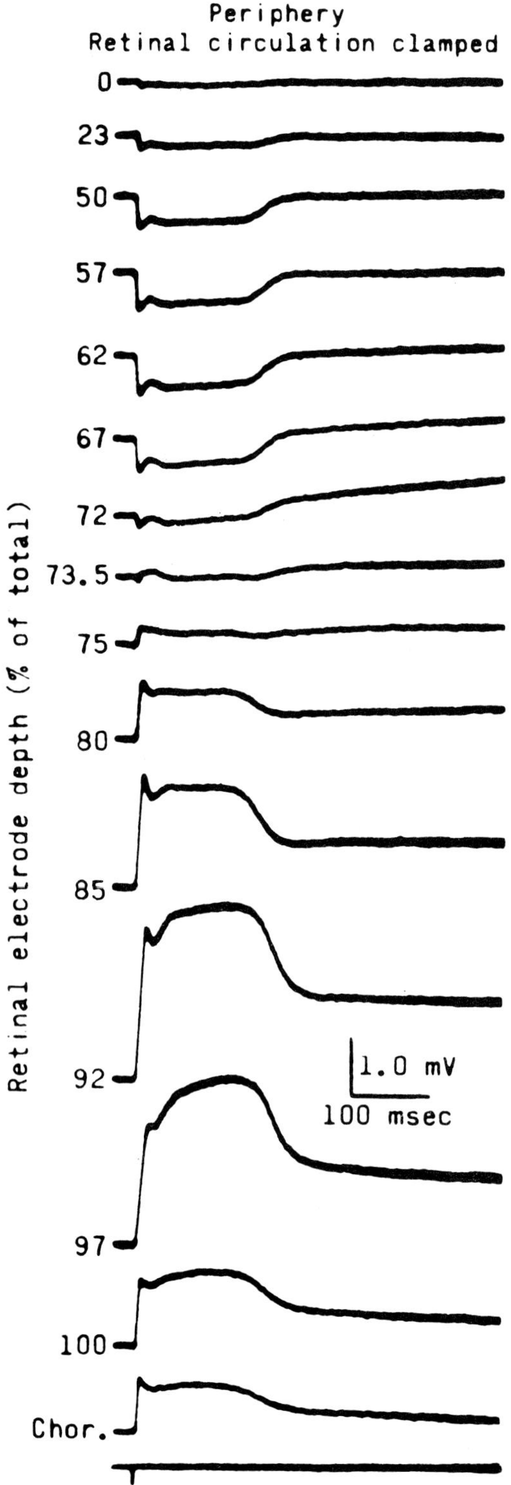

Figure 158. The late RP of the cynomolgus monkey, isolated by clamping the retinal circulation and recorded as a function of depth of a tungsten microelectrode in the peripheral retina. The reference electrode was a chlorided silver wire in the vitreous humor. Electrode depth is expressed as a percentage of the total distance along the electrode track from the retinal surface to the pigment epithelium; thus the 100 per cent record was obtained adjacent to the retinal side of the pigment epithelium. The record marked "Chor." was from the choroid. Responses were recorded by a tape recorder with flat frequency response from 0–5000 cps and were photographed later. The stimulus was a 20 μsec. flash from a Grass photo-stimulator operated at maximum intensity. This stimulus was carried to the animal's eye by a flexible fiber optics bundle (Amer. Opt. type LG5-36), one end of which was directly against the light source and the other directly over the animal's eye. The stimulus was repeated every 10 sec., and the time of the stimulus is shown in the bottom record. (From Brown, Watanabe & Murakami, 30.)

our purposes the delay is helpful, since it permits both the onset and decay of the cone late RP to be seen, although it is elicited by a very brief flash.

Figure 158 shows that, as the electrode was withdrawn from the retinal side of the pigment epithelium, the response of positive polarity increased in amplitude and attained a maximum at about 92 per cent of the total depth. Thus when the late RP is isolated, and when large responses are evoked by intense stimuli, the amplitude maximum of the positive late RP proves not to be against the retinal side of the pigment epithelium, as indicated by early experiments on the cat's a-wave, but more proximally in the region of the inner segments (30). With further withdrawal the response declined and disappeared, and then the cone late RP inverted. The negative response increased to a maximum at about the 62 per cent level, after which it declined and disappeared when the electrode approached the retinal surface. The initial portions of the positive and negative responses in Figure 158 have quite similar time-courses, and the latencies of these positive and negative responses are not detectably different (30). Hence these responses of opposite polarity are not generated by two different cells which are separated by a chemical synapse. On the contrary, they must represent the source (maximum positivity) and sink (maximum negativity) of extracellular current which flows axially along the photoreceptor during the late RP. The percentage depth values of Figure 158 are artificially large, due to edema of the surface layers of the retina after clamping the retinal circulation, and the maximum negativity appears to occur at or very near the receptor axon terminals (30).

Figure 159 shows a similar experiment in the fovea of the same animal. Since the stimulus spot was large and not confined to the fovea, a marked slow decay phase is present. But the rapid decay phase represents a larger proportion of the total response than in the peripheral records of Figure 158, which is typical when foveal and peripheral responses to large stimulus spots are compared. In the fovea the late RP of positive polarity was recorded, but there was no polarity inversion during electrode withdrawal, although a response was detected almost all the way to the retinal surface. Thus the source of extracellular current flow is present in the fovea, but the sink is absent.

In this work there are three types of evidence which seem especially crucial for identifying the late RP as generated by the receptors. First, the results of Figure 158 show that the generating cells must be oriented radially through the retina, and must extend through essentially the entire deeper half of the peripheral retina, to account for the observed locations of the source and sink of extracellular current flow during this response. Second, the generating cells must be strongly represented in the fovea, to account for the especially large responses recorded in that area. Third, the generating cells must be modified in the fovea in a manner which explains that the source of current flow is found in the fovea while the sink is absent. In the case of foveal receptors, the axons proceeding from the cell bodies turn laterally and course outward to the parafovea, where the cone pedicles synapse with second order neurons; this means that an electrode traversing the fovea passes all portions of the receptors except for the axon terminals, where the sink of current appears to occur during peripheral penetrations. Thus all three of

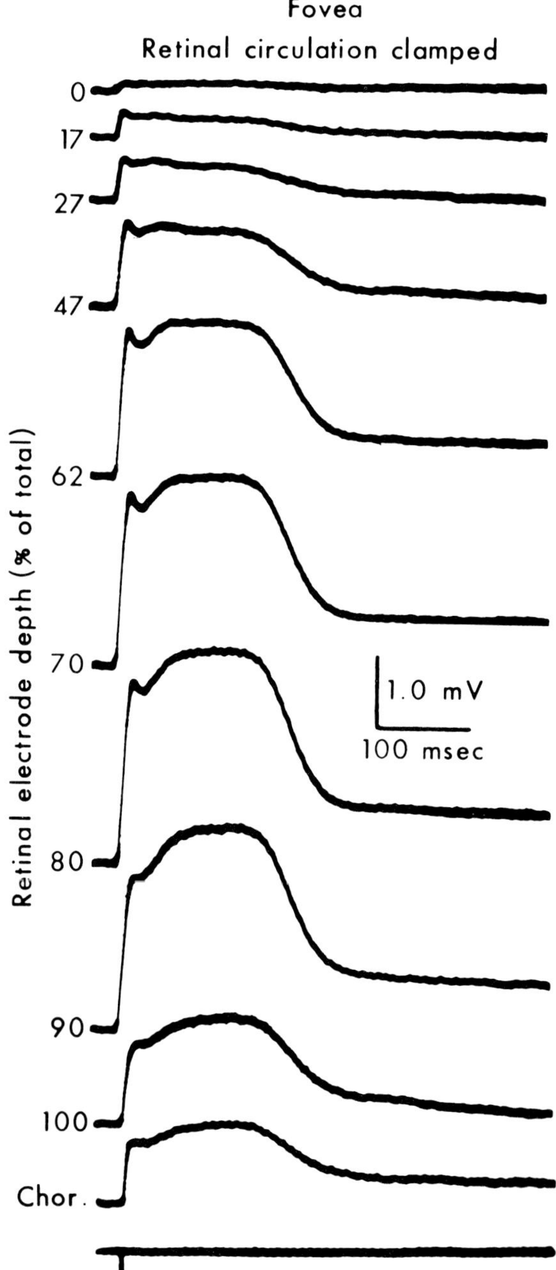

Figure 159. The late RP of the cynomolgus fovea, recorded as a function of electrode depth after its isolation by clamping the retinal circulation. This series of records was obtained from the same animal as the peripheral series of Figure 158, and the conditions of stimulating and recording were as described in Figure 158. (From Brown, Watanabe & Murakami, 30.)

these observations are adequately explained by the receptors, but not by any other type of cell. A more detailed account of this evidence has been given previously (30). It is supported by many observations which do not identify the specific generating cells, but agree with this identification, and which have been discussed in earlier reviews (34,46,49). Support is also provided now from certain findings in retinas of cold-blooded vertebrates, to be discussed later in this paper. Thus identification of the mammalian PIII as a response of the retinal receptors seems satisfactory.

Analysis of the d-Wave

With regard to component analysis, it remains to show more clearly how the d-wave is formed. Flash stimulation has also proved useful for evoking the d-wave of the cynomolgus monkey and for studying it as a function of electrode depth. Figure 160 shows this type of experiment in the peripheral retina, keeping the retinal circulation normal to maintain the d-wave. In the record at the 76 per cent electrode depth the major deflections are labeled. When elicited by an intense flash, the negative intraretinal d-wave is large and is shown to occur after a delay. Since the decay of the cone late RP is delayed with this type of stimulation, the decay of the d-wave suggests that its onset phase is contributed by decay of the cone late RP. Since the *entire* d-wave is delayed, this also suggests that decay of the cone late RP triggers decay of the D.C. component, which contributes the falling phase of the d-wave. These suggestions are supported by the effects of reducing stimulus intensity. This procedure causes the delay of decay of the isolated cone late RP to decrease and disappear, and the entire d-wave likewise moves forward in time (25). In other words, when the time of decay of the cone late RP is varied by means of stimulus intensity, the timing of the entire d-wave varies in the predicted manner.

Figure 160 also shows that the relative amplitudes of the onset and falling phases of the d-wave vary with electrode depth. As the electrode was withdrawn from the pigment epithelium, the amplitude of the onset phase of the d-wave increased and reached a maximum at about the 87 per cent level, where the amplitude of the a-wave was also maximum. With further electrode withdrawal, both the onset phase of the d-wave and the a-wave declined in amplitude. But the falling phase of the d-wave increased in amplitude until the electrode was at about the 56 per cent level, where the amplitude of the b-wave was maximum, and these responses then decreased as the electrode approached the retinal surface. Thus the amplitude of the d-wave's onset phase varies similarly to that of the a-wave, while the amplitude of its falling phase varies similarly to that of the b-wave. Since the onset and falling phases of the d-wave can vary independently, the d-wave must result from two different components of opposite polarity. Furthermore, the onset phase appears to result from decay of the cone late RP, while the falling phase appears to result from decay of the D.C. component from the inner nuclear layer.

Further evidence for this has been obtained by recording from the fovea, and by clamping the retinal circulation. Figure 161 shows that in the fovea the onset phase of the d-wave is larger than the falling phase through the deeper half of the

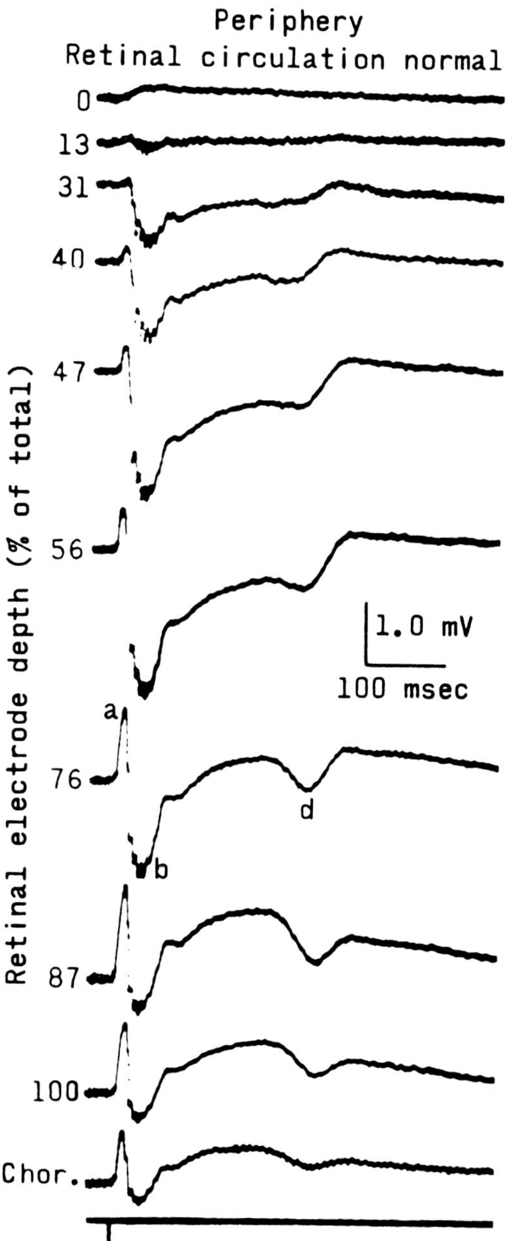

Figure 160. The normal LERG recorded as a function of electrode depth from the peripheral retina of cynomolgus. The major deflections are labeled in the record at the 76 per cent depth. Conditions of stimulating and recording were as described in Figure 158.

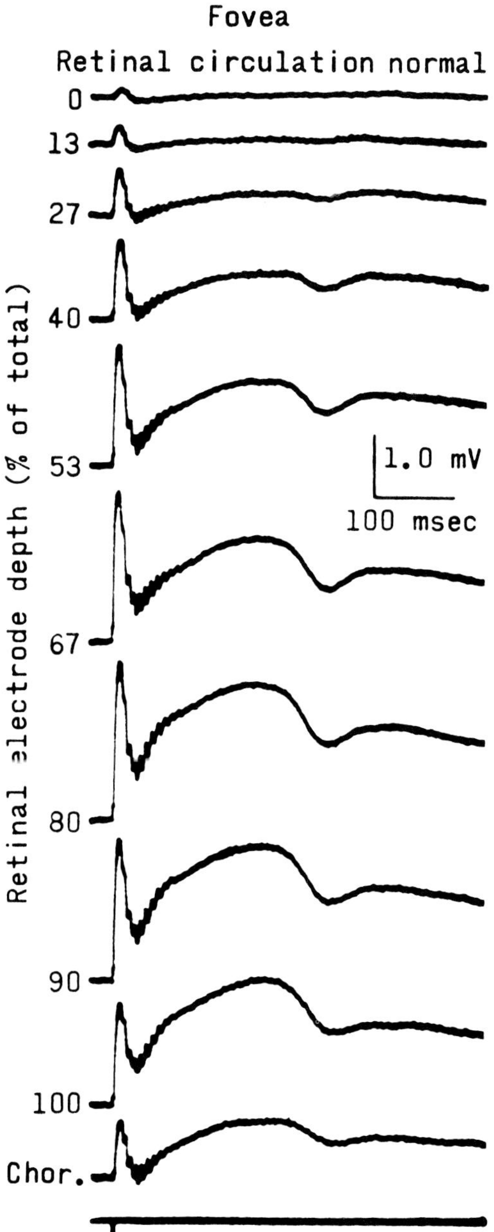

Figure 161. The normal LERG recorded as a function of electrode depth from the fovea of cynomolgus. The conditions of stimulating and recording were as described in Figure 158.

penetration, and at shallow electrode locations the falling phase does not become larger than the onset phase. Since the D.C. component is recorded at reduced amplitude in the fovea, and since its site of generation is not traversed in the fovea, these results are as expected.

The timing of off-responses before and after clamping the retinal circulation cannot be compared accurately with intense flash stimuli, since edema of the surface layers of the retina causes reduced stimulus intensity at the receptors, which causes earlier decay of the isolated cone late RP (25,30). But the timing may be compared by using longer stimuli of lower intensity. This is because the longer stimulus elicits a distinct off-response even in a lower intensity range where stimulus intensity does not appreciably affect the time at which the cone late RP decays. It has been shown that with intraretinal recording the d-wave of cynomolgus is more distinct in the dark-adapted state (29). Thus the top record of Figure 162 is a dark-adapted response with the retinal circulation normal, and the lower record is a similarly dark-adapted response after clamping the retinal circulation. A constant time line shows that the onset of the normal d-wave coincides with onset of the rapid decay of the cone late RP. In this case the falling phase of the d-wave appears not to be entirely abolished by clamping the retinal circulation; this may mean that a portion of the D.C. component is sometimes

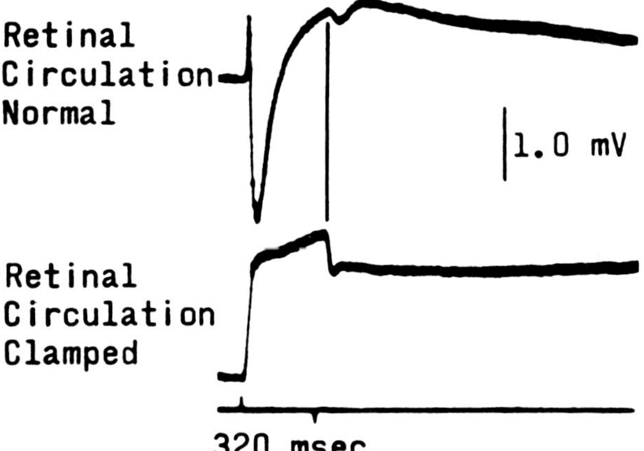

Figure 162. The effect of clamping the retinal circulation upon the dark-adapted LERG of cynomolgus. Both responses were recorded from the same region of the peripheral retina of the same animal, using a tungsten microelectrode against the retinal side of the pigment epithelium. The reference electrode was a chlorided silver wire in the vitreous humor, and amplification was direct-coupled. Prior to each record the retina was first light-adapted by repetitive stimulation at 5 sec. intervals until the responses were stable in form and amplitude. Then the retina was dark-adapted for 15 min., and a record was taken immediately after this period of dark adaptation. The stimulus spot was centered upon the electrode. It had a retinal diameter of 2.72 mm and gave a retinal illumination of 3.28 log lumen/m^2. (After Brown & Watanabe, 29.)

supported by the choroidal circulation, or the small deflection in this record may not be part of the D.C. component. In other experiments the falling phase of the d-wave has been completely abolished by clamping the retinal circulation, as may be seen by comparing Figures 160 and 161 with Figures 158 and 159. Thus the falling phase of the d-wave, like the D.C. component, is supported primarily by the retinal circulation, while the onset phase is well supported from the choroidal circulation alone. In short, all of these lines of evidence indicate that the d-wave results from decay of the cone late RP, followed by decay of the D.C. component.

Summary of Analyses of Mammalian Rod and Cone ERGs into Major Components

Schematic analysis of the mammalian ERG into its major neural components is summarized in Figure 163, which shows separate analyses for predominantly rod and for pure cone retinas. Analysis of the rod ERG is based primarily upon work in the cat and night monkey. The form of the pure cone ERG is based mainly upon records from diurnal squirrels, which are the only mammals known to have pure cone retinas (7,75), and the analysis of the cone ERG is based primarily upon work in the cynomolgus monkey. For purposes of illustration, certain simplifications have been made which are described in the legend. The most important of these is omission of the c-wave from the rod ERG, to show more clearly how the remaining response is an algebraic summation of the three neural components which have been identified.

In the predominantly rod ERG the a-wave is shown to result from the onset of the rod late RP. The b-wave and D.C. component of the inner nuclear layer begin after an additional delay, which probably results mainly from transmission time. Since these later components are of opposite polarity to the late RP, and since the b-wave is relatively large, they drive the summated response upward and give rise to the b-wave. The steady level of negativity, which occurs after the b-wave, is presumably due to the rod late RP having larger amplitude than the D.C. component. When the stimulus terminates, the D.C. component decays, giving a simple negative deflection which is the typical off-response in rod ERGs, being found not only in the cat and night monkey, but also in the bush baby (40) and rat (38). There is then a slowly decaying negativity, referred to in the literature as "remnant negativity" (48). This may now be understood from the very slow decay of the rod late RP.

In Granit's analysis of the cat ERG, PIII was shown as decaying more slowly than in the cone ERG, but sufficiently fast to account for a deflection which he labeled the d-wave. In his work this deflection seems to have been evoked only with intense stimuli having durations of two seconds or more; I have also found it only under these conditions, and an explanation is now evident. With increased stimulus duration, the isolated rod late RP has been found to decay more rapidly, probably because of the strong light adaptation which develops during long stimuli. This more rapid decay of the rod late RP seems to account for the upward deflection labeled as a d-wave in Figure 144. It now appears that this is not a true

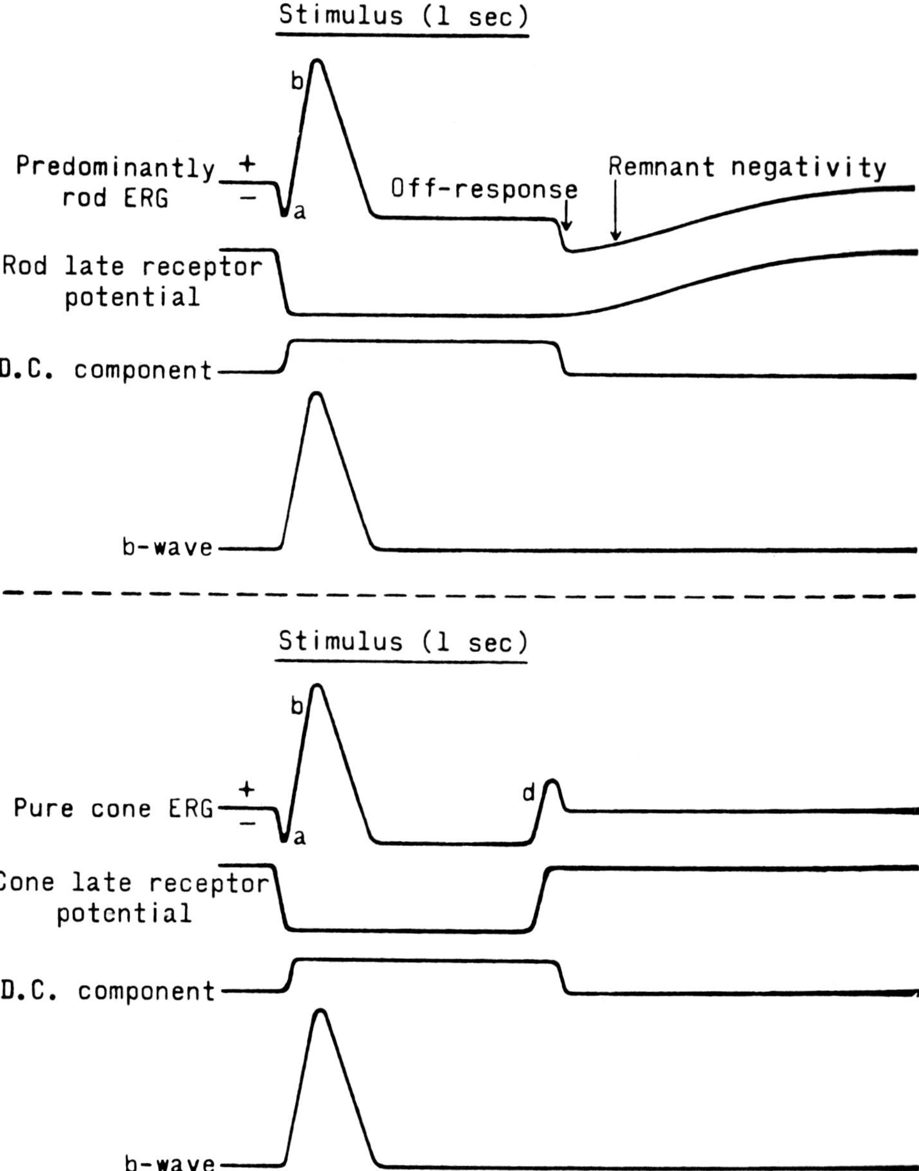

Figure 163. Schematic component analyses of light-adapted mammalian ERGs from predominantly rod eyes and from pure cone eyes. Conventional recording is assumed, with the active electrode in front of the retina and the reference electrode behind the eye. In the predominantly rod ERG the c-wave from the pigment epithelium has been omitted to show more clearly how the remaining response is formed as a simple algebraic sum of the three major neural components. For purposes of illustration, the time-courses of the a- and b-waves are broader than normal. Certain simplifications have also been made. In both the rod and cone late receptor potentials, complexities which follow the rapid initial rise have been omitted, and the responses are shown as flat during the remainder of the stimulus. The b-wave and D.C. component are shown with similar latencies; the exact latency relation is not known, and any existing latency difference would be negligible on the time scale of this illustration. For further explanation, see text.

d-wave, since it occurs *after* decay of the D.C. component, but is a special case resulting from more rapid decay of the rod late RP following a long stimulus.

The general form of the pure cone ERG is similar to that of the rod ERG, prior to termination of the stimulus, as shown by Figures 142 and 143. In the pure cone ERG of Figure 163, a steady negativity is shown during the later part of the stimulus. This facilitates comparison with the rod ERG, and this negativity has been shown by Chaffee & Sutcliffe (35) in the pure cone ERG of the horned toad. It is not shown in the squirrel ERG of Figure 143, but this may be a consequence of condenser-coupled amplification, which is suggested by the recorded form of the calibration pulse in that figure. In the case of the cone ERG, termination of the stimulus is followed first by decay of the cone late RP, which gives the onset phase of the d-wave. Decay of the D.C. component occurs somewhat later, because of this component being generated at a later stage of the retinal pathway, and this gives the falling phase of the d-wave. In Figure 163 the decay of the D.C. component is shown as beginning after the cone late RP has decayed to the base-line; this is done to illustrate how the d-wave is formed, but several observations indicate that the two decays overlap in time. For example, in Figure 162 the onset phase of the d-wave has a slower time-course than decay of the cone late RP, apparently because the D.C. component is also decaying during most of the onset phase of the d-wave. Also, in Figure 160 the recorded onset of decay of the D.C. component occurs earlier at shallow levels of the retina than at the deeper levels. This is apparently because the late RP is smaller at shallow retinal levels, so that the early portion of decay of the D.C. component is more completely revealed. Although overlap occurs, the cone late RP appears to have decayed to the base-line by the time the d-wave is completed. Thus the rapid decay of the cone late RP accounts for both the presence of a d-wave and the absence of remnant negativity in cone ERGs.

In summary, both rod and cone ERGs appear to consist of three major neural components, which are fundamentally similar. But the cone late RP decays rapidly, while the rod late RP decays much more slowly, and these different decay rates account for the different forms of off-responses in cone and rod ERGs. The c-wave from the pigment epithelium is a fourth major component of the rod ERG, but its amplitude varies greatly among predominantly rod species. No c-wave has been found from the squirrel retina, even after dark adaptation (7,39), or from the pure cone retina of the horned toad (35), so in the cone ERG the c-wave must be very small or absent. Retinas containing strong contributions from both rods and cones, such as those of cynomolgus and the human, seem to represent intermediate cases which yield ERGs with both rod and cone characteristics. In these cases the well-known stimulus factors which selectively activate primarily the rod or cone systems are of special importance in determining the form of the recorded ERG.

The Generality of These Component Analyses

Light-Adapted and Dark-Adapted ERGs

Evidence for the component analyses of Figure 163 was obtained primarily in the light-adapted state, which permits most experiments to be performed more conveniently, but dark adaptation does not seem to reveal any additional components. The pure cone ERG of the squirrel shows no distinct changes of form after dark adaptation (7,39). In mixed rod-cone eyes the ERG tends to be like that of a predominantly cone eye in the light-adapted state; with dark adaptation a c-wave appears and the d-wave usually becomes less prominent (49). In cynomolgus the effects of adaptation have been demonstrated with intraretinal recording (29), and in this case the amplitudes of all deflections are larger after dark adaptation. The increase of the a-wave seems due largely to a longer latency of the b-wave, and the more prominent d-wave is not understood. But the isolated cone and rod late RPs were found to be little affected by dark adaptation, although the b-wave is greatly increased. Thus all components are not affected to the same extent, which must cause minor changes of response form. In the cat retina, dark adaptation likewise increases the amplitudes of all deflections and alters certain details, as shown in Figure 164. In this experiment the eye was first dark-adapted for 30 minutes; then the retina was light-adapted by stimulating every 10 seconds, and the response to each stimulus was recorded. The first response, at zero time after dark adaptation, shows neither steady negativity during the later part of the stimulus nor remnant negativity after the stimulus. This is because the c-wave begins shortly after onset of the stimulus, as shown by Figure 146, and the c-wave is especially enlarged by dark adaptation. As the eye was light-adapted the c-wave declined, and in the response after 30 seconds the potential levels just before and just after termination of the stimulus are near the baseline level. After 120 seconds the response shows both steady negativity during the later part of the stimulus, and remnant negativity after the stimulus, and responses to subsequent stimuli showed no further effects of light adaptation. Thus the state of adaptation is crucial in determining whether the phases of slow negativity appear in the cat ERG. In the night monkey, where the c-wave is much smaller, the phases of slow negativity appear even after dark adaptation, which increases the ERG but has little effect upon its form. Thus the component analyses of Figure 163 seem to apply equally well to dark-adapted conditions, but in some animals the dark-adapted ERG shows changes in form because of unequal increases in amplitude of the different components.

The ERG of Cold-Blooded Vertebrates

It may also be asked whether these analyses of the mammalian ERG may be extended to other vertebrate groups. Since the general form of the ERG is very similar in retinas of cold-blooded vertebrates, most aspects of the mammalian analyses probably apply also in those cases. In fish and frog retinas, Tomita (77) has localized the b-wave to the inner nuclear layer by microelectrode methods. Until recently, PIII was also localized entirely to the inner nuclear layer by these methods (77), but new evidence has been obtained on that subject (78). Murakami & Kaneko (63) have now shown that part of PIII is generated by the receptors; they designate this the distal PIII, and believe it is identical with the mammalian late RP. This portion of PIII was isolated by applying ammonia vapor to the retina, and was identified with the receptors by electrode depth

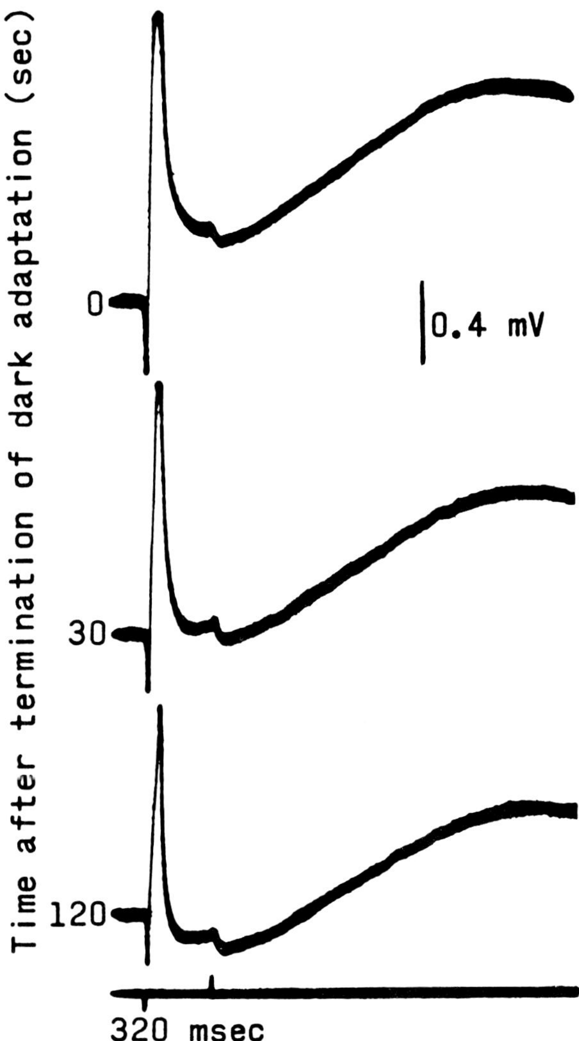

Figure 164. Effect of light adaptation upon the cat ERG. Responses recorded between a chlorided silver wire in the vitreous humor and a chlorided silver reference electrode in the orbit behind the eye, using direct-coupled amplification. Following a 30 min. period of dark adaptation, the eye was light-adapted by stimulating every 10 sec. The response to each stimulus was recorded, and records are shown at representative times after terminating dark adaptation. The stimulus was a 2.18 mm spot delivered in the area of the tapetum, and the retinal illumination in the focused spot was 4.6 log lumen/m^2.

studies. This confirms the result first obtained by these methods in the work of Mitarai et al. (61), in which the isolated PIII was also reported to decay much more slowly after dark adaptation than in the light-adapted state. Thus it seems likely that the late RP occurs in cold-blooded vertebrates, and that the different decay rates of cone and rod late RPs apply in those animals. This conclusion is also supported by preliminary reports of intracellular recording. In the inverted fish retina, Tomita (78) has obtained intracellular responses from close to the receptor surface by using exceptionally fine micropipettes and imparting a rapid motion to the retina. These responses are tentatively identified as from the inner segments of cones, and have a general form similar to that of the mammalian cone late RP. Also Bortoff (10) has taken advantage of the especially large photoreceptors of *Necturus* to obtain intracellular records by direct penetrations. In this work the recording site was identified as the inner segment by electrode marking, and the intracellular response appears to correspond with the extracellularly recorded PIII (11).

Murakami & Kaneko (63) also describe a proximal PIII, which has a distinctly longer latency and higher sensitivity to ammonia vapor than the distal PIII, and they localize the proximal PIII to the inner nuclear layer. In agreement with these findings, the dual origin of the a-wave in cold-blooded animals was demonstrated by Brown (17) and by Yonemura & Hatta (85). We found in toad and frog retinas, respectively, that a brief high-intensity flash evokes an a-wave which rises in two separate phases. There is first a relatively slow rise, followed by a much more rapid rise. In the toad retina, tetrodotoxin abolished the rapidly rising second phase of the a-wave, and the b-wave was also abolished, but the initial slowly rising phase of the a-wave was not abolished (17). Thus the slowly and rapidly rising phases of the a-wave must be generated by separate mechanisms. In the frog retina the second phase of the a-wave was blocked by anoxia or KCN, and evidence from depth recording indicated that the first phase is from the receptors while the second phase is from the inner nuclear layer (85). Hence these two phases of the a-wave probably correspond to the distal and proximal PIIIs.

In the human retina a notch has been observed in the a-wave, which has been postulated to result from a photopic response followed after a slight delay by a scotopic response (8). It is not clear whether these results are due to different rates of rise of the cone and rod late RPs, or to components occurring sequentially in the retinal pathway. Thus a proximal PIII has not been identified in mammals, and a splitting of the a-wave like that found in cold-blooded animals has not been observed with intense flashes. But this problem should be studied in mammals with higher flash intensities and lowered temperatures, to obtain conditions comparable to those which have pertained in studies of cold-blooded animals. On the other hand, no counterpart of the mammalian D.C. component has been found in cold-blooded vertebrates. Thus clear differences between results from mammals and from cold-blooded animals now pertain only to components of the inner nuclear layer. This is a complex layer of the retina, and studies by electron microscopy have shown important differences in its structure between mammals and cold-blooded vertebrates (83). Hence it would not be surprising if ERG components generated by cells of this layer showed some differences between these widely separated vertebrate groups. But it also seems possible that the observed differences result only from incomplete analyses of responses of that layer, so further work is needed on this subject.

The Nature of an ERG Component

A further problem of special importance is the general nature of an ERG component and how it is recorded. It has long been proposed that each component must be generated by a dipole which is radially oriented through the retina (79), as indicated by the polarity inversion between a given component of the gross ERG and the same component of the LERG. But the time-courses of these responses are different and they are generated in different retinal areas (33), so direct confirmation of this concept seemed to require that the *local* response be shown to invert polarity without any distinct change of time-course as an electrode traverses the retina (34). This type of experiment was first successful for the isolated late RP, as shown in Figure 158. The receptors are relatively long cells, which are precisely oriented in a radial direction through the peripheral retina, and which give a dipole of the late RP with considerable separation between the two poles. Hence the late RP was an especially favorable case for demonstration of the local dipole.

Since the positive and negative late RPs of Figure 158 are local responses, the polarities of these potentials are independent of the position of the reference electrode. This was shown by Arden & Brown (3) who found similar polarity inversions for the a-wave of the cat when the reference electrode was effectively behind the eye. The situation for recording these local responses is similar to that for recording extracellular impulses from a single cell; in both cases the response polarity is independent of the position of a remote reference electrode. These findings for the local late RP, combined with earlier work comparing a component of the LERG with the same component recorded in the gross ERG (33), provide an explanation for the polarity at which the late RP or a-wave is recorded under different conditions. With conventional recording the active electrode is in front of the retina and the reference electrode is behind the eye. With this orientation the active electrode will become negative with respect to the reference electrode during the late RP, which will be a gross response resulting from the summated activity of all of the local dipoles. If the active electrode is a penetrating microelectrode, and the reference electrode is kept behind the eye, the negative response will increase in amplitude as the microelectrode approaches the negative end of a local dipole, where the response will result primarily from the local activity. Then the response will decline and invert with further penetration, and a local positive response will reach maximum amplitude at the other end of the dipole. Beyond that point the response will decline, dropping sharply when the R-membrane is penetrated. If the reference electrode is in the vitreous humor, the penetrating electrode will initially record nothing, but a local negative response will be detected with increasing depth which will become maximum at the negative end of the dipole. This response will then decline and invert, and a local positive response will reach maximum amplitude at the other end of the dipole. This response will then decline as the R-membrane is approached. After penetration of the R-membrane the electrodes will be oriented oppositely from conventional recording, and a summated response will be recorded from the entire retina which is positive in polarity.

In Figure 158 a negative slow decay phase of the rod late RP was not recorded at the level of the axon terminals, but the rod late RP shows a similar polarity inversion to that of cones. In the cynomolgus periphery this is readily demonstrated with small stimulus spots, which have yielded depth recordings of the slowly decaying rod late RP which are similar to those of the rapidly decaying cone late RP (30). Polarity inversions similar to that of Figure 158 have also been demonstrated for the rod late RP in the night monkey (28,30), and in the cat. Hence the cone and rod late RPs are generated by dipoles which are similarly oriented, and which have their positive and negative poles at comparable levels of the retina. Since current flows from positive to negative, by convention, the extracellular current during the late RP is flowing from the distal to the proximal end of the cell. Thus the late RP must have a different function from that of potentials which serve in other types of receptors as generator potentials for nerve impulses (30).

Since the local cone and rod late RPs invert polarity as the receptors are traversed, these responses seem to provide models which show how an ERG component is generated and recorded. In early intraretinal work it was uncertain whether the c-wave shows a true polarity inversion across the R-membrane (33). But an intense brief flash evokes a large c-wave, which inverts polarity without any distinct change of time-course when the R-membrane is penetrated. This result provides further evidence that the c-wave is generated by cells of the pigment epithelium, which are the only cells traversed when the R-membrane is penetrated. In this case the radial dipole must be quite short, not exceeding the thickness of the pigment epithelium cells.

Cellular Origins of Components of the Inner Nuclear Layer

The inner nuclear layer is complex, consisting of bipolar cells, horizontal cells, amacrine cells, and the glial cells of Müller. Hence positive identification of the type of cell which generates a given response from this layer is especially difficult, and has not been achieved for either the b-wave or D.C. component. There are, however, some noteworthy points. When the retinal circulation is clamped, all impulse activity of the retina is quickly abolished. Thus all cells which fire impulses appear to be supported by the retinal circulation. There are also single cells which generate only the slow potentials which were discovered by Svaetichin (74), and which have come to be called S-potentials. Although originally identified with the receptors, these potentials have now been shown by electrode marking to be generated by cells of the inner nuclear layer in both cold-blooded animals (59) and mammals (26). In acute experiments the mammalian S-potentials are not abolished by clamping the retinal circulation (30); hence the generating cells must be well supported by the choroidal circulation. In this respect the S-potentials are unique among responses of the inner nuclear layer. The generating cells have not been positively identified, but the horizontal cells have been most strongly implicated (59). Since the b-wave and D.C. component are both abolished by clamping the retinal circulation, these components are probably generated by cells of the inner nuclear layer other than those which generate S-potentials. Furthermore, ammonia vapor abolishes the S-potentials from isolated retinas of cold-blooded animals without abolishing PIII (61). Thus the S-potentials appear not to contribute any portion of the ERG which has been identified to date in mammals.

The locally recorded b-wave has also been shown to invert polarity as the retina is penetrated. Since the b-wave is positive when recorded by conventional methods, the positive pole of the b-wave dipole should be closer to the retinal surface than the negative pole. But when local responses are recorded by placing the reference electrode in the vitreous humor, only the negative response has been detected (33,34). It was reasoned that this may be because the positive pole is so close to the retinal surface that under these conditions there is not enough electrical resistance between the electrodes to detect it. Thus a method was needed for recording local responses without placing the reference electrode in the vitreous humor. In the work of Arden & Brown (3), this was done by replacing the vitreous humor of the cat with a heavy oil (Pantopaque) having a specific gravity of 1.27. The oil was injected through one needle, and the vitreous was extruded through another needle. Because of its high density, the oil sank and became closely apposed to the retinal surface. A microelectrode was then inserted through the oil for penetration of the retina. The non-conducting oil prevents current generated at remote retinal areas from reaching the site of the microelectrode. Hence only local responses are recorded, regardless of the position of the reference electrode, which was placed effectively behind the eye. It was then found that the local b-wave inverted polarity during penetration, with no distinct change of time-course, the maximum negativity occurring near the outer margin of the inner nuclear layer and the maximum positivity near the inner margin of the inner plexiform layer. The results of five separate penetrations are shown in Figure 165 on a percentage depth scale, compared with a histological section of the cat retina. These findings indicate that the cells which generate the b-wave are radially oriented through the retina, and must extend from about the outer margin of the inner nuclear layer to the inner margin of the inner plexiform layer. The bipolar cells have frequently been suggested as generators of the b-wave, and this suggestion now has some support, since the bipolar cells are the only ones which can readily explain this result. Although the b-wave and D.C. component are separately generated, it is not clear whether these are different responses of the same cell or are generated by two different cell types. Further methods are strongly needed for positive identification of the types of cells which generate the various responses of the inner nuclear layer.

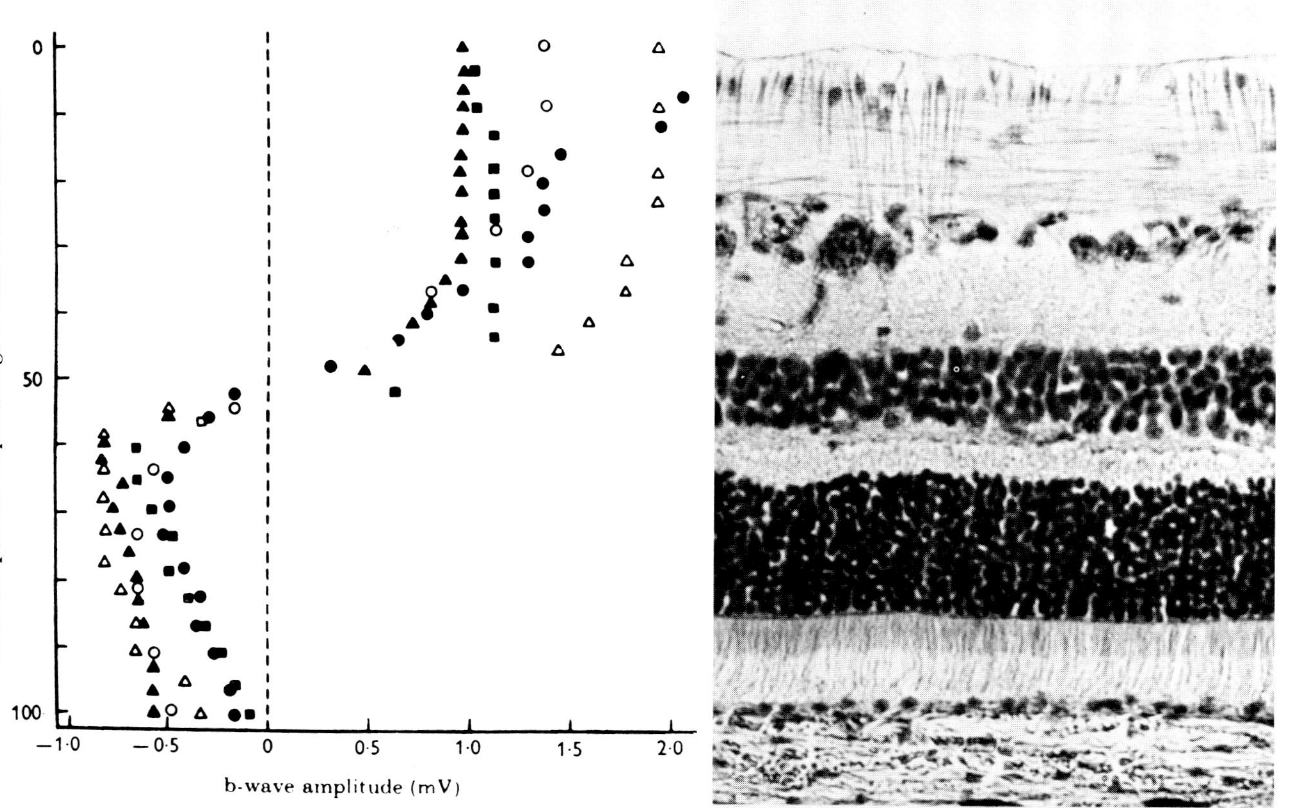

Figure 165. Amplitude of the local b-wave of the cat as a function of electrode depth. Responses were recorded by a tungsten microelectrode with the reference electrode in the mouth, after replacement of the vitreous humor with a heavy oil. Results from five separate penetrations are plotted on a scale of percentage electrode depth. For comparison, a histological section of the peripheral retina of the cat, in the region of the tapetum where all the penetrations were made, is shown on the right. Histological technique as described in Figure 149. No background illumination was used. The stimulus duration was 350 msec. and the stimulus was repeated every 10 sec.; the stimulus spot had a diameter of 1.14 mm and was centered upon the tip of the microelectrode. The stimulus intensity was constant in any given depth series, but varied between series from 4.5 to 5.5 log units below the maximum stimulus intensity of 4.72 log lumen/m². (From Arden &

THE EFFECTS OF STIMULUS INTENSITY UPON LOCALLY RECORDED RESPONSES

It has often been considered puzzling that reduction of stimulus intensity should abolish the a-wave of the ERG prior to the b-wave, as shown in Figure 145, if the a-wave is due to receptor activity which is a precursor of the b-wave. But failure to record an electrical response does not show that it is not generated, and this is particularly true when recording summated extracellular responses such as ERG components. It seemed more likely that with conventional recording reduced stimulus intensity simply makes the a-wave undetectable before the b-wave disappears (34), and this interpretation has now been confirmed by results of local recording under oil (3). The amplitude of the locally recorded b-wave was found to summate over a larger receptor area than is true for the a-wave; thus the cells

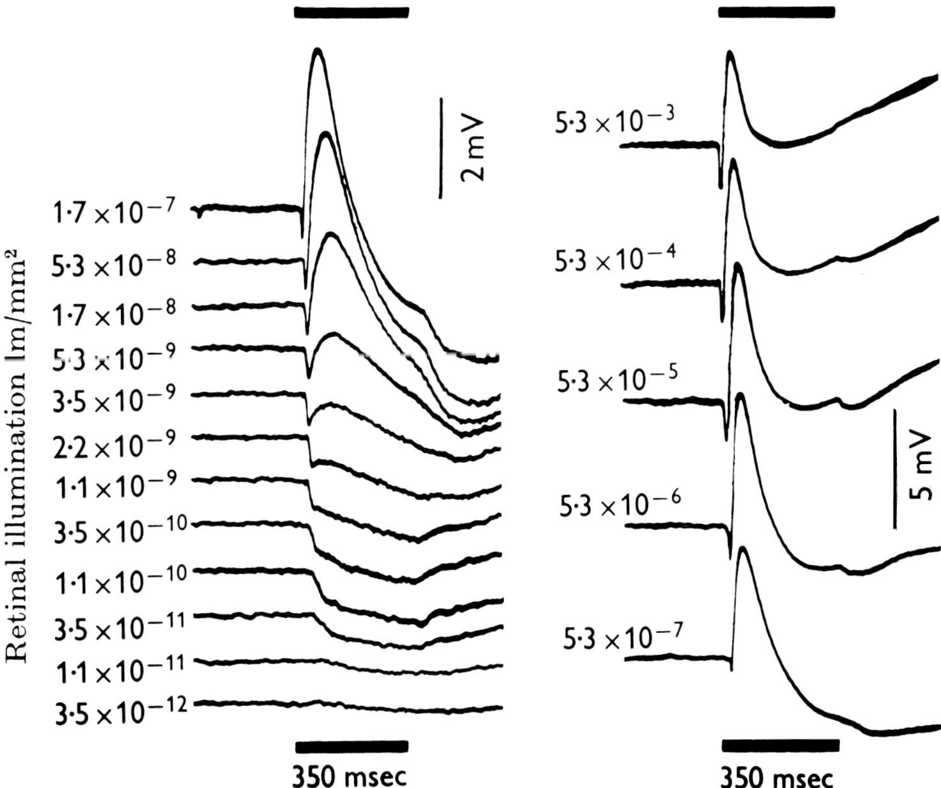

Figure 166. The effect of stimulus intensity upon the LERG of the cat, recorded by a tungsten microelectrode on the retinal surface after replacing the vitreous humor with a heavy oil. The reference electrode was in the mouth, and amplification was direct-coupled. This series of records was begun after 90 min. of dark adaptation. The stimulus spot was centered upon the microelectrode and had a diameter of 1.14 mm. The sequence of records was from the bottom left (lowest intensity used) to the upper right (maximum intensity available). Stimuli were separated by one min. intervals to reduce the effect of light adaptation by the stimuli. Note that amplification was reduced for the records of the right column. (From Arden & Brown, 3.)

which generate the b-wave are subject to considerable convergence of pathways from the receptors. When responses are evoked by large stimulus areas, as required to give responses of useful amplitude by conventional recording methods, this convergence of retinal pathways causes an amplification of the b-wave from any unit area of the retina, relative to the a-wave from that same unit area. Hence these recording conditions are more favorable for the b-wave than for the a-wave. When local responses are evoked by relatively small stimulus spots, this advantage of the b-wave is reduced. Also, recording under oil gives exceptionally large responses, and hence improved sensitivity for detecting responses to weak stimuli. Figure 166 shows the effects of stimulus intensity upon the LERG of the cat, when evoked by a relatively small stimulus spot and recorded by a surface electrode under oil. The stimulus intensity increases from the lower left to the upper right, and the lowest intensity is only about one log unit above the absolute dark-adapted human threshold. At this intensity a late RP is already distinct, and at higher intensities the rising phase of the late RP becomes the rise of the a-wave. In this experiment the late RP was detected at a lower stimulus intensity than required to detect other electrical responses of the visual system in either this experiment or in other studies. Ganglion cell discharges appeared only at higher intensities, and Figure 166 shows that more than 2.5 log units of additional intensity were required to detect the b-wave. Hence these results are consistent with evidence that the late RP is a receptor response, while the b-wave is generated by cells of the inner nuclear layer.

Perhaps it should be emphasized that although there are many methods for abolishing the b-wave and D.C. component, while still recording the late RP, there is no method which shows that the late RP may be abolished while still recording responses of the inner nuclear layer. Thus there is no critical finding which is contrary either to the origin of the late RP from the receptors, or to a causal role of the late RP in evoking later responses from the inner nuclear layer. Evidence along these lines prior to 1961 has been reviewed previously (34). Although a recent paper concludes that the rod late RP may be selectively abolished (38), these results are readily understood from limitations of the methods used (25). There is also evidence which strongly suggests that decay of the cone late RP serves to trigger decay of the D.C. component (25).

Minor Components of the ERG

Minor Components Subsequent to the a-Wave

In addition to the major components, a number of other components contribute to the detailed form of the ERG. A subcomponent of the b-wave has been described which was first discovered in the human retina by Motokawa & Mita (62), and which they designated the x-wave. As shown in Figure 167, the peak of the x-wave is quite sharp and occurs prior to the more prolonged main portion of the b-wave. Since Motokawa & Mita found that the x-wave was most readily elicited by red light, they identified it as dependent upon the cone system of receptors. This response was also discovered later but independently by Adrian (1), who showed by systematic studies that the x-wave is photopic while the

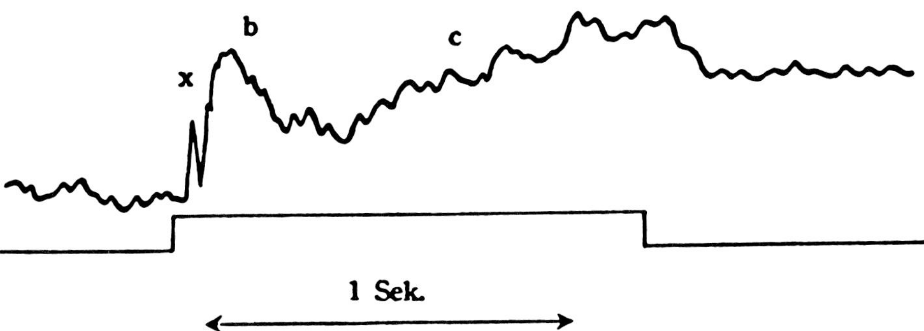

Figure 167. The x-wave of the human electroretinogram, which closely precedes the b-wave. The c-wave is also labeled, and the lower trace shows the duration of the red light stimulus. (From Motokawa & Mita, 62.)

slower part of the b-wave is scotopic. But Crescitelli (39) has shown that in the pure cone squirrel retina the b-wave also has two subcomponents, both of which appear to be dependent upon cone activity.

At high stimulus intensities rapid oscillations may be seen on the b-wave, as first described by Cobb & Morton (36) in responses of the human retina. Similar oscillations have since been found in many species, and have been designated the "oscillatory potential" by Yonemura, Masuda & Hatta (87). In the monkey retina these oscillations are very prominent in response to high-intensity flashes. Figure 168 shows these oscillations from both the peripheral retina and fovea, and the effects of clamping the retinal circulation. With the retinal circulation normal, the rather large oscillations of the peripheral retina begin on the rising phase of the b-wave and then diminish and disappear during the later part of the b-wave. In the normal foveal response these oscillations, like the b-wave, are recorded at

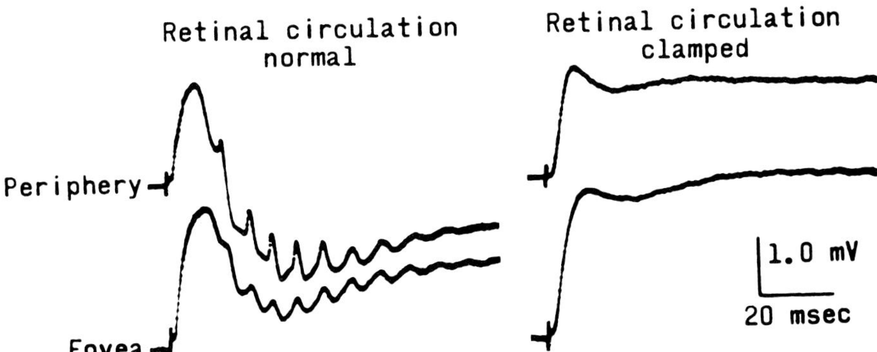

Figure 168. Oscillations on the local b-waves recorded from the peripheral retina and fovea of cynomolgus, and the abolition of these oscillations by clamping the retinal circulation. All records were taken from the same animal by a tungsten microelectrode at the level of maximum amplitude of either the a-wave or the isolated positive late RP. The reference electrode was a chlorided silver wire in the vitreous humor. Responses were recorded by a tape recorder, with flat frequency response from 0–5000 cps and were photographed later. The stimulus was an intense brief flash, as described for Figure 158. The timing of the stimulus flash is shown by a stimulus artifact shortly after the beginning of each record, and a relatively high sweep is used to resolve the oscillations.

smaller amplitude. Since receptor responses are consistently recorded at larger amplitude in the fovea (30), the oscillations must arise from cells proximal to the receptors. When the retinal circulation is clamped, recordings from both the fovea and periphery show that the oscillations, like the b-wave, are abolished. Yonemura et al. (87) noted similar effects of restricted retinal circulation in human clinical cases. Thus the oscillations are critically dependent upon the retinal circulation, which means they probably do not arise from either the receptors or from the cells which generate S-potentials.

In Figure 169 the oscillations are recorded from the peripheral retina of cynomolgus as a function of electrode depth. They increase in amplitude until about 16 per cent of the retinal depth, after which there is no distinct change in

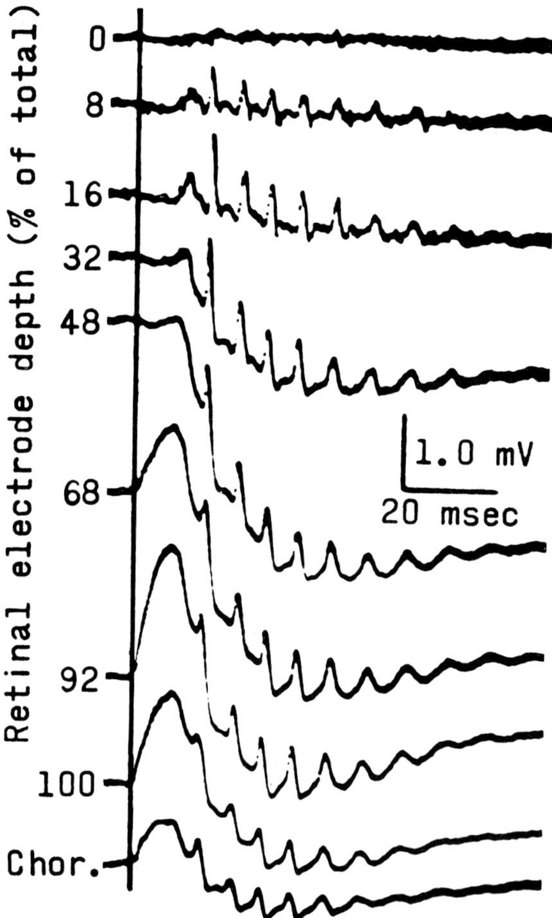

Figure 169. Oscillations on the local b-wave as a function of depth of a tungsten microelectrode in the peripheral retina of cynomolgus, with the reference electrode in the vitreous humor. Stimulating and recording conditions as described in Figure 158, except for an increased sweep speed to resolve the oscillations on the b-wave. A vertical line has been drawn which passes through all the stimulus artifacts.

amplitude until about 92 per cent, beyond which they are reduced. Thus in Figure 169 the oscillations do not pass through an amplitude maximum where the b-wave is maximum, in the range of 48–68 per cent, or in the range where the a-wave is maximum at about 92 per cent. These results make it very unlikely that the oscillations arise from either the receptors or from cells of the inner nuclear layer. Depth studies in the monkey retina by Ogden* have now demonstrated a small but distinct peak of the oscillations which is superficial to the inner nuclear layer. Ogden (65) has also shown that sectioning the optic tract abolishes the oscillations of the pigeon retina, but only after sufficient time for retrograde degeneration of the ganglion cells; hence the ganglion cells appear to be involved in generating the oscillations. But Doty & Kimura (42) find in cats and monkeys that antidromic stimulation does not reset the rhythm of the oscillations, from which they infer that the pacemaker for the oscillations is not in the ganglion cells. Somewhat different results have been obtained in the frog, where Yonemura et al. (87) find the oscillations to be maximum in the inner nuclear layer. Hence the possibility of species differences arises again at this point. This is not surprising, since oscillations probably depend upon neural feedback circuits, the details of which could well vary between species.

A further minor component is a slow potential described by Arden & Brown (3), which has negative polarity when recorded by an electrode on the surface of the cat retina. By comparison with the late RP, which has the same polarity, this new component has a slower rise and is enhanced by light adaptation. Also, it is best elicited by annular stimuli which are too large to elicit a local a-wave, so it was designated "surround negativity". It was found to have maximum amplitude near the retinal surface, so the ganglion cells are also candidates for the generators of surround negativity. The usual statement that ganglion cells make no contribution to the ERG refers to the major components, for which evidence seems in agreement, but there is no evidence that this applies to all of the minor components. Stimulation of the retina can either depolarize the ganglion cell membrane, which increases its firing rate, or cause a hyperpolarization which inhibits firing, as first shown with intracellular recordings from ganglion cells of the cat by Brown & Wiesel (31,32). Since ganglion cells generate slow potentials, they could give rise to ERG components if the recording methods were sufficiently sensitive.

The Early Receptor Potential

When the latency of the late RP had been reduced to 1.7 msec., it became evident that it was closely approaching an absolute minimum. This order of latency seemed too long for a response which is triggered directly by one of the rapid molecular events known to follow absorption of light in a photopigment molecule and believed crucial for excitation (56,80). Thus a separate response was predicted to intervene between the excitatory molecular event in the photopigment and the onset of the late RP (28). When the higher stimulus intensity of a condenser-discharge flash was used, Brown & Murakami (22) found such an earlier

* Personal communication.

response in the monkey retina, which proved biphasic in form (23). This response was found by microelectrode methods and identified as generated by the receptors; hence it was designated the early RP. Figure 170 shows the early RP elicited from the monkey retina by a 20 μsec. flash and recorded by a microelectrode at about the level of the inner segments of the receptors. In the upper record the stimulus artifact caused only a break in the baseline, which is marked by an arrow. Immediately following this flash there is a positive early RP which appears as a foot preceding the rising phase of the a-wave. The latency of the a-wave in this record is about 1.5 msec., which is the shortest recorded to date. When artificial respiration was terminated at the end of the experiment, followed quickly by death of the animal, the a-wave declined without affecting the amplitude of

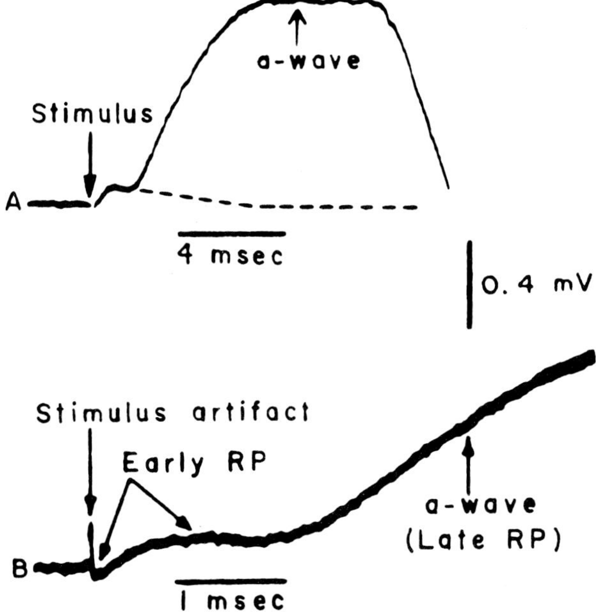

Figure 170. The early receptor potential of the cynomolgus monkey. Responses were recorded by a tungsten microelectrode at about the level of the inner segments, with the reference electrode in the vitreous humor, and the frequency response of the recording system was flat from 1.6 to above 10,000 cps. The stimulus was an intense 20 μsec. flash, as described in Figure 158, and the sweep speeds were much higher than used in conventional ERG work. In record *A*, from the peripheral retina, the early response may be seen to intervene between the stimulus flash and the rising phase of the a-wave. The time-course of decay of this early response, when isolated by cessation of artificial respiration, is shown by the dashed line which has been drawn in. Record *B* is from the fovea, where the response is larger, with an even more expanded time scale to resolve details of its onset. In this record the stimulus artifact consists only of the positive pip which is labeled. Thus the early RP is biphasic, and is followed by the late RP, which gives the rising phase of the a-wave. (Combined from Brown & Murakami, 22,23.)

the early RP. After about 24 minutes the a-wave was completely abolished and the early RP was isolated (22,30). The time-course of decay of the early RP, when isolated by this method, is shown by the dashed line in the upper record of Figure 170. This procedure shows that the early RP is not merely an initial portion of the a-wave, but is generated in a different manner, since it is much more resistant to ischemic anoxia. The lower record shows a response from the monkey fovea, where the early RP is larger than in the periphery, and with a faster time scale to resolve further details of the response. In this record the stimulus artifact gave only the vertical positive pip which is labeled, as shown by control experiments. Thus the early RP is biphasic, consisting of an initial phase of opposite polarity from the a-wave, followed by a second phase with the same polarity as the a-wave.

Both phases of the early RP were identified with the receptors by similar criteria (22,23,30). Since the response proved larger in the fovea than in the periphery, it could not be generated by any type of cell proximal to the receptors. Generation by the pigment epithelium cells was also excluded by this observation, and by the fact that the early RP increased amplitude over a distinct range as the electrode was withdrawn from the pigment epithelium. Maximum amplitudes of both phases of the early RP have now been found at essentially the same retinal level as the maximum late RP of positive polarity (30).

With even higher stimulus intensities, Cone (37) showed that the early RP may be recorded with gross electrodes by conventional ERG methods. This type of recording has revealed a similar early RP from the human eye (5,86) and from a variety of mammals and lower vertebrates (16,37,69), so it seems to occur in all vertebrate eyes. Also, similar biphasic responses have been obtained from pure cone and from essentially pure rod eyes, although the time-course of the cone response may be slightly faster (69).

Since the early RP is remarkably resistant to anoxia, and even to death of the animal, it may be studied in isolated eyes and retinas without sacrificing normality of the response. Studies in such preparations have shown that the two phases of the early RP may be separated, and hence are generated by somewhat different mechanisms. When the temperature of the excised albino rat eye was reduced, the second phase of the early RP was abolished and the first phase thereby isolated (68). Hence the second phase is more temperature-dependent than the first phase. The second phase has also been selectively abolished by light adaptation (16), as shown in Figure 171. In this experiment a toad retina was removed from the eyecup, the dissection being conducted under dim red light, and it was visually verified that pigment epithelium cells did not remain with the retina. Responses were then recorded by cotton wicks on either side of the retina. The usual ERG convention was used, so the upward first phase of the early RP results from positivity of the electrode on the vitreous side of the retina, while the second phase is a negative deflection of slower time-course. The response to the first stimulus flash shows first and second phases which are about equal in amplitude, so the toad retina is favorable for observing the different effects of light adaptation upon the two phases of the response. When the retina was light-adapted

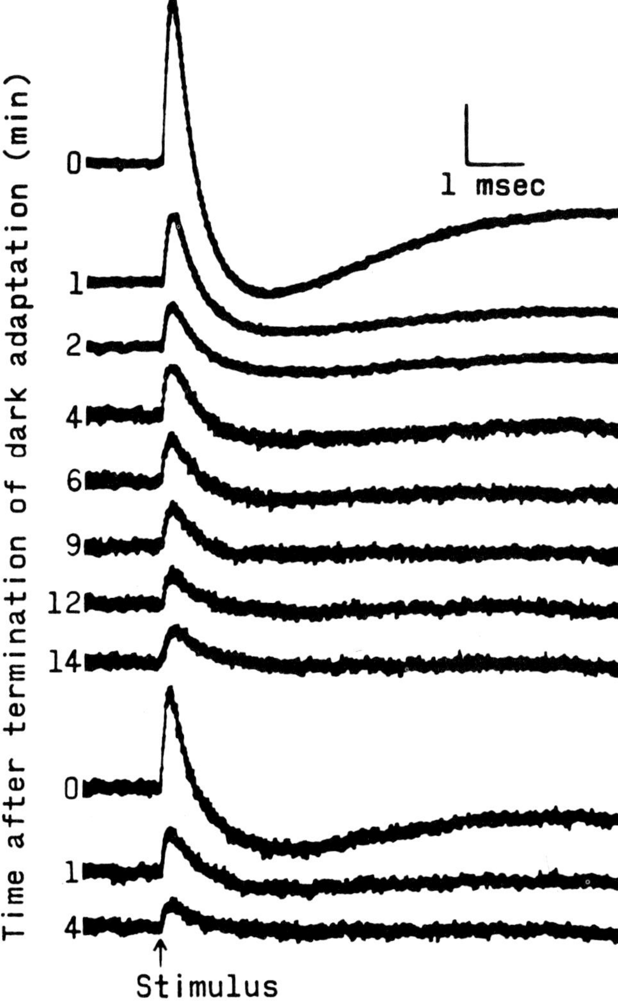

Figure 171. The effects of light adaptation upon the early receptor potential of the isolated toad retina. The retina was removed from the eye under dim red lighting and placed upon a cotton wick, which served as the active electrode. The receptors were facing upward, and a second cotton wick on the receptor surface served as the reference electrode. The frequency response of the recording system was flat from about 6–60,000 cps, which was sufficient to give undistorted responses. The stimulus was a condenser-discharge flash from a photographic lamp (Honeywell's Strobonar 65C), which has a total duration of about 1 msec. Stimulus artifacts were abolished by placing the light source outside the electrically shielded recording room, and the onset of the stimulus flash is indicated in the bottom record. The light was led to the preparation by a fiber optics bundle (Amer. Opt. type LG5-36), one end of which was close to the flash tube and the other directly over the retina. The preparation was light-adapted by 15 flashes at one min. intervals, followed by 15 min. of dark adaptation, and was then light-adapted again by five more flashes at one min. intervals. The calibration marker indicates 100 μV for the top three records and 50 μV for all other records.

by successive flashes, separated by one-minute intervals, the second phase was reduced more rapidly than the first phase. After about ten minutes the first phase was completely isolated by this procedure, and showed no further changes during the series of light-adapting stimuli. When the preparation was again dark-adapted, considerable recovery occurred. Thus the preceding effects were not due to deterioration of the preparation, but to light adaptation, which has a greater effect upon the second phase of the early RP than upon the first phase.

Although the functional significance of the early RP is not known, it must be closely associated with very rapid events which occur in the photopigment molecule after absorption of a light quantum. The latency of the first phase is extremely short, and in the isolated toad retina it cannot exceed a few microseconds (16). Hence the first phase must represent an essentially instantaneous end-product of a biological transduction. In the predominantly rod retina of the rat, Pak & Cone (68) have shown that the spectral response curves of both phases of the early RP are in good agreement with the absorption spectrum of rhodopsin, so the early RP results from absorption of light by the photopigment of the outer segments. Also, Arden & Ikeda (4) have shown that an inherited retinal dystrophy in rats, which at a certain stage affects the inner segments more than the outer segments, reduces the late RP but not the early RP. Thus the early RP is probably generated in the outer segments. The upper record of Figure 170 shows that the total duration of the early RP is about 6 msec., and that the late RP begins soon after the second phase of the early RP has reached its peak. Hence the early RP bridges the time gap between rapid photochemical events and the late RP, and provides a type of link between photochemical and neurophysiological studies of retinal photoreceptors.

Direct Light-Evoked Responses of Pigment Epithelium Cells

When the retina was removed from the toad's eyecup, leaving only the pigment epithelium-choroid complex supported by the sclera, experiments with this eyecup preparation showed that it also gave responses to light (16). At room temperatures the response consists of a rapid negative phase, followed by a much slower positive phase, as shown by the top record of Figure 172. It was readily demonstrated that this response was not due to receptor outer segments which remained with the eyecup, since the eyecup response proved insensitive to light adaptation. At room temperatures the negative phase has a latency of 25–30 μsec., so it seemed likely that there was an even earlier phase of this response. This was revealed by Brown & Gage (21) with two methods. When the temperature of the preparation was lowered, the slow positive phase was most strongly affected, but the rapid negative phase was also reduced, revealing a small positive initial phase with no detectable latency. Next the initial positive phase was isolated, at room temperature, by filling the eyecup with a Ringer's solution containing polyethylene glycol (Carbowax). This large molecule is biologically inactive and does not penetrate cell membranes, providing a stable hyperosmotic external medium which dehydrates the generating cells. Figure 172 shows that after this procedure the slow positive third phase is most quickly affected, and in

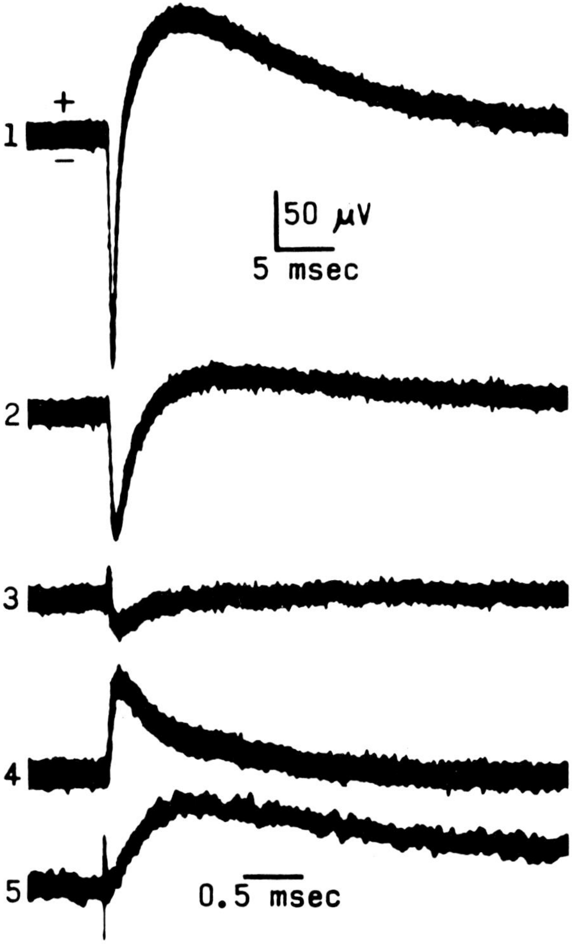

Figure 172. Responses evoked by light from the pigment epithelium of the toad's eye. The retina had been removed from the eyecup, leaving only the pigment epithelium-choroid complex, supported by the sclera. A cotton wick electrode was placed in the solution in the eyecup, and the reference electrode was a second cotton wick under the eyecup. The frequency response of the recording system was flat from about 6–60,000 cps. The stimulus was delivered as described in Figure 171, and was repeated every 15 sec. Record 1 is a control response with Ringer's solution in the eyecup; then the Ringer's solution was sucked out and a Ringer's solution containing Carbowax was introduced to provide a hyperosmotic medium. Record 2 was taken about 20 sec. after this procedure, and record 3 after 170 sec. Record 4 shows the final effect of this procedure, after the second and third phases of the normal response had been abolished and the positive first phase had been isolated. Record 5 shows this isolated first phase at higher sweep speed. In this case a stimulus artifact was introduced for timing purposes; it was recorded as a vertical line, and is followed immediately by the rise of the response. (From Brown & Gage, 21.)

record 3 has been abolished; at this time the negative second phase is greatly reduced, and the positive first phase is becoming evident. In record 4 the initial positive phase is isolated, and record 5 shows this isolated first phase at higher sweep speed to illustrate that it has no detectable latency. After isolating the first phase by this method, it is stable for an hour or more and may be studied systematically (19,21). Thus the response of the eyecup preparation consists of three phases, which must be separately generated, since they show different sensitivities to both lowered temperature and hyperosmotic external media.

Since the pigment epithelium cells are at the surface of the eyecup preparation, the first membrane penetrated is that of a pigment cell; hence intracellular responses of these cells may be positively identified. In this type of work, conducted with micropipette electrodes in frog eyecups, Brown & Crawford (18,19) found that the pigment cells are the primary generators of the light-evoked response. All three phases are generated across structures which are penetrated when the electrode passes directly through the pigment cells. Also the first two phases invert polarity as the electrode penetrates the front membrane of the pigment cell, and this appears to be true for the third phase as well.

Since the pigment cells generate the responses of the eyecup preparation, they must be regarded as very primitive photosensitive cells, by comparison with the highly differentiated retinal photoreceptors. Thus it is of special interest that the responses of these two preparations show strong similarities. In both cases there are three phases, of which the first two are very rapid and of opposite polarity, while the third phase is much slower. Also in both cases the three phases show the same order of temperature-dependence (21). Most striking, perhaps, is that in both preparations the third phase appears to be generated by a transmembrane ion flux, being abolished by sufficient lowering of the external sodium concentration (21,44,53), while the first two rapid phases are very insensitive to the ionic composition of the external medium (13,21,67).

The similarities between responses of retinal photoreceptors and pigment cells strongly suggest that a fundamental sequence of electrical responses has been found which occurs in many or all types of photosensitive cells. This is now supported by the finding of a rapid response from *Limulus* photoreceptors (72). Rapid potentials have also been reported now from pigmented frog skin and from the iris (6,9). Of special interest is the green leaf, where such potentials have now been found by Arden, Bridges, Ikeda & Siegel (2). Here also the response is biphasic, with distinct similarities to the early RP and pigment cell response. It has long seemed likely that there are steps which are common to the processes of photoreception and photosynthesis, and it now seems possible that the rapid electrical responses fulfill this expectation.

Although the functional significance of the photosensitivity of pigment epithelium cells is unknown, these responses are mediated by melanin. They have been demonstrated in the eyes of pigmented rats, but are not present in albinos (6,18,20). Also, Brown & Crawford (18,20) have shown in the frog that the spectral response curves of all three phases of the response are quite flat throughout the central portion of the visible spectrum. This excludes the possibility that these responses are mediated by rhodopsin or any of the other retinal photopigments, and is as expected for responses mediated by melanin. By contrast, the spectral response curve for the c-wave has been shown to be similar to that of rhodopsin in both frog (50) and rabbit (41). This may well account for why the c-wave has not been recorded from eyecup preparations after removal of the retina. Present evidence suggests that the c-wave may be initiated by absorption of light in the retinal receptors, rather than from an intrinsic photosensitivity of the pigment cells, and further work is needed on this subject.

The time-course of the directly evoked pigment cell response overlaps that of the retinal photoreceptors, so these responses summate in recordings from the whole eye of the toad (16). All three phases of the pigment cell response have also been demonstrated from the eyecup of the guinea pig, after removal of the retina, so similar principles pertain in mammalian eyes (6). Thus the isolated retina, and the eyecup after removing the retina, offer special promise for studying responses of photosensitive cells in future work. The whole eyes of albino animals are likewise favorable for studying the responses of retinal photoreceptors.

A final point of special interest is that after penetrating a pigment epithelium cell the membrane potential declines, owing to damage by the microelectrode, and as this occurs the second phase of the response decreases more rapidly than the first phase. This indicates that the second phase is especially dependent upon the integrity of the cell membrane. Hence the second phase must be generated as an alteration of charge across the cell membrane, and cannot be accounted for solely by a photochemical alteration of a light-absorbing molecule which is located in the cell cytoplasm. This same principle may apply to the first phase as well, since both phases invert polarity after penetrating the front membrane of the pigment cell. This involvement of the cell membrane in rapid responses, as first reported in pigment cells (18,19), seems to increase the possibility that the rapid responses serve a role in excitation. And a similar principle seems to hold in *Limulus* photoreceptors, where the rapid response found by Smith & Brown (72) was shown to be related to the amplitude of the membrane potential.

Some Present Perspectives

The ERG has often been regarded as posing problems, rather than offering solutions to problems, and in balance it is both. But there now seems sufficient progress on the problems that the opportunities offered merit increasing attention. These opportunities may now be understood from general principles of neurophysiology, and from the problems which are becoming critical in retinal physiology. In studying complex nervous structures, such as the retina, we must deal primarily with the electrical signals by which nerve cells transmit information. Although self-evident, this is worth emphasis because the use of neurophysiological techniques in retinal physiology has tended to lag behind other methods, such as those of photochemistry and psychophysics. The now-classical method of analyzing nervous activity is to record the extracellular impulse activity of a single cell. In the retina this was first applied to ganglion cells by Hartline's technique of fiber dissection (54) and by the use of a glass-insulated wire to record impulses from ganglion cells near the retinal surface (52). This general method was extended by the development of microelectrodes, which permit impulse activity to be recorded from a cell which is buried in a mass of nervous tissue. If a retinal cell does fire impulses, they are rather readily detected by an extracellular microelectrode, identified by constant size as being from a single cell, and recorded for long periods under stable conditions (32). Hence in the cat this method has revealed impulse activity from cells of unidentified type in the inner nuclear layer (26,32). But nerve impulses constitute a special method utilized by nerve cells for transmitting signals over long distances. The initiation or inhibition of impulse activity is controlled by slow potentials which depolarize or hyperpolarize the cell membrane, and which have been studied intensively by neurophysiologists in recent years. If cells are sufficiently short, they have no need for impulses, since they can conduct entirely by means of slow potentials. This appears to be the case for early stages of retinal activity, since there is no sign of impulse activity from the cells which generate S-potentials, or from the retinal photoreceptors. In recording the activity of such cells, the technical problems are quite different. It appears possible to record a slow potential from a single cell by extracellular methods, providing that the electrode is pressing upon the membrane, but the potential cannot be identified as from a single cell unless it is of large amplitude and recorded from a highly restricted locus; in the retina this method has thus far been useful only for S-potentials (32). If an intracellular response can be obtained, it is obviously from a single cell, but intracellular responses from small cells are exceptionally difficult to obtain. Good success has been achieved with S-potentials from cold-blooded retinas, where the generating cells are very large (59,61,74,78,79). But even S-potentials are quite difficult to record by this method in mammals (32). With the possible exception of work in *Necturus* (10,11), intracellular records from retinal photoreceptors are rarely obtained, small in amplitude, and deteriorate rapidly (78). Similar limitations hold for intracellular responses from pigment epithelium cells (19,34). Thus different methods seem required for systematic studies of electrical activity from retinal receptors and pigment epithelium cells.

For many problems it is not necessary to record the response of a single cell, but only a response resulting from the activity of many cells of a given type. This is especially true when recording slow potentials from cells of a given class at an early stage of retinal activity, since the responses of the individual cells may be assumed to be well synchronized by the stimulus. In other words, the form and general characteristics of a summated response of this type must be typical of the single cell responses of which it is composed. This would not be true if the response of each cell consisted of impulse discharges, for which synchrony among the various cells could not be expected. Hence this is a characteristic of slow potentials which may be taken advantage of in solving the technical problem of recording them. The term "slow potential" is used here to mean activity other than nerve impulses, and includes responses such as the early RP which are actually quite rapid. As thus defined, methods are now available for using the ERG to record several types of slow potentials from retinal rods and cones, and also from pigment cells, under stable and relatively normal conditions. Hence the ERG now seems uniquely valuable for studying a large variety of problems concerning excitation, transmission, and processing of signals in the retinal photoreceptors.

SUMMARY

Three major neural components of the mammalian ERG have been demonstrated, including the late RP (receptor potential), b-wave, and D.C. component. These give an adequate explanation of all main features of the cone ERG. Main features of the rod ERG are accounted for by these same three components, plus the c-wave from the pigment epithelium. Different forms of the off-responses in cone and rod ERGs are now readily understood from the rapid decay of the cone late RP, compared with the much slower decay of the rod late RP. The generating cells have been identified for the late RP and c-wave, and the b-wave and D.C. component have been localized to the inner nuclear layer, but the cell types which generate these latter components have not been identified. In addition to the major components, a number of minor components have been found which contribute to the detailed form of the ERG. Such components are still being discovered, and this process may continue. Among these, only the biphasic early RP and the directly evoked triphasic response of the pigment epithelium cells have been positively identified with particular cell types. In addition to analyzing the ERG into components, and determining the cellular origin of each component, it is especially important to determine the role of each component in retinal functions. This further phase of ERG work is just beginning, since we now have components which are identified with both the receptors and cells of the pigment epithelium.

REFERENCES

1. Adrian, E. D., The electric response of the human eye. *J. Physiol.* (London), 1945, **104**: 84–104.
2. Arden, G. B., Bridges, C. D. B., Ikeda, H., and Siegel, I. M., Rapid light-induced potentials common to plant and animal tissues. *Nature* (London), 1966, **212**: 1235–1236.
3. Arden, G. B., and Brown, K. T., Some properties of components of the cat electroretinogram revealed by local recording under oil. *J. Physiol.* (London), 1965, **176**: 429–461.
4. Arden, G. B., and Ikeda, H., Effects of hereditary degeneration of the retina on the early receptor potential and the corneo-fundal potential of the rat eye. *Vision Res.*, 1966, **6**: 171–184.
5. ———, Electrophysiological findings in congenital retinal degeneration in rats. *Jap. J. Ophthal.*, 1966, **10**, Supp.: 222–230.
6. Arden, G. B., Ikeda, H., and Siegel, I. M., New components of the mammalian receptor potential and their relation to visual photochemistry. *Vision Res.*, 1966, **6**: 373–384.
7. Arden, G. B., and Tansley, K., The spectral sensitivity of the pure-cone retina of

the grey squirrel (*Sciurus carolinensis leucotis*). *J. Physiol.* (London), 1955, **127**: 592–602.

8. Armington, J. C., Johnson, E. P., and Riggs, L. A., The scotopic *A*-wave in the electrical response of the human retina. *J. Physiol.* (London), 1952, **118**: 289–298.
9. Becker, H. E., and Cone, R. A., Light-stimulated electrical responses from skin. *Science*, 1966, **154**: 1051–1053.
10. Bortoff, A., Localization of slow potential responses in the *Necturus* retina. *Vision Res.*, 1964, **4**: 627–635.
11. Bortoff, A., and Norton, A. L., Simultaneous recording of photoreceptor potentials and the P III component of the ERG. *Vision Res.*, 1965, **5**: 527–533.
12. Brindley, G. S., The passive electrical properties of the frog's retina, choroid and sclera for radial fields and currents. *J. Physiol.* (London), 1956, **134**: 339–352.
13. Brindley, G. S., and Gardner-Medwin, A. R., The origin of the early receptor potential of the retina. *J. Physiol.* (London), 1966, **182**: 185–194.
14. Brindley, G. S., and Hamasaki, D. I., The properties and nature of the R membrane of the frog's eye. *J. Physiol.* (London), 1963, **167**: 599–606.
15. Brown, K. T., Optical stimulator, microelectrode advancer, and associated equipment for intraretinal neurophysiology in closed mammalian eyes. *J. Opt. Soc. Amer.*, 1964, **54**: 101–109.
16. ———, An early potential evoked by light from the pigment epithelium-choroid complex of the eye of the toad. *Nature* (London), 1965, **207**: 1249–1253.
17. ———, The analysis of ERG and the origin of its components. *Jap. J. Ophthal.*, 1966, **10**, Supp.: 130–140.
18. Brown, K. T., and Crawford, J. M., Intracellular recording of rapid light-evoked responses from pigment epithelium cells of the frog eye. *Physiologist*, 1966, **9**: 146.
19. ———, Intracellular recording of rapid light-evoked responses from pigment epithelium cells of the frog eye. *Vision Res.*, 1967, **7**: 149–163.
20. ———, Melanin and the rapid light-evoked responses from pigment epithelium cells of the frog eye. *Ibid.*: 165–178.
21. Brown, K. T., and Gage, P. W., An earlier phase of the light-evoked electrical response from the pigment epithelium-choroid complex of the eye of the toad. *Nature* (London), 1966, **211**: 155–158.
22. Brown, K. T., and Murakami, M., A new receptor potential of the monkey retina with no detectable latency. *Nature* (London), 1964, **201**: 626–628.
23. ———, Biphasic form of the early receptor potential of the monkey retina. *Nature* (London), 1964, **204**: 739–740.
24. ———, Receptive field organization of S-potentials and receptor potentials in light and dark adapted states. *Fed. Proc.*, 1964, **23**: 517.
25. ———, Delayed decay of the late receptor potential of monkey cones as a function of stimulus intensity. *Vision Res.*, 1967, **7**: 179–189.

25a. ———, Rapid effects of light and dark adaptation upon the receptive field organization of *S*-potentials and late receptor potentials. *Vision Res.*, 1968, **8**: 1145–1171.

26. Brown, K. T., and Tasaki, K., Localization of electrical activity in the cat retina by an electrode marking method. *J. Physiol.* (London), 1961, **158**: 281–295.

27. BROWN, K. T., and WATANABE, K., Isolation and identification of a receptor potential from the pure cone fovea of the monkey retina. *Nature* (London), 1962, **193**: 958–960.

28. ———, Rod receptor potential from the retina of the night monkey. *Nature* (London), 1962, **196**: 547–550.

29. ———, Neural stage of adaptation between the receptors and inner nuclear layer of monkey retina. *Science*, 1965, **148**: 1113–1115.

30. BROWN, K. T., WATANABE, K., and MURAKAMI, M., The early and late receptor potentials of monkey cones and rods. *Sympos. Quant. Biol.*, 1965, **30**: 457–482.

31. BROWN, K. T., and WIESEL, T. N., Intraretinal recording in the unopened cat eye. *Am. J. Ophthal.*, 1958, **46**(3/2): 91–98.

32. ———, Intraretinal recording with micropipette electrodes in the intact cat eye. *J. Physiol.* (London), 1959, **149**: 537–562.

33. ———, Analysis of the intraretinal electroretinogram in the intact cat eye. *J. Physiol.* (London), 1961, **158**: 229–256.

34. ———, Localization of origins of electroretinogram components by intraretinal recording in the intact cat eye. *Ibid.*: 257–280.

35. CHAFFEE, E. L., and SUTCLIFFE, E., The differences in electrical response of the retina of the frog and horned toad according to the position of the electrodes. *Am. J. Physiol.*, 1930, **95**: 250–261.

36. COBB, W. A., and MORTON, H. B., A new component of the human electroretinogram. *J. Physiol.* (London), 1954, **123**: 36–37*P*.

37. CONE, R. A., Early receptor potential of the vertebrate retina. *Nature* (London), 1964, **204**: 736–739.

38. CONE, R. A., and EBREY, T. G., Functional independence of the two major components of the rod electroretinogram. *Nature* (London), 1965, **206**: 913–915.

39. CRESCITELLI, F., The electroretinogram of the antelope ground squirrel. *Vision Res.*, 1961, **1**: 139–153.

40. DARTNALL, H. J. A., ARDEN, G. B., IKEDA, H., LUCK, C. P., ROSENBERG, M. E., PEDLER, C. M. H., and TANSLEY, K., Anatomical, electrophysiological and pigmentary aspects of vision in the bush baby: an interpretative study. *Vision Res.*, 1965, **5**: 399–424.

41. DODT, E., Ein Doppelinterferenzfilter-Monochromator besonders hoher Leuchtdichte. *Bibl. Ophthal.*, 1957, **48**: 32–37.

42. DOTY, R. W., and KIMURA, D. S., Oscillatory potentials in the visual system of cats and monkeys. *J. Physiol.* (London), 1963, **168**: 205–218.

43. FOODEN, J., Rhesus and crab-eating macaques: intergradation in Thailand. *Science*, 1964, **143**: 363–365.

44. FURUKAWA, T., and HANAWA, I., Effects of some common cations on electroretinogram of the toad. *Jap. J. Physiol.*, 1955, **5**: 289–300.

45. GRANIT, R., The components of the retinal action potential in mammals and their relation to the discharge in the optic nerve. *J. Physiol.* (London), 1933, **77**: 207–239.

46. ———, *Sensory Mechanisms of the Retina*. Hafner, New York, 1947.

47. ———, *Receptors and Sensory Perception*. Yale Univ. Press, New Haven, 1955.

48. ———, Neural activity in the retina. In: *Handbook of Physiology; Neurophysiology I* (J. Field, H. W. Magoun and V. E. Hall, Eds.). American Physiological Society, Washington, D.C., 1959: 693–712.

49. Granit, R. Neurophysiology of the retina. In: *The Eye, Vol. 2: The Visual Process* (H. Davson, Ed.). Academic Press, New York, 1962: 575–691.
50. Granit, R., and Munsterhjelm, A., The electrical responses of dark-adapted frogs' eyes to monochromatic stimuli. *J. Physiol.* (London), 1937, **88**: 436–458.
51. Granit, R., and Riddell, L. A., The electrical responses of light- and dark-adapted frogs' eyes to rhythmic and continuous stimuli. *J. Physiol.* (London), 1934, **81**: 1–28.
52. Granit, R., and Svaetichin, G., Principles and technique of the electrophysiological analysis of colour reception with the aid of microelectrodes. *Upsala Läkaref. Förh.*, 1939, **45**: 161–177.
53. Hamasaki, D. I., The effect of sodium ion concentration on the electroretinogram of the isolated retina of the frog. *J. Physiol.* (London), 1963, **167**: 156–168.
54. Hartline, H. K., The response of single optic nerve fibers of the vertebrate eye to illumination of the retina. *Am. J. Physiol.*, 1938, **121**: 400–415.
55. Holmgren, F., Method att objectivera effecten av ljusintryck pa retina. *Upsala Läkaref. Förh.*, 1865, **1**: 177–191.
56. Hubbard, R., and Kropf, A., Molecular aspects of visual excitation. *Ann. N.Y. Acad. Sci.*, 1959, **81**: 388–398.
57. Kolmer, W., Zur Kenntnis des Auges der Primaten. *Zschr. Anat. Entwicklungsgesch.*, 1930, **93**: 679–722.
58. Kuffler, S. W., Discharge patterns and functional organization of mammalian retina. *J. Neurophysiol.*, 1953, **16**: 37–68.
59. MacNichol, E. F., Jr., and Svaetichin, G., Electric responses from the isolated retinas of fishes. *Am. J. Ophthal.*, 1958, **46**(3/2): 24–46.
60. Michaelson, I. C., *Retinal Circulation in Man and Animals*. Thomas, Springfield, 1954.
61. Mitarai, G., Svaetichin, G., Vallecalle, E., Fatehchand, R., Villegas, J., and Laufer, M., Glia-neuron interactions and adaptational mechanisms of the retina. In: *The Visual System: Neurophysiology and Psychophysics* (R. Jung and H. Kornhuber, Eds). Springer, Berlin, 1961: 463–481.
62. Motokawa, K., and Mita, T., Über eine einfachere Untersuchungsmethode und Eigenschaften der Aktionsströme der Netzhaut des Menschen. *Tohoku J. Exp. Med.*, 1942, **42**: 114–133.
63. Murakami, M., and Kaneko, A., Subcomponents of *P*III in cold-blooded vertebrate retinae. *Nature* (London), 1966, **210**: 103–104.
64. Noell, W. K., The origin of the electroretinogram. *Am. J. Ophthal.*, 1954, **38**: 78–90.
65. Ogden, T. E., Oscillatory potentials of the pigeon ERG. *Physiologist*, 1966, **9**: 256.
66. Ottoson, D., and Svaetichin, G., Electrophysiological investigations of the frog retina. *Sympos. Quant. Biol.*, 1952, **17**: 165–173.
67. Pak, W. L., Some properties of the early electrical response in the vertebrate retina. *Sympos. Quant. Biol.*, 1965, **30**: 493–499.
68. Pak, W. L., and Cone, R. A., Isolation and identification of the initial peak of the early receptor potential. *Nature* (London), 1964, **204**: 836–838.
69. Pak, W. L., and Ebrey, T. G., Early receptor potentials of rods and cones in rodents. *J. Gen. Physiol.*, 1966, **49**: 1199–1208.
70. Polyak, S., *The Vertebrate Visual System* (ed. by H. Klüver). Univ. of Chicago Press, Chicago, 1957.
71. Sickel, W., Respiratory and electrical responses to light stimulation in the retina of the frog. *Science*, 1965, **148**: 648–651.

72. SMITH, T. G., JR., and BROWN, J. E., A photoelectric potential in invertebrate cells. *Nature* (London), 1966, **212**: 1217–1219.

73. STONE, J., A quantitative analysis of the distribution of ganglion cells in the cat's retina. *J. Comp. Neurol.*, 1965, **124**: 337–352.

74. SVAETICHIN, G., The cone action potential. *Acta Physiol. Scand.*, 1953, **29**: 565–600 (Suppl. 106).

75. TANSLEY, K., Comparative anatomy of the mammalian retina with respect to the electroretinographic response to light. In: *The Structure of the Eye* (G. K. Smelser, Ed.). Academic Press, New York, 1961: 193–206.

76. TOMITA, T., Studies on the intraretinal action potential. Part I. Relation between the localization of micro-pipette in the retina and the shape of the intraretinal action potential. *Jap. J. Physiol.*, 1950, **1**: 110–117.

77. ———, Electrical activity in the vertebrate retina. *J. Opt. Soc. Amer.*, 1963, **53**: 49–57.

78. ———, Electrophysiological study of the mechanisms subserving color coding in the fish retina. *Sympos. Quant. Biol.*, 1965, **30**: 559–566.

79. TOMITA, T., MURAKAMI, M., and HASHIMOTO, Y., On the R membrane in the frog's eye: its localization, and relation to the retinal action potential. *J. Gen. Physiol.*, 1960, **43**(6): 81–94.

80. WALD, G., BROWN, P. K., and GIBBONS, I. R., The problem of visual excitation. *J. Opt. Soc. Amer.*, 1963, **53**: 20–35.

81. WALLS, G. L., *The Lateral Geniculate Nucleus and Visual Histophysiology*. Univ. of California Publications in Physiology, Vol. 9. Univ. of California Press, Los Angeles, 1953.

82. ———, *The Vertebrate Eye and Its Adaptive Radiation.* Hafner, New York, 1963.

83. YAMADA, E., and ISHIKAWA, T., The fine structure of the horizontal cells in some vertebrate retinae. *Sympos. Quant. Biol.*, 1965, **30**: 383–392.

84. YAMASHITA, E., Some analyses of slow potentials of toad's retina. *Tohoku J. Exp. Med.*, 1959, **70**: 221–233.

85. YONEMURA, D., and HATTA, M., Localization of the minor components of the frog's electroretinogram. *Jap. J. Ophthal.*, 1966, **10**, Supp.: 149–154.

86. YONEMURA, D., KAWASAKI, K., and HASUI, I., The early receptor potential in the human ERG. *Acta Soc. Ophthal. Jap.*, 1966, **70**: 766–768.

87. YONEMURA, D., MASUDA, Y., and HATTA, M., The oscillatory potential in the electroretinogram. *Jap. J. Physiol.*, 1963, **13**: 129–137.

TOPOGRAPHY OF THE ADULT HUMAN RETINA

BRADLEY R. STRAATSMA, MAURICE B. LANDERS, ALLAN E. KREIGER and LEONARD APT*
UCLA School of Medicine
Los Angeles, California

The topography of the human retina has become increasingly important since the principles of ophthalmoscopy were presented by Helmholtz (17,18) more than a century ago. This epochal discovery introduced an era that continues to the present time. It has been marked by the development of diverse and ingenious methods for visualizing and recording the appearance of the living human retina. Reduced to their essentials, these methods for *in vivo* evaluation of the retina provide for its illumination and for observation of the illuminated area. In addition, whenever appropriate, these methods enable structures under observation to be selectively modified and permit the appearance of the retina to be documented.

TABLE 9

Illumination of the Retina

Source
Sunlight
Generated white light
Polarized light
Restricted visible and infrared light
Mercury vapor lamp
Sodium vapor lamp
Absorption filter
Interference filter
Laser
Direction
Direct illumination
Retroillumination
Focus
Diffuse
Proximal (indirect)
Slit (focal)

* The authors wish to acknowledge the assistance of Miss Jill Penkhus and Miss Gwynn Gloege with the illustrations, Miss Alice Arvin with the histologic preparations, and Dr. Morton B. Brown and Mr. John Shahinian with statistical analyses.

One of the fundamental requirements, illumination of the retina, may be achieved by a variety of sources that reach the retina directly or by retroillumination and are focused diffusely, indirectly on a proximal area, or as a sharp slit (3,5,12,14,32,34,36,40,46,49) (Table 9). The other requirement, observation of the illuminated area, may be accomplished by the unaided eye, vision that is assisted by optical and electronic devices and by systems that permit all or only a part of the source to be transmitted (54) (Table 10).

TABLE 10

OBSERVATION OF THE RETINA

Observation System
Unaided vision
Direct ophthalmoscopy
Monocular
Binocular
Indirect ophthalmoscopy
Monocular
Binocular
Stereoscopic slit lamp biomicroscopy
Precorneal concave lens
Precorneal convex lens
Corneal contact lens
Television ophthalmoscopy
Source Transmission
Unmodified
Polarized
Restricted

While under observation, the retina can be modified mechanically by scleral depression, its circulation altered by pressure and its appearance changed by injections of substances such as intravenous fluorescein (6,15,19,23–26,28,37,50) (Table 11). Furthermore, its appearance may be documented by a comparison of fundus structures or graticule measurements and recording methods such as drawings, photographs, holograms, and television procedures (1,8–10,12,23,27, 28,39,54) (Table 12). Thus, there is an enormous array of methods for observing and recording the appearance of the entire retina. With increasing precision, these methods have been applied to the evaluation of retinal characteristics.

TABLE 11

MODIFICATION OF THE RETINA

Mechanical Movement
Scleral depression
Pressure to Alter Circulation
Ophthalmodynamometry
Ophthalmodynamography
Injection to Alter Appearance
Intravenous fluorescein

TABLE 12

RECORDING OF RETINAL APPEARANCE

Dimension
- Comparison of fundus structures
- Graticule measurements

Recording Method
- Drawing
- Photography
  - Technique
    - Reflexless photography
    - Stereophotography
    - Motion picture photography
  - Film
    - Black and white
    - Color
    - Special
- Television
- Hologram

Clinical studies of the optic disk (obviously closely related to the retina proper), the macula, the peripheral fundus, and the retina as a whole have supplied information of genuine value (2,3,7,12,13,16,20,22,26,29,37,38,41,42,45,52).

For optimum scientific progress, however, *in vivo* evaluation of the retina must be correlated with an accurate and detailed understanding of retinal topography. In essence, the ideal application of methods for clinical evaluation of the retina must be related to knowledge of the size, shape, and gross morphology of the retina. Recognizing this, we are surprised to note that information concerning topography of the human retina is limited. Much of what is known stems from the excellent general anatomical description of the retina by Salzmann in 1912 (35) and the monumental work of Polyak published in 1941 (31). These authors do not record the exact source or extent of material studied, but do estimate that the optic disk is about 1.5 mm in diameter, that the temporal disk margin is about 3.5 mm from the foveola (fovea centralis), and that "the total expanse of the human retina in the horizontal meridian is . . . 43 mm, more or less" (31). They also describe the irregular anterior termination of the retina as the ora serrata and emphasize that it is closer to the corneal limbus and more jagged on the nasal side, while temporally it is further from the limbus and smoother in contour.

Unfortunately, Polyak used the term "ora serrata" to describe both the grossly visible anterior edge of the retina and a microscopically discernible retinal zone, synonymous with the extreme periphery, that included the most peripheral 0.7–0.8 mm nasally and 2.1 mm temporally. This concept of the ora serrata as the gross border and a microscopically distinct zone has been perpetuated in several contemporary texts (11,33); however, other anatomical descriptions and virtually all clinical accounts use the term ora serrata to denote the scalloped anterior edge of the retina (4,43,51,55). This anterior edge of the retina is distinct and well defined both clinically and grossly. In this study, therefore, the ora serrata is defined as the most anterior macroscopically visible portion of the sensory retina.

In the years since Polyak's work, other investigators have reviewed the dimensions of the optic disk and the relationships of the ora serrata. Ishii (21), for example, reported that the optic disk has an average horizontal diameter of 1.618 mm and a vertical diameter of 1.796 mm. Several authors recognized the importance of establishing the relationship of the ora serrata to the limbus (44,47,53); in 1955, Thiel (48) studied 89 eyes obtained at autopsy and 11 eyes removed surgically. Infants and adults were included in this material and the location of the ora serrata was established by transillumination rather than by direct inspection. A wide range of measurements was obtained, but interestingly, in one small group of adult eyes removed surgically, the distance from the limbus to the ora serrata was 7.4 mm superiorly, 6.9 mm inferiorly, 6.6 mm nasally, and 7.5 mm temporally.

Although these and other studies provide valuable information, the diversity of material examined and methods employed prevents the formation of an overall concept of retinal topography. Moreover, significant details are often lacking and there is much concerning the ora serrata that is frankly unknown. Therefore, this investigation was undertaken on a sizable group of adult human eyes obtained at autopsy or surgery, fixed in a manner that produced a volume change of less than two per cent,* and processed systematically to: (*a*) determine the general size and shape of the adult human retina; (*b*) provide quantitative data concerning the optic disk, the foveola, and the ora serrata; and (*c*) supply a direct correlation between clinical and anatomical observations.

Material and Methods

Material incorporated in this study consisted of 200 autopsy eyes on which topographic studies were performed, and six surgically enucleated eyes on which direct clinicopathologic correlation was carried out.

The 200 postmortem eyes were obtained from 183 autopsies conducted at the UCLA Center for the Health Sciences, Los Angeles, and the Veterans Administration Hospital, Long Beach. All patients in the series were 20 years of age or more at the time of death, and were distributed according to age and sex as noted in Figure 173. Autopsies were consecutive, except for the exclusion of cases with significant gross retinal disease. In 17 autopsy cases, both eyes were studied to compare symmetry. In each of the remaining 166 postmortem examinations, a single eye was incorporated in the study and the second eye was processed in the routine manner. The laterality of material was randomized and, consequently, the series included 98 right eyes and 102 left eyes. The eyes were removed as soon as possible after death, fixed in formalin for seven days and maintained in 50 per cent alcohol for three days prior to examination.

The anteroposterior diameter of the eye was measured with calipers and, using the muscle insertions and long ciliary arteries and nerves as guides, the equator

* R. Foos, personal communication.

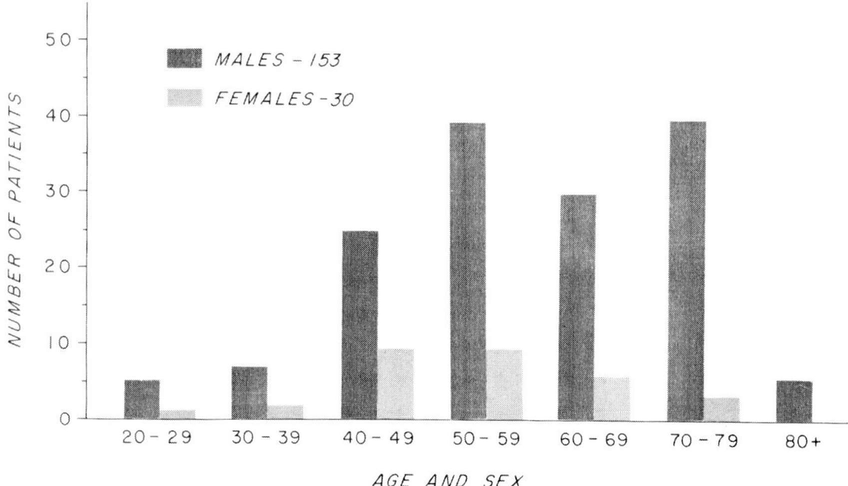

Figure 173. Age and sex distribution of the 183 autopsy subjects from whom 200 eyes were obtained. The preponderance of male subjects reflects the fact that a significant portion of this material was obtained from a Veterans Administration Hospital.

(i.e., the circumference of greatest dimension in the frontal plane) was marked at the superior, inferior, nasal, and temporal meridians. The vertical and horizontal diameters of the equator were then measured with calipers, and the globe was sectioned at the equator.

With the aid of engineering calipers equipped with a vernier scale, the dimension of the retina was measured, as a chord, from the margin of the optic disk to the equator in the superior, inferior, nasal, and temporal meridians. The same instrument was then used to measure the vertical and horizontal diameters of the retina (from its internal surface) at the equator and to make comparable measurements of the vertical and horizontal diameters at the ora serrata.

A stereoscopic microscope with a calibrated graticule providing 10× magnification was then employed to measure the vertical and horizontal dimensions of the optic disk and the distance from the temporal horizontal margin of the disk to the foveola. Some thickening of the retina in the posterior pole area was almost invariably present, but this did not significantly interfere with the identification of the foveola.

The anterior calotte was placed, corneal surface down, in a molded silastic device marked to divide the circumference into sectors of 30 degrees corresponding to the 12 conventional clock hours. The ora serrata was then inspected with the graticule-equipped stereoscopic microscope, and dentate processes, large dentate processes, giant dentate processes, meridional folds, meridional folds with posterior retinal abnormalities, ora bays, large ora bays, partly enclosed ora bays, enclosed ora bays, doubled ora bays, and retinal tags in ora bays were tabulated according to the definitions and criteria cited in the following section. All tabulations were made in a clockwise direction so that the 12:00 o'clock tabulation included all features between 12:00 and 1:00, the 1:00 o'clock tabulation included all features between 1:00 and 2:00, and so on. These tabulations were made, as previously noted, with the eye positioned so that the ora serrata was viewed from its posterior aspect. Therefore, the "clock hours" that were recorded do not correspond to the conventional clinical designations, which are derived from viewing the ora serrata from its anterior aspect. Consequently, after all tabulations were completed, the "clock hours" were reassigned to correspond with the customary clinical usage.

The lens and iris were then removed and, with the graticule-equipped microscope, the dimension of the retina from the equator to the ora serrata was measured, as a chord, in the superior, inferior, nasal, and temporal meridians. Concurrently, the distance from the ora serrata to Schwalbe's line, which constitutes the posterior border of the limbus, was measured in the same principal meridians.

Microscopic sections incorporating the ora serrata were made whenever necessary to confirm the nature of a macroscopic feature of the ora. In addition, to correlate gross and microscopic anatomy, representative examples of each characteristic macroscopic feature of the ora were photographed, serially or step-sectioned, and examined histologically.

The six surgically enucleated eyes were from four males and two females ranging in age from 40 to 62 years, with an average age of 51 years. Each eye contained an intraocular tumor (five were malignant melanomas of the choroid and/or the ciliary body, and one was a large leiomyoma of the ciliary body) which necessitated removal. Prior to enucleation, however, a complete ocular examination, including appraisal of the retina with opththalmoscopy, contact lens biomicroscopy and scleral depression, was performed, and appropriate fundus photographs and drawings were obtained. Gross and microscopic studies of the enucleated eyes provided direct correlation between clinical observations and anatomical features.

Results

In the series of 200 topographically studied eyes, the overall dimensions were as noted in Table 13. For all eyes the average anteroposterior diameter and standard deviation were 24.75 ± 0.74 mm, the vertical equatorial diameter was 24.12 ± 0.86 mm, and the horizontal equatorial diameter was 24.26 ± 0.82 mm.

TABLE 13

Dimensions of the Eye*

	Anteroposterior Diameter	Equatorial Diameters Vertical	Horizontal
Right Eye	24.73 ± 0.74	24.12 ± 0.89	24.33 ± 0.79
Left Eye	24.77 ± 0.75	24.13 ± 0.83	24.19 ± 0.89
All Eyes	24.75 ± 0.74	24.12 ± 0.86	24.26 ± 0.82

*In this and the subsequent tables, all dimensions are in millimeters, with standard deviations as noted.

The dimensions of the retina (measured as chords) from the corresponding margin of the optic disk to the equator were as recorded in Table 14. The average retinal dimension was 14.71 ± 1.08 mm in the superior meridian, 14.51 ± 1.01 mm inferiorly, 13.27 ± 1.11 mm nasally, and 17.29 ± 1.60 mm temporally. From the equator to the ora serrata, the average retinal dimensions, measured as chords, were 5.07 ± 1.11 mm superiorly, 4.79 ± 1.22 mm inferiorly, 5.81 ± 1.12 mm nasally, and 6.00 ± 1.22 mm temporally (Table 15). Thus the overall average chord dimensions of the retina were as noted in Figure 174.

TABLE 14

Dimensions of the Retina from the Disk Margin to the Equator
(Chord measurements)

	Superior	Inferior	Nasal	Temporal
Right Eye	14.73 ± 1.07	14.56 ± 0.99	13.30 ± 0.93	16.62 ± 1.06
Left Eye	14.70 ± 1.09	14.46 ± 1.02	13.23 ± 1.25	17.94 ± 1.75
All Eyes	14.71 ± 1.08	14.51 ± 1.01	13.27 ± 1.11	17.29 ± 1.60

TABLE 15

Dimensions of the Retina from the Equator to the Ora Serrata
(Chord measurements)

	Superior	Inferior	Nasal	Temporal
Right Eye	5.17 ± 1.08	4.79 ± 1.16	5.77 ± 1.07	6.11 ± 1.17
Left Eye	4.98 ± 1.12	4.8 ± 1.26	5.84 ± 1.17	5.90 ± 1.27
All Eyes	5.07 ± 1.11	4.79 ± 1.22	5.81 ± 1.12	6.00 ± 1.22

In regard to shape, the retina expanded from the optic disk to line the posterior pole and reach the equator. At the equator, the retina (measured from its internal surface) had an average diameter of 24.08 ± 0.94 mm in the vertical meridian, and 24.06 ± 0.80 mm in the horizontal meridian (Table 16). At the ora serrata, the average internal diameter of the retina was 20.41 ± 1.09 mm in the vertical direction, and 20.03 ± 1.04 mm in the horizontal direction. As depicted in Figure 175, the retina had the shape of a cup expanded to its greatest diameter at the equator and considerably reduced in diameter at its serrated anterior margin.

TABLE 16

Diameters of the Retina

	Diameter at Equator		Diameter at Ora	
	Vertical	Horizontal	Vertical	Horizontal
Right Eye	24.04 ± 0.97	24.17 ± 0.92	20.35 ± 1.17	19.95 ± 1.04
Left Eye	24.11 ± 0.94	23.97 ± 0.81	20.47 ± 1.02	20.11 ± 1.04
All Eyes	24.08 ± 0.94	24.06 ± 0.80	20.41 ± 1.09	20.03 ± 1.04

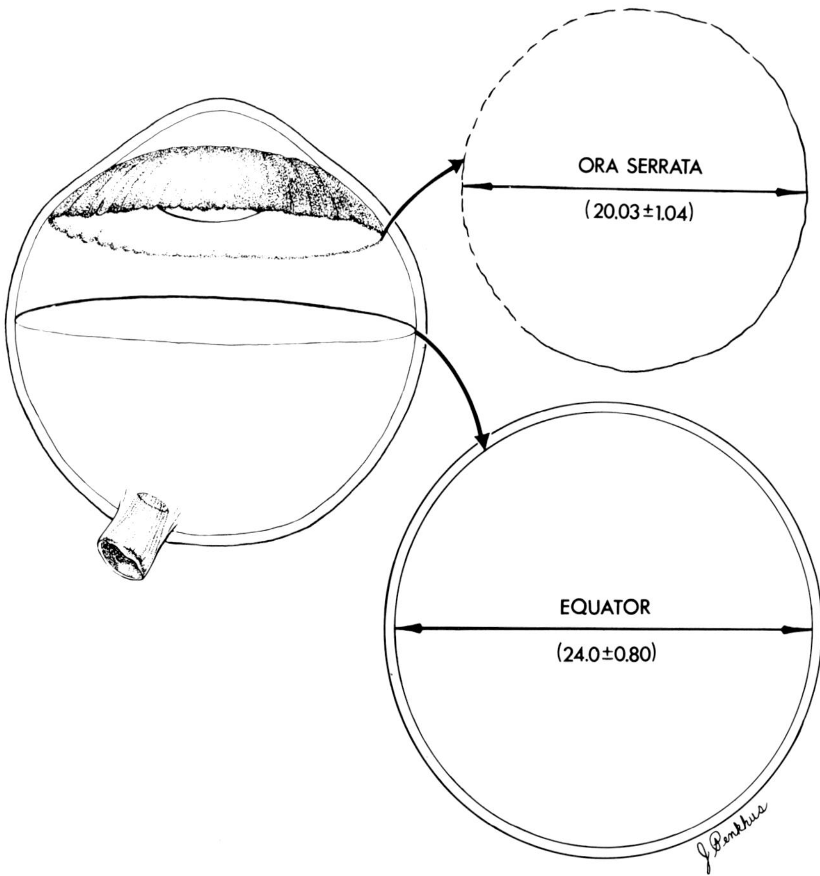

Figure 175. In shape, the retina resembles a cup that is expanded to its greatest diameter at the equator and is considerably reduced in diameter at its serrated anterior margin. Measurements and standard deviations in millimeters.

In the retina and the closely related optic disk, three areas assume particular topographic significance. Consequently, these areas—the optic disk, the foveola, and the ora serrata—were statistically evaluated.

The optic disk had an average vertical diameter of 1.86 ± 0.21 mm and an average horizontal diameter of 1.75 ± 0.19 mm (Table 17). Interestingly, the disk was round (i.e., the vertical and horizontal diameters were equal) in 56 eyes;

TABLE 17

DIAMETERS OF THE OPTIC DISK

	Vertical	Horizontal
Right Eyes	1.85 ± 0.19	1.73 ± 0.19
Left Eyes	1.88 ± 0.21	1.76 ± 0.18
All Eyes	1.86 ± 0.21	1.75 ± 0.19

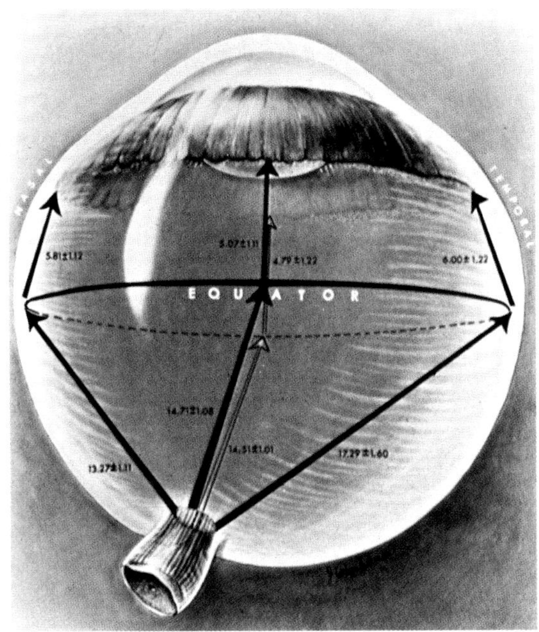

Figure 174. Average measurements from the disk margin to the equator and from the equator to the ora serrata in four principal meridians for 200 adult human eyes. Measurements and standard deviations in millimeters.

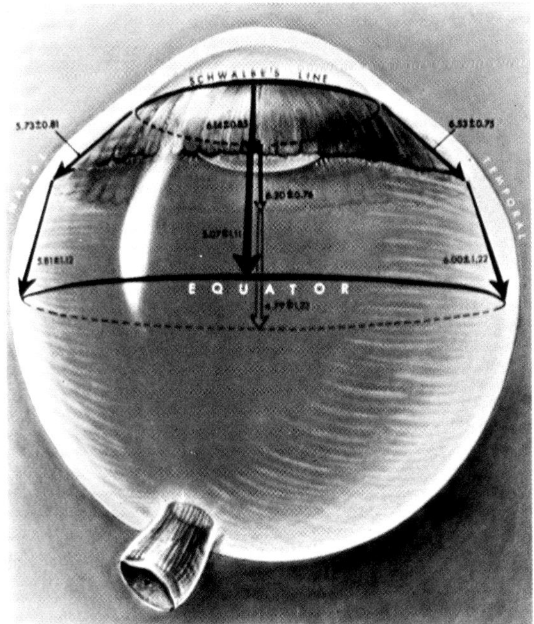

Figure 177. Diagram of the relationship of the ora serrata to Schwalbe's line and to the equator in 200 adult human eyes. Average measurements and standard deviations for the four principal meridians in millimeters.

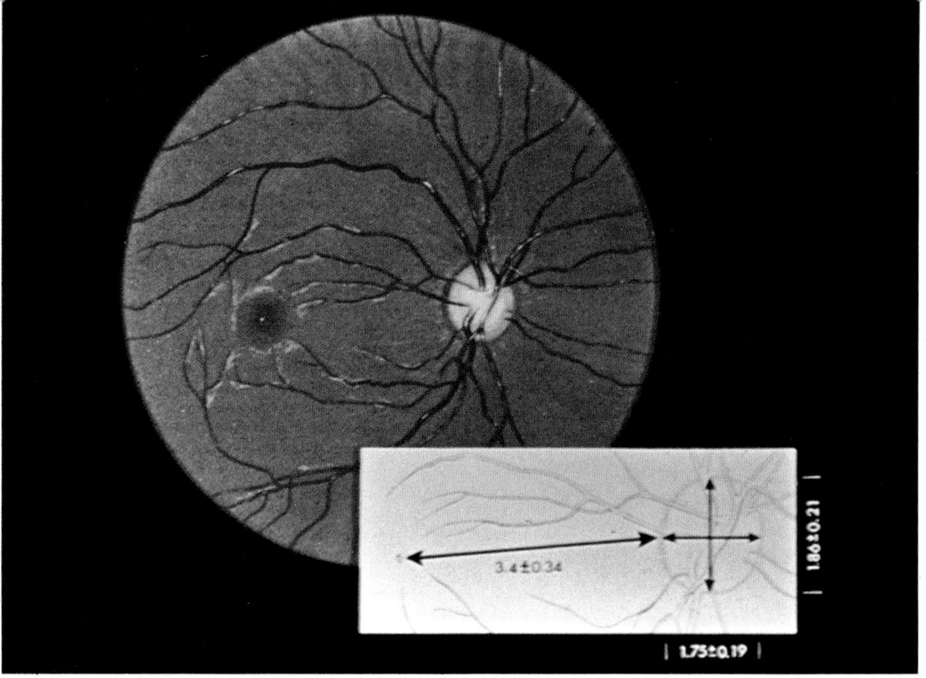

Figure 176. Average dimensions of the optic disk and the relationship between the disk and foveola in 200 adult human eyes. Measurements and standard deviations in millimeters. (From Penkhus, 30.)

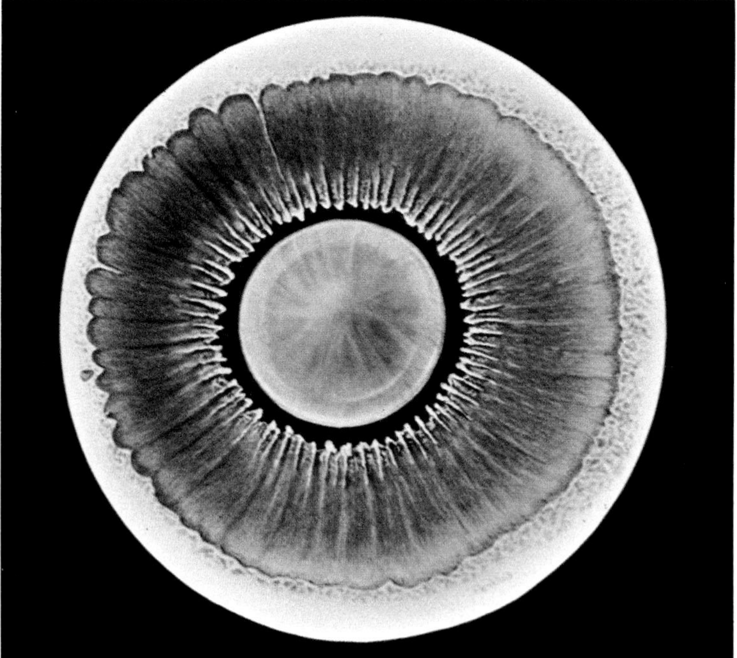

Figure 178. Composite scale drawing of the right eye, depicting the peripheral retina, the ora serrata and the anterior ocular tissues as viewed from the posterior aspect. The lens is shown in its characteristically slightly eccentric position within the circle formed by the ciliary processes. There are approximately 70 ciliary processes which blend with the relatively smooth and striated pars plana. The overall anteroposterior extent of the ciliary body is least nasally, greater superiorly and inferiorly, and greatest temporally. The ciliary body merges with the ora serrata. The ora serrata is irregularly scalloped with variations in contour that are more pronounced nasally than temporally. Dentate processes extend anterior to the main contour of the ora serrata, and ora bays extend posterior to the main contour. In addition to the rather common dentate processes and ora bays, this illustration portrays a large dentate process in the 10:00 o'clock meridian, a giant dentate process in the 11:00 o'clock meridian, a retinal tag projecting from the margin of an ora bay in the 10:30 o'clock meridian and an enclosed ora bay in the 9:00 o'clock meridian.

The disk was somewhat oval with the long axis vertical in 120 eyes and somewhat oval with the long axis horizontal in only 24 eyes.

The center of the fovea (i.e., the foveola) was located temporal to the optic disk and slightly inferior to the horizontal diameter of the disk. From the horizontal meridian of the temporal disk margin to the foveola the average dimension, measured as a chord, for all eyes of the series was 3.42 ± 0.34 mm (Table 18). The average dimensions of the optic disk and the relationship between the disk and the foveola are depicted in Figure 176.

TABLE 18

DIMENSIONS FROM THE OPTIC DISK TO THE FOVEOLA
(Chord measurements)

Right Eyes	3.45 ± 0.35
Left Eyes	3.38 ± 0.34
All Eyes	3.42 ± 0.34

The ora serrata received particular attention in this study because of its importance, the lack of quantitative information in the literature, and its morphologic variations. This anterior limit of the retina was located anterior to the equator and, as previously noted in Table 15, the distance from the equator to the ora serrata was 5.07 ± 1.11 mm in the superior meridian, 4.79 ± 1.22 mm inferiorly, 5.81 ± 1.12 mm nasally, and 6.00 ± 1.22 mm temporally. Furthermore, the distance from the ora serrata to Schwalbe's line, which constitutes the posterior border of the limbus, was 6.14 ± 0.85 mm superiorly, 6.20 ± 0.76 mm inferiorly, 5.73 ± 0.81 mm nasally, and 6.53 ± 0.75 mm temporally (Table 19). On the basis of these measurements, the relationships of the ora serrata to the equator and to Schwalbe's line are illustrated in Figure 177.

TABLE 19

DIMENSIONS FROM THE ORA SERRATA TO SCHWALBE'S LINE

	Superior	Inferior	Nasal	Temporal
Right Eyes	5.97 ± 0.88	6.12 ± 0.75	5.65 ± 0.76	6.47 ± 0.78
Left Eyes	6.30 ± 0.80	6.27 ± 0.76	5.80 ± 0.84	6.60 ± 0.71
All Eyes	6.14 ± 0.85	6.20 ± 0.76	5.73 ± 0.81	6.53 ± 0.75

This relationship of the ora serrata to structures in the anterior segment of the eye can be further appreciated by viewing the peripheral retina, ora serrata, and anterior ocular tissues as they appear from the posterior aspect (Figure 178). Illustrated in a composite scale drawing depicting the right eye, the lens is shown in its characteristic, slightly eccentric position within the circle formed by the ciliary processes. There are approximately 70 ciliary processes which blend with the relatively smooth and striated pars plana. The overall anteroposterior extent of the ciliary body is least on the nasal aspect of the eye, greater superiorly and inferiorly, and greatest temporally. The ciliary body merges abruptly with the ora serrata.

In general configuration, the ora serrata was irregularly scalloped (Figure 178). Irregularities in contour of the ora serrata were more pronounced nasally than temporally, and the overall contour presented marked fluctuations and extreme variations. Dentate or tooth-like processes extended anteriorly to the main contour of this border, and bays or indentations extended posteriorly to the main contour of the ora serrata. At the ora serrata, projections of the retina toward the vitreous body were termed meridional folds or retinal tags. Significant variations, degenerations, and other abnormalities beyond the scope of this study were often present in the adjacent retina, choroid, ciliary body, and vitreous.

For topographic evaluation, definite although obviously somewhat arbitrary classification of the morphologic features of the ora serrata was necessary. Therefore, to ensure appropriate categorization of these characteristics, the following definitions and criteria for classification were employed in this study.

Dentate process: An anterior extension of the retina that projects from 0.5 to 2.5 mm anterior to the adjacent retina on both sides. To be distinguished from a fluctuation in the contour of the ora, this projection must occur in a circumferential (i.e., parallel to the ora serrata) distance of 1.0 mm or less (Figure 179A).

Large dentate process: An anterior extension of the retina that projects onto the pars plana of the ciliary body more than 2.5 mm anterior to the adjacent retina on both sides (Figure 179B).

Giant dentate process: An anterior extension of the retina that projects to or onto the pars plicata of the ciliary body and is markedly anterior to the retina on each side (Figure 179C).

Meridional fold: A ridge-like projection of the retina toward the vitreous body that is located at and perpendicular to the ora serrata (Figure 179D). Immediately posterior to some meridional folds there is a localized retinal abnormality, usually an area of retinal thinning (Figure 179E).

Ora bay: A posterior indentation in the retina that extends from 0.5 mm to 2.5 mm posterior to the adjacent retina on both sides. To be distinguished from a fluctuation in the contour of the ora, this indentation must occur in a circumferential distance of 2.0 mm or less (Figure 179F).

Large ora bay: A posterior indentation in the retina that extends more than 2.5 mm posterior to the adjacent retina on both sides (Figure 179G).

Partially enclosed ora bay: A posterior indentation in the retina that extends more than 0.5 mm posterior to the adjacent retina on both sides and has a width anteriorly that is less than half its maximum width posteriorly.

Enclosed ora bay: A posterior indentation in the retina that is completely separated from the pars plana anteriorly by retinal tissue (Figure 179H).

Doubled ora bay: A posterior indentation in the retina that extends from 0.5 to 2.5 mm posterior to the adjacent retina on both sides; it is divided by an abbreviated anterior extension of the retina that projects less than 0.5 mm. The entire doubled bay must occur within a circumferential distance of 4.0 mm or less (Figure 179I).

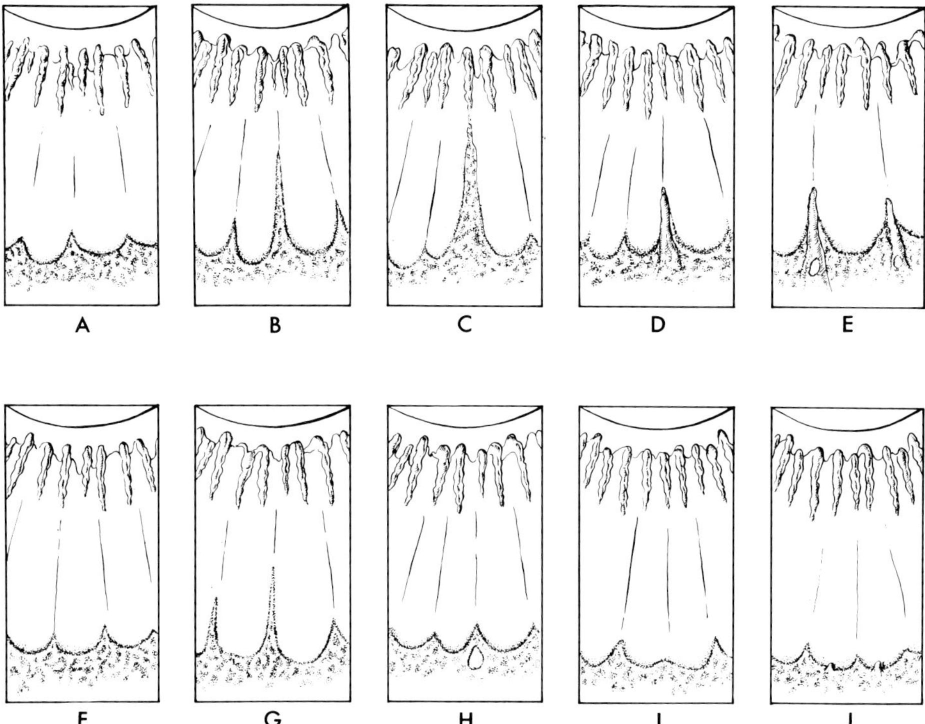

Figure 179. Schematic scale drawings of morphologic features of the ora serrata. *A:* Dentate process; *B:* large dentate process; *C:* giant dentate process; *D:* meridional fold; *E:* meridional fold with localized posterior retinal defect; *F:* ora bay; *G:* large ora bay; *H:* enclosed ora bay; *I:* doubled ora bay; *J:* retinal tag in an ora bay. See text.

Retinal tag in an ora bay: A projection of the retina which originates at the posterior margin of an ora bay and extends anterior to and internal to the immediately adjacent retina (Figure 179J).

A tabulation of these morphologic features was made for each 30-degree sector or "clock hour" of the 200 eyes in the study. Recorded according to clinical convention, which views the ora serrata from its anterior aspect, and arranged so that corresponding quadrants of the right and left eye, such as the superior nasal quadrants, are superimposed, the results of this analysis are listed in Table 20.

In overall incidence, the most common morphologic features of the ora serrata were the dentate processes and the ora bays (Table 20). Generally less common were doubled ora bays, retinal tags in ora bays, giant dentate processes, meridional folds, large dentate processes, and large ora bays. Least common were the meridional folds with posterior anomalies, enclosed ora bays, and partly enclosed ora bays.

An analysis of distribution demonstrated that dentate processes (Figure 180) and ora bays (Figure 181) were significantly most frequent in the superior nasal quadrant, less frequent in the inferior nasal quadrant, even less frequent in the superior temporal quadrant, and least frequent in the inferior temporal quadrant.

TABLE 20

TOPOGRAPHIC FEATURES OF THE ORA SERRATA

200 Eyes		Superior Nasal Quadrant			Inferior Nasal Quadrant			Inferior Temporal Quadrant			Superior Temporal Quadrant			
98	O.D.	12–1	1–2	2–3	3–4	4–5	5–6	6–7	7–8	8–9	9–10	10–11	11–12	Total in
102	O.S.	11–12	10–11	9–10	8–9	7–8	6–7	5–6	4–5	3–4	2–3	1–2	12–1	200 Eyes
Dentate Processes	O.D.	152	157	202	198	167	86	15	18	50	74	70	104	2573
	O.S.	159	174	191	213	181	82	13	20	31	55	70	91	
Large Dentate Processes	O.D.	2	6	4	8	–	–	–	–	1	1	3	–	64
	O.S.	–	3	11	13	1	–	2	1	–	4	3	1	
Giant Dentate Processes	O.D.	2	2	12	9	–	–	–	3	2	5	2	7	109
	O.S.	10	8	17	9	4	2	–	–	2	5	3	5	
Meridional Folds	O.D.	–	12	17	3	6	1	–	1	1	4	1	1	80
	O.S.	1	6	14	7	1	–	1	–	–	2	1	–	
Meridional Folds with Posterior Retinal Abnormalities	O.D.	–	1	2	3	–	–	–	–	–	–	1	1	25
	O.S.	2	4	6	3	–	–	–	–	1	1	–	–	
Ora Bays	O.D.	127	129	149	166	137	58	6	13	36	52	61	76	2037
	O.S.	123	132	173	210	140	48	15	12	22	32	53	67	
Large Ora Bays	O.D.	1	4	7	4	–	–	–	2	1	5	1	4	63
	O.S.	3	3	7	7	3	–	1	1	–	5	2	2	
Bays Partly Enclosed	O.D.	–	–	2	1	–	–	–	–	–	1	–	–	10
	O.S.	–	–	–	–	–	–	–	–	1	3	1	1	
Bays Completely Enclosed	O.D.	1	1	2	3	–	–	–	–	–	2	1	–	16
	O.S.	1	2	2	–	–	–	–	–	1	–	–	–	
Doubled Ora Bays	O.D.	6	15	21	10	6	7	1	–	2	9	4	9	185
	O.S.	16	23	19	12	4	4	3	1	3	7	2	1	
Retinal Tags in Ora Bays	O.D.	4	15	34	13	7	5	1	–	2	3	–	2	174
	O.S.	6	15	25	21	5	6	–	1	2	6	–	1	

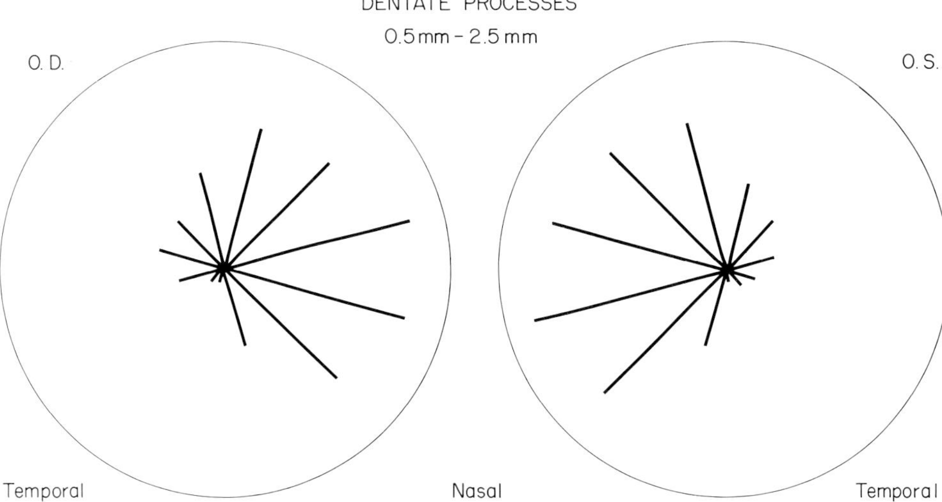

Figure 180. The meridional incidence of dentate processes in 200 adult human eyes.

Moreover, a statistical regression pattern established that the peak incidence of dentate processes and ora bays was in the superior nasal quadrant and within one clock hour of the horizontal meridian (i.e., between 2:00 and 3:00 o'clock in the right eye and between 9:00 and 10:00 o'clock in the left eye). From this point, progression clockwise or counterclockwise was associated with a decreasing incidence of processes and bays.

Other topographical features of the ora serrata were, as previously noted, encountered far less frequently than the dentate processes and ora bays (Table 20). From the standpoint of distribution, these less frequent processes, bays, folds,

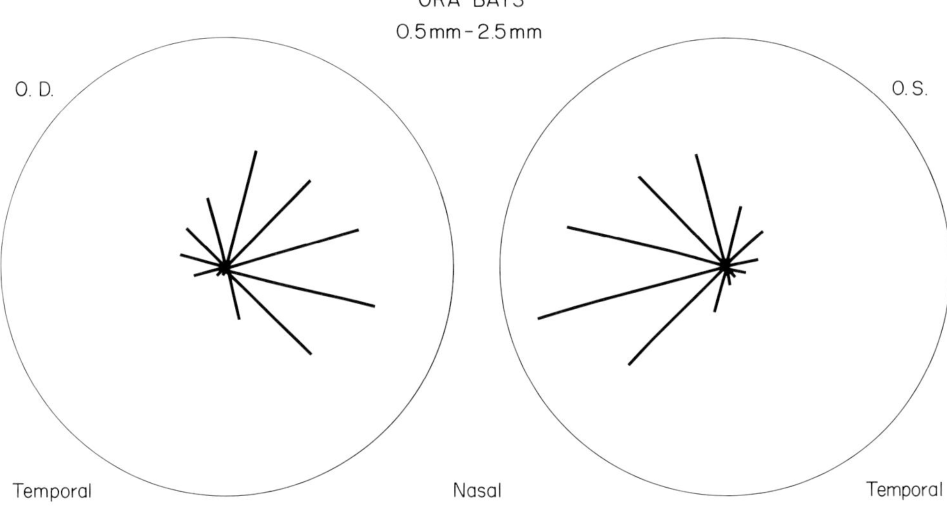

Figure 181. The meridional incidence of ora bays in 200 adult human eyes.

and tags were as a group most common in the superior nasal quadrant, and present in decreasing frequency in the inferior nasal, superior temporal, and inferior temporal quadrants.

Thus, the overall topography of the ora serrata is characterized by the highest incidence of processes and bays in the superior nasal quadrant, and a progressively smaller incidence of these features in the inferior nasal, the superior temporal, and the inferior temporal quadrants. This pattern is remarkably consistent, but it should be emphasized that marked variations in the contour of the ora were encountered. In some eyes, the ora serrata was extremely irregular and in others it was remarkably smooth. Both eyes of 17 cases were examined and, not unexpectedly, these cases demonstrated a general symmetry in the configuration of the ora in the two eyes.

To correlate gross topographic features of the ora serrata with microscopic findings, serial or step sections of representative areas were made. Dentate processes that projected from 0.5 to 2.5 mm anterior to the adjacent retina often demonstrated a slight thinning of the retina, a rather broad area of firm attachment between retina and pigment epithelium, and a pronounced degree of peripheral cystoid degeneration (Figure 182).

Dentate processes of large or giant size obviously extended for an appreciable distance onto the ciliary body. Microscopic serial sections reflected this change in retinal contour and demonstrated a large area of retinal union with the pigment epithelium in the anterior portion of the process. In addition, the retina usually became progressively thinner as it approached its anterior termination, and the process generally presented an advanced degree of cystoid change and general retinal degeneration (Figure 183).

In association with dentate processes, particularly those of large or giant size, a meridional fold was not uncommon. This projection of the inner surface of the retina toward the vitreous was related to an increase in the thickness of the degenerated and cystoid retina (Figure 184). As an extension of this degeneration, there often was an area of retinal thinning at the posterior extremity of the meridional fold. Occasionally, this abnormality was severe enough to interrupt the continuity of the retina and a through-and-through retinal hole occurred at this site (Figure 185).

In contrast to the retinal thickening and localized accentuation of retinal degeneration in the dentate process, sectors of relatively smooth ora, devoid of dentate processes or ora bays, usually were characterized by an abrupt termination of the retina, a localized firm attachment of the retina to the pigment epithelium, and variable cystoid degeneration of the peripheral retina (Figure 186). The retina corresponding to an ora bay usually terminated abruptly as well, unless a retinal tag was present, and the degree of retinal degeneration was comparable to adjacent areas (Figure 187). This microscopic pattern was also consistently observed in large and doubled ora bays. Enclosed ora bays were confirmed by microscopic sections, which demonstrated an island of pars plana epithelium completely surrounded by extensions of the sensory retina. Significant abnormalities in the retina bordering an enclosed bay were not usually present,

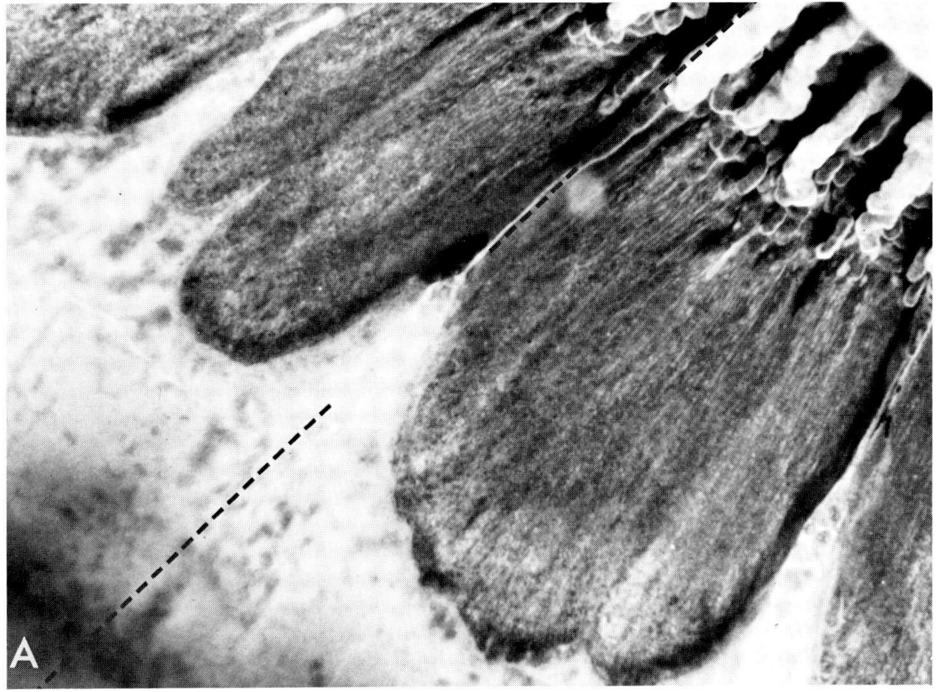

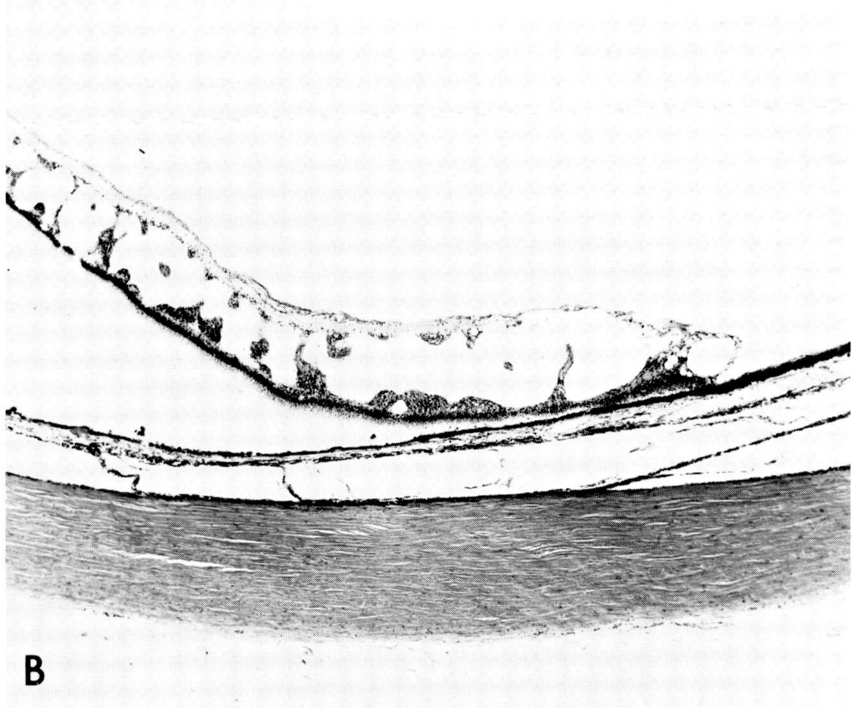

Figure 182. *A:* Gross appearance of dentate process is triangular or awl-shaped; dotted line indicates site depicted in B. *B:* Microscopically, the retina in this process is somewhat thinned, markedly degenerated, and firmly attached to the pigment epithelium; $\times 35$.

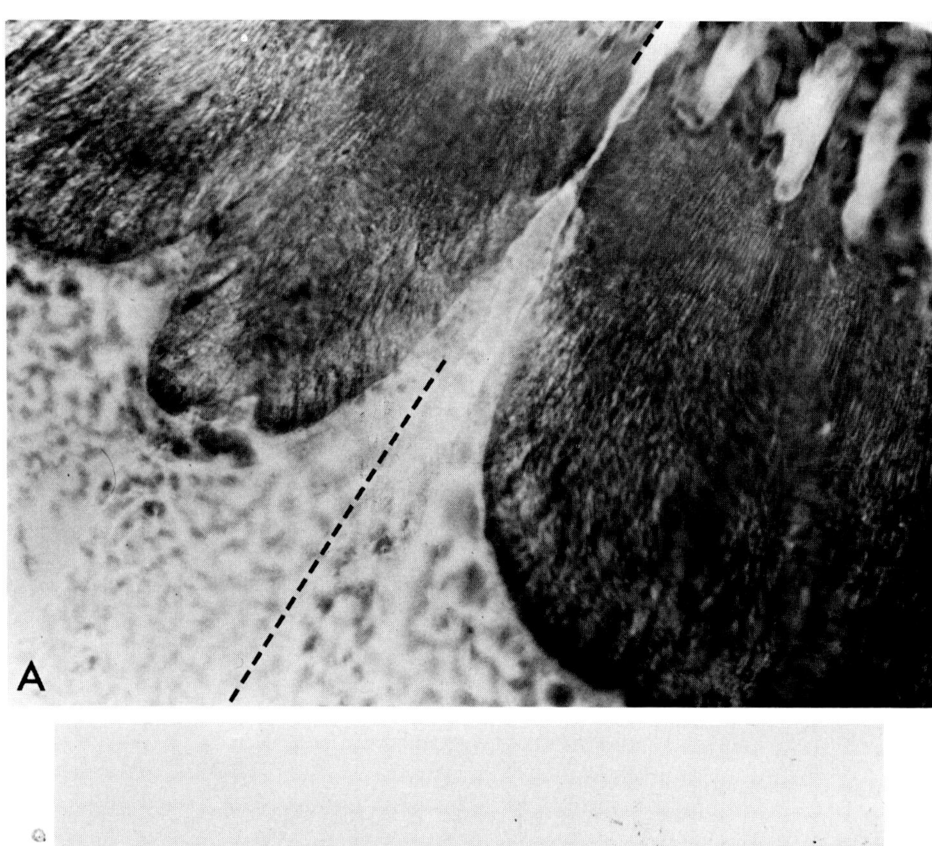

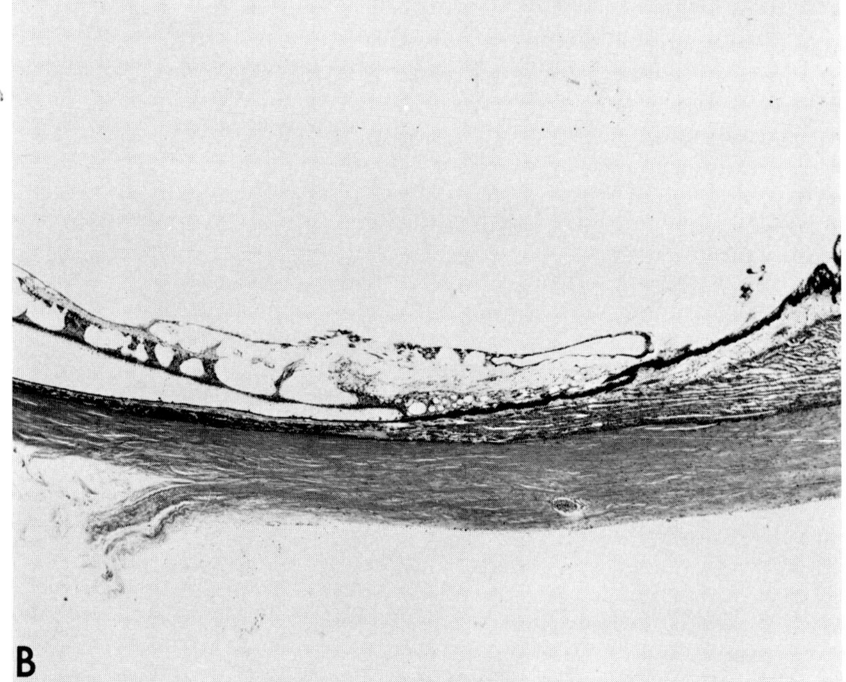

Figure 183. *A:* Large or giant dentate process extending onto the ciliary body for an appreciable distance; dotted line indicates site depicted in B. *B:* Microscopic features of this process include mild thinning of the retina, an advanced degree of cystoid degeneration, and a broad attachment between retina and the adjacent pigment epithelium; ×25.

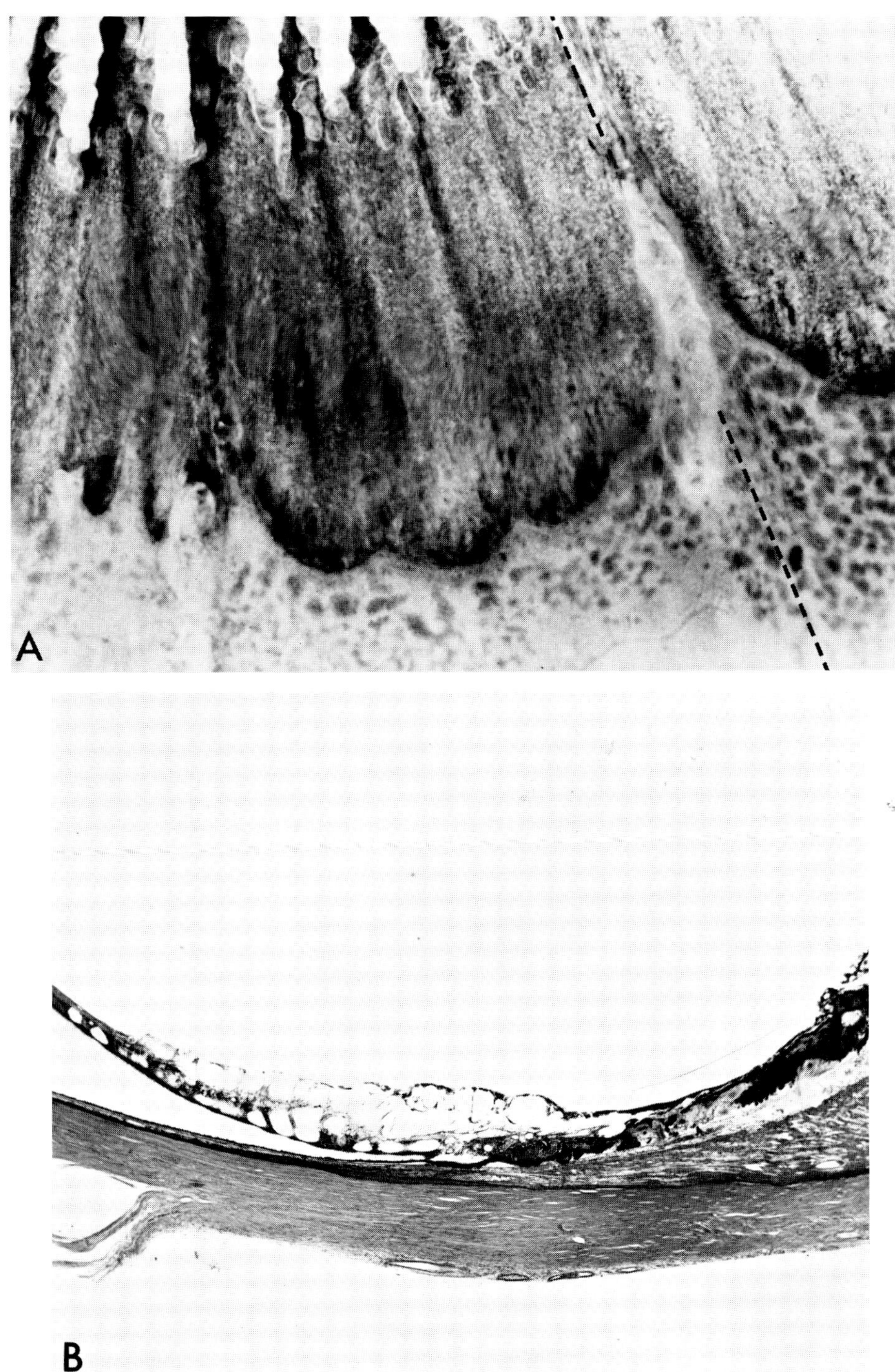

Figure 184. *A:* A meridional fold associated with this large dentate process; dotted line indicates site depicted in B. *B:* Microscopically, this projection of the inner surface of the retina toward the vitreous is related to an increase in the thickness of the degenerated and cystoid retina; ×25.

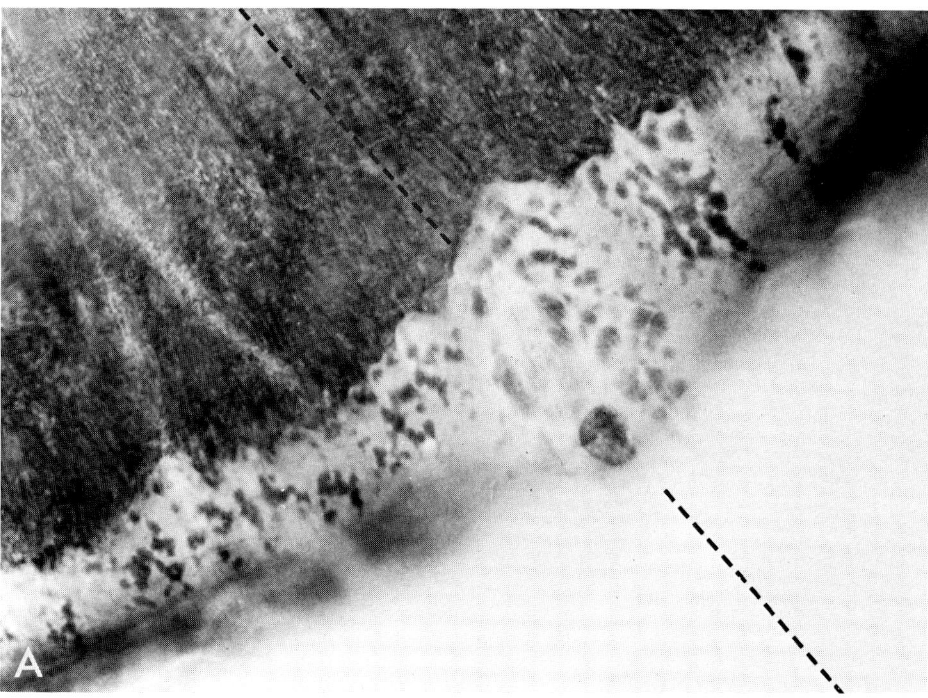

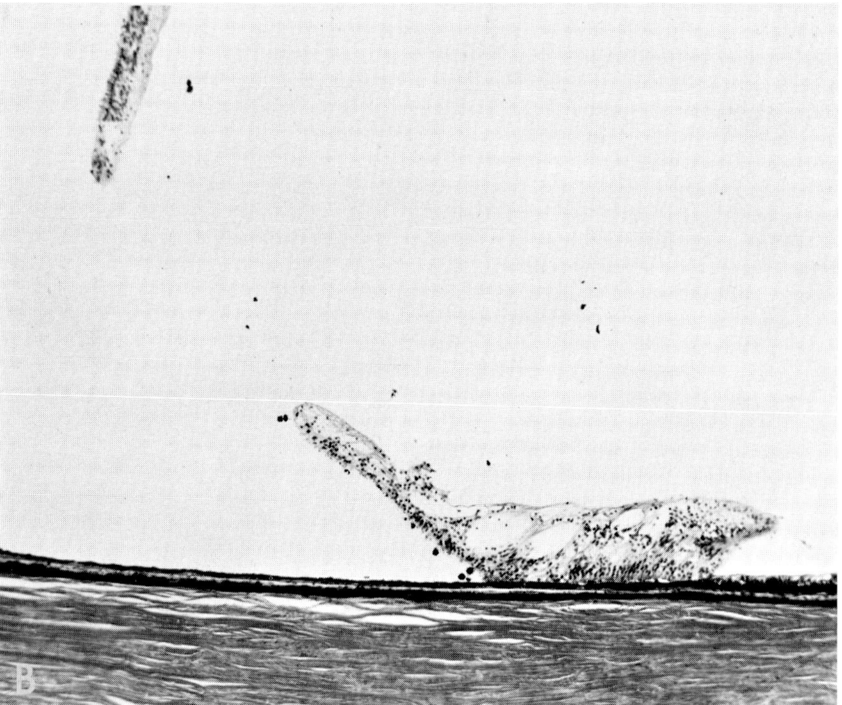

Figure 185. *A:* Definite retinal abnormality at the posterior extremity of this meridional fold; dotted line indicates site depicted in B. *B:* Histologic study of this abnormality reveals a thru-and-thru retinal break; $\times 75$.

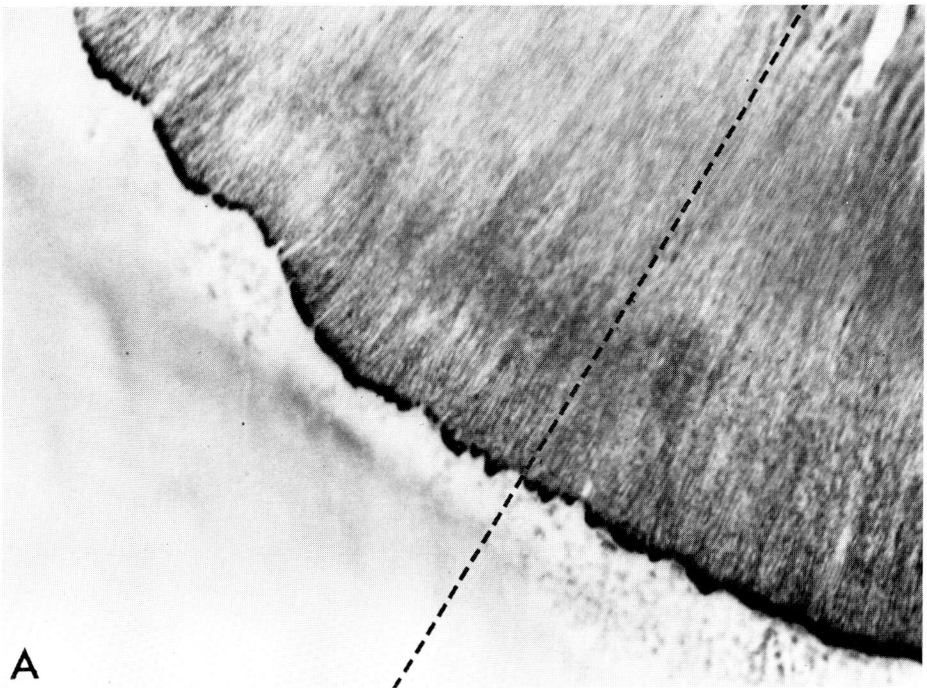

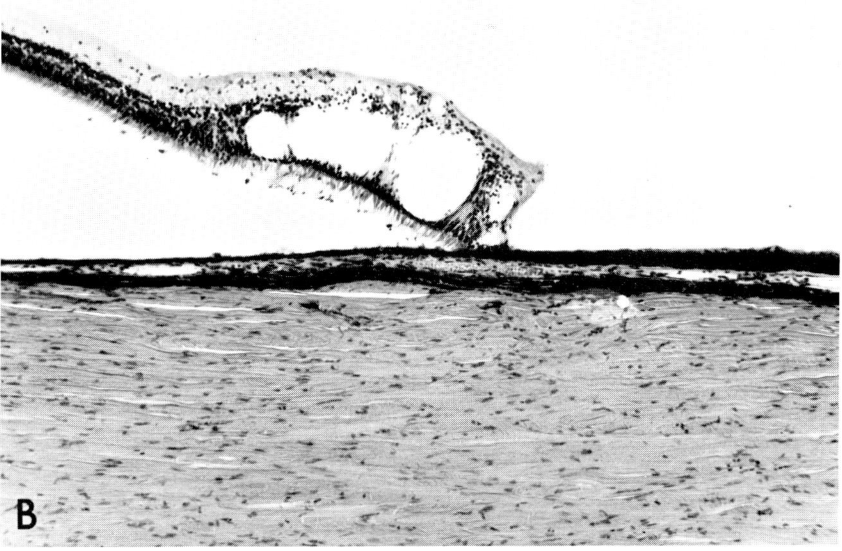

Figure 186. *A:* A sector of smooth ora serrata from the inferior temporal quadrant; dotted line indicates site depicted in B. *B:* Microscopically, this area is characterized by an abrupt termination of the retina, mild cystoid degeneration, and a localized firm attachment of the retina to the pigment epithelium; × 75.

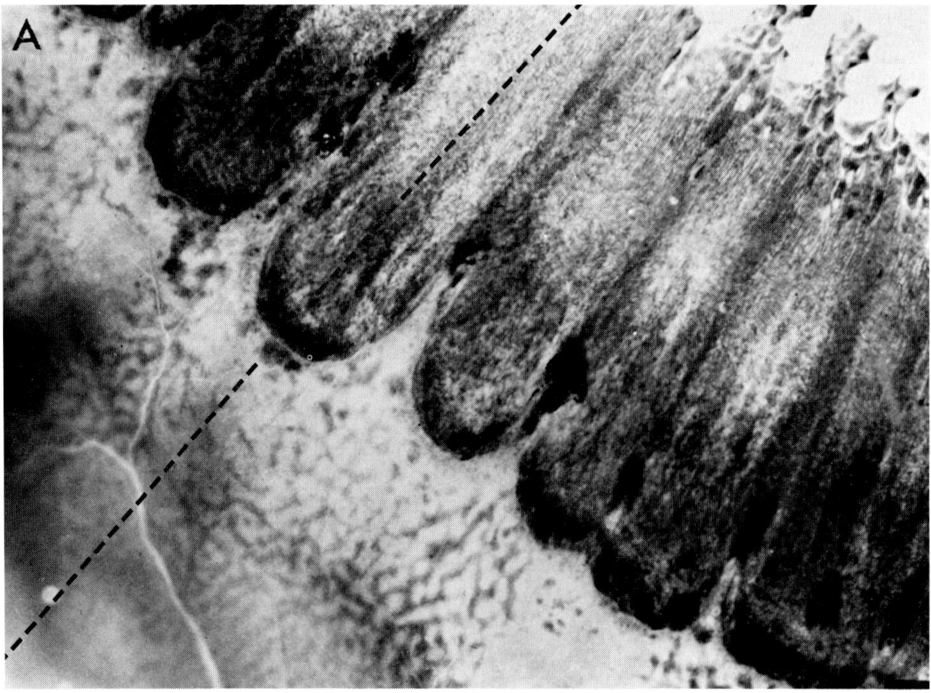

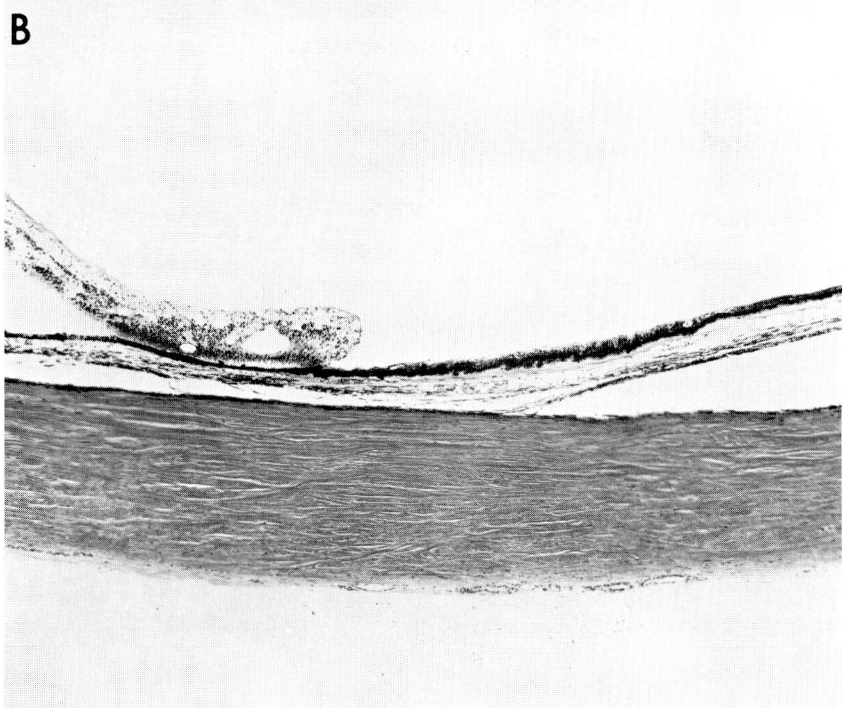

Figure 187. *A:* Several ora bays present in this sector of the retina; dotted line indicates site depicted in B. *B:* Microscopically, the retina demonstrates an abrupt termination and only mild cystoid retinal degeneration.

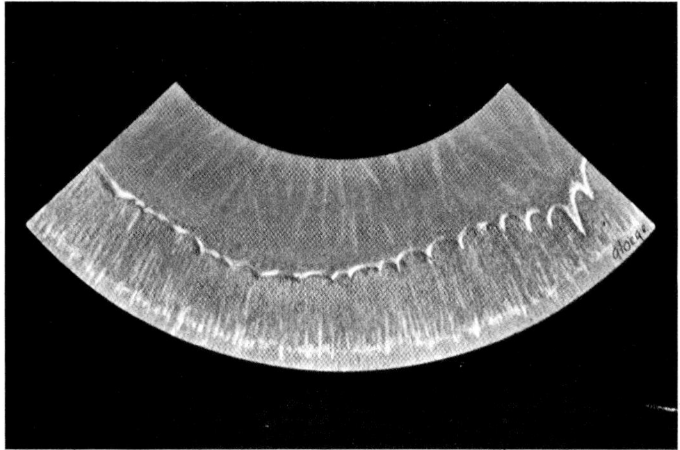

Figure 189. Sector of the ora serrata and adjacent structures, visualized clinically. The prominent dentate processes in the inferior nasal sector contrast markedly with the relatively smooth ora serrata in the inferior temporal sector.

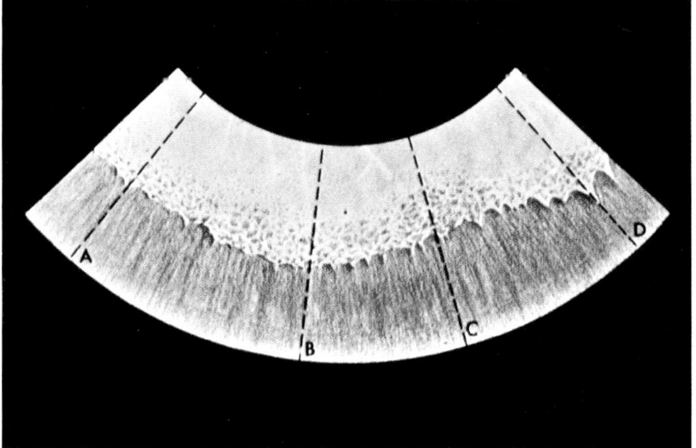

Figure 190. Sector of ora serrata portrayed in Figure 189, drawn after enucleation and fixation of the eye. Contour is unaltered, but the retina is grayish white in color. Microscopic sections were obtained through the ora serrata at *A*, *B*, *C*, and *D* (see Figure 191).

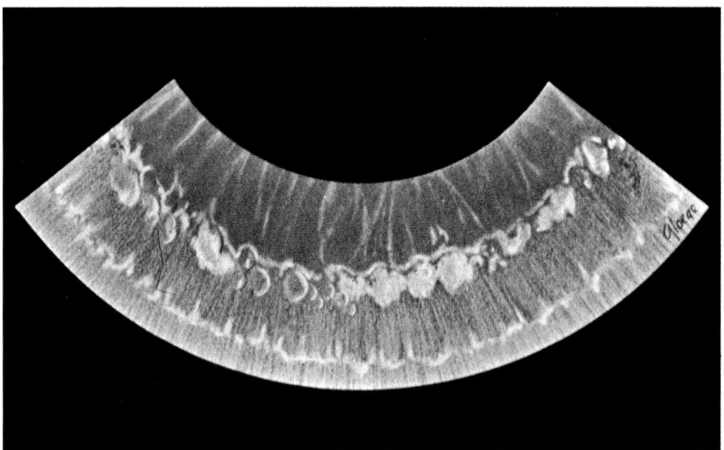

Figure 192. Inferior temporal sector of the ora serrata and adjacent structures, visualized clinically. Retinal cystoid degeneration, numerous pars plana cysts, and the anterior margin of the vitreous base were noted.

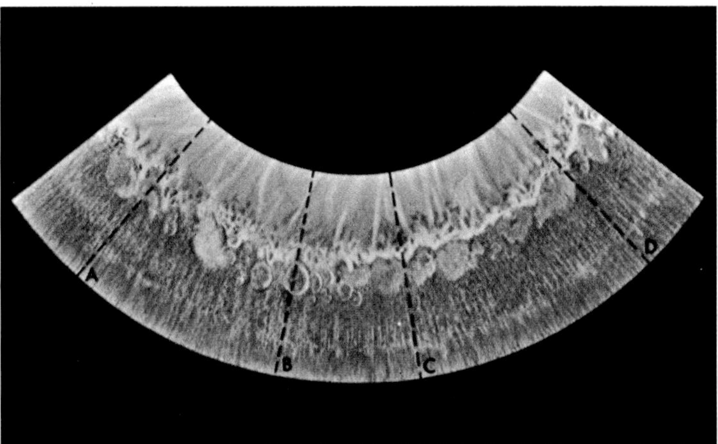

Figure 193. Opacification of the retina and general mild color change after enucleation and fixation of the eye, (compare with Figure 192). Microscopic sections were prepared at *A*, *B*, *C*, and *D* (Figure 194).

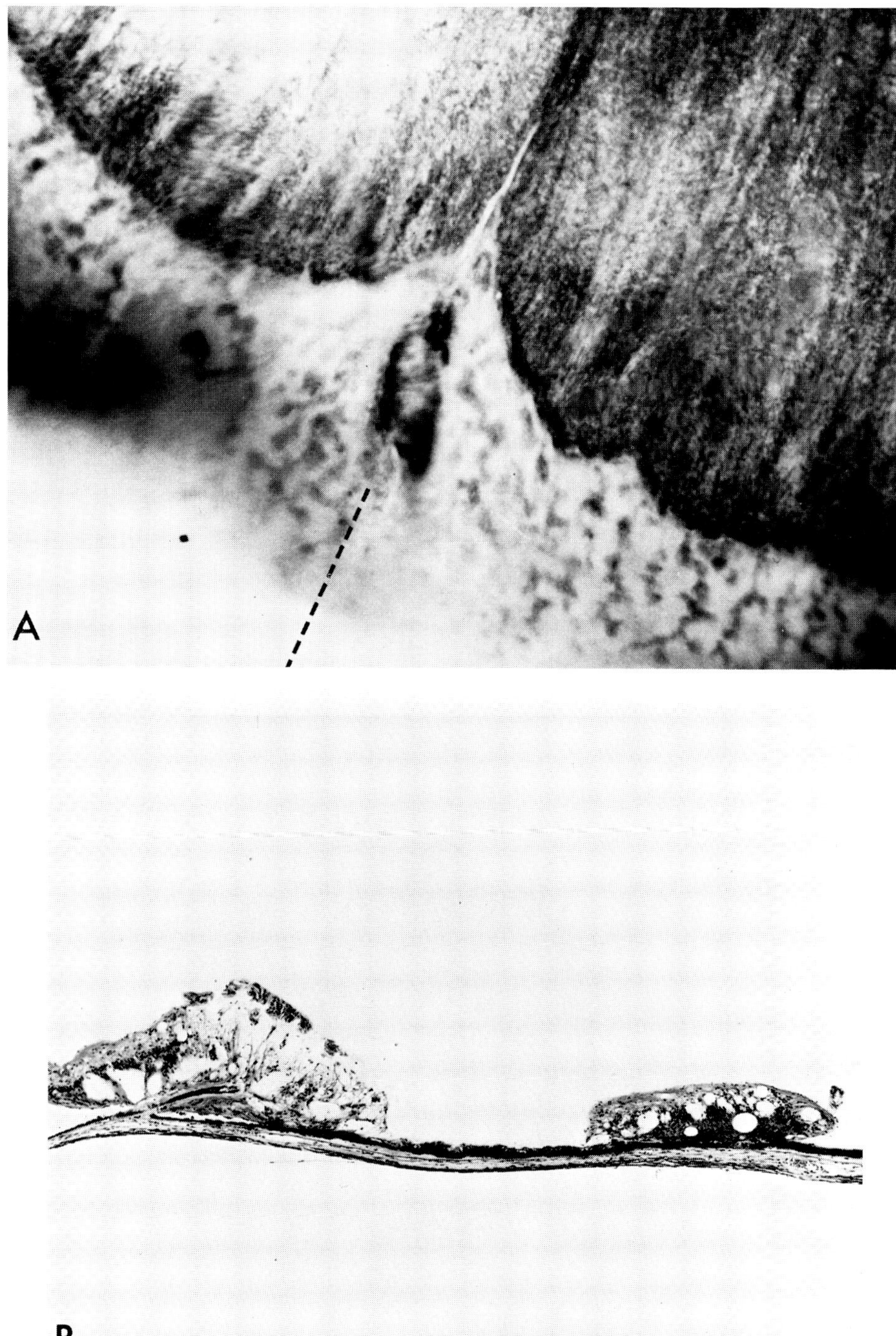

Figure 188. *A:* An enclosed ora bay; dotted line indicates area depicted in B. *B:* A section through this bay demonstrates ciliary body epithelium in the area corresponding to the enclosed bay; the adjacent posterior retina presents degeneration and proliferation of the pigment epithelium; ×45.

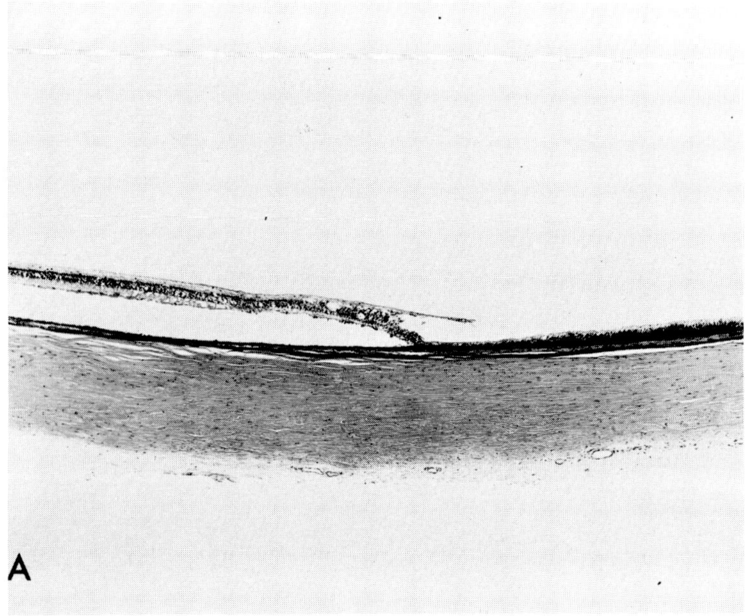

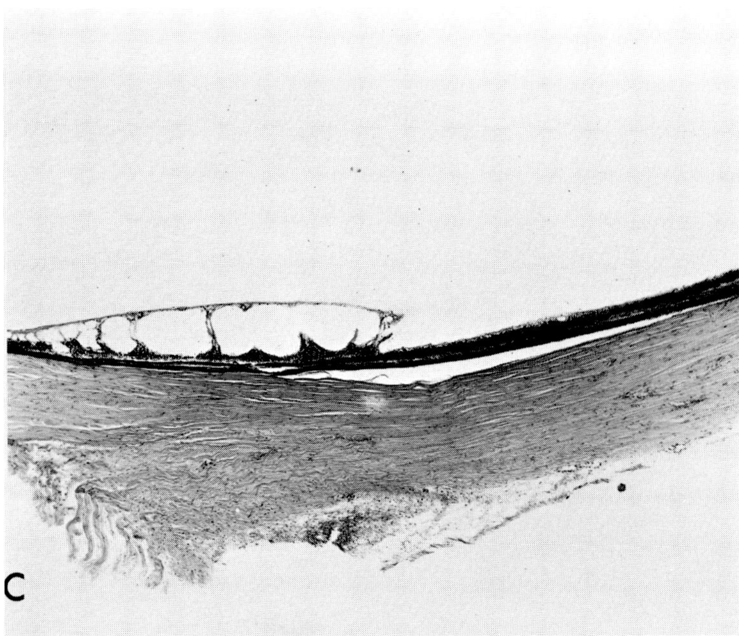

Figure 191. *A, B, C, D:* Corresponding to the lines of section noted in Figure 190, microscopic sections prepared and photographed at ×35.

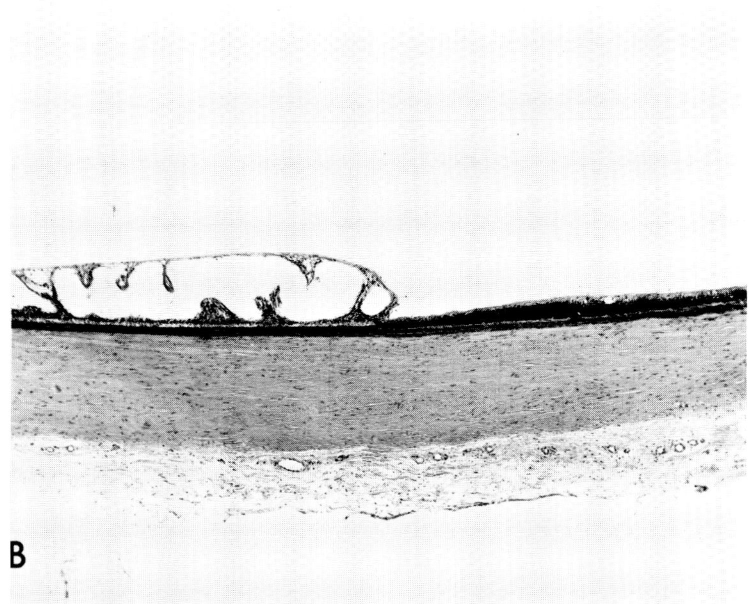

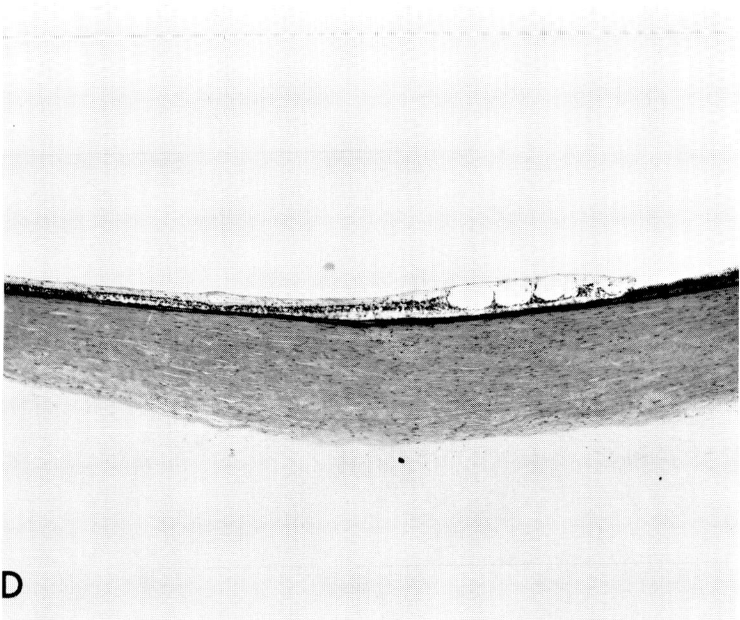

magnification. *A* is of interest because it demonstrates the not uncommon extension of a thin strand of tissue anterior to a prominence of the ora serrata, which probably indicates traction at this site.

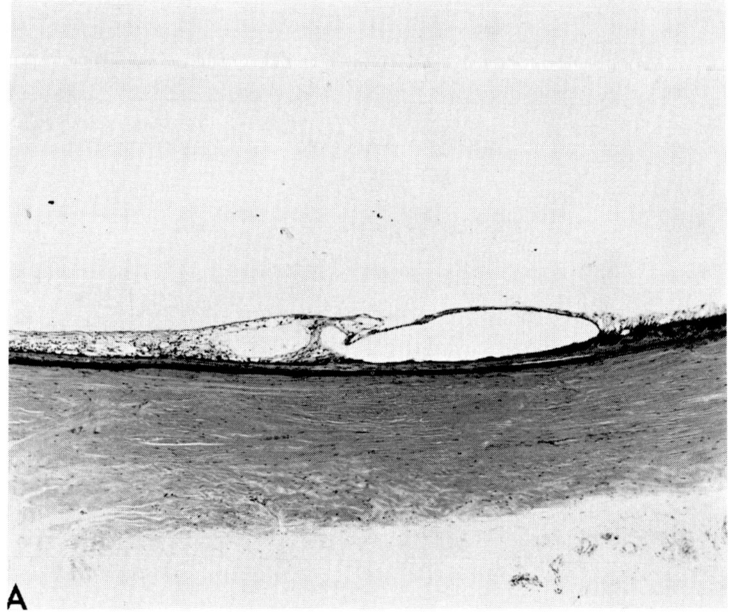

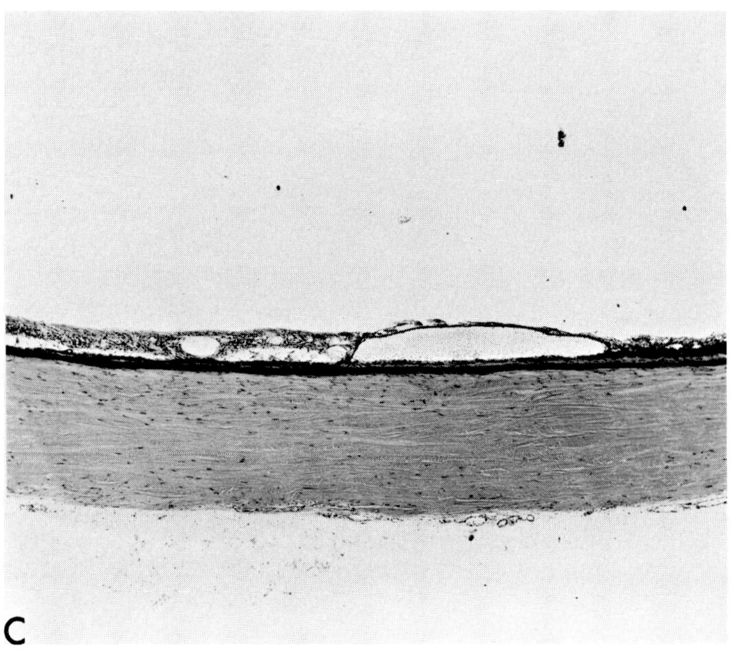

Figure 194. *A, B, C, D:* Sections prepared through the corresponding areas shown in Figure 193; ×39.

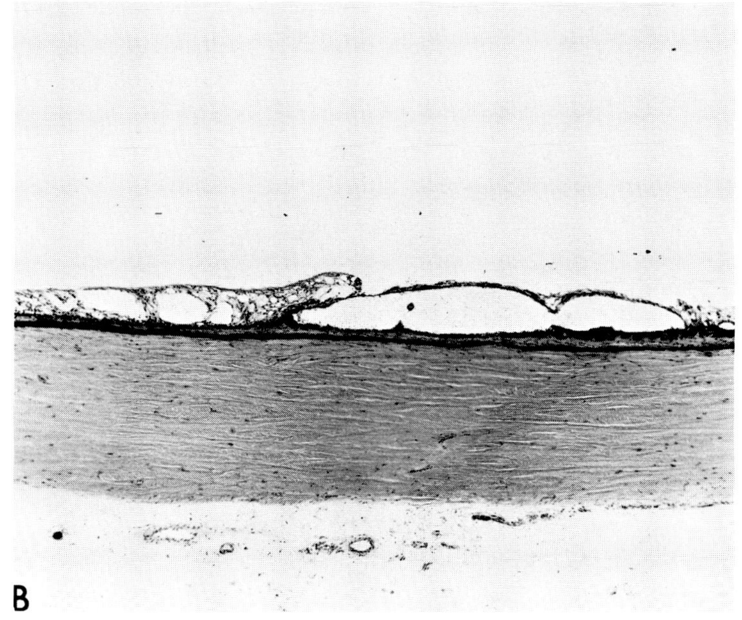
B

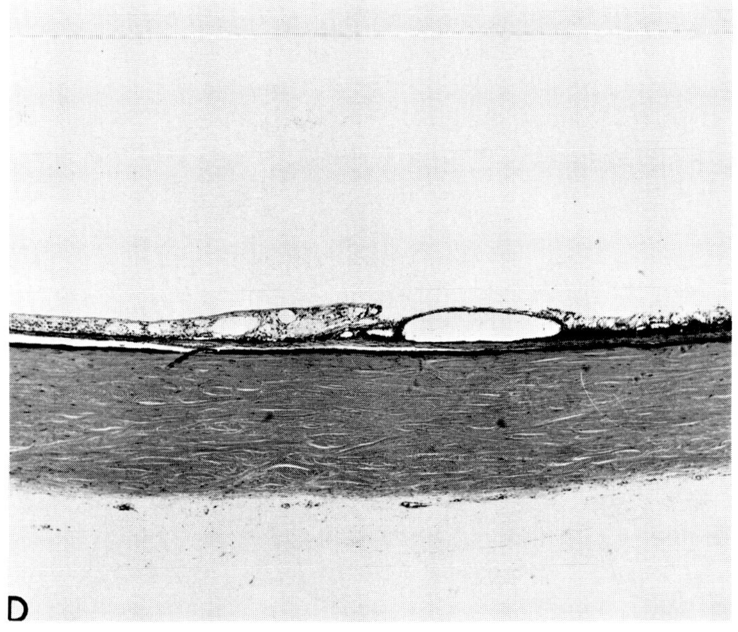
D

but occasionally pronounced retinal degeneration and even proliferation of the contiguous pigment epithelium were evident (Figure 188).

Representative Cases

A direct correlation between clinical observations and tissue findings was achieved in a select group of eyes. Two cases illustrate this correlation as it pertains to the ora serrata.

Case 1 (B.G.). A 40-year-old Caucasian woman, referred with a history of decreased vision in the right eye for one year. Ocular, general, and family history revealed no other pertinent findings. General examination revealed no significant abnormalities.

Upon ocular examination, positive pertinent findings were confined to the right eye. Visual acuity in this eye was 20/30 with +3.25 +1.75 × 72. The visual field was essentially intact, the iris was dark brown; a solid pigmented tumor mass projected into the vitreous from the ciliary body. The posterior segment of the eye was essentially unremarkable. A sector of uninvolved ora serrata in the inferonasal and inferotemporal quadrants was diagrammed and drawn (Figure 189).

After enucleation of the eye, pathologic studies established the diagnosis of malignant melanoma of the ciliary body. The clinically evaluated sector of ora serrata was subjected to further examination and again drawn (Figure 190). Morphologic features noted clinically were readily identified during gross examination, although changes in tissue color and transparency associated with death and fixation were clearly evident.

Microscopic sections through representative and preselected portions of the ora serrata revealed the histologic characteristics of the tissue (Figure 191). For example, a section through *A* demonstrated a thin strand of tissue anterior to the ora serrata and suggested traction at this site. Other sections demonstrated variations in retinal cystoid degeneration and changes in contour associated with dentate processes.

Case 2 (A.K.). A 57-year-old Caucasian male, examined with a history of decreased vision in the right eye for about eight years. Six years prior to examination a ciliary body mass and a cataract were noted in this eye. Five years prior to examination a cataract extraction was performed; the intraocular mass had slowly increased in size thereafter. Ocular, general, and family history revealed no other pertinent findings. General examination did not demonstrate any significant abnormalities.

Upon ocular examination, positive pertinent findings were confined to the right eye. Visual acuity in this eye was 20/25 with +11.00 +1.00 × 150. The visual field was moderately restricted, a superior limbal scar was present, a sector iridectomy had been performed in the brown iris, and lens remnants were present. A large, lightly pigmented solid mass, which fluoresced only minimally after intravenous fluorescein, extended into the vitreous from the ciliary body, but the posterior segment demonstrated no abnormality of significance. A sector of uninvolved and clearly visualized ora serrata in the inferior temporal quadrant was diagrammed and drawn (Figure 192). Pathologic studies performed after enucleation indicated a leiomyoma of the ciliary body. Thereafter, the clinically documented sector of ora serrata was again drawn, to reflect the color and appearance in the postmortem state and to serve as a guide for microscopic studies (Figure 193).

The histology of representative preselected sites demonstrated advanced peripheral retinal degeneration and irregularities in the pigment epithelium of both the retina and the ciliary body. Also evident were numerous pars plana cyst (Figure 194).

Analysis

Many aspects of this investigation of retinal topography merit consideration. Recognizing, however, that a primary purpose of this study is to supply information of particular value to the clinician, this discussion will be confined to a review of the changes that alter the postmortem appearance of the retina and to a notation of some of the practical aspects of this topographical appraisal.

To aid the clinician accustomed to evaluate the remarkably transparent sensory retina during life, it is pertinent to note that when death occurs the retinal arteries become very attenuated, the veins assume a darker color and, if the patient is supine, the blood in the veins becomes segmented or beaded within a few seconds after circulation ceases. These beaded segments of venous blood often move slowly toward the disk for several minutes and then become stationary. At the same time, the optic disk turns pale, white and avascular. Within five or ten minutes after death the retina becomes translucent and grayish white. This process continues and the entire retina is white and opaque about an hour after death (12,31).

If the eye is enucleated and sectioned at this stage, the relatively fresh, unfixed, and unstained retina can be examined. Fresh tissue, however, does not maintain its relationships satisfactorily or lend itself to further processing and staining. It is customary, therefore, to fix the specimen as soon as possible after death. In this series, fixation was accomplished with formalin and 50 per cent alcohol; this sequence results in only a minimal change in the measured volume of the eye* and no appreciable alteration in general size, shape, appearance, or relationships.

Macroscopically, in the fixed eye the optic disk is white and usually undistorted, although sectioning of the optic nerve close to the eye can force myelin into the optic nervehead. The boundaries of the disk can be readily identified even though the adjacent retina is white and opaque. In the macular area, the retina is thickened and to some degree distorted in eyes obtained postmortem. Primarily related to an accumulation of fluid in the prominent external plexiform layer, this macular artifact does not discernably alter the peripheral retina, which maintains its distinct white color, form, and relationship until it terminates abruptly at the ora serrata. Without question, the postmortem opacification of

---

* R. Foos, personal communication.

the retina, which contrasts with the retained transparency of the ciliary body epithelium, greatly facilitates the postmortem evaluation of anterior retinal topography.

Viewed as a whole, this study supplies practical information concerning the size and shape of the adult human retina, as well as quantitative data pertaining to the optic disk, foveola and ora serrata. The concept of retinal size and shape derived from this investigation is, of course, influenced by the manner in which the measurements were taken. For example, the similarity between external and internal diameters at the equator (Tables 13 and 16) probably reflects a slight collapse or change in shape in the eye after sectioning of the specimen at the equator. In addition, the measurement of chords rather than arcs affects the information provided by the study, although the difference between chord and arc measurements is rather insignificant for small segments and the overall form of the retina is revealed by the measurements that were obtained. This concept of retinal size and shape (Figures 174–177) is likely to be of value to clinicians and to investigators who almost invariably must conceive of the retina without actually visualizing its structure.

As one facet of this concept, it should be stressed that the retina is considerably smaller in diameter and in circumference at the ora serrata than at the equator (Figure 175). Thus, the conventional charts of the ocular fundus (Figure 195), which depict the ora serrata as having a diameter and circumference greater than the equator, are inaccurate. In essence, these charts should be considered as diagrammatic projections in which the retina anterior to the equator is disproportionately expanded. Stated another way, features of the peripheral retina and ora serrata are actually closer together than they appear to be in the conventional fundus diagram.

Quantitative data on the size and shape of the optic disk and its relationship to the foveola are comparable to other measurements in the wide range cited in the literature (11,31,55). The disk measurements of 1.86 $\pm$ 0.21 mm vertically and 1.75 $\pm$ 0.19 mm horizontally are, nevertheless, helpful general standards for establishing other dimensions and distances in the ocular fundus.

The topography of the ora serrata constitutes probably the most useful body of information derived from this study because of the paucity of data on this anterior edge of the retina. In general, this study demonstrated that the ora serrata has extraordinary variations. There is a tendency to symmetry in the appearance of a subject's two eyes, the overall range is great. This range in the configuration of the ora serrata makes it difficult and somewhat misleading to describe a "typical" ora. Nonetheless, to present schematically an "average" anterior edge of the retina, it is necessary to consider the localization and incidence of the topographical features. In localization there is a concentration, statistically significant at the P 0.01 level, of dentate processes, ora bays, meridional folds, doubled ora bays, and retinal tags in the superior nasal quadrant. Generally, these and other features progressively decrease in incidence in the inferior nasal, superior temporal, and inferior temporal quadrants. In the full circumference of the eye, the "average" ora serrata presents approximately sixteen

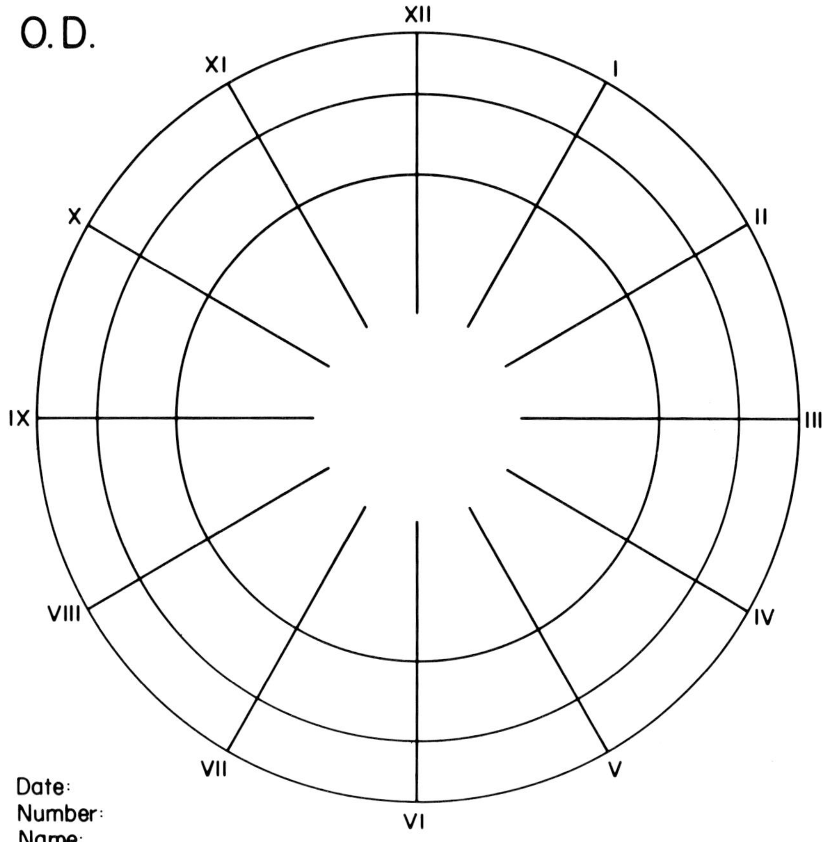

Figure 195. Conventional chart for drawing the retina, representing the anterior margin of the pars plana at the largest circle, the ora serrata at the middle circle, and the equator of the eye at the smallest circle. Compare with Figure 175.

dentate processes, one large or giant dentate process, ten ora bays, one double ora bay, and one retinal tag in an ora bay. Also to be expected are features such as a meridional fold in approximately 40 per cent of eyes, a retinal abnormality posterior to a meridional fold in 12 per cent of eyes, and a completely closed ora bay in 8 per cent of eyes.

The clinical importance of meridional folds and the occurrence of retinal defects and holes posterior to these have been stressed by several authors. It is obvious that many defects and holes of this type are asymptomatic and unassociated with clinical retinal disease. However, they may also be associated with retinal detachment, as indicated by a recent report of 100 eyes with symptomatic retinal breaks, which noted 18 meridional folds in 11 of the eyes and clinically diagnosed a retinal break at the posterior extremity of the fold in 13 of the 18 meridional folds (13).

Also to be emphasized is the not uncommon occurrence of closed ora bays—usually in the superior nasal quadrant. Clinically, these would simulate the appearance of a retinal break near the ora serrata, and therefore the existence of this topographical feature of the peripheral retina must be appreciated by the clinician. In fact, all information pertaining to the ora serrata, as well as to the disk, foveola, and retina as a whole, attains full usefulness only when combined with knowledge derived from *in vivo* and *in vitro* studies of many types. From this combination a concept of the retina, optimum for investigation and clinical practice, is formed.

SUMMARY

Many methods for observing and recording the *in vivo* appearance of the retina are available. For optimum utilization, however, these methods require an accurate understanding of retinal topography.

Retinal topography was therefore systematically evaluated in a series of 200 adult human eyes obtained at autopsy, and a direct clinico-anatomical correlation was established in six surgically enucleated eyes. This analysis revealed the general size and shape of the retina, the dimensions of the optic disk, and the relationship between the disk and the foveola.

In addition, the gross morphology of the ora serrata was evaluated. The incidence and the meridional distribution of the dentate processes, ora bays, meridional folds, retinal tags and other topographic features were recorded. To provide further information, the gross morphologic features of the ora serrata were correlated with microscopic findings and, in selected instances, clinical observations.

In the discussion of these findings, particular attention is given to postmortem changes that alter retinal appearance and to the practical aspects of retinal topography.

REFERENCES

1. Allen, L., Stereoscopic fundus photography with the new instant positive print films. *Am. J. Ophthal.*, 1964, **57**: 539–543.
2. Allen, R. A., and Straatsma, B. R., Ocular involvement in leukemia and allied disorders. *Arch. Ophthal.* (Chicago), 1961, **66**: 490–508.
3. Ballantyne, A. J., and Michaelson, I. C. (Eds.), *Textbook of the Fundus of the Eye.* Livingstone, Edinburgh, 1962.
4. Bedrossian, E. H., *The Eye.* Thomas, Springfield, 1958.
5. Behrendt, T., and Wilson, L. A., Spectral reflectance photography of the retina. *Am. J. Ophthal.*, 1965, **59**: 1079–1088.
6. Brockhurst, R. J., Modern indirect ophthalmoscopy. *Am. J. Ophthal.*, 1956, **41**: 265–272.
7. Byer, N. E., Clinical study of lattice degeneration of the retina. *Trans. Am. Acad. Ophthal. Otolaryng.*, 1965, **69**: 1064–1081.
8. Christensen, R. E., and Nursall, J. F., Motion picture photography of the inner eye; technique and apparatus. *Arch. Ophthal.* (Chicago), 1963, **70**: 540–545.
9. Clinical Trends, 3-D camera captures inner eye, baring hidden pathology. *Clin. Trends*, 1966, **5**(4): 1, 4–5.
10. Donaldson, D. D., A new camera for stereoscopic fundus photography. *Arch. Ophthal.* (Chicago), 1965, **73**: 253–267.

11. DUKE-ELDER, S. (Ed.), *System of Ophthalmology, Vol. II: The Anatomy of the Visual System*. Kimpton, London, 1961.
12. ———, *System of Ophthalmology, Vol. VII: The Foundations of Ophthalmology*. Kimpton, London, 1962.
13. DUMAS, J., and SCHEPENS, C. L., Chorioretinal lesions predisposing to retinal breaks. *Am. J. Ophthal.*, 1966, **61**: 620–630.
14. GOLDMAN, H., *Two Lectures on Biomicroscopy of the Eye*. Berne, 1954.
15. GOLDMAN, H., and SCHMIDT, T., Ein Kontaktglas zur Biomikroskopie der Ora serrata und der Pars plana. *Ophthalmologica*, 1965, **149**: 481–483.
16. GONIN, J., *Le Décollement de la Rétine; Pathogenie—Traitement*. Payot, Lausanne, 1934.
17. HELMHOLTZ, H., *Beschreibung eines Augen-Spiegels zur Untersuchung der Netzhaut im lebenden Auge*. Förstner, Berlin, 1851.
18. ———, *Arch. Physiol. Heilk.*, 1852, **11**: 827.
19. HILL, D. W., DALLERY, C. T., HODGE, J. V., and SCOTT, D. J., Fluorescein studies of the choroidal circulation. *Proc. Roy. Soc. Med.*, 1964, **57**: 500–502.
20. HOWARD, G. M., and ELLSWORTH, R. M., Findings in the peripheral fundi of patients with retinoblastoma. *Am. J. Ophthal.*, 1966, **62**: 243–251.
21. ISHII, K., The diameter of the optic disc in the Japanese. *Ophthal. Lit.*, 1951, **5**: 529.
22. KORNZWEIG, A. L., The eye in old age. V. Diseases of the macula: a clinico-pathologic study. *Am. J. Ophthal.*, 1965, **60**: 835–843.
23. LINHART, J. W., MCINTOSH, H. D., HEYMAN, A., and HART, L. M., Clinical experience with fluorescence retinal cinematography. *Circulation*, 1964, **29**: 577–582.
24. LOBSTEIN, A., BRONNER, A., and NORDMANN, J., De l'intérêt de la dynamométrie dans le glaucome simple. *Ophthalmologica*, 1960, **139**: 271–275.
25. MACLEAN, A. L., and MAUMENEE, A. E., Hemangioma of the choroid. *Am. J. Ophthal.*, 1960, **50**: 3–11.
26. NORTON, E. W. D., GASS, J. D., SMITH, J. L., CURTIN, V. T., DAVID, N. J., and JUSTICE, J., JR., Fluorescein in the study of macular disease. *Trans. Am. Acad. Ophthal. Otolaryng.*, 1965, **69**: 631–642.
27. NORTON, H. J., Photographic analysis of the retinopathy accompanying adrenal pheochromocytoma. *Am. J. Ophthal.*, 1964, **57**: 967–973.
28. NOVOTNY, H. R., and ALVIS, D. L., A method of photographing fluorescence in circulating blood in the human retina. *Circulation*, 1961, **24**: 82–86.
29. O'MALLEY, P., ALLEN, R. A., STRAATSMA, B. R., and O'MALLEY, C. C., Paving-stone degeneration of the retina. *Arch. Ophthal.* (Chicago), 1965, **73**: 169–182.
30. PENKHUS, J., *The Ora Serrata and Its Anatomical Variations*. M.S. Thesis, Univ. of California, Los Angeles, 1966.
31. POLYAK, S. L., *The Retina*. Univ. of Chicago Press, Chicago, 1941.
32. REESE, A. B., *Tumors of the Eye* (2nd ed.). Hoeber, New York, 1963.
33. RENARD, G., LEMASSON, C., and SARAUX, H., *Anatomie de l'Oeil et de ses Annexes*. Masson, Paris, 1965.
34. RUBIN, M. L., The optics of indirect ophthalmoscopy. *Survey Ophthal.*, 1964, **9**: 449–464.
35. SALZMANN, M., *The Anatomy and Histology of the Human Eyeball in the Normal State*. Univ. of Chicago Press, Chicago, 1912.

36. Schepens, C. L., A new ophthalmoscopic demonstration. *Trans. Am. Acad. Ophthal. Otolaryng.*, 1947, **51**: 298–301.
37. ———, Examination of the ora serrata region: its clinical significance. In: *Acta XVI Concilium Ophthalmologicum (Britannia)*, 1950 Vol. II: 1384–1393.
38. Schepens, C. L., and Marden, D., Data on the natural history of retinal detachment; further characterization of certain unilateral nontraumatic cases. *Am. J. Ophthal.*, 1966, **61**: 213–226.
39. Schirmer, K. E., Microfilm photography in ophthalmology. *Brit. J. Ophthal.*, 1965, **49**: 76–79.
40. Serr, H., Das monochromatische Licht der Natriumdampflampe als Lichtquelle für Augenspiegeluntersuchungen. *Graefe Arch. klin. exp. Ophthal.*, 1937. **137**: 636–647.
41. Smolin, G., Statistical analysis of retinal holes and tears. *Am. J. Ophthal.*, 1965, **60**: 1055–1059.
42. Snydacker, D., The normal optic disc; ophthalmoscopic and photographic studies. *Am. J. Ophthal.*, 1964, **58**: 958–964.
43. Sorsby, A. (Ed.), *Modern Ophthalmology, Vol. I: Basic Aspects.* Butterworth, London, 1963.
44. Stein, R., Beiträge zur Topographie und Anatomie der Ora serrata und des Orbiculus ciliaris. *Arch. Augenheilk.*, 1932, **106**: 145–184.
45. Straatsma, B. R., and Allen, R. A., Lattice degeneration of the retina. *Trans. Am. Acad. Ophthal. Otolaryng.*, 1962, **66**: 600–613.
46. Straatsma, B. R., and Christensen, R. E., Ophthalmoscopy of infants and children. *Int. Ophthal. Clin.*, 1963, **3**: 919–932.
47. Thiel, H.-L., Beiträge zur Anatomie der Ora serrata. *Ber. Deutsch. Ophth. Ges.*, 1953, **58**: 249–256.
48. ———, Zur topographischen und histologischen Situation der Ora serrata. *Graefe Arch. klin. exp. Ophthal.*, 1955, **156**: 590–629.
49. Thiel, R., Verwendung von Metalldampflampen beim Augenspiegeln. *Ber. Deutsch. Ophth. Ges.*, 1934, **50**: 290–291.
50. Trantas, A., Moyens d'explorer par l'ophtalmoscope—et par translucidité—la partie antérieure du fond oculaire, le cercle ciliaire y compris. *Arch. Ophtal.* (Paris), 1900, **20**: 314–326.
51. Trevor-Roper, P. D., *Ophthalmology; a Textbook for Diploma Students.* Year Book Publishers, Chicago, 1955.
52. Vogt, A., *Die operative Therapie und die Pathogenese der Netzhautablösung.* Enke Stuttgart, 1936.
53. Wagner, H., Bestimmung der linearen Masse auf der Bulbusoberfläche vom Limbus zur Ora serrata, zum hinteren Pol und zur Papille. *Graefe Arch. klin. exp. Ophthal.*, 1931, **127**: 103–136.
54. Williams, G. R., and Schwartz, J. T., Television ophthalmoscopy. In: *Proceedings of the National Institute of Neurological Diseases and Blindness.* U.S. Government Printing Office, Washington, D.C., 1965.
55. Wolff, E., *Anatomy of the Eye and Orbit*, 5th ed. (R. J. Last, Rev.). Lewis, London, 1961.

RETINAL BLOOD VESSELS AND OCULAR BLOOD FLOW

ROBERT E. CHRISTENSEN, THOMAS H. PETTIT and ARNOLD L. BARTON
UCLA School of Medicine
Los Angeles, California

This paper's purpose is to review some of the clinical characteristics of the normal retinal vessels and report some observations on the physiology of ocular blood flow. The first section will describe studies of the retinal vessels in 100 normal patients; the second section presents observations on the physiology of ocular blood flow in patients studied by a variety of techniques.

RETINAL STUDIES

Anatomical Considerations

The blood supply to the eye comes directly from branches of the ophthalmic artery, which takes origin from the internal carotid artery as it emerges from the cavernous sinus. The uveal tract is supplied by numerous anterior and posterior ciliary arteries, while the retina is supplied by a single vessel, the central retinal artery. The central retinal artery takes origin from the ophthalmic artery near the optic foramen and runs into the orbit under the optic nerve to penetrate the dura and arachnoid 10–15 mm behind the globe (56); it then courses 12 mm through the substance of the optic nerve, giving off small nutrient twigs to the substance of the nerve before it penetrates the cribiform plate to enter the eye (28).

The retinal arteries and arterioles are distinguished from their corresponding retinal veins and venules by lighter red color and smaller caliber. The color differential reflects the difference in oxygenation of arterial and venous blood. The retinal vessels have a shiny linear central reflex stripe, thought to be produced by light reflecting from the convex cylindrical surface of either the blood column within the vessel (24) or the internal limiting membrane of the retina (35). This reflex is sharp and uniform in normal arteries and arterioles and can be observed even in the smallest branches.

In the veins, the central reflex is less consistent and narrower and usually more glittering, suggesting that it is of a different origin than the arteriolar reflex. It has been proposed that the reflex on the veins corresponds to the watered silk reflex from the surface of the retina (3).

As the central retinal artery enters the eye, it divides into superior and inferior retinal arteries, which subsequently divide dichotomously with considerable variation to supply the nasal and temporal quadrants of the retina. The pattern of the retinal vessels on the disk and the number of major retinal vessels that cross the disk margin depend on the number of bifurcations occurring in or on the disk, and also on the level at which these bifurcations take place relative to the cribiform plate.

Since bifurcations hidden in the substance of the optic nerve or behind the cribiform plate cannot be visualized directly, the origin of the vessels appearing in an isolated fashion on the nervehead is not clear. Most are assumed to be branches of the central retinal artery, with the exception of the cilioretinal arteries, derived from the circle of Zinn. These usually appear in the temporal half of the optic nerve and course onto the retina either as a small insignificant twig or, in some cases, as a major vessel supplying the macula. The recent development of fluorescein angiography has made it possible, as reported by Norton et al. (42), to demonstrate that certain arteries appearing on the nervehead take origin from the posterior ciliary arteries, since they fill with fluorescein during the initial choroidal phase and before the central retinal artery fills with fluorescein.

Method of Clinical Study

The retinal vessels in 100 patients between the ages of 20 and 40 years were judged to be normal on the basis that the patients were in good health and without histories of systemic vascular disease or any ocular abnormality except for correctable refractive errors. Eighty of the patients studied were seen on several occasions over a two-year period; they had an initial eye examination, followed by interval examinations every six to nine months. Examinations consisted of thorough direct and indirect ophthalmoscopic studies of the retina with the pupil well dilated, supplemented by color fundus photographs of the optic nervehead, vessels, and macula. This group of patients was being observed primarily as part of another study to determine if persons engaged in research work involving the use of lasers sustain discernible retinal or choroidal damage as the result of exposure in the research situation. The group of 80 patients was supplemented by 20 volunteer subjects who, in addition to the ocular examination and routine fundus photography, had fluorescein angiography performed.

Of the 100 patients studied, 85 were male. The distribution of refractive errors was as follows: 38 patients with myopia ranging from −1.0 to −8.0; 10 with hyperopia with errors of greater than +1.0, and 52 with emmetropia or refractive errors of less than 1 diopter.

Fundus photographs were taken with the Zeiss fundus camera. Fluorescein angiography was performed as previously described (34), with the exception that the Baird-Atomic interference filter type B-4, as described by Hodge & Clemett (32), was used for fluorescein excitation.

The clinical characteristics studied in this group of normal patients included the distribution of the retinal vessels on the disk and about the macula, the variations in the arteriovenous crossings, the characteristics of the central avascular foveal area, and the arterial-venous ratio as an index of generalized arteriolar narrowing.

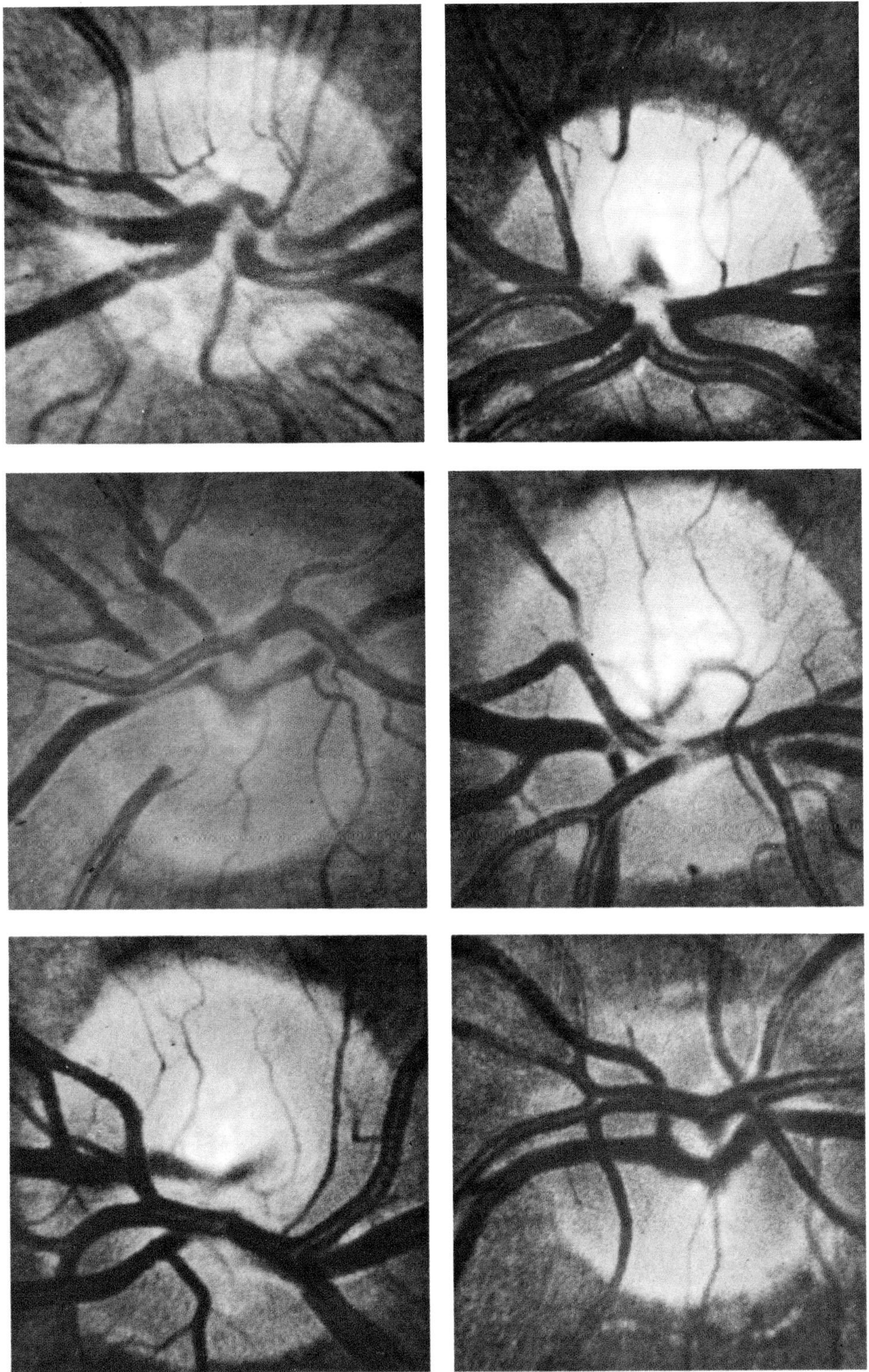

Figure 196. Optic nerveheads showing variable distribution of major vessels in normal eyes.

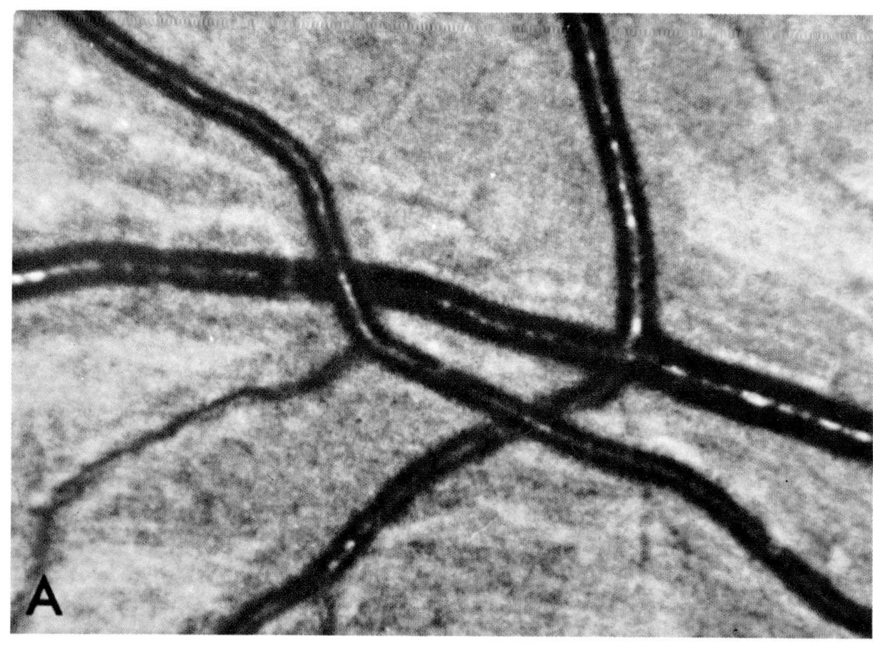

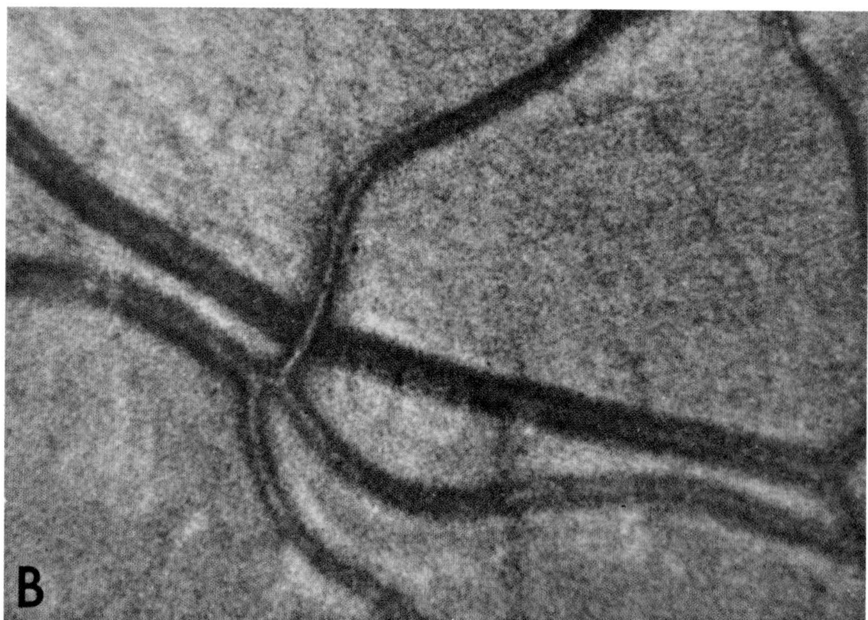

Figure 197. *A:* Trichotomous division of a retinal vein. *B:* Trichotomous division of a retinal arteriole.

the fovea in these conditions. Stereoscopic fluorescein angiography (2) or biomicroscopic observation of the macula (22) at the peak of fluorescein passage help differentiate the choroidal and retinal vessels.

As part of this study, an attempt was made to estimate the size of the avascular foveal area, as demonstrated by fluorescein angiography in photos showing both the optic nervehead and the fovea. By measuring the optic nervehead and the avascular foveal area and assuming the optic nervehead to be approximately 1.5 mm in diameter, the avascular area was estimated to be 0.2 to 0.3 mm in diameter; this is only slightly less than the 0.4–0.5 mm diameter reported from *in vitro* studies (3).

Other capillary-free areas, 50–120 μ in width, are present in the retina, surrounding the retinal arterioles down to the precapillary level. First demonstrated histologically in 1880 by His (31), their presence has since been confirmed by others (36,38), although they cannot ordinarily be appreciated clinically. (Figures 201 and 202.) Recent fluorescein angiography studies of the retinal vessels do appear to demonstrate these capillary-free areas around the arterioles (Figure 203).

Study of the distribution of the larger vessels around the macula revealed that the largest vessels approaching it were usually arteriolar in origin, although considerable variation occurred. In this study of 200 normal eyes it was found that in 80 per cent (160 eyes) the major arterioles supplying branches to the macula followed a course that placed them closer to the macula than their corresponding venous counterparts. This distribution did not relate to refractive error or type of

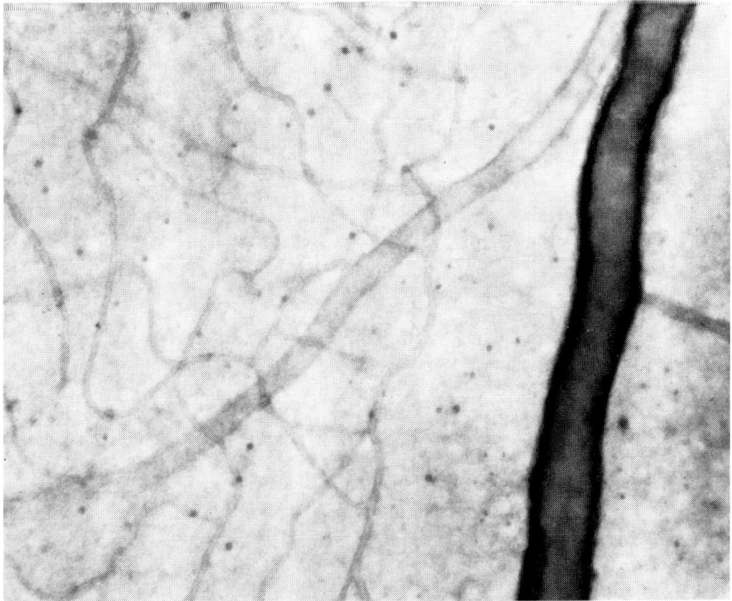

Figure 202. Flat preparation of human retina demonstrating capillary-free area around arteriole and network of capillaries surrounding the adjacent venule.

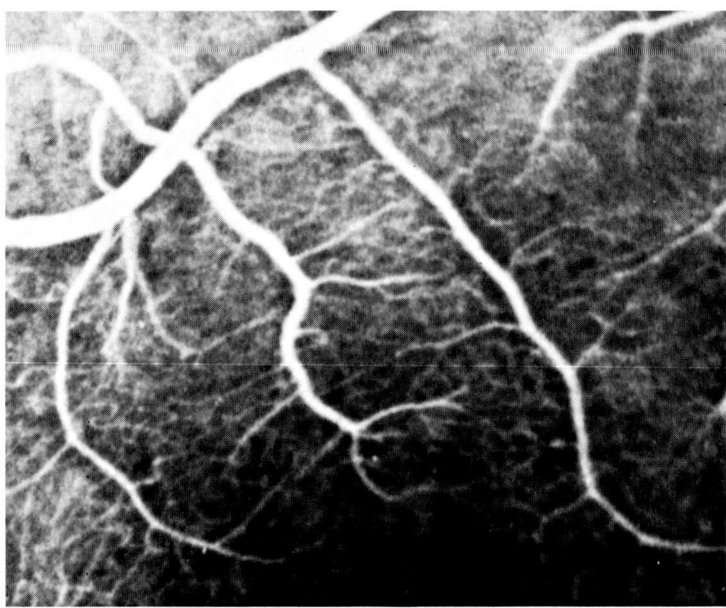

Figure 203. Retinal fluorescein angiography showing capillary network between retinal arterioles and venules. The largest vessel is an arteriole with two major branches. The capillary network does not appear as dense around the arterioles.

optic nerve entry into the eye. In three eyes examined, a single arteriole divided to supply both a superior and an inferior branch to the macula.

As the vessels of the retina course from the nervehead to the periphery, the arteries and veins cross each other a number of times. The arterioles usually maintain their level in the nerve fiber layer, while the veins pass behind them by coursing posteriorly into the deeper layers of the retina. Infrequently, the vein passes in front of the artery at the crossing; this was observed only 59 times in 486 major crossings studied (approximately 12 per cent), although it was reported to occur at a higher rate in one previous study (33). When the vein passed in front of the artery, the artery maintained its level in the retina and the vein humped forward in varying degrees to get over it. The retinal vessels crossed each other at a variety of angles and, although the veins gave way to the arterioles by passing behind or in front, both vessels appeared to be significantly affected by the crossing, as they frequently demonstrated a rather abrupt change in direction near the crossing (Figure 204).

Histologic studies of ophthalmoscopically normal vessel crossings in healthy young adults have been reported by a number of authors (48,51). The usual finding is a common glial and advential sheath shared by the arteriole and vein, with a fusion of the vessel walls at the crossing. There is also not infrequently a thinning of the common vascular wall and an apparent narrowing of the vein to about two-thirds its pre- and postcrossing lumen size under the crossing. In the present study there were several young adult eyes examined which had no other

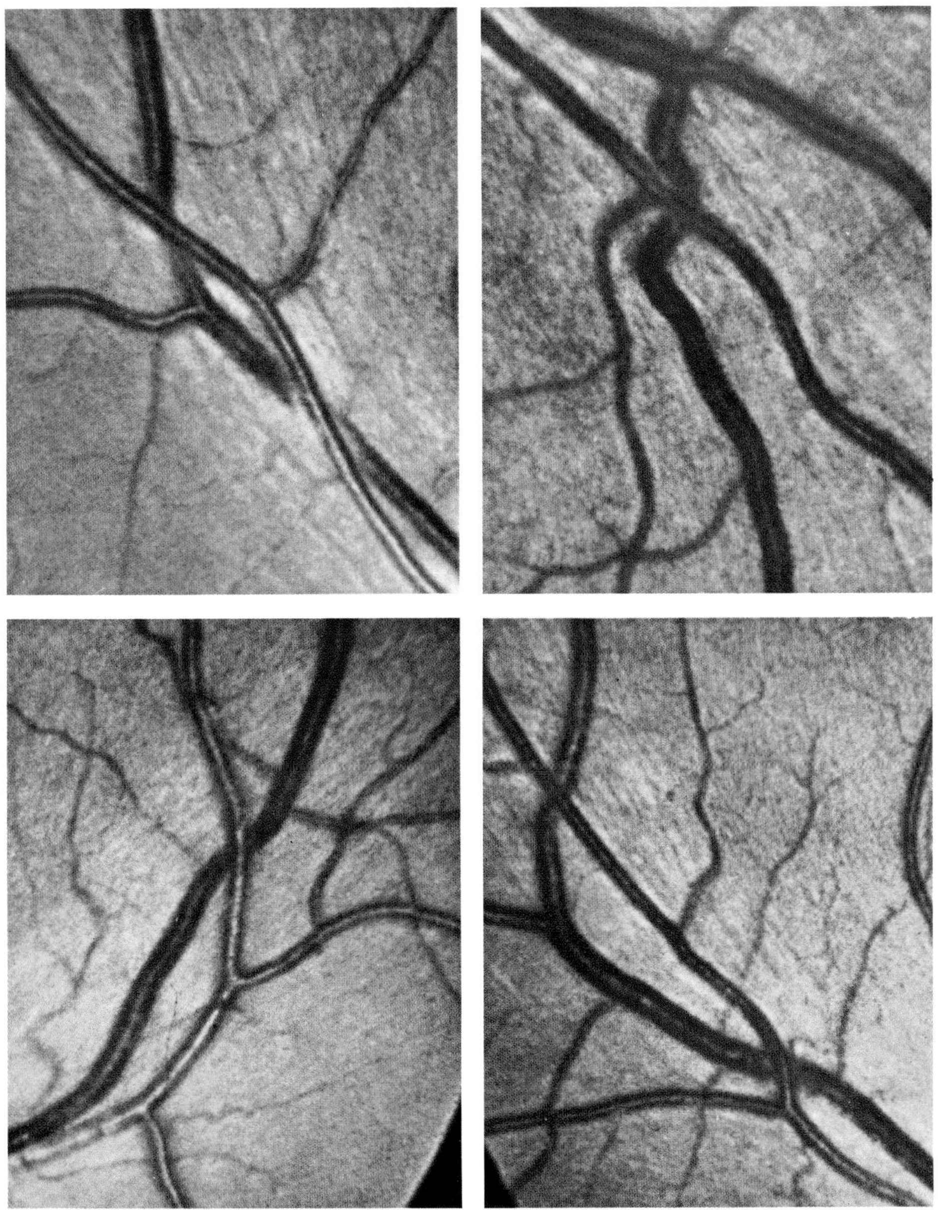

Figure 204. Some variations in the arteriovenous crossings as seen in the normal human eye.

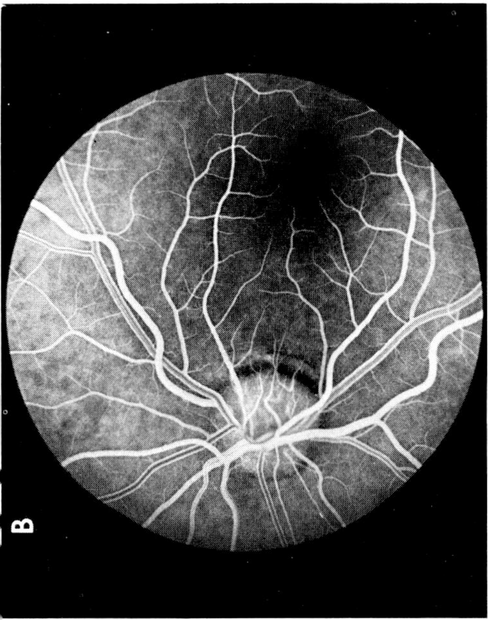

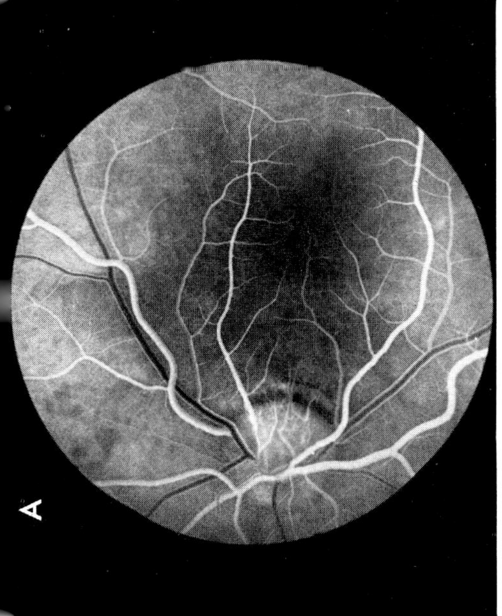

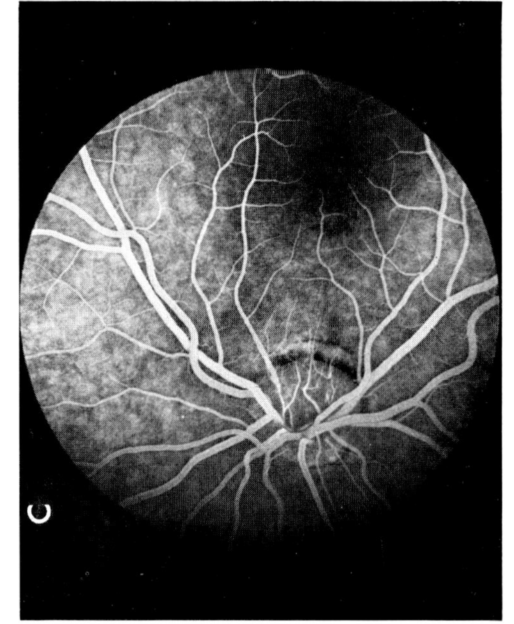

Figure 205. *A:* Fluorescein angiography of normal ocular fundus, arterial phase. *B:* Fluorescein angiography, arteriovenous phase; note laminar flow in the veins. *C:* Fluorescein angiography, venous phase.

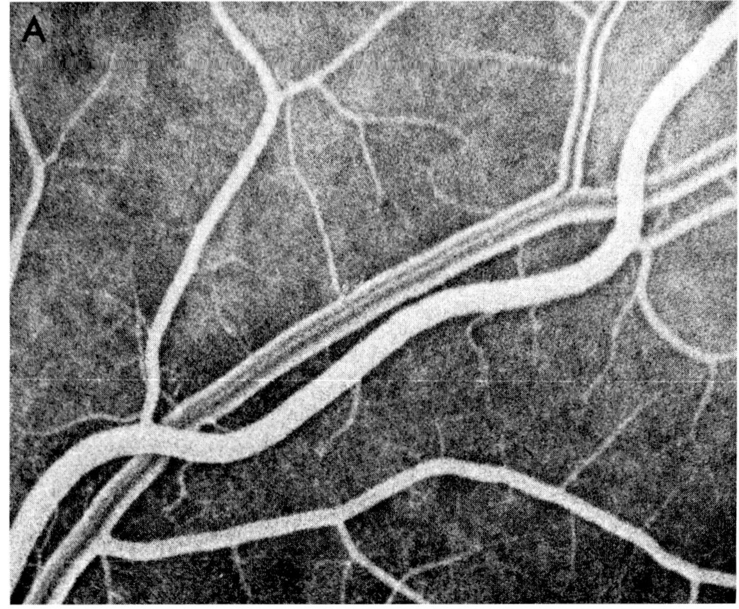

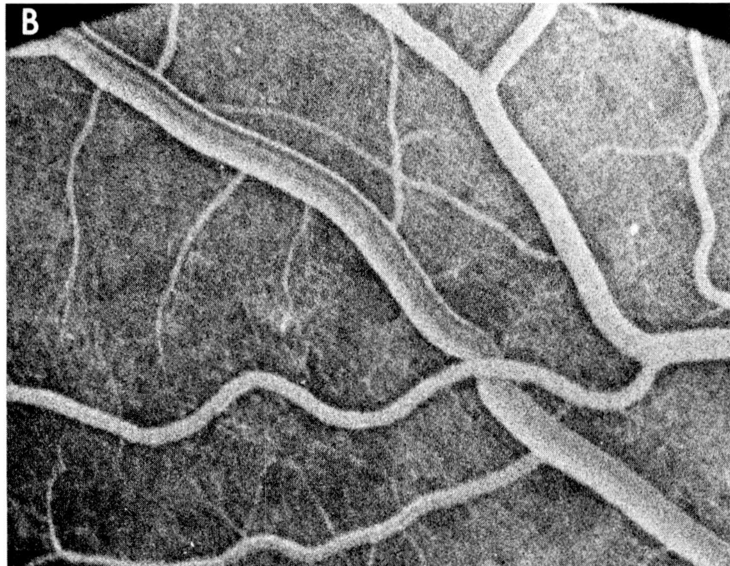

Figure 206. Arteriovenous phase of fluorescein angiography. *A:* Laminar flow and its undisturbed flow under an arteriovenous crossing. *B:* Note the laminar flow in the vein that disappears at the arteriovenous crossing; this suggests the presence of sufficient narrowing and compression of the vein to produce turbulence in the venous flow with mixing of the separate streams of fluorescein at the crossing.

evidence of vascular disease, but showed varying degrees of apparent venous narrowing and possible compression at the crossings (Figure 204).

A recently published study of the retinal vessels by Seitz (48) has pointed out that what may appear ophthalmoscopically to be attenuation and compression of the veins at the vessel crossings may in fact be only adventitial and glial opacification about the vessel that obscure visualization of the blood column and in actuality have no effect on the caliber of the vessel.

A preliminary study of the arteriovenous crossings with fluorescein angiography suggests that it is possible to obtain a better view of the changes occurring at the crossings with this technique than with conventional ophthalmoscopy. The glial and adventitial changes are not opaque to the fluorescein, and thus one may observe the crossing more accurately (Figure 205). During the early arteriovenous phase of fluorescein angiography, the laminar characteristics of the blood flow in the veins can be seen (Figure 205B). Study of the arteriovenous crossings during this phase of angiography and the changes in the venous laminar flow occurring at the crossings can give information about narrowing or compression of the venous blood column at the crossings (Figure 206). If one is fortunate enough to have laminar flow occurring prior to a crossing, any disturbance in that flow seen at the crossing suggests true narrowing or compression with induced eddy currents that produce mixing of the fluorescein. It appears that some narrowing of the vein and turbulence in the venous flow may occur at the retinal vessel crossings even in the apparently normal young adult (Figure 206B).

THE PHYSIOLOGY OF OCULAR BLOOD FLOW

Studies of retinal and choroidal blood circulation *in vivo* may be made by a variety of techniques in addition to direct observation of the ocular vessels with ophthalmoscopy and still photography (43). The dynamics of human ocular blood flow may be visualized and monitored by color motion picture photography utilizing the Zeiss operating microscope and a Goldman corneal contact fundus lens, as previously described (12). Spontaneous venous compression may be easily seen on the optic disk; serpentine motion, pulsatile flow, and color changes of the ocular fundus during systole and diastole are noted. The ocular venous pressure end-point may be recorded, as well as the diastolic and systolic ophthalmic artery occlusion pressures during ophthalmodynamometry (50). It has been shown that oxygen inhalation in greater than normal concentrations decreases retinal vessel caliber and the arteriovenous color differential (16). This vascular constriction, and the opposite effect produced by carbon dioxide inhalation (19), may also be demonstrated by color motion picture photography.

While fluorescein angiography is not practical with color motion picture film (12), satisfactory results may be obtained by using the Zeiss semi-automatic fundus camera (2) and appropriate filters with black-and-white motion picture film (27).

Recent attempts to quantitate changes in retinal blood flow by photographic means show promise. Hickam & Frayser (30) have utilized a difficult photographic method for estimating the mean retinal circulation time in man: using intravenous fluorescein injections and serial fundus photographs, and subsequent densitometric measurements on the photographic images of the retinal vessels, concentration curves are derived from the relative concentration of fluorescein in arterial and venous blood at the time of each picture; arterial and venous retinal circulation times are then calculated by formulae. The authors have found the mean retinal circulation time in normal males to be 4.7 ± 1.1 seconds. The technique is applicable to the study of the circulatory effects of inhaled gases (19,25,30); such studies report that retinal circulation time is prolonged by inhalation of 100 per cent oxygen and by sublingual administration of nitroglycerin, and is shortened by the inhalation of 7 per cent carbon dioxide and 21 per cent oxygen.

The eye, supplied by the first branch of the internal carotid artery, must certainly mirror the cerebral blood flow. Voluminous research has been done on the cerebral circulation, utilizing electromagnetic flow meters, color indicators, photoelectric devices, inert gas analysis, and radioactive scan techniques (44,55). Such studies have indicated that, in spite of various stimuli, the cerebral blood flow is remarkably consistent; ocular blood flow is probably similarly consistent. The difficulties encountered in measuring and interpreting changes in ocular blood flow have been summarized by Walsh (55), and are numerous. Although direct measurements of ocular blood flow would be desirable, such determinations by cannulation are rarely feasible (29), and most of our knowledge concerning ocular blood flow must therefore be gained from indirect methods of measurement.

Photometric estimations of ocular blood flow have been performed for many years. In 1936, Schubert (47) measured the amount of light leaving the pupil of albino rabbits whose globes were subluxated and illuminated diasclerally. In 1956, Rushton (46), using reflectance photometry, plotted absorption curves for the various ocular pigments. Niedermeier (40) performed photographic experiments of choroidal blood thickness using diascleral illumination with yellow-green light. In 1961, Broadfoot (9) used reflectance photometry and Rushton's principles concerning visual pigments; his experiments utilized an ophthalmoscopic system with a photoelectric pickup, which allowed simultaneous recording of the amounts of light of three different wavelengths reflected through the pupil when the ocular fundus was illuminated by a light source projecting three different colors; this in turn allowed measurement of the blood oxygenation in the fundus and the effects of changes in blood pressure and intraocular pressure upon the choroidal blood color and blood volume. Cristini (15) adapted this photometric technique to the slit lamp by transilluminating the globe and measuring the light leaving the pupil with a photocell mounted in the applanation tonometer prism.

Trokel (52) has recently adapted the reflection densitometry techniques of previous investigators to the binocular ophthalmoscope. Using a photomultiplier and dichroic filters, a 7.5 mm area of the retina and choroid is illuminated and the reflected light is analyzed. This photometric device allows simultaneous comparison of the mean ocular blood flow in the two eyes as affected by changes in blood oxygen saturation, CO_2 concentration, systemic blood pressure, and specific pharmacologic stimuli. Another technique for the quantitative measurement of pulsatile and other volume changes in the cardiovascular pulse wave is photoelectric plethysmography; it involves the principle of reflectance plethysmography, in which color changes reflect blood volume changes in the tissue (41). With suitable devices for attaching the photoelectric sensing device, the measurements may be taken from the finger, toe, arm, leg, or neck.

Ophthalmodynamometry, tonometry and tonography, orbital tonometry and oscillometry, and ophthalmodynamography, are all accepted clinical methods for recording the ocular pulse (37). Unfortunately, each of them increases the intraocular pressure significantly. An attempt has therefore been made to develop a method for the study of the ocular pulse wave in as nearly an undisturbed state as possible, and to compare it with the pulse wave formed in other parts of the peripheral vascular system. The technique involved is that of photoelectric ocular plethysmography (P.E.P.). As part of this investigation, an instrument has been developed for sensing the pulse wave from the retina and iris of the human eye (6,11).

Clinical Studies

Method 1

In this study a Kenelco KE-72 photoelectric plethysmograph transducer coupled to a KE-68 plethysmograph amplifier and recorder was used to sense and indicate (as an electric signal) the cardiovascular pulse pressure wave in the index finger. For detection of the ocular pulse wave by photometrics, a special corneal contact lens mounting, 12 mm in diameter, was devised with a self-contained light source, photocell, and low vacuum attachment for suction when desired (11) (Figure 207); the total weight of the instrument is approximately 4 g. The

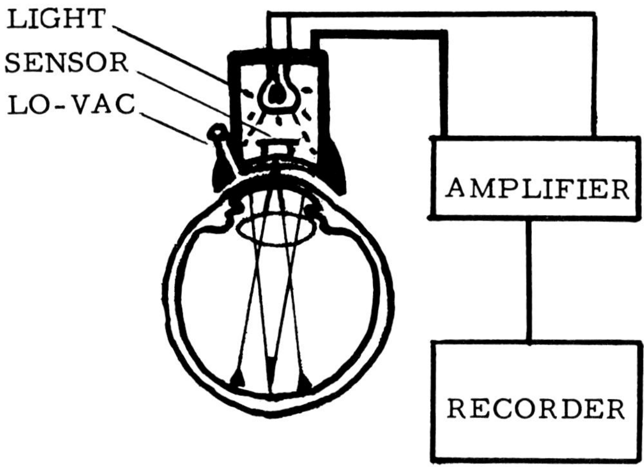

Figure 207. Ocular photoelectric plethysmography device utilizing a corneal contact lens with self-contained light source and photosensor.

spectral response curve of the sensor peaks at 7350 Å, a desirable sensitivity range for hemoglobin pigment study. This instrument makes use of the optical principle of reflectance photometry, in which both incident and reflected light pass through the dilated pupil. A diffuse light from an incandescent lamp source passes through the contact lens into the eye and interacts with the vascular layers by being absorbed, transmitted, or reflected. Since the photosensor is most sensitive in a spectral zone of minimal absorption for hemoglobin, incident light is either reflected directly from the vascular space or transmitted to the sclera, from which it is reflected back through the vascular media (53). At systole, the volume pulse increases momentarily the density of the near infrared reflective media, which in turn is recorded as an increase in the output of the photoelectric system. In the individual patient, changes in blood volume (optical density) are recorded as changes in the baseline level of the pulse record, and with stable blood pressure (brachial, carotid, or ocular) this change in volume would also indicate a change in mean blood flow.

Observations. The ocular pulse wave demonstrated by photoelectric plethysmography (P.E.P.) is of low amplitude and coincides with cardiac systole (Figure 208). The wave form is similar to that obtained during nasal septum photoelectric plethysmography (Figure 209). The shape and height of the pulse wave varies from patient to patient, and the sensitivity is such that even differences between volume pulses are evident. The photosensor is responsive to changes in systemic blood pressure such as occur in cardiac arrhythmias (Figure 210). The ocular pulse wave (P.E.P.) may also be recorded from the undilated iris, in which case the pulse amplitude is greater than that recorded from retina and choroid (Figure 211); there are, however, superimposed effects of pupillary constriction and dilation which vary the amount of light reflection from the iris. It is hoped that, with further refinements in instrumentation and amplification, this technique will be useful for the clinical investigation of pulsatile ocular blood flow. With this approach, patient cooperation is less essential than with some other photometric techniques, and examinations may also be performed on eyes of patients under general anesthesia.

The pulsatile nature of ocular blood flow may be observed in a variety of other ways. Occasionally, ocular pulsations are visible to the unaided eye. During slit lamp biomicroscopy and with exophthalmometry, corneal pulsations are noted which are coincident with the carotid pulse. During ophthalmoscopy, spontaneous venous pulsations are often visible, and arteriolar pulsations may be elicited by digital or dynamometric pressure upon the globe (26). Applanation and Schiotz tonometry also demonstrate the presence and the amplitude of the ocular pulse. It is obvious that the less the method of measurement disturbs the ocular steady state, the more nearly the measurement should approximate the true ocular pulsation. For example, increasing the intraocular pressure from the undisturbed level (P_0) to the tonometric pressure (P_t) during tonometry undoubtedly affects the ocular hemodynamics. With fixed gain amplification during tonography, however, comparisons may be made of the ocular pulse amplitudes of various

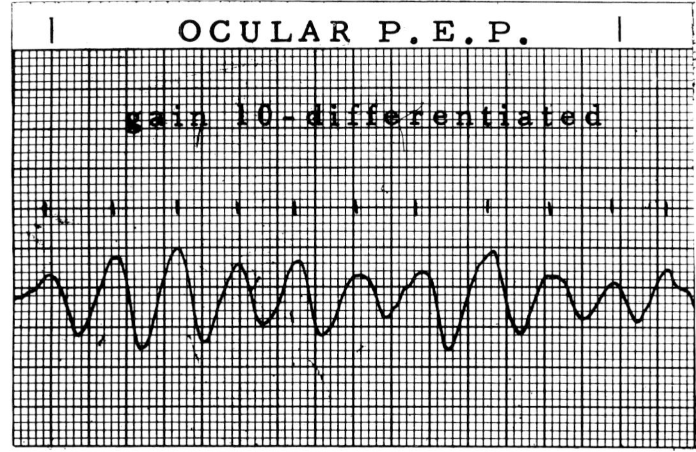

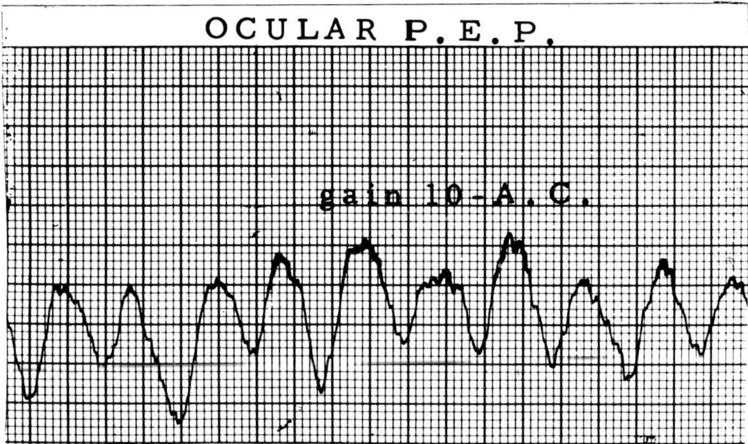

Figure 208. Ocular photoelectric plethysmographic tracing; normal subject with dilated pupil. *Above:* differentiated tracing; *below:* undifferentiated tracing (A–C).

individuals, or between the pulse amplitudes of the same individual in experimental situations.

The ocular pulse amplitude depends upon many factors. Moses (39) has mentioned among these the systolic and diastolic blood pressure levels, the pulse rate, the peripheral resistance associated with episcleral venous pressure, the scleral rigidity (E) or the scleral distensibility (1/E), the level of the intraocular pressure (P_0), the coefficient of aqueous outflow facility (C), and phasic respiratory and systemic blood pressure changes. It has been stated that the ocular pulse amplitude is related to the level of intraocular pressure (21). There have been suggestions that the pressure pulse in the eye is caused entirely by a change in volume equivalent to the pressure change. As previously mentioned, tonographic tracings may be evaluated for data concerning the amplitude of the ocular pulse. Analysis of such data from normal patients in our laboratory would indicate that, particularly

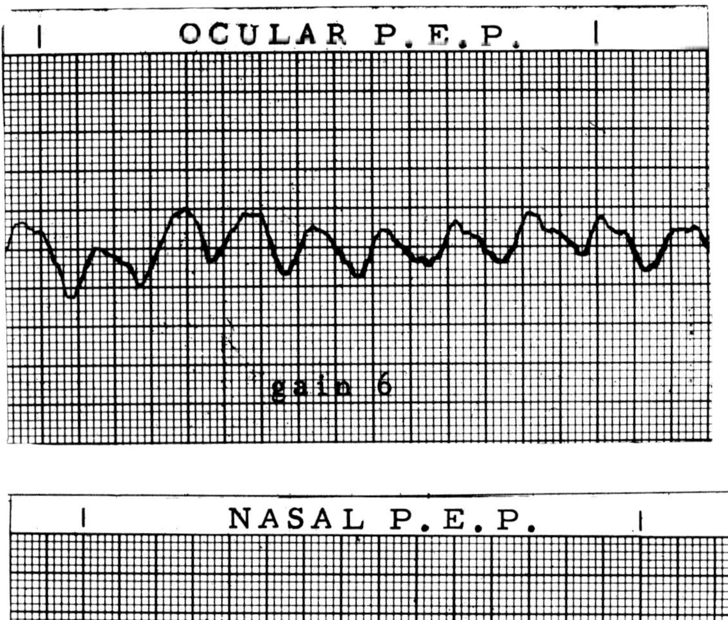

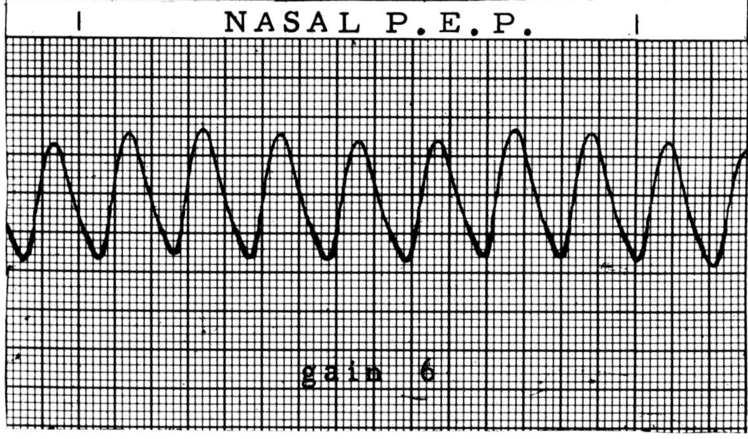

Figure 209. Photoelectric plethysmographic tracing from eye (above) and nasal septum (below).

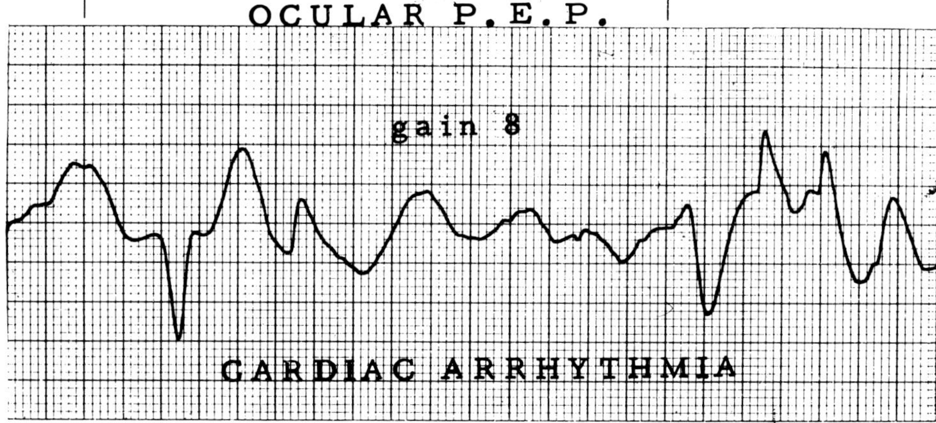

Figure 210. Ocular photoelectric plethysmographic tracing from patient with cardiac arrhythmia.

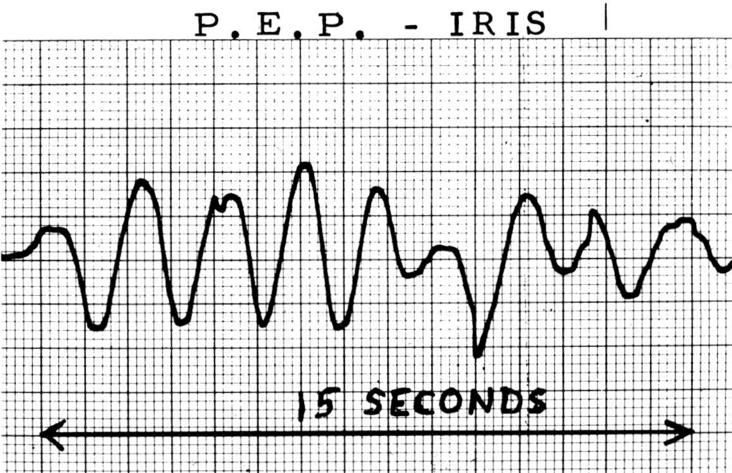

Figure 211. Ocular photoelectric plethysmographic tracing from normal subject with undilated pupil.

at normal levels of intraocular pressure, other factors are also involved in the amplitude of the ocular pulse.

Method 2

For comparative purposes, a series of 45 normal eyes were subjected to tonography utilizing fixed gain amplification and the appropriate tonometric weight. Intraocular pressure, tonometric pulse amplitude, systemic blood pressure, pulse pressure, and pulse rate are compared in Table 22. In this group of patients with small variations of intraocular pressure, the tonometric pulse amplitude is variable and only casually related to the level of intraocular pressure. A comparison of the tonographic pulse amplitude of patients with the same level of intraocular pressure shows no consistent relationship in this study or in previous ones (13). The pulse amplitude does not seem to be correlated directly with systolic, diastolic, or mean systemic blood pressure, pulse pressure, or pulse rate.

Conventional tonographic paper roll speeds are relatively slow (120 inches per hour) and yield a spike-type of ocular pulse wave (10) (Figure 212). An attempt has been made to compare as closely as possible the wave form of the tonometric ocular pulse with that obtained by other measurements, including photoelectric digital plethysmography and the newly developed technique of ocular photoelectric plethysmography described earlier (Figure 208). To accomplish this comparison, the tonographic paper roll speed was doubled (240 inches per hour); at this speed, the ocular pulse wave form parallels closely the digital wave form (Figure 213), and even reflects volume pulse changes with respiration (Figure 214). The rapid tonogram wave form is also similar to the wave form obtained by ocular photoelectric plethysmography. Tonographic pulsations reflect faithfully changes in the vascular pulsations in the fingers, even in transient (Figure 215) or constant (Figure 216) cardiac arrhythmias. There is a slight difference in contour

TABLE 22

TONOGRAPHIC DATA FROM FORTY-FIVE NORMAL EYES

P_0	Pamp	B.P.	P.P.	P.R.	P_0	Pamp	B.P.	P.P.	P.R.
12.00	2	122/54	68	80	12.00	3	112/76	36	72
16.50	4	130/68	62	72	16.00	2	174/110	64	72
10.00	4	100/60	40	68	12.00	2	138/70	68	92
16.50	2	154/90	64	80	14.75	4	170/100	70	76
13.00	4	140/62	78	68	19.00	2	120/80	40	84
12.00	3	140/70	70	64	11.00	2	98/70	28	56
15.50	2	200/110	90	80	11.00	3	110/60	40	64
12.50	3	144/82	52	76	13.00	3	112/70	42	64
14.00	2	120/70	50	72	14.75	4	124/70	54	64
13.00	3	180/90	90	76	17.00	4	120/70	50	56
13.00	2	90/70	20	64	11.50	4	118/72	46	60
12.00	3	100/70	30	68	9.50	2	134/90	44	64
12.50	2	122/70	52	60	14.00	3	150/70	80	64
14.75	2	160/104	56	82	14.75	8	110/54	56	48
14.75	6	154/72	82	68	15.50	6	160/80	80	76
14.75	3	130/88	42	72	13.00	1	130/70	60	88
13.00	3	100/80	20	72	9.50	2	118/68	50	68
17.00	3	120/70	50	72	10.00	1	116/78	38	84
13.00	3	100/80	20	72	12.50	3	110/60	50	84
17.00	3	120/70	50	72	14.00	4	118/80	38	80
16.50	3	132/74	58	72	12.50	3	98/70	28	80
10.00	4	138/80	58	92	15.50	3	128/68	60	68
					12.00	3	162/72	90	72

P_0: Intraocular pressure; Pamp: tonometric pulse amplitude; B.P.: brachial blood pressure; P.P.: brachial pulse pressure; P.R.: pulse rate.

of the ocular pulse wave, which may be secondary to the inertia of the measuring method. It seems apparent, however, that the ocular pulse wave, although smaller in amplitude, does resemble closely the pulse wave form noted in other parts of the peripheral vascular system, and that it reflects changes in respiration and blood pressure rapidly.

Walsh and others (44,55) have emphasized that the rate of cerebral blood flow is essentially constant. The total cerebral blood pool has been calculated to be

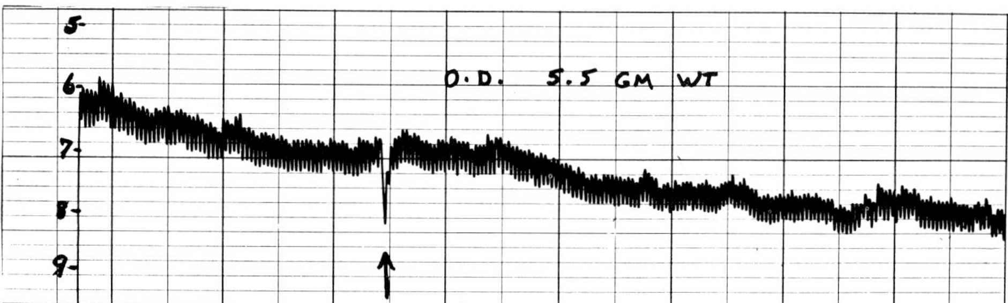

Figure 212. Conventional tonogram (120 inches/hour), demonstrating spike type of ocular pulse wave. Vertical arrow indicates single ectopic heart beat reflected on tonographic tracing.

70 ml, and the usual exchange rate for cerebral blood is found to be 54 ml/100 g of brain tissue/minute; since the average brain weight is 1500 g, the calculated average cerebral blood flow rate is approximately 810 ml/minute (44). Cerebral blood flow differs in some respects from that in other areas of the body due to the

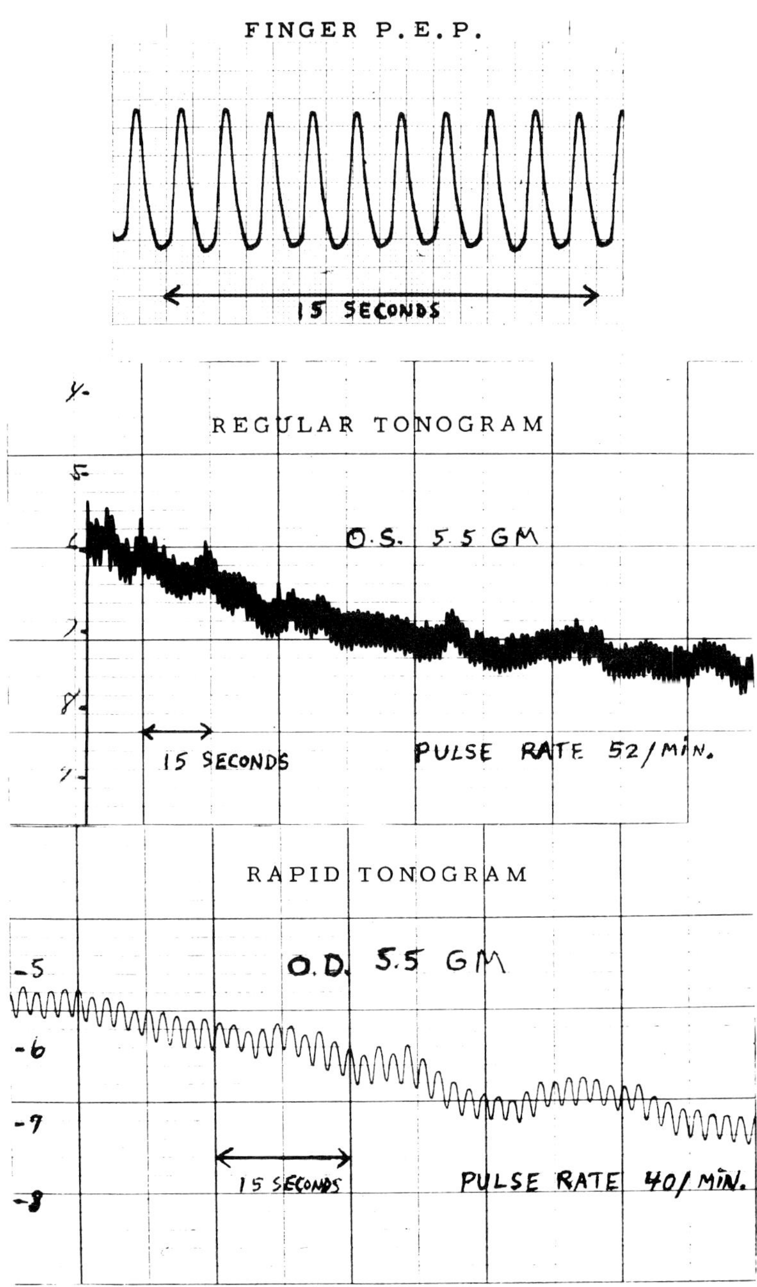

Figure 213. Finger photoelectric plethysmogram (above), regular tonogram (middle), and rapid tonogram (below). All tracings from same patient.

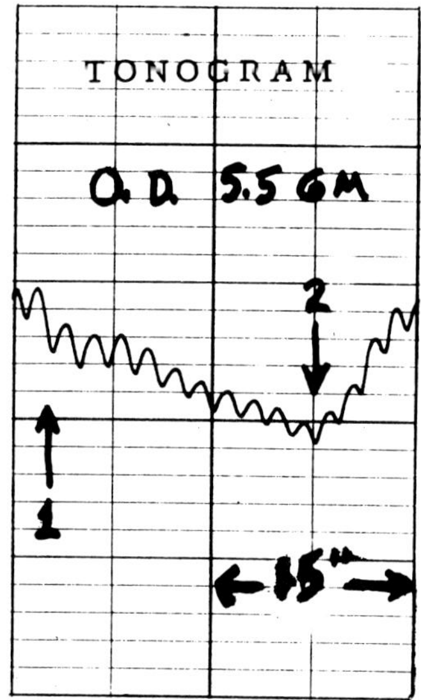

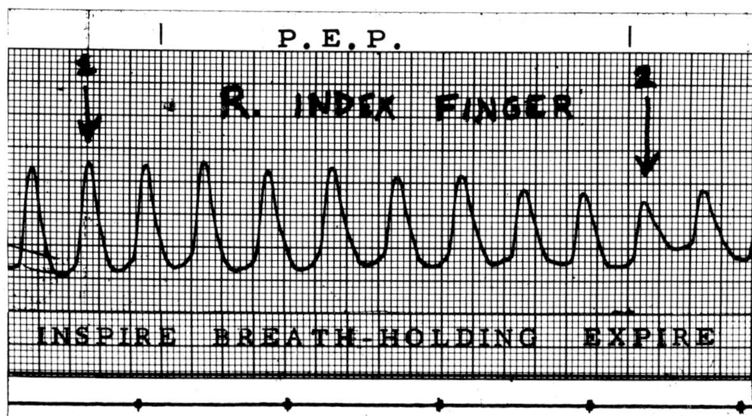

Figure 214. *Above:* rapid tonogram at paper speed of 240 inches/hour. *Below:* finger photoelectric plethysmogram from same patient. Arrow 1: inspiration; arrow 2: expiration.

closed vault in which the brain lies. However, the extracranial factors of greatest significance in maintaining cerebral blood flow are, as elsewhere, the cardiac output and the systemic blood pressure.

Estimates of ocular blood flow and blood volume are difficult and inaccurate due to the inaccessibility of the organ and to the cross circulation between the external carotid system through the ophthalmic artery (55). An exact measurement of the human ocular blood volume has never been made; Becker & Friedenwald (4) estimated it to be 200 mm^3 from a study of histological sections. In recent years, it has been shown that changes in intraocular pressure are accompanied by changes in intraocular blood volume; furthermore, the intraocular

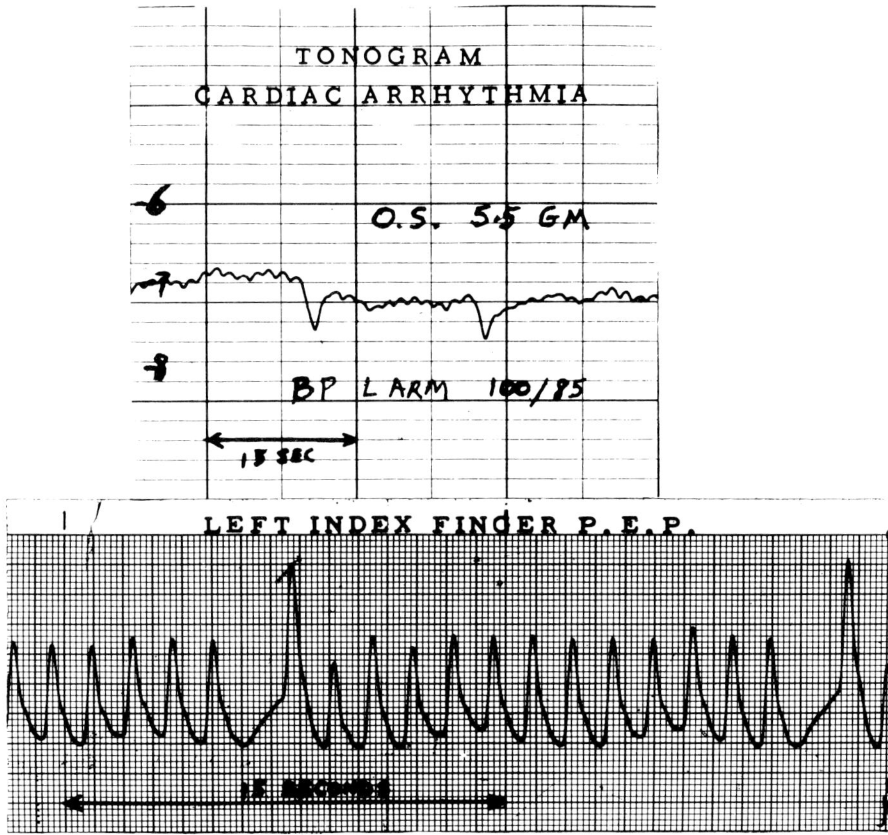

Figure 215. Rapid tonogram (above) and finger photoelectric plethysmogram (below) of patient with transient cardiac arrhythmia.

blood volume depends upon systemic blood pressure. Moses (39) has stated that, as the arterial pulse wave enters the eye, the volume of blood within the eye is momentarily increased; this augmentation of intraocular volume produces an increase of intraocular pressure amounting to 2–3 mm Hg. The ocular volume change is reflected in a pulsatile pressure change within the eye which may be observed tonometrically. Studies on human patients performed by Becker & Friedenwald (4) showed that variations in systemic blood pressure and respiration influenced the intraocular pressure and possibly influenced blood flow and content. Bettman and coworkers (8) studied the effects of tonography upon the ocular blood volume of animals, utilizing radioactive tracer substances injected intravascularly and increasing the intraocular pressure of cannulated eyes by stepwise increments; they concluded that tonography performed with the 5.5 g weight resulted in no significant change in ocular blood volume.

We have compared the peripheral pulse in the index finger, monitored by a photoelectric plethysmographic device, with the tonographic tracing of the same patient. Numerous tracings have shown without question that conventional tonograms faithfully record variations in cardiac output, including respiratory

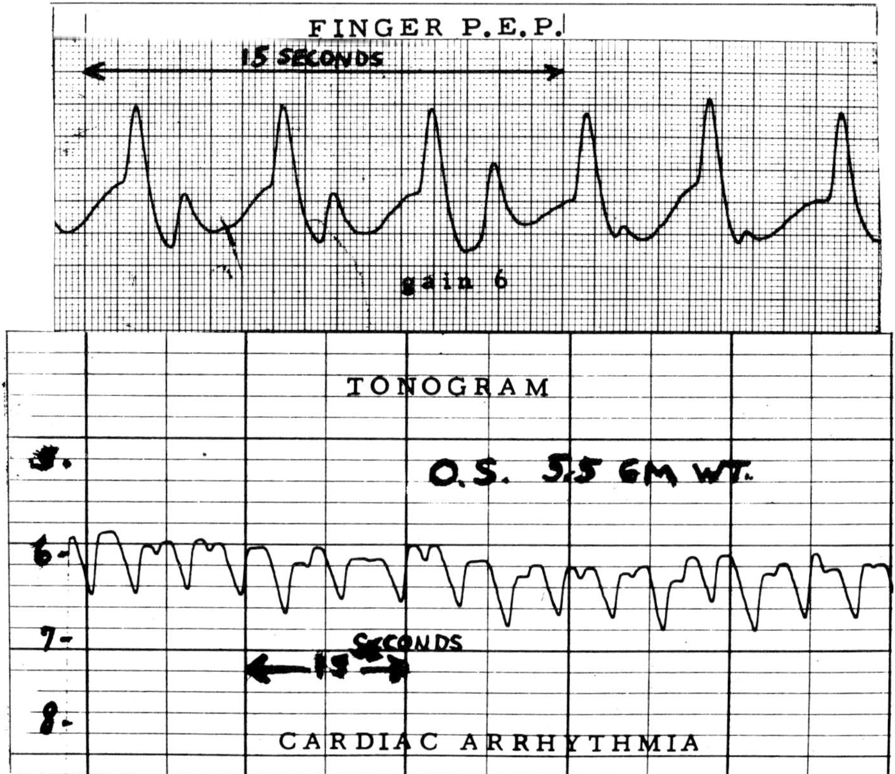

Figure 216. Finger photoelectric plethysmogram (above) and rapid tonogram (below) in patient with constant cardiac arrhythmia.

changes, cardiac arrhythmias, and premature (ectopic) heartbeats with their attendant compensatory pause. Whenever the electrocardiogram demonstrates a premature (ectopic) heartbeat sufficient to result in a change in the digital pulse wave, the tonographic pulse wave is similarly affected.

It occurred to us that information concerning ocular blood flow could be obtained by analyzing tonographic data from humans during transient changes in cardiac output, i.e., premature heartbeats (Figure 215). Thus, an estimate of ocular minute blood flow could be made by measuring reflected tonographic volume changes occurring during single premature cardiac beats and relating them to the pulse rate and to relevant data concerning pressure changes within the carotid artery, obtained from other (cardiac catheterization) studies (7).

Premature heartbeats may occur as an isolated phenomenon. Their occurrence during tonography may be related to posture, since they are known to be much more common in the recumbent position. The ultimate effect of a cardiac arrhythmia depends in part upon the rapidity of the heartrate and the effect of the arrhythmia upon the systemic blood pressure (7). The depression in systemic blood pressure accompanying a premature beat is a direct result of reduced stroke output.

Comment should be made concerning the effect of a premature heartbeat and

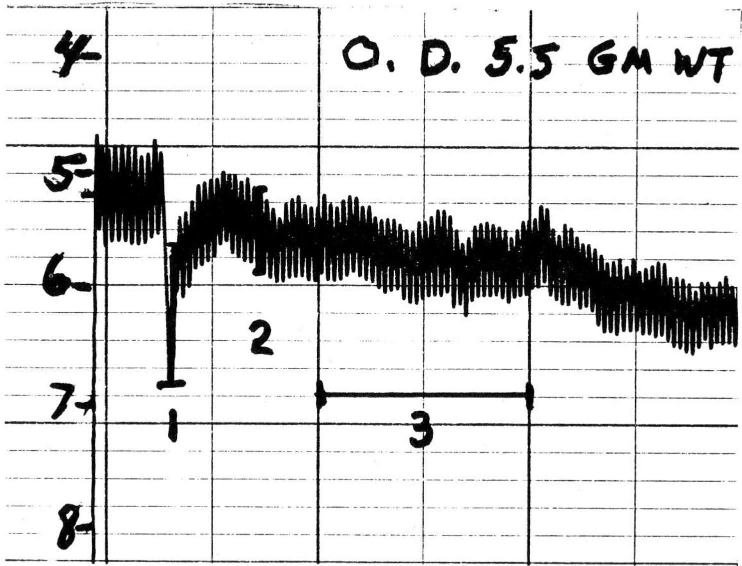

Figure 217. Tonogram in cardiac arrhythmia. Tonographic pulse following compensatory pause (#1) is roughly twice the usual pulse amplitude (#2). Time scale (#3) is 30 seconds.

the following compensatory pause upon the general configuration of the tonographic tracing (Figure 217). The ectopic beat is usually not reflected. Following the premature beat there is a rapid decrease in intraocular pressure; this reflects the carotid artery pressure-volume change during the missed beat (compensatory pause). The initial tonometric pulse amplitude after the compensatory pause is considerably larger than the average (compare #1 and #2 in Figure 217); after three to four more pulses the tonographic tracing resumes its normal slope. In patients tested repeatedly, the effect of single or several cardiac premature beats upon the validity of the tonogram is negligible (Figure 218). Relating the premature heartbeat to Starling's law, the tonometric pulse amplitude reflects the ventricular stroke volume finding of cardiac catheterization (7) in that the pulse

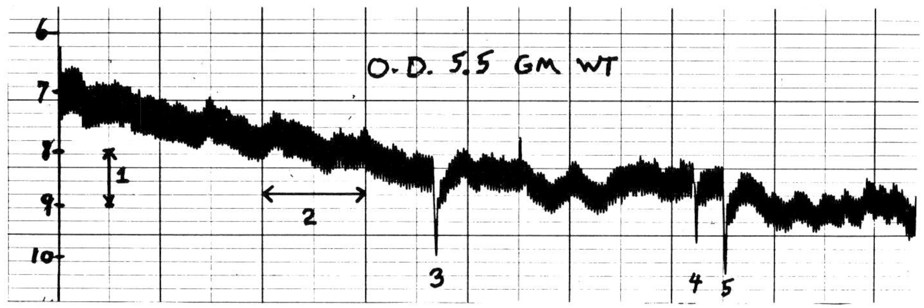

Figure 218. Tonogram in cardiac arrhythmia; 1 scale unit (#1) = 14 mm; time interval (#2) = 30 sec. Ectopic cardiac beats at #3, #4, and #5.

amplitude immediately following the compensatory pause is, in almost all instances, considerably greater than the normal pulse amplitude. With few exceptions the slow paper speed of 120 inches per hour used for tonography does not allow differentiation between premature auricular and ventricular contractions. It is assumed that most recorded premature beats are ventricular, since no increase in the tonometric pulse amplitude is noted prior to the compensatory pause.

Method 3

To investigate the relationship of tonographic data and ocular blood flow, 250 conventional tonograms of 150 normal patients who demonstrated single or multiple ectopic cardiac beats were carefully evaluated. As in previous investigations, all tonographic studies were performed using a Mueller electronic tonometer coupled to a fixed gain Leeds and Northrup Speedomax H Recorder (10). To minimize measurement error, only technically good tonographic tracings were used, and the initial ectopic (premature) cardiac beat was analyzed (Figure 219). The data recorded for statistical review included the patient's age, intraocular pressure, aqueous outflow facility value (C), tonographic pulse amplitude (Pamp), the tonographic pulse change occurring during a compensatory pause after an ectopic beat (PVC), the systemic blood pressure when available, the pulse rate, and the calculated tonometric pulse change due to blood loss from the

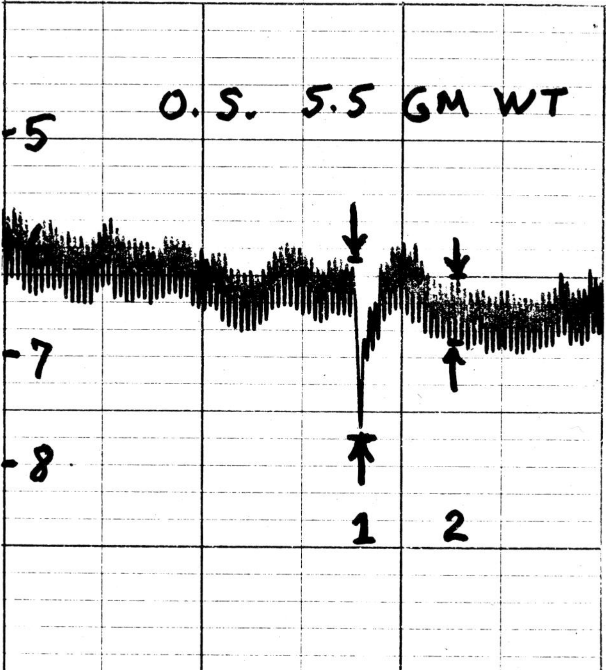

Figure 219. Tonogram in cardiac arrhythmia, comparing total ocular volume decrement (PVC) after ectopic beat (#1) with usual pulse amplitude (Pamp) (#2).

eye during the compensatory pause (PVC-Pamp). To correlate tonographic data with volume change within the eye, one must make reference to the Friedenwald tables (20) of intraocular volume change (ΔV) during tonometry (Table 23).

TABLE 23

INTRAOCULAR VOLUME CHANGES DURING TONOMETRY*

Intraocular Pressure (P_0 = mm Hg)	Tonometer Scale Reading (R)	Change in Ocular Volume (ΔV = mm^3)
22	3.5	12.4
21	4.0	14.14
19	4.5	15.87
17	5.0	17.61
16	5.5	19.35
15	6.0	21.09
13	6.5	22.86
12	7.0	24.63
11	7.5	26.41
10	8.0	28.21
9	8.5	31.87

*After Friedenwald (20).

Between tonometric scale readings of 4/5.5 g weight to 10/5.5 g weight, the volume change of corneal indentation equivalent to 0.5 scale reading varies between 1.73 mm^3 at higher levels of intraocular pressure to 1.84 mm^3 at lower intraocular pressure levels. In our tonographic technique, the vertical deflection of one tonometric scale reading equals 14 mm Hg, and is equivalent to 3.50 mm^3 intraocular volume change (Table 24). In order to assume that the change in ocular volume (ΔV) reflecting a volume change in the eye during an ectopic beat is proportional to a volume of blood change within the eye during the same missed beat, we must also assume that scleral rigidity (R), aqueous flow rate (F), aqueous outflow facility (C), and episcleral venous pressure (Pv) remain stable during the very transient change in ocular status. This assumption seems reasonable. The amount of aqueous humor expressed during one heartbeat in the average patient (heart rate 70/min. and C value of 0.28 mm^3/min./mm Hg pressure applied) would be so minimal as to require no correction. (At P_0 = 16 mm Hg, C = 0.28,

TABLE 24

TONOGRAPHY IN CARDIAC ARRHYTHMIA
250 NORMAL EYES
Conversion of scale reading to intraocular volume change

Scale Reading (R)	Vertical Deflection *mm*	Volume Change (ΔV) *mm^3*
0.5	7	3.50
1.0	14	1.75

and F = 2.0 mm^3/min., the calculated aqueous loss during one pulse beat would be 0.03 mm^3 and is therefore an insignificant amount compared to the blood loss during the same period.)

Results. The 150 patients in this study were sedentary, hospitalized males who ranged in age from 38 to 84 years, with an average age of 66 years. Some were cardiac patients, but the majority were hospitalized for surgical diseases. Although they probably do not reflect the normal population distribution in some respects, in others they would be considered average normal. None of the patients had glaucoma or other eye disease, with the exception of cataract. Tables 25 and 26 show the average and range values obtained for the study group.

TABLE 25

Tonography in Cardiac Arrhythmia
(250 Eyes)

	Average	Range
Intraocular Pressure (P_0)	13.7 mm Hg	8.25–19 mm Hg
Aqueous Facility (C)	0.25	0.13–0.51
Pulse Rate	71/min.	42–92/min.

The calculated minute ocular blood volume change from this study has limited significance concerning the total ocular blood flow unless reference can be made to blood pressure changes within the carotid artery during premature (ectopic) heartbeats. Furthermore, blood flow is more directly related to mean arterial pressure than to systolic, diastolic or pulse pressure. Cardiac catheterization studies (7,14), in which aortic pressure-volume flow measurements have been determined at the time of premature heartbeats reveal helpful information. In these studies the effective mean pressure was either measured directly or was calculated using the formula, mean arterial pressure = diastolic pressure plus $\frac{1}{3}$ pulse pressure; the data revealed that the mean carotid arterial pressure decreases

TABLE 26

Tonography in Cardiac Arrhythmia
Volume Change (ΔV) of Ectopic Beat
(250 normal eyes)

	Average	Range
Vertical Deflection	3.5 mm	1–11 mm
Pulse Amplitude (Pamp)	0.87 mm^3	0.25–2.8 mm^3
ΔV with Ectopic Beat (PVC)	3.36 mm^3	0.98–4.76 mm^3
ΔV of Missed Beat (PVC – Pamp)	2.49 mm^3	1.5–7.0 mm^3
Calculated ΔV/min. PR (PVC – Pamp)	177 mm^3/min.	70–328 mm^3/min.

10 to 15 per cent as a result of a premature beat. Applying this correction factor to the data from this study, the average ocular volume change per minute of 177 mm³ represents 0.1 to 0.15 of the total minute blood flow. The calculated human ocular minute blood flow would vary between 1770 mm³ (30 mm³/sec.) to 1133 mm³ (19 mm³/sec.).

Tonography may also be used to estimate the patency of the carotid artery when used in conjunction with carotid artery compression. The principle involved is that of unilateral digital compression of one carotid artery during tonography, which, in the normal patient, causes a sudden and rather marked decrease of intraocular pressure on the side of carotid compression (Figure 220). The 4- to 6-second period of carotid compression apparently does not allow compensatory filling of the ipsilateral ophthalmic artery through the circle of Willis (37,44). Following release of the carotid pressure the intraocular pressure rapidly returns to its previous level. Contralateral compression of the carotid artery causes no decrease of intraocular pressure of the eye undergoing tonography. This test demonstrates graphically the effect of systemic blood pressure changes upon the

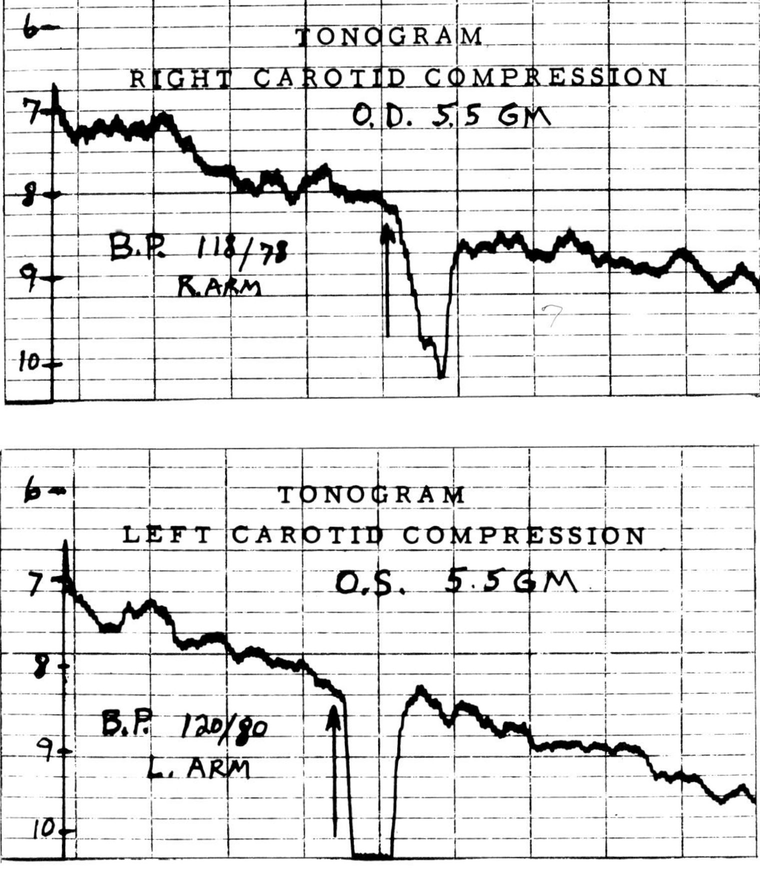

Figure 220. Carotid compression tonogram of right eye (above) and left eye (below).

eye pressure. Although purportedly avoiding the inaccuracies of ophthalmodynamometry, the tests need considerable standardization, however, for variable results may be obtained in the same individual on repeated tests. The carotid artery is difficult to palpate and compress in many patients, particularly those with muscular or obese necks. Also, there is no current method for quantitating the exact amount of direct pressure placed upon the carotid artery. A paradoxical result may even be obtained when jugular vein compression is performed without sufficient pressure being applied to produce carotid artery compression, in which case the intraocular pressure actually rises on the side of purported carotid compression; a false-positive test could thus be obtained. In spite of these limitations, the technique may aid in the diagnosing of occlusive carotid artery disease.

Ocular hemodynamics and pulsatile blood flow may also be evaluated by the technique of ocular oscillometry, which utilizes a sensitive pressure transducer connected to a perilimbal suction cup (37). Differences in the pulse amplitudes between the two eyes, responses of the ocular pulse to changes in intraocular pressure, and the effects of unilateral and bilateral carotid compression are easily recorded in the amplified pulse wave.

Recent improvements in the technique of ophthalmodynamometry (18) utilize ipsilateral mean brachial blood pressure, intraocular pressure levels, and mean ophthalmic artery occlusion pressures. With suitable correction factors, more consistent clinical correlations are thus possible.

Ophthalmodynamography (26) allows estimation of the ocular pulse, amplitude, and the ocular blood pressure in the ophthalmic artery and retinal artery. This refinement of orbital oscillometry (37) uses a sensitive pressure transducer and a technique for compression of the globe and orbital contents within the bony orbit.

SUMMARY

This presentation reviews the clinical characteristics of the normal human retinal vasculature. The ophthalmoscopic appearance of these vessels as recorded by color fundus photography is described and compared with the results obtained by fluorescein angiography, spectral reflectance, and monochromatic light photography.

The dynamics of ocular blood flow may be monitored by motion picture fundus photography. Attempts at comparative blood flow studies utilize fluorescein appearance times, radioactive tracer substances, and ophthalmodynamometry with and without carotid compression. Semiquantitative estimates of ocular blood flow are possible through the use of tonography, ocular oscillometry, and various photometric techniques.

REFERENCES

1. Adler, F. H., *Textbook of Ophthalmology* (7th ed.), Saunders, Philadelphia, 1962.
2. Allen, L., Kirkendall, W. M., Snyder, W. B., and Frazier, O., Instant positive photographs and stereograms of ocular fundus fluorescence. *Arch. Ophthal.* (Chicago), 1966, **75**: 192–198.

3. Ballantyne, A. J., and Michaelson, I. C. (Eds.), *Textbook of the Fundus of the Eye.* Williams & Wilkins, Baltimore, 1962.

4. Becker, B., and Friedenwald, J. S., Clinical aqueous outflow. *Arch. Ophthal.* (Chicago), 1953, **50**: 557–571.

5. Behrendt, T., and Wilson, L. A., Spectral reflectance photography of the retina. *Am. J. Ophthal.*, 1965, **59**: 1079–1088.

6. Beintema, D. K., Mook, G. A., and Worst, J. G. F., Arm-retinacirculatietijd met behulp van fundusreflectometrie. *Nederl. T. Geneesk.*, 1964, **108**: 1099–1100.

7. Bellet, S., *Clinical Disorders of the Heart Beat.* Lea & Febiger, Philadelphia, 1963.

8. Bettman, J. W., Fellows, V., Chao, P., and Johnson, J. P., The effect of tonography and other pressures on the intraocular blood volume. *Arch. Ophthal.* (Chicago), 1958, **60**: 230–236.

9. Broadfoot, K. D., Gloster, J., and Greaves, D. F., Photoelectric method of investigating the amount of oxygenation of blood in the fundus oculi. *Brit. J. Ophthal.*, 1961, **45**: 161–182.

10. Christensen, R. E., A tonographic recorder; for research and office practice. *Am. J. Ophthal.*, 1963, **56**: 302–307.

11. ———, Ocular photoelectric plethysmography. In preparation.

12. Christensen, R. E., and Nursall, J. F., Motion picture photography of the inner eye; technique and apparatus. *Arch. Ophthal.* (Chicago), 1963, **70**: 540–545.

13. Christensen, R. E., and Pearce, I., Homatropine hydrobromide: effect of topical administration upon the intraocular pressure and aqueous facility values of normal and chronic simple glaucomatous eyes. *Ibid.*: 376–380.

14. Corday, E., and Irving, D. W., Effect of cardiac arrhythmias on the cerebral circulation. *Am. J. Cardiol.*, 1960, **6**: 803–808.

15. Cristini, G., and Fiorenzi, G., Misura in vivo dello spessore sanguigno uveale con il nostro metodo bio-emo-fotometrico. *Minerva Oftal.*, 1961, **3**: 4–6.

16. Dollery, C. T., Hill, D. W., Mailer, C. W., and Ramalho, P. S., High oxygen pressure and the retinal blood-vessels. *Lancet*, 1964, **2**: 291–292.

17. Erbaugh, J. K., *Principles of Ophthalmoscopy.* Thomas, Springfield, 1958.

18. Evans, P. Y., Oberhoff, P., Young, P. W., and Finnerty, F. A., Jr., Standardized ophthalmodynamometry; current concepts, pitfalls, and potentials. *Georgetown Univ. Med. Cent. Bull.*, 1964, **18**: 83–105.

19. Frayser, R., and Hickam, J. B., Retinal vascular response to breathing increased carbon dioxide and oxygen concentrations. *Invest. Ophthal.*, 1964, **3**: 427–431.

20. Friedenwald, J. S., Tonometer calibration; an attempt to remove discrepancies found in 1954 calibration for Schiotz tonometers. *Trans. Am. Acad. Ophthal. Otolaryng.*, 1956, **61**: 108–126.

21. Garrison, L., Christensen, R. E., and Allen, R. A., Angle-closure glaucoma from metastatic carcinoma. *Am. J. Ophthal.*, 1967, **63**: 503–507.

22. Gass, J. D. M., Pathogenesis of disciform detachment of the neuroepithelium. *Ibid.*: 587–615.

23. Gifford, S. R., *A Textbook of Ophthalmology.* Saunders, Philadelphia, 1941.

24. Gowers, W. R., *A Manual and Atlas of Medical Ophthalmology.* Blakiston, Philadelphia, 1882.

25. Haddad, H. M., and Leopold, I. H., Effect of hyperbaric oxygenation on microcirculation: use in therapy of retinal vascular disorders. *Invest. Ophthal.*, 1965, **4**: 1141–1151.

26. Hager, H., Objektive elektrische Dinamometrie mit Hilfe des Bulbus-Orbita-Pulses. In: *Acta XVIII Councilium Ophthalmologicum (Belgica)*, 1958 Vol. II:1302–1306.
27. Hart, L. M., Heyman, A., Linhart, J. W., McIntosh, H., and David, N. J., Fluorescence motion picture photography of the retinal circulation; a description of technique and normal retinal blood flow. *J. Lab. Clin. Med.*, 1963, **62**: 703–709.
28. Hayreh, S. S., The central artery of the retina; its role in the blood supply of the optic nerve. *Brit. J. Ophthal.*, 1963, **47**: 651–665.
29. Hedges, T. R., Ophthalmic artery cannulation. *Trans. Am. Ophthal. Soc.*, 1963, **61**: 560.
30. Hickam, J. B., and Frayser, R., A photographic method for measuring the mean retinal circulation time using fluorescein. *Invest. Ophthal.*, 1965, **4**: 876–884.
31. His, W., Abbildungen über das Gefässsystem der menschlichen Netzhaut und derjenigen des Kaninchens. *Arch. Anat. Physiol.*, 1880: 224–231.
32. Hodge, J. V., and Clemett, R. S., Improved method for fluorescence angiography of the retina. *Am. J. Ophthal.*, 1966, **61**: 1400–1404.
33. Jensen, V. H., Studies on the branchings of the retinal blood-vessels. *Acta Ophthal.* (Kobenhavn), 1936, **14**: 100–109.
34. Kimura, S. J., and Caygill, W. M. (Eds.), *Retinal Diseases: A Symposium.* Lea & Febiger, Philadelphia, 1966.
35. Kreiker, A., Ueber die Entstehungsweise des Lichtreflexes auf den Netzhautgefässen. *Klin. Mbl. Augenheilk.*, 1924, **72**: 621–628.
36. Kuwabara, T., and Cogan, D. G., Studies of retinal vascular patterns. I. Normal architecture. *Arch. Ophthal.* (Chicago), 1960, **64**: 904–911.
37. Lester, H. A., Ocular oscillometry in cerebrovascular disease. *Arch. Ophthal.* (Chicago), 1966, **76**: 391–398.
38. Michaelson, I. C., and Campbell, A. C. P., The anatomy of the finer retinal vessels, and some observations on their significance in certain retinal diseases. *Trans. Ophthal. Soc. UK*, 1940, **60**: 71–112.
39. Moses, R. A., Intra-ocular circulation and pressure. In: *Modern Ophthalmology, Vol. I: Basic Aspects* (A. Sorsby, Ed.). Butterworths, London, 1963: 290–303.
40. Niedermeier, S., Spektrofotografische Aderhautmessung. *Klin. Mbl. Augenheilk.*, 1958, **132**: 828–839.
41. Nieveen, J., van der Slikke, L. B., and Reichert, W. J., Photoelectric plethysmography using reflected light. *Cardiologia* (Basel), 1956, **29**: 160–173.
42. Norton, E. W. D., Gass, J. D., Smith, J. L., Curtin, V. T., David, N. J., and Justice, J., Jr., Fluorescein in the study of macular disease. *Trans. Am. Acad. Ophthal. Otolaryng.*, 1965, **69**: 631–642.
43. Novotny, H. R., and Alvis, D. L., A method of photographing fluorescence in circulating blood in the human retina. *Circulation*, 1961, **24**: 82–86.
44. Oldendorf, W. H., and Crandall, P. H., Bilateral cerebral circulation curves obtained by intravenous injection of radioisotopes. *J. Neurosurg.*, 1961, **18**: 195–200.
45. Oosterhuis, J. A., and Lammens, A. J. J., Fluorescein photography of the ocular fundus. *Ophthalmologica*, 1965, **149**: 210–220.
46. Rushton, W. A. H., The difference spectrum and the photosensitivity of rhodopsin in the living human eye. *J. Physiol.* (London), 1956, **134**: 11–29.
47. Schubert, B., Untersuchung des Blutsauerstoffgehaltes und der Durchblutung des

Auges auf lichtelektrischem Wege. *Graefe Arch. klin. exp. Ophthal.*, 1936, **135**: 558–560.

48. Seitz, R., *The Retinal Vessels; Comparative Ophthalmoscopic and Histologic Studies on Healthy and Diseased Eyes* (F. C. Blodi, Transl.). Mosby, St. Louis, 1964.
49. Stokoe, N. L., and Turner, R. W. D., Normal retinal vascular pattern; arterio-venous ratio as a measure of arterial calibre. *Brit. J. Ophthal.*, 1966, **50**: 21–40.
50. Swan, K. C., and Bailey, P., Jr., Cinematography of the retinal vessels. *Trans. Am. Ophthal. Soc.*, 1959, **57**: 210–220.
51. Tominaga, Y., and Ikui, H., The fine structure of the arterio-venous crossing parts in the human retina (the preliminary report). *Acta Soc. Ophthal. Jap.*, 1964, **68**: 148–150.
52. Trokel, S., Photometric study of ocular blood flow in man. *Arch. Ophthal.* (Chicago), 1964, **71**: 528–530.
53. ———, Quantitative studies of choroidal blood flow by reflective densitometry. *Invest. Ophthal.*, 1965, **4**: 1129–1140.
54. Vogt, A., Herstellung eines gelbblauen Lichtfiltrates, in welchem die Macula centralis in vivo in gelber Färbung erscheint, die Nervenfasern der Netzhaut und andere feine Einzelheiten derselben sichtbar werden, und der Grad der Gelbfärfund der Linse ophthalmoskopisch nachweisbar ist. *Graefe Arch. klin. exp. Ophthal.*, 1913, **84**: 293–311.
55. Walsh, F. B., Some considerations regarding occlusive vascular disease. *Am. J. Ophthal.*, 1963, **55**: 1–18.
56. Wolff, E., *Anatomy of the Eye and Orbit*, 5th ed. (R. J. Last, Rev.). Lewis, London, 1961.

VISUAL ACUITY *

KENNETH N. OGLE †
Mayo Clinic and Mayo Foundation
Rochester, Minnesota

The term "visual acuity" usually conveys the idea of sharpness of vision—a somewhat vague phrase which perhaps should be left so. I shall use "visual acuity" to indicate the degree to which the eye is able to discriminate small details within and between objects. The basic underlying capacity of the eye in this respect is the visual discrimination of contrast,‡ and this leads to the major aspect of visual acuity, namely visual resolving power. With certain types of test details, it is impossible to differentiate between contrast discrimination and visual resolution. For the most part, visual resolution pertains to a person's ability to discriminate whether adjacent contours appear as one or two.

Since some of the significant facts and problems of visual acuity have recently been considered by Le Grand (34), Adler (1), Pirenne (54), Riggs (59), Westheimer (70) and others, it will be unnecessary to treat each topic in great detail in this review.

Visual Direction Sense of the Eye

It is important to reiterate the common experience that separate objects in the field of view are perceived in different visual directions (48). The difference is certainly related to the actual angular separations of the objects subtended at the eye, which in turn must correspond to a separation of the objects' images on the retina. We must attribute the discrimination of differences in visual direction, first, to the discrete character of the organization of the retinal receptors, an organization that consists of a mosaic of separated and effectively insulated light-sensitive elements, and second, to the continued topographical identity of those

* This investigation was supported in part by Research Grant NB-1637 from the National Institute of Neurological Diseases and Blindness, U.S. Public Health Service.

† Dr. Ogle passed away February 22, 1968.

‡ Contrast is defined as the difference in luminance of the test details, above or below the background luminance, divided by the background luminance. That is, $C = (I_s - I_b)/I_b$, in which I_s is the luminance of the test details and I_b that of the background or adaptation level. This ratio, when multiplied by 100, gives the percentage of contrast. If the luminance of the test details, I_s, is higher than that of the background (as with point light sources), C is positive; if I_s is lower than I_b (as with the Landolt ring), C is negative. The contrast threshold of the eye, as determined experimentally, would be the least difference between the luminance of the stimulus and the luminance of the background ($I_s - I_b$) that the eye can detect.

elements in the organization of nerve fibers connecting them to the terminal areas in the occipital cortex of the brain.

It logically follows that associated with each stimulated receptor (or receptor unit in the periphery) there emerges a specific subjective visual direction—a local sign—which differs from the direction of any other receptor (or receptor unit) when stimulated. This conclusion seems inescapable. The principal question is, are these relative visual directions—these local signs—stable? The evidence suggests that they are, or that at least they maintain their ordinal values of relative subjective direction. Visual acuity, in its broadest sense, and resolving power in particular, depend on the least difference in visual direction that can be discriminated.

Visual acuity would also include the smallest details with barely identifiable shapes or forms. This, like visual resolution, depends on the direction sense associated with receptor elements of the retina.

Resolving power alone, however, may not be a complete measure of the absolute ability of the eye to discriminate the fine aspects of visual space. For example, the minimum angle of resolution at the 50 per cent level of probable resolution of two point light sources arranged in the horizontal meridian is about 56 seconds of arc, with a standard deviation of about 10 seconds of arc. The discrimination of the minimum horizontal displacement of the central of three vertically separated point light sources is more precise, the accuracy varying with the separation of the outer lights. At the 75 per cent level of probable discrimination, the threshold displacement at the minimum was found to be about 2 seconds of arc for a separation of the outer points of light of 15 minutes of arc (37) (see also the discussion of Figure 235*). Although this precision is definitely an aspect of the ability of the eye to discriminate differences in visual direction, visual resolution cannot account directly for it.

Blur Disk on the Retina

Every discussion of resolving power is confronted with the fact that the dioptric image on the retina of even a point of light in space, with sharpest focus, is a blur disk, within which there is a variation in illuminance (Figure 221A). The distribution of light in the disk is known as the "spread function", and is essentially the older concept of irradiation. Such a disk usually falls on a number of retinal receptors or receptor units. *Herein lies the critical problem in visual acuity: how can we account for the delicacy of visual detection and resolution when the images on the retina are so relatively large?*

For an extended luminous surface, the image on the retina is also larger than that to be expected on the basis of geometric optics (Figure 221B), but for a small black area on an illuminated surface the contrast is reduced because of the filling in of the geometric image (Figure 221C). The size of the blur disk will depend on the pupil size, accuracy of the eye's focus, the particular distribution of light wavelengths, and scattering of light by retinal tissues. In the case of small pupils (less

---

* Page 459.

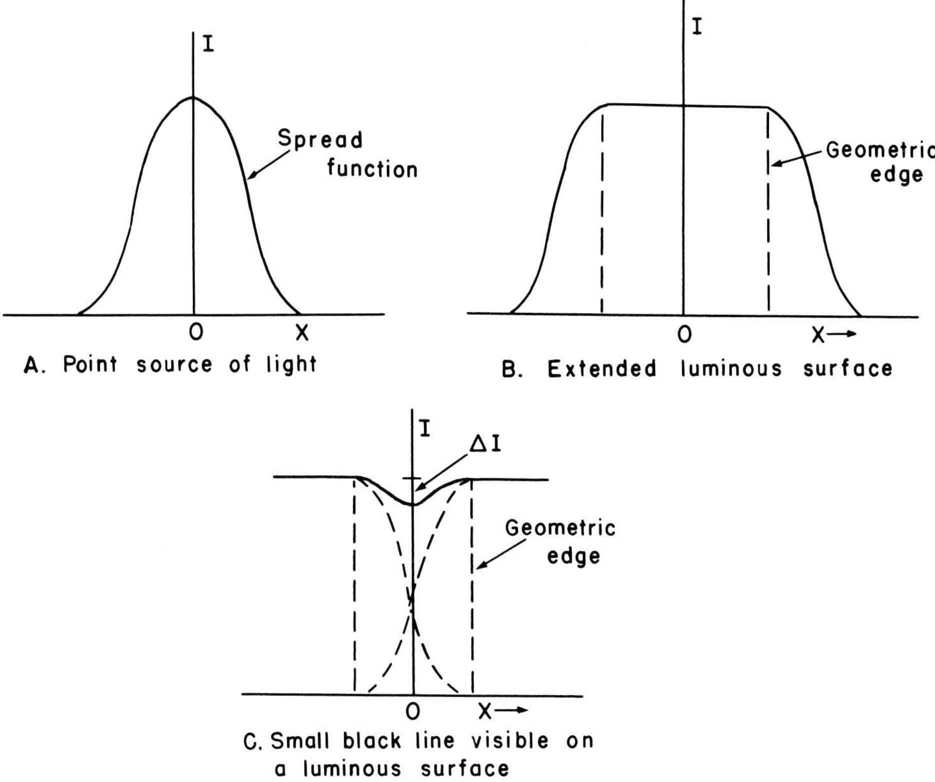

Figure 221. Schematic representation of the distribution of illuminance in the dioptric image falling on the retina for three types of test targets (*A*, *B*, *C*).

than 1.5 mm in diameter), the size of the disk will be due solely to diffraction and chromatic aberration; for large pupils, spherical aberration plays the greater role in the formation of the blur disk.

The visual or subjective size of the disk will depend on a number of factors, especially on the spread function, the contrast threshold of the retina (ΔI, the least difference in illuminance that can be detected), and therefore on the light adaptation level (I), because the outer portions of the lightspread will generally be below contrast threshold, the finite areas (cross section) of the receptors, and probably on neurologic interactions between retinal receptors associated with stimulation and with lateral inhibition. Under critical conditions, the threshold of resolution will depend on the contrast threshold of the eye.

Consider the problem posed by the familiar Landolt ring (Figure 222): how small can we make the ring and still perceive the gap? There is general agreement that in the image of the ring on the retina there must be at least one receptor element (or group of elements), corresponding to the center of the gap image, which is more highly illuminated than are the neighboring elements corresponding to the dark portions forming the gap. The difference in these illuminances will diminish as the size of the gap decreases. The smallest size which allows detection

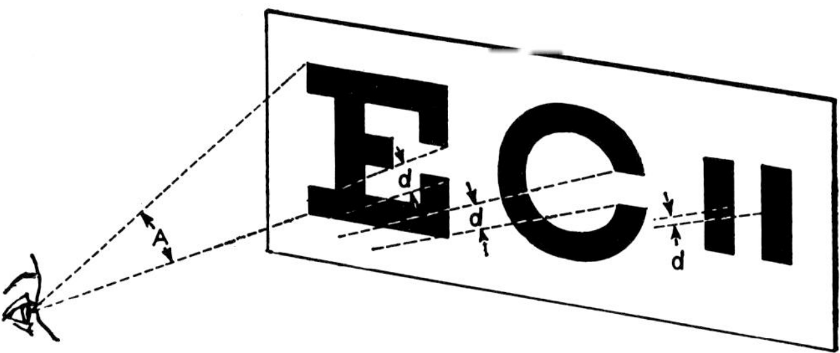

Figure 222. Method of specifying the angle of resolution for three types of test targets. (From *IES Lighting Handbook*, 29.)

of this difference will determine the threshold of resolution. Though the detection of the separation of contours per se is clearly not involved in this example, the minimum angle of resolution is defined as the angle, α, subtended by the gap to the eye. This minimum angle of resolution will vary with test conditions, especially with the relative luminance between the background and the dark ring.

Traditionally, this minimum angle of resolution, α, is expressed in minutes of arc. Under test conditions, resolving power of the eye is defined as the reciprocal of α (RP $= 1/\alpha$), when α is expressed in minutes of arc.

Meaning of a Threshold

It should be emphasized that even under constant test conditions the minimum angle of resolution of the eye, like all other physiologic processes, is subject to random variations. These variations, often with no apparent cause, may include physical fluctuations in number of light quanta absorbed, differences in discharge rates of adjacent receptor cells of the retina, and perhaps oscillations in the activity of cells in the central nervous system. They also may include optical factors such as fluctuations in the accommodation, uneven tearing on the surface of the cornea, and so forth.

The definition of a *threshold* must therefore deal with a statistical quantity. For a particular angular size of the Landolt ring, for example, the gap may never be perceived, whereas for a somewhat larger ring the gap can always be apprehended. There is a certain probability that any given size of gap between these rings will be detected. In painstaking laboratory experiments using the method of constant stimuli, this probability can be determined for each of a sequence of sizes (usually five). When the probability of detection is plotted against the angular size of the ring gap, the usual psychophysical sigmoid curve is obtained, from which a threshold size corresponding to any selected level of probability can be found.

The most accurate threshold size is that which has a 50 per cent probability of being perceived. The rate of change in probability of detection with change in stimulus size (the slope of the central portion of the curve) is a measure of the variability. Thus, the criterion used in determining visual acuity must always be stated. Often we are effectively speaking of a mean value, which is a variable measure.

Even with the letter test chart, the examiner, in asking the patient to read the letters in successive lines, may be using a crude constant stimulus method by selecting as the threshold the letter size corresponding roughly to perhaps a 90 per cent level of probable identification.

Basic Considerations

The classic and basic test object for studying visual resolution consists of two point sources of light. This type of test is important in laboratory studies seeking the basic characteristics of visual resolution; it is not suitable for general acuity testing. As stated previously, the dioptric image on the retina of a point light source is spread over a small area within which the illuminance decreases rapidly from the center. An estimate of the distribution of the illuminance within the area has been made by means of instrumentation which measures the light reflected from this area from the retina (32,71) (actually, luminous lines rather than point sources are commonly used). Except at the exact center, this distribution of the spread can be described approximately by $I = I_0 \exp(-a|x|)$, where I is the illuminance at a point at an angular distance x from the center of the area, and a is approximately unity for point light sources. Although knowledge of this spread function describing the illuminance of the image is important, we are more interested subsequently in a *sensation* spread function. The size of this spread will depend on the luminous intensity of the point source of light, the luminance of the background, the pupil size, the degree to which the dioptric image is focused sharply on the retina, and probably on certain neurologic processes.

Data on the foveal contrast threshold (whether the light is perceived or not) for a point source of light for different amounts of blurring of the dioptric image on the retina are illustrated graphically in Figure 223 (45); the graph shows that, as the image is blurred by being made out of focus, the threshold rapidly increases. A theoretical study of these data suggested that, even under these threshold conditions with 20 msec. exposure, there is effectively a minimum diameter of the sensation spread area, or neural unit, of about 5 minutes of arc.

Data on the foveal contrast threshold for two point sources of light, the separation of which can be changed from zero (superposition) to 6 minutes of arc, are shown graphically in Figure 224 (47). The subject reported only whether he perceived light from the sources, not whether he saw one or two lights. These results show that, with a natural pupil, an interaction appears to occur between the two point sources, in the sense of a partial summation of the luminous energy, until the separation becomes 3 to 4 minutes of arc; this critical separation varies somewhat between subjects. With momentary exposures we find no evidence that the stimulation from one source inhibits the response from the other, because the threshold levels off at 0.3 log unit (*two times*) above that detected when the two sources are superposed. There is evidence that, had one of the two point sources of light been exposed continuously, and the threshold of the second then determined with brief exposure, an inhibitory effect might have been found. This supposition

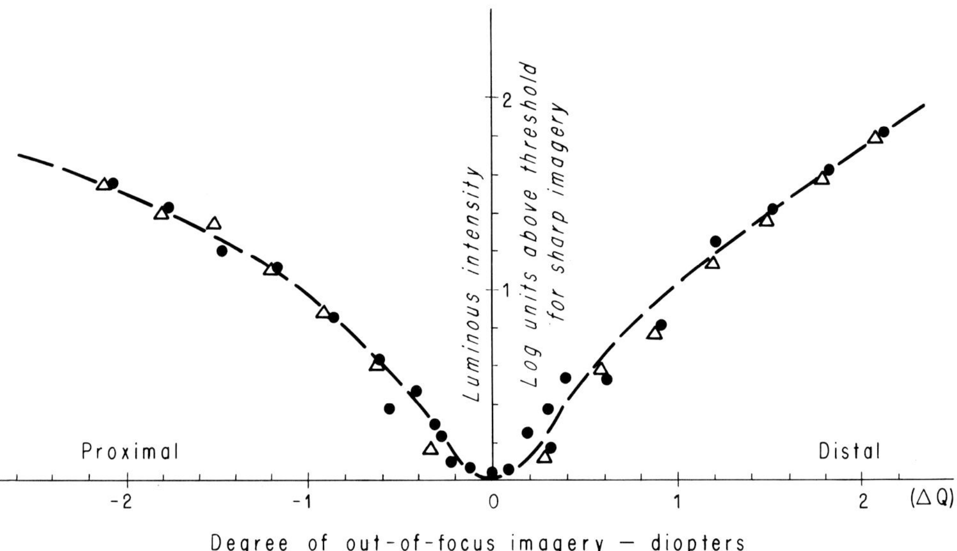

Figure 223. Contrast thresholds for a point light source with different degrees of out-of-focus blurring (in diopters). (From Ogle, 45.)

is based on the concept that the effect of inhibition may increase spatially with time.

The minimum angle of resolution for point light sources is smaller than the critical angle shown in these graphs. This means that there is some mutual enhancement or interaction between the images, even though they may appear resolved.

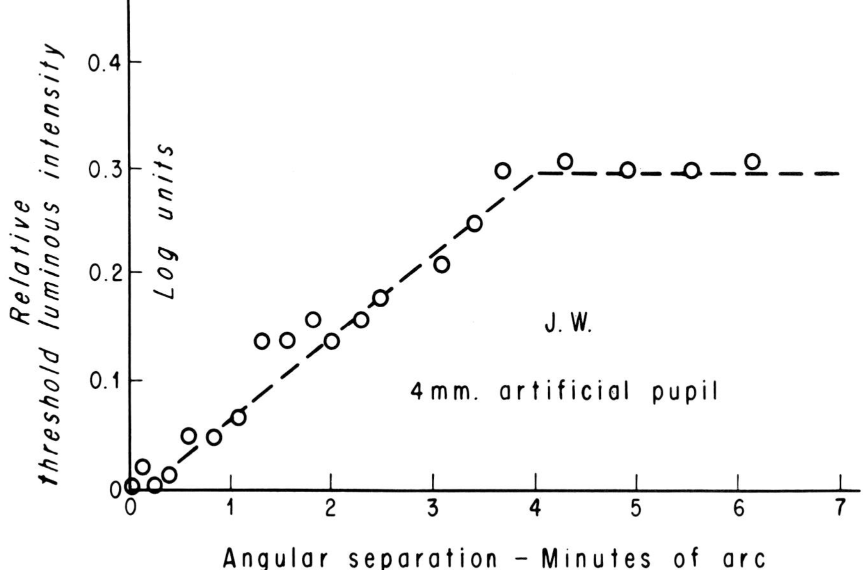

Figure 224. Contrast threshold for two point light sources with increasing separations, exposed for 20 msec. (From Ogle, 47.)

At this point we could perhaps inject some pragmatism, and ask why we are interested in visual acuity and its measurement from such a scientific point of view. Ordinarily, the ophthalmologist is content to use a letter chart with which he can arrive at a refractive correction to give the patient 20/20 (6/6) visual acuity; he may also use his letter chart to obtain an approximate idea of the reduction of visual acuity in pathologic conditions or changes therein. For these purposes, the ordinary Snellen letter chart (provided it is clean and properly illuminated) is sufficient. The ophthalmologist becomes very familiar with his own chart and it serves his purposes adequately. Problems arise, however, when clinicians have to compare their findings as, for example, to establish eligibility of patients for benefits or for admission to sight-saving classes. More important, accurate measurement of visual acuity may be necessary to establish fitness for particular job placements in industrial organizations, and especially in the military services. It behooves us, therefore, to determine the most reliable and meaningful test, even though no single test may ever be adequate in all situations nor will any one test meet all requirements.

Visual Acuity Test Targets

Nearly all visual acuity targets make use of one or a combination of several basic types of task details. Figure 225 illustrates the important ones, together with several more complex tasks; certain tests that depend on contrast discrimination alone have been excluded. All the tests of resolving power require suprathreshold contrasts, but targets are sometimes designed with reduced contrast, such as gray instead of black letters.

It should be mentioned that visual acuity is relatively good for monochromatic test objects which differ from their backgrounds in hue but not in brightness (15);

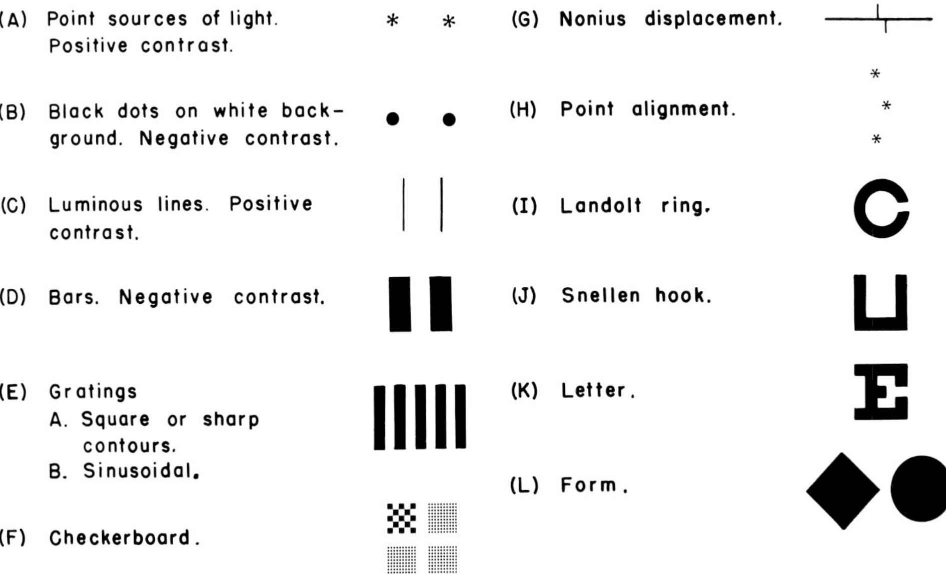

Figure 225. Basic types of details for testing visual acuity.

better acuity is obtained from highly saturated hues with large wavelength differences, even complementary hues. These findings are important in the design of anaglyphs with which stereoscopic depth from photographs or drawings can be obtained.

Point Light Sources

The visual resolution of point light sources is often considered the basic test because of its simplicity. The theoretical implications of the test, however, may be far from simple. The resolving power of the point light sources cannot be found consistently at contrast thresholds determined for the 50 per cent level of probable perceptibility, so that measurements of the minimum angle of resolution must be made at luminous intensities of the point sources considerably above threshold—at least above the 99 per cent level of probable visibility. At these levels there may be some interaction (a summation or inhibition) between the responses from the two sources, even though resolvable.

Determination of resolving power with point light sources involves the problem of criterion. As the separation of the two sources is slowly increased from superposition, the resultant image appears circular, then oblong, then dumbbell-shaped, and finally as two fully separated images. One may say that, if the image appears as an ellipse or (certainly) as a dumbbell, the points must be resolved; this, however, is only an inference. The minimum angle of resolution measured from center to center of the sources would be smaller in these cases than if the criterion of absolute separation were demanded. (It is highly probable that many of the early reports of resolution of double stars of the order of 1 minute of arc sprang from inferred resolution based on image shapes.) In the experiments reported herein, complete separation was the criterion. Figure 226 shows a schematic distribution of the illuminance of separated images of point light sources in the central meridian. The illuminance difference (ΔI) at the center must be greater than the contrast threshold if the point sources are to appear

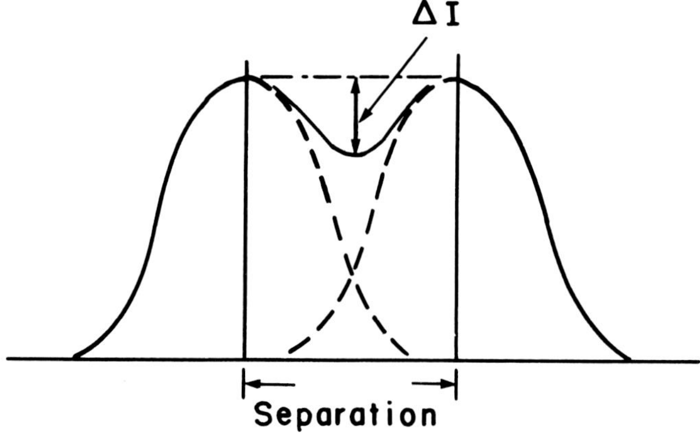

Figure 226. Scheme of the addition of illuminances of the images of separated point light sources.

separated. It must be remembered that the illuminance distribution is over an area. The perceptual response to the luminance energy represented by the difference in illuminance (ΔI) will depend also on the separations and the cross section areas of the retinal receptors.

Three results from resolving power experiments with point light sources should be recognized.

a. With a given luminance of the background, an *increase* in the luminous intensity of the point light sources results in a *larger* minimum of resolution, that is, a decrease in resolving power.

b. If the ratio of the luminous intensity of the point light sources to the luminance of the background is kept *constant*, the resolving power is the same, independent of changes in intensities of the sources or the background luminance. This means that the resolving power of point light sources depends only on the contrast (Figure 227) (43). These data also show that the minimum angle of resolution *increases* with contrast, which would be consistent with *a*.

c. For low contrasts, the minimum angle of resolution was found to remain almost constant for a contrast range of about 1 log unit (49) (Figure 228). However, the precision with which the data for resolution could be obtained diminished with the decrease in contrast, i.e., the standard deviations of the measurements increased with decrease in contrast.

To explain these results, the existence of integrative areas in the fovea has been postulated, their size decreasing with increase in intensity of the point light sources. The concept of integrative areas whose size decreases with illuminance of the retinal image could also be interpreted as an increase in extent of an inhibition surrounding the image (58) (see Figure 243).

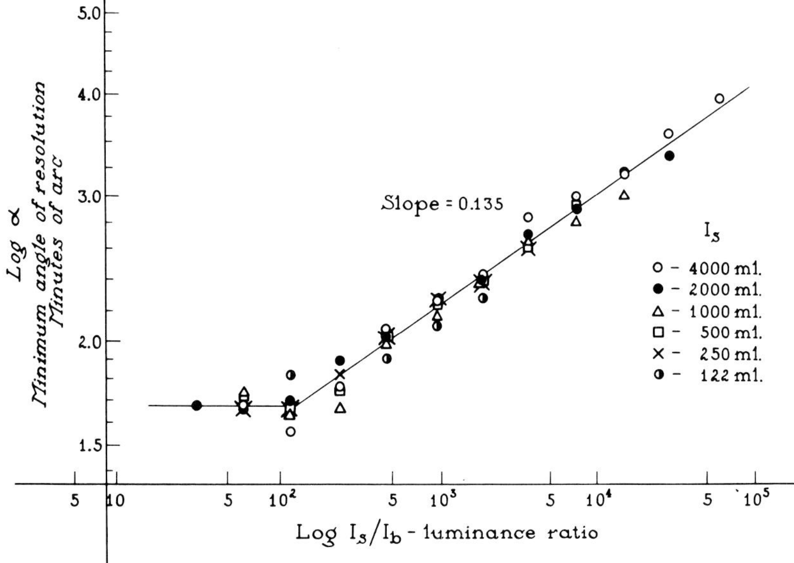

Figure 227. Data showing that the minimum angle of resolution of point sources of light is dependent on contrast. (From Ogle, 43.)

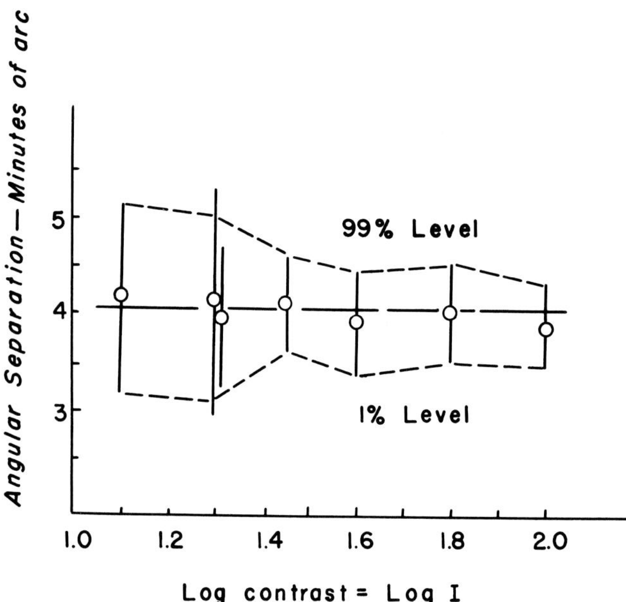

Figure 228. Data showing a relatively constant minimum angle of resolution for increases in contrast for a range of low contrasts. (From Ogle, 49.)

There is increasing evidence from electrophysiological as well as psychophysical studies supporting the concept of inhibition. This has also proved to be a possible explanation for the apparent sharpening of contours or borders between light and dark areas and for the appearance of Mach bands near the lines of discontinuities in graded illuminance patterns. The apparent sharpening of borders surrounding the images of the objects may be an important aspect in the discrimination of form (23). Whether or not it plays a role in visual acuity, where the discrimination is so near threshold, is not clear. On the other hand, there seems to be a mutual enhancement of contiguous images in the contours perceived; a luminous line appears brighter than a point source of light of the same luminous intensity.

Black Dots

Small black dots with various separations on a white background provide a resolution task similar to the points of light but with negative contrast. This test is rarely applied in resolution experiments, but is sometimes useful in "push up" tests to estimate the effect of retinal image blurring on resolution and visibility.

Narrow Luminous Lines

Narrow luminous lines have been used for resolution experiments principally in the laboratory to test optical theories of dioptric image formation on the retina and visual responses, since calculation of distribution of illuminance from diffraction theory is somewhat simpler for line targets.

Black Lines or Bars on Light Background

Black bars printed on a white background in a series of rows with decreasing separation have been used occasionally in wall charts. At a fixed distance, the minimum angle of visual resolution could be estimated from the row for which the gap could no longer be detected. The standard design of these bars specifies them as five units high, one unit wide, and separated by one unit. Increasing the length of the bars up to a limit tends to improve visual resolution.

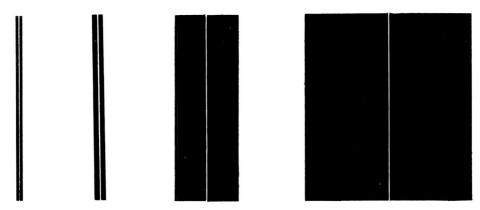

Figure 229. Illustration of the effect of increasing and decreasing the width of the bar test pattern on "visual acuity". The spacing between the bars is the same in all four patterns. (After Wilcox & Purdy, 73.)

Modifying the width and separation of the bars brings out pointedly the problem of distinguishing between resolution per se and simple contrast discrimination. Figure 229 illustrates this clearly: the bars in each of the four patterns are equally separated; at the left they are essentially narrow lines equal in width to the separation; at the right they are very wide. The detection of the space in the left pattern might be considered a resolution problem, but on the right it is purely a matter of contrast discrimination. It is also readily evident that the space between the wide bars can be seen from much greater distances than that between the narrow bars. These effects are usually explained in terms of the spread function, wherein the resultant central difference in illuminance between the bars at the left is small, while that between the bars at the right is pronounced. This problem is obviously important in the design and standardization of optotypes or test figures.

The Grating

The grating—a series of equidistant parallel black and white stripes—is an important extension of the two-bar test idea, and has been used extensively in determining the resolution of optical systems and photographic films. With the eye, it is proving to be useful, although it complicates the light-dark illuminance image pattern on the retina and the sensory responses to that pattern, for it implicates a larger number of retinal receptors than do the simpler targets. Grating test targets of various designs have been proposed over the years, and instruments using the grating principle, such as the Ives acuity meter, have been built for clinical use to measure visual acuity.

The use of the grating leads to a revised specification of visual acuity measurements in terms of the "spatial frequency response of the eye". Ordinarily, when the spacing (usually equal) of the light and dark bands of a given grating is such that the bands are just resolvable, the minimum angle of resolution would be defined as the angle subtended by the light band. The reciprocal of this angle in minutes would be the usual measure of the visual acuity; thus, if the angle subtended by the light band was 0.8 minute of arc, the visual acuity would be 1.25.

The angular distance from the edge of one dark band to the next dark band (the sum of the angular widths of one light and one dark band) is called a "cycle". The spatial frequency of a given grating would be the reciprocal of this angular subtense, that is, cycles per unit of angle. Thus, in the example just given, a cycle would be 1.6 minutes of arc, whence the spatial frequency would be 0.62 cycle per minute of arc, or 37 cycles per arc degree. For a low-frequency grating—wide separations of the bars—the bars are easily resolved visually; as the frequency increases (the separation of the bars decreases), a frequency is attained at which the lines of the grating can barely be resolved. In simplest terms, we might represent the spatial frequency response of the eye in terms of the probability of resolution (percentage of the times the subject can resolve the bars out of a number of exposures) as a series of different grating frequencies, perhaps as shown in Figure 230. The frequency at which the grating spaces become so small that they cannot be resolved, i.e., where the curve intersects the abscissa, is said to be the

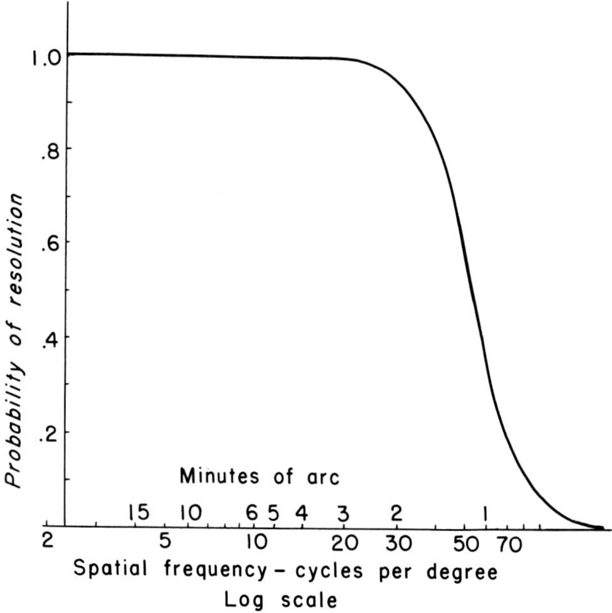

Figure 230. Schematic representation of the spatial frequency of a grating test target and the probability of visual resolution for one contrast and one mean luminance.

"frequency cutoff point"; this would be a critical measure of visual acuity with the grating test target.

Most grating targets are designed with sharp edges or contours between the light and dark spaces, to achieve abrupt contrast changes. Recent studies have been made with grating targets in which the contrast between light and dark spaces varies sinusoidally, that is, the transitions between the lighter and the darker contrasts are gradual, like the curve of a sine function. Such grating patterns can be obtained on a cathode-ray oscilloscope. Figure 231 illustrates the modulation transfer frequencies from recent data (52) obtained with sinusoidal gratings for four mean retinal illuminances. For a given grating frequency, the contrast—difference in luminances between the light and dark stripes—is found for visual resolution thresholds; these thresholds are plotted in terms of percentage of contrast. For the mean retinal illuminance of 100 trolands, the cutoff spatial frequency is about 50 cycles per arc degree. This, then, corresponds to a visual angle of 0.02 arc degree per cycle, or to a visual angle between the light stripes of 0.01 degree (or 0.6 minute) of arc; the visual acuity in usual units would then be 1.67. One advantage of the frequency modulation curves is that peculiarities in the resolution response become evident in departures from smooth curves. Even more recently, a sinusoidal grating has been designed (11) with increasing frequency to the right and with an overall increase in contrast from the top to the bottom of the target; by observing this target under adequate lighting, one can almost trace the contrast-frequency response curve.

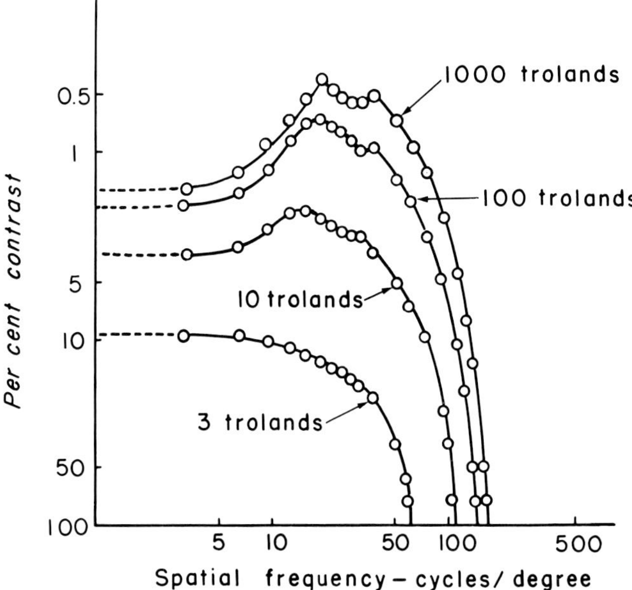

Figure 231. Illustration of frequency modulation transform curves for expressing visual sensitivity for resolution of sinusoidal gratings for different mean retinal illuminances and grating frequencies. (Data from Patel, 52.)

A further extension of the grating method of visual acuity measurement was the determination of the visual resolution of the *retina* independent of the optical system of the eye, by producing Young's interference fringes at the retina. This concept originated with Le Grand (33), and has been used variously by other investigators, most recently by Campbell & Green (13), who used the coherent light from a continuous gas laser. Two beams of nearly monochromatic light are projected into the eye, the frequency of the two beams differing in phase depending on the difference in the lengths of the two paths. By varying the phase difference, the spatial frequency of the interference pattern falling on the retina can be varied also, and the threshold frequency for visual resolution can easily be found. Le Grand (33) compared the resolution of the retinal interference pattern and the normal resolution of an equivalent grating presented to the whole eye by using an artificial pupil 3 mm in diameter. Some of his results (Table 27) show that for high luminances resolution depends on retinal structure, while for low luminances it is influenced by optical aberrations of the eye.

TABLE 27

Resolution of Retinal interference Patterns Compared with Normal Resolution of an Equivalent Grating Presented to the Whole Eye *
(Artificial pupil, 3 mm in diameter)

Mean Illuminance	Minimum Angle of Resolution Retinal	Whole Eye
50 Lux	75″	78″
0.01 Lux	87″	120″

* Data from Le Grand (33).

These grating experiments are of considerable theoretical interest. On the basis of their results, efforts have been made to derive the excitation and inhibition spread functions, both optical and physiological. The cumulative results of the studies in this area are not complete enough to establish their ultimate usefulness. Neither are they particularly helpful as yet in solving the problem of visual resolution in its more microscopic aspects, since too many retinal elements are involved in the perception of the grating. There is also evidence that with blurred

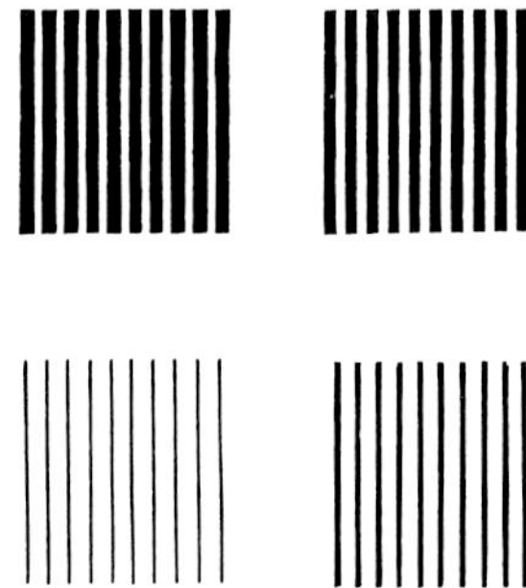

Figure 232. Series of grating targets having the same spatial frequency but varying widths of the dark and white stripes, all of which give approximately the same visual resolution. (After Lehmann, 35.)

imagery the grating type test target can lead to spurious resolution; uncorrected astigmatism may also influence the degree of visual resolution in these tests.

One of the interesting results found in the visual resolution of grating targets was described many years ago by Lehmann (35), to the effect that, for a series of gratings with the same spatial frequency but with varying widths of light and dark bars (the sum of the widths of the light and dark bars is kept constant), the visual resolution is approximately the same. Four gratings of such a series are shown in Figure 232. Thus it appears that, with the grating target, visual resolution does not depend on the width of either the dark or the light bands, but only on the spatial frequency.

The Checkerboard

The checkerboard design of a visual acuity test type has been subject to much research. With careful design, it has been declared to provide the purest measure of visual resolution. In part originally suggested by Goldmann (26) as an optokinetic test target, the useful chart consists of four squares of equal size, one of which is a black and white checkerboard (Figure 233); each of the other three squares is variously composed of closely spaced black dots arranged in rows. Ideally, when the angular size of the target is too small for the checkerboard to be discriminated, all four squares appear equally and uniformly gray.

In the test the chart is oriented at random, but so that the checkerboard square is always either up or down; when the target is exposed, the observer is asked to state the position of the checkerboard. When the threshold of discrimination of a given chart is attained from progressively smaller charts, the minimum angle of resolution is taken as the visual angle subtended by the width of one of the squares in the checkerboard; the visual acuity would be the reciprocal of this angle when expressed in minutes of arc. Great care must be taken in the actual construction of the target, for secondary cues unrelated to visual resolution may make one of the squares appear different, which would make the checkerboard identifiable.

When a given chart has been validated, it is most useful in the determination of small changes in visual acuity with greater precision than is possible with other charts (42). This target has been used in measuring visual acuity at extremely low levels of illumination. Although for highest precision psychophysical methods should be used, the chart has been incorporated into instruments for machine

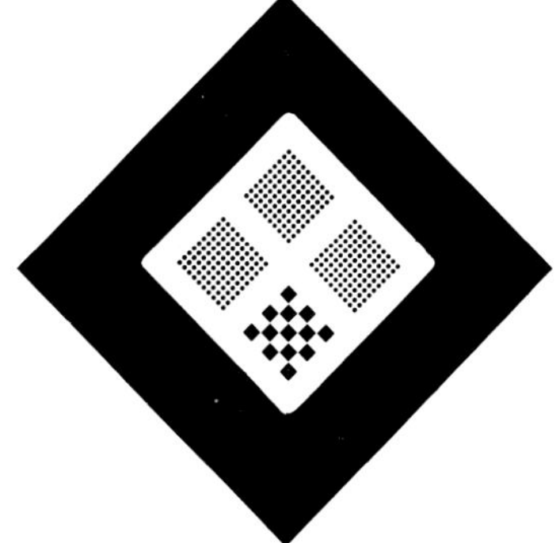

Figure 233. The checkerboard visual resolution test target.

testing of visual acuity when no greater precision than that corresponding to the ordinary measures of visual acuity is desired.

The Nonius (Vernier) Acuity Test

The nonius (vernier) acuity test (Figure 234) for the discrimination of a break or discontinuity in alignment has been of great theoretical and practical interest. With it, displacement can be detected with higher precision than with any of the other visual acuity test details.* Many experiments record that under adequate lighting and with high contrast the break can be discriminated when the angular displacement of the lines is perhaps 2 to 5 seconds of arc. It is sometimes difficult to interpret the thresholds reported since it is not always clear to what they refer.

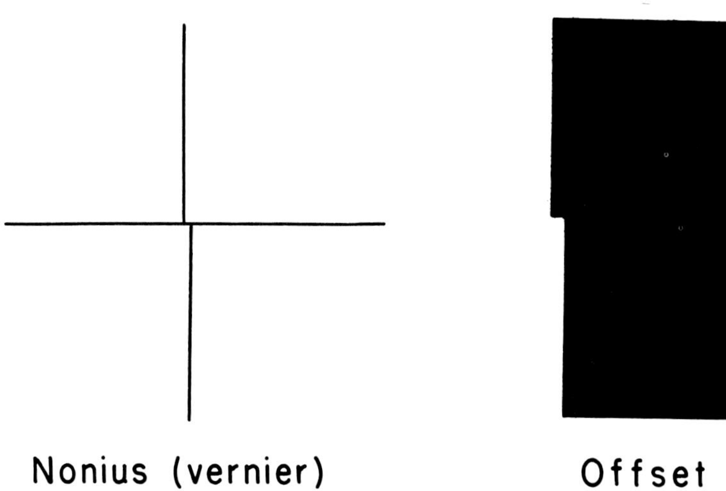

Figure 234. The nonius (vernier) and offset tests for the discrimination of a break in alignment.

It must be pointed out that the nonius acuity does not depend on the discrimination of contrast, as do most of the other acuity tests, but rather on the underlying mechanism of visual directional localization. The nonius acuity probably plays a role in letter discrimination. The accuracy with which the break can be discriminated also increases with the lengths of the lines—up to a certain asymptotic limit of about 20 minutes of arc. The high precision achieved by this visual resolution test, though ascribed to an averaging process of the visual directions of many retinal elements, has nevertheless made possible the design of the vernier scale, by which fractions of divisions of the main scale can be read with accuracy.

Point Alignment

The high precision with which three vertically separated point light sources can be aligned has been described. Figure 235 illustrates the data of Ludvigh (37),

* Exception must be made for stereoscopic acuity test, which also shows very high precision.

showing a maximal precision of 2 seconds of arc for a separation of the reference points of 15 minutes of arc. For this type of acuity task, contrast discrimination is also not involved; precision must depend on an averaging of the directional values of retinal receptors.

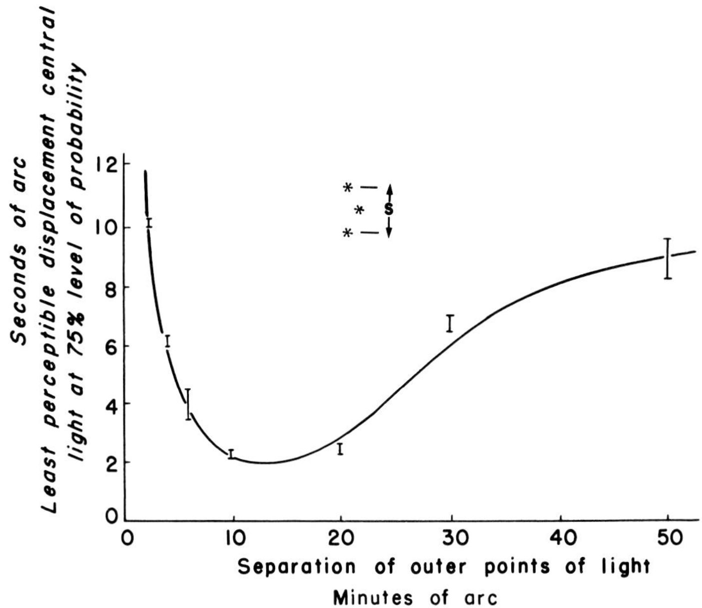

Figure 235. Data of Ludvigh (37) showing the high degree of precision in the discrimination of the displacement of a central point light source with respect to two outer points, for different separations.

The Landolt Ring

The Landolt ring is one of the best known and the most studied of all the visual acuity test designs. Also known sometimes as the "split-ring" or the "C" test, the pattern consists of a black ring with a small gap on one side (Figure 222) printed on a white background. The usual design calls for a ring diameter of five units, with a width of one unit and a gap of one unit. In the visual acuity test, the ring is oriented at random, preferably in two meridians—up or down, right or left (though often all four meridians are used)—and, if the subject discriminates the gap, he is able to state its orientation. In precision tests, allowance must be made for guessing.

The Landolt ring was adopted as an international standard test target in 1909. It does not depend on language or literacy; it is simple to construct and easy to administer. When the angular size of the gap subtending one minute to the eye is just discriminable, the visual acuity is written as 1.0; when the angular size of the gap is twice as large, but is also just discriminable by another subject, the visual acuity is said to be 0.50.

Wall charts showing sequential rows of rings of increasing size from bottom to top are available. When the chart is viewed from a fixed observation distance, the visual acuity is based on the proportion of rings in which the orientation of the gap is correctly perceived in each successive row; the visual acuity measured corresponds to the last row of rings in which the orientation of the gap is correctly discriminated. If desired, the visual acuity can be converted readily to the Snellen notation.

The Snellen Hook

The Snellen hook or test device (Figure 222) is a variation of the double bar test. It is used less often, except perhaps in testing the visual acuity of very young children or of illiterates.

Letter Charts—Optotypes

The history of the use of letters as visual acuity test types is so well known that only certain aspects need to be discussed here. The fact that a suitable chart provides a simple, rapid, and easily understood method of estimating visual acuity has accounted for its general acceptance.

Sloan (66) published in 1951 an excellent critical review of the measurement of visual acuity with letters, and quoted Emsley, who had stated that, for determining the visual acuity in subjects with uncorrected refractive errors, the test should consist "of as complicated form as is clinically convenient in order to subject the eye to a test comparable with the varied tasks imposed upon it in everyday life. At the same time, however, the test should permit simple questions to and simple answers from the subject; and his answers should be capable of rapid checking. To make the test precise the characters should quickly become unrecognizable when not seen clearly" (66). Such ideal test characters should have horizontal, oblique, vertical, and curved contours. When complex test characters are employed as measures of acuity, the assumption is usually made that the recognition of a familiar letter or symbol requires only the visual resolution of its component parts. Acuity therefore has been measured by the visual angle subtended by the constituent parts of the test letter.

Design

The letters selected by Snellen in 1862 for his acuity test chart were designed so that the black lines and the white spaces were equal in width. "The letters are enclosed in a square whose sides are five times the width of the letter strokes. Serifs are added to the longer strokes in order to maintain the unit separation of black and white areas throughout the letter" (66). A difficult problem encountered in the design and selection of letters for a test chart is that all letters should be equally legible or, possibly, equally difficult to recognize; the Snellen letters are certainly not equally legible. A great deal of work has gone into determining the relative legibility of various letter designs and of different letters. The results reported by many investigators (7) show little consistency. Attempts have been made to alter the basic design of the various letters in order to make their legibility comparable (55). In general, nearly all investigators have recommended letters without serifs.

Sloan (66) suggested the use of ten familiar nonserif letters which, according to her experiments, did not differ greatly in legibility; these are, in order of increasing difficulty, Z N H R V K D C O S. By designing a chart in which the same group of letters would be used on each line, she argued that "the average difficulty of each line as a whole will vary only with the size of its letters."

In each line's design, the separation of the letters presents a problem. Apart from the effect of uncorrected astigmatism on the legibility of a row of letters, the phenomenon of contour interference (24) and its influence on the acuity, as demonstrated by Landolt rings, surely applies with letters (21). There seems little question that separated letters are more readily identifiable than those crowded together. This is especially evident in amblyopic eyes. For the identification of words in general reading, however, the optimal separation of the letters is about 2 minutes of arc for letters that are about 5 minutes of arc high and 5 minutes of arc wide. In the majority of acuity charts, the separation of the letters is about the same as the width of the letters themselves. Some care should be taken in the choice of letters to be used at the beginning and at the end of each line.

Gradation

The much-debated problem of the desirable gradation in size of the letters in successive lines on the visual acuity chart revolves on whether the progression should be arithmetic or geometric. Suppose the angular size of the letters in one of the lower lines of the chart, regarded as the standard or normal, is A_0 minutes of arc. Then, for an arithmetic progression, the angular size A_N for the letters in the Nth line above the first would be equal steps of visual angle, $A_N = A_0 + k(N - 1)$, in which k is additional increment of size.

For the geometric progression, $A = A_0R^{(N-1)}$, in which R is the ratio of the size of the angles subtended by the letters in any line to that of the preceding line (44). For most of the charts available, geometric progression is used, as in the well-known chart of Green, where $R = 1.26$.

TABLE 28

EXAMPLES OF ARITHMETIC AND GEOMETRIC PROGRESSIONS IN VISUAL ACUITY LETTER CHARTS

Line	Arithmetic $k = 0.5$			Geometric $R = 1.26$		
N	A	Snellen		A	Snellen	
1	1.0	6/6	20/20	1.00	6/6	20/20
2	1.5	6/9	20/30	1.26	6/7.5	20/25
3	2.0	6/12	20/40	1.59	6/9.5	20/32
4	2.5	6/15	20/50	2.00	6/12	20/40
5	3.0	6/18	20/60	2.52	6/15	20/50
6	3.5	6/21	20/70	3.18	6/19	20/63
7	4.0	6/24	20/80	4.00	6/24	20/80
8	4.5	6/27	20/90	5.03	6/30	20/100
9	5.0	6/30	20/100	6.33	6/45	20/125

Table 28 gives examples of the letter sizes of successive lines of a visual acuity letter chart, computed for an arithmetic ($k = 0.5$) and a geometric ($R = 1.26$) progression.

Data obtained from checkerboard target experiments testing the depth of eye focus based on the loss of visual acuity with blurring of the retinal image show a linear relationship between logarithm of visual acuity and degree of out-of-focus imagery (Figure 236). This proportionality supports the design of the Snellen-type visual acuity test charts, for which the size of the letters on each line bears a constant ratio to the size of the letters on the adjacent line, that is, a geometric progression of letter size.

There is evidence that, beyond a certain threshold, the number of errors subjects make in reading charts varies inversely with the logarithm of the visual angle. On this basis, visual acuity test charts would be most reliable with a logarithmic gradation with R between 1.17 and 1.40 (19).

Charts would be advantageous for refraction determination if the successive

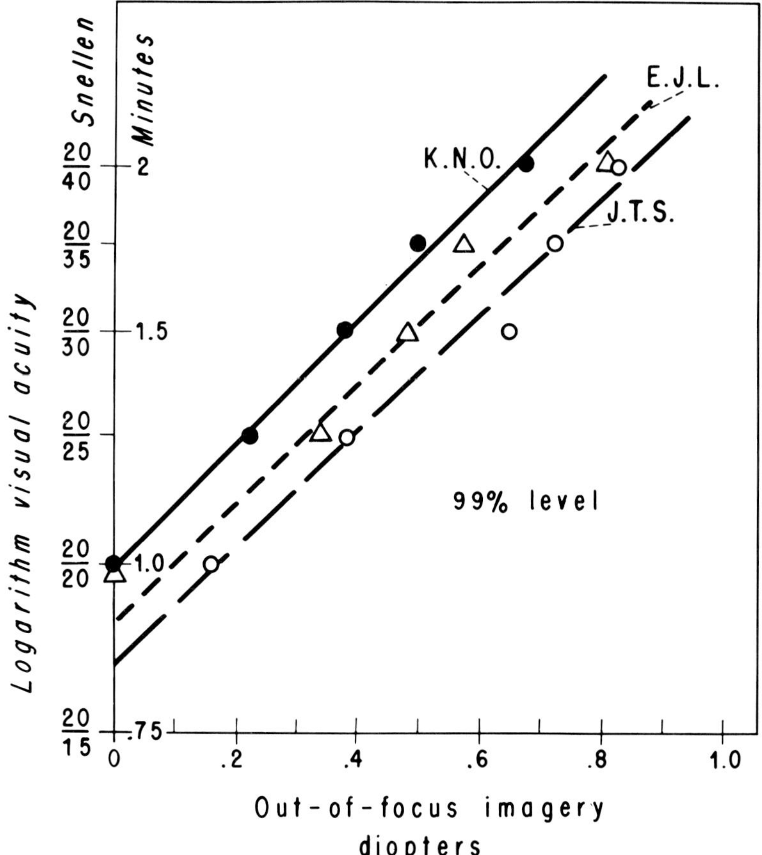

Figure 236. Relationship between half of the depth of focus at the 99 per cent level of probable resolution (corresponding to uncorrected myopia) and the visual angle subtended by the details of the test target. (From Schwartz & Ogle, 62.)

lines on the chart were related to fixed steps of the uncorrected ametropia and, in particular, uncorrected myopia. There is some evidence (44) that charts designed with $R = 1.30$ closely approximate this type of chart; each succeeding line would correspond to an increase of 0.25 diopter uncorrected myopia.

Notation

Finally, there is the problem of how visual acuity should be specified when determined from letter charts. The classic Snellen notation generally used is the fractional designation $V = d/D$, in which d is the visual distance at which letters of a certain size can be barely discriminated (the test distance) and D is the standard distance at which those same letters would subtend a visual angle of 1.0 minute of arc. This designation of visual acuity implies a standard against which the visual acuity of a subject is compared. This so-called standard (for example, 20/20) has become a fetish and is misleading in that it is called the "normal acuity", whereas a considerable proportion of the population has better acuities. This standard has also led to the use of a similar notation to indicate the acuity in tests made at other distances, for example, at near vision.

Decimal visual acuity is defined as the reciprocal of the visual angle in minutes of arc subtended by the component parts of the letters expressed as a decimal fraction equal to the numerical value of the Snellen fraction. Thus, $V = 20/40 = 0.5$. This decimal designation of visual acuity is used rather generally, especially as an international notation. The principal objection to it is that it tends to suggest a percentage of useful vision (the difference from unity as a percentage loss of vision), an erroneous concept. It has been suggested* that, to avoid any false connotations, the word *Snellen* should always accompany this decimal notation, as, for example, Snellen 0.5.

It has also been suggested (44) that the visual acuity be designated directly and simply as the visual angle subtended by the component parts of the letters used—or of any other visual acuity test target. Thus, $A = 1.5$, or 1.5 minutes of arc, would—if a comparison were needed—correspond to a Snellen 0.66 or Snellen fraction $V = 20/30 = 6/9$. Such a notation could be easily converted into any system, and at the same time it avoids more easily the fetish of 20/20 or 6/6 vision.

Discrimination of Form

The discrimination, or identification, of familiar geometric figures has been used infrequently for estimates of visual acuity. Examples include the identification of such forms as circles, squares, trapezoids, hexagons, and modified shapes of these forms, such as a Maltese cross with a rounded edge, bars with parallel and nonparallel edges, etc. One of the more successful studies of form discrimination was that of Aulhorn (3), who used a circle and square (see Figure 242, discussed on pp. 468–469).

---

*J. E. Lebensohn, personal communication.

Effect of Astigmatism

Uncorrected astigmatism may have a pronounced effect on an evaluation of visual acuity by means of any of the test types described herein. Spurious acuities may often be obtained when the axis of astigmatism is parallel to or perpendicular to the predominant direction of the letter strokes or line details of the target (55,56). No test is free from this effect. With repeated patterns, spurious resolution may even be found with uncorrected spherical errors. The evidence suggests, however, that relatively *small* (perhaps subclinical) uncorrected astigmatic errors play only a minor role in the spurious estimates of visual acuity obtained from most of these tests.

Depth of Focus of the Eye

The degree to which the image falling on the retina can be thrown out of focus without causing a loss of visual acuity is a measure of the eye's depth of focus. This plays a role in all testing of visual acuity as it relates to refraction.

The characteristics of the blur on the human retina due to an out-of-focus image cannot be compared directly to the characteristics of blur of the out-of-focus image in a centered photographic lens system. Small irregular refractive and astigmatic errors, decentration of optical elements, and the asphericity of the refractive eye surfaces complicate the character of the blurred image in the eye. Consequently, anomalous effects sometimes occur in that the blurred image—for example, of a luminous line against a dark background—will appear as multiple sharp images with minute separations, and these effects will influence the measurement of depth of focus.

Although there are other criteria for determining the depth of focus, we shall restrict this discussion to loss of visual acuity.

Suppose the eye fixates point *C* (Figure 237) and the accommodation remains constant for this stimulus distance (50,62). If a test target is moved along the axis,

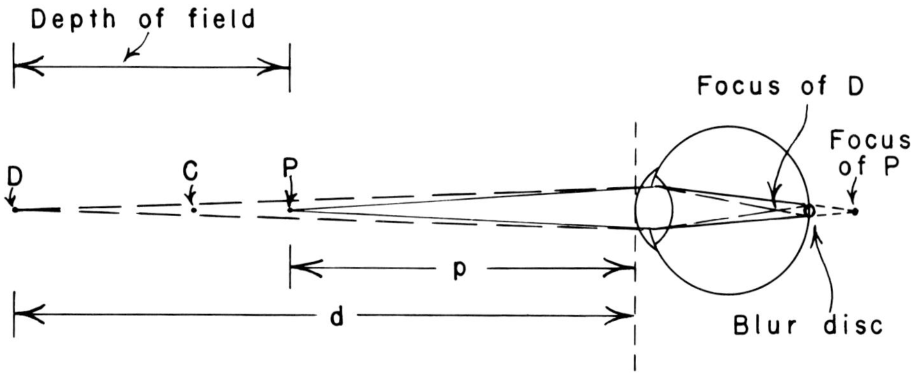

Depth of focus = 1/p − 1/d

Figure 237. Quantities used to define the eye's depth of field and depth of focus, corresponding to a maximal tolerable blur of the retinal image. See text. (From Schwartz & Ogle, 62.)

nearer to or farther from the eye than point *C*, the image falling on the retina becomes blurred because the geometric image of the test target initially falls in front of the retina and then behind it, respectively. The out-of-focus image of a point appears on the retina as a blur disk; the more the image is out of focus, the larger is the blur disk. If the target is a visual acuity chart, then at a certain degree of blurring the details on the chart can no longer be discriminated. Corresponding to the maximal amount of blurring without deterioration of visual acuity, there would be a *proximal* position, *P*, and a *distal* position, *D*, of the test target, at distances *p* and *d*, respectively, from the eye. The total depth of focus (in diopters) then is defined as $1/p - \frac{1}{3}$ (when *p* and *d* are expressed in meters). The actual spatial interval between *P* and *D* is the "depth of field".

In an experiment to determine the depth of focus by using the criterion of loss of visual acuity for out-of-focus images, the checkerboard test was used under controlled constant conditions (50,62). Obviously, the degree to which the image of the target can be thrown out of focus before there is a loss of visual resolution will depend on the size of test details, the luminance of the target, and the pupil size. Data for one observer are shown in Figure 238. The abscissas are the *diopters* out of focus of the image of the test target. The "distal blurring" (right of the graph)

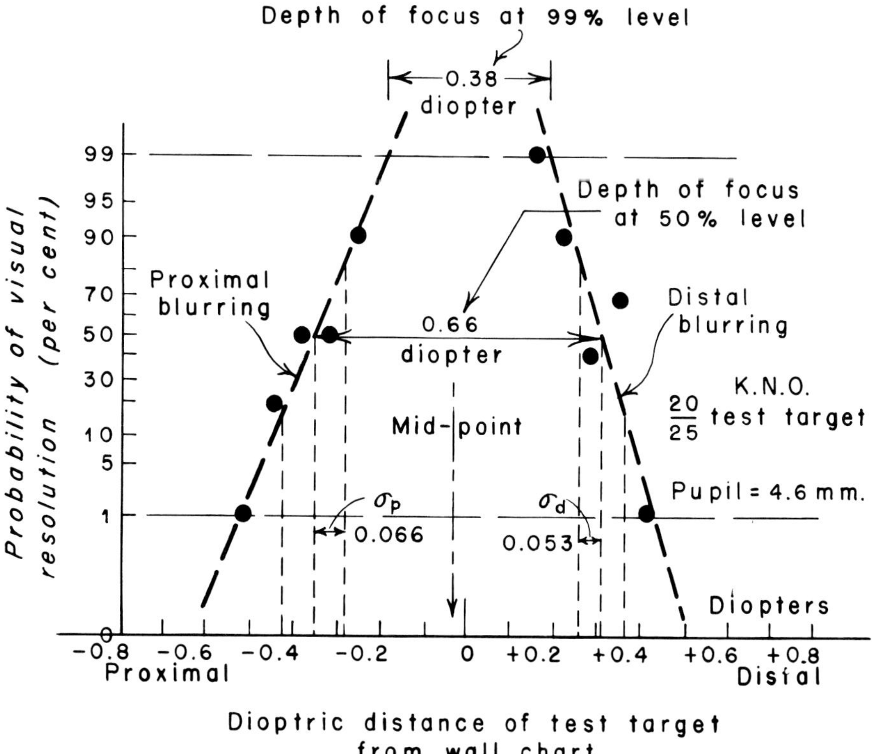

Figure 238. Typical data of proximal and distal limits of the depth of focus of the eye, plotted on probability ordinate scale and showing the proximal and distal loss of visual resolution with increased out-of-focus imagery, for a target corresponding to V = 20/25. (From Schwartz & Ogle, 62.)

corresponds to the kind of blur experienced by a subject with uncorrected myopia, and the "proximal blurring" (left) corresponds to the kind of blur experienced, for example, by the presbyope for a near object. On the ordinates is plotted the percentage of probability for the detail of the checkerboard target to be discriminated and therefore visually resolved. The subject's ability to discriminate the details of the checkerboard chart decreases somewhat rapidly beyond a certain degree of out-of-focus blurring of the image.

TABLE 29

SUMMARY OF DATA FOR THE DEPTH OF FOCUS FOR DIFFERENT SIZES OF TEST DETAILS

	Size of Test Target				
	20/20	20/25	20/30	20/35	20/40
Mean size of entrance pupil, mm	3.7	3.9	4.0	3.8	4.0
Depth of focus, 50% level, D	0.71	1.04	1.71	1.95	2.24
Depth of focus, estimated at 99% level, D	0.33	0.76	1.31	1.45	1.65
σ for proximal distribution, D	0.10	0.06	0.10	0.11	0.13
σ for distal distribution, D	0.08	0.07	0.08	0.10	0.12

Table 29 summarizes the results for one subject. The mean total depth of focus, obtained with the checkerboard test with resolvable details of angular size equivalent to 20/25 Snellen notation, was found to be 0.94 *D* at the 50 per cent level and estimated to be 0.63 *D* at the 99 per cent level of probable visual resolution of the target details. The degree to which the image of the target can be thrown out of focus before losing resolution would, of course, be only half of the total depth of focus.

VISUAL ACUITY AND ILLUMINATION

It is common knowledge that visual acuity for dark test figures on an illuminated background increases with illumination. The classic sigmoid curve describing this relationship is that of Koenig (1897), as recalculated by Hecht (27). The data plotted in Figure 239 were obtained with an opaque Snellen hook seen against a uniformly transilluminated background, with an artificial pupil before the subject's eye. In the middle range of luminance the visual acuity increases in almost direct proportion to log luminance, reaching a maximum at higher luminances and increasing only gradually at lower luminances. A graph of these same data plotted on log-log coordinates is shown in Figure 240; the curves are theoretical, computed by Shlaer (64). The graph suggests that the data should be described by two curves, with a transition between 1 and 0.1 mL. The lower curve is thought to represent the retinal rod response, and the upper the response of the retinal cones. Some evidence has also been found to indicate that the visual acuity may decrease slightly from a maximum when the luminances are exceedingly high—greater than 1000 mL (22).

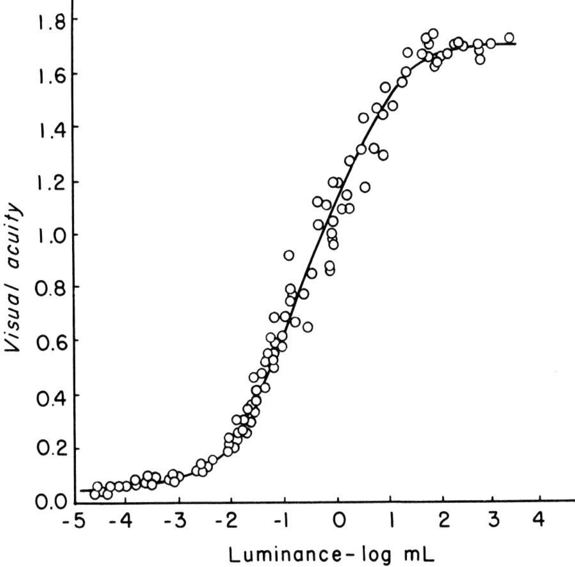

Figure 239. The classic curve of the data of Koenig, showing the relationship between visual acuity and illumination (with an artificial pupil).

In carefully conducted experiments using both a Landolt ring and a grating with maximum contrast (transparencies), Shlaer (64) studied the relationship between visual acuity and illumination; his results are shown in Figure 241. The curves were obtained theoretically on the basis of Hecht's photochemical stationary-state equation. The striking aspect of these results is the difference

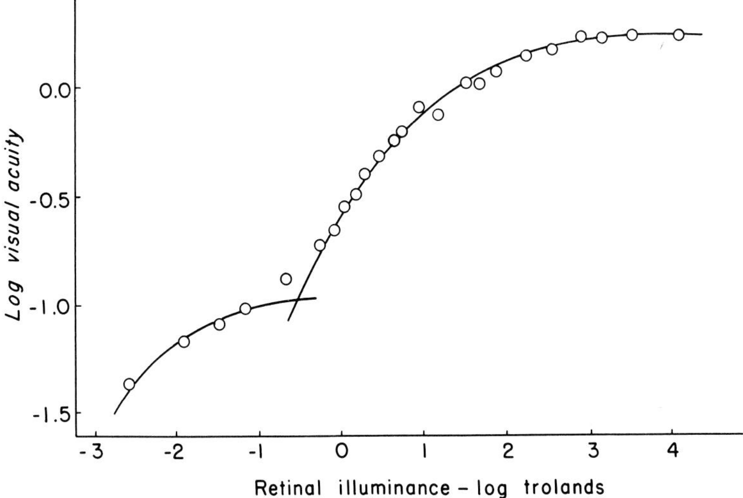

Figure 240. The data of Koenig plotted on a log-log graph. (After Shlaer, 64.)

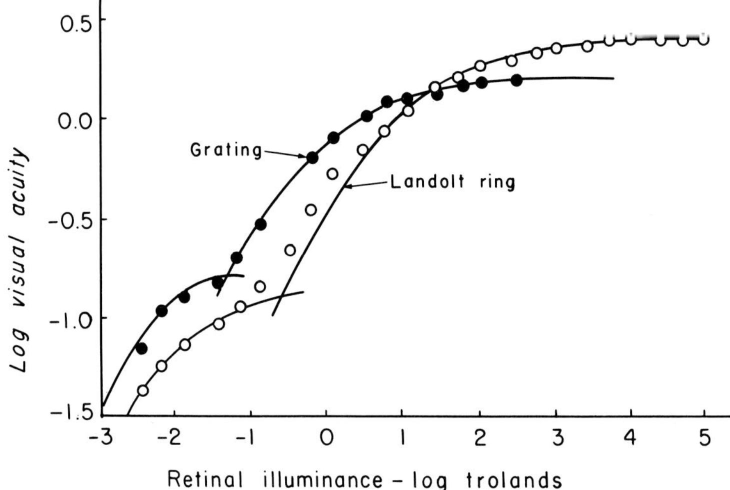

Figure 241. Results of measurements by Shlaer (64) on visual acuity and illumination, for a Landolt ring and a grating with maximum contrast.

between the acuity obtained with the ring and with the grating. It appears that the maximum visual acuity obtainable with the grating is 30 per cent lower than that with the Landolt ring for higher luminances of the background, but the acuity with the grating is higher for lower luminances. The difference between these two types of targets illustrates one of the problems of determining the basic nature of visual resolution, as well as the inadequacy of specifying that resolution exclusively by grating targets.

Theoretical attempts to relate visual acuity to contrast thresholds and both of these, in turn, to change in illumination, have needed reference to data which more often than not were obtained under different experimental conditions and from different types of test stimuli. Aulhorn (3) undertook to study both visual acuity and contrast thresholds using the same test targets under the same experimental conditions. Her measurements of visual acuity depended on the form discrimination between the square and the circle. For the contrast or detection thresholds, either a circle or a square could be used, for their areas were the same. Figure 242 illustrates one set of data from her results. In her test, she defined visual acuity as the reciprocal of the visual angle subtended by a small imaginary circle in the square target, which was tangential to the sides of the square at a corner and to an inscribed circle in the square (Figure 242). Thus, if d is the angular diameter of the circle whose area is equal to that of the square, the angular diameter of this small circle used by Aulhorn to define the minimum angle of resolution would be $\alpha = 0.15\, d$. The visual acuity so defined would be $1/\alpha$.

The data illustrated in Figure 242 were obtained for a light circle and square visible against a gray background having a constant luminance of 1 mL. The detection data—contrast thresholds—show the relationship between the diameter of the circle and its luminance above that of the background for detection. The

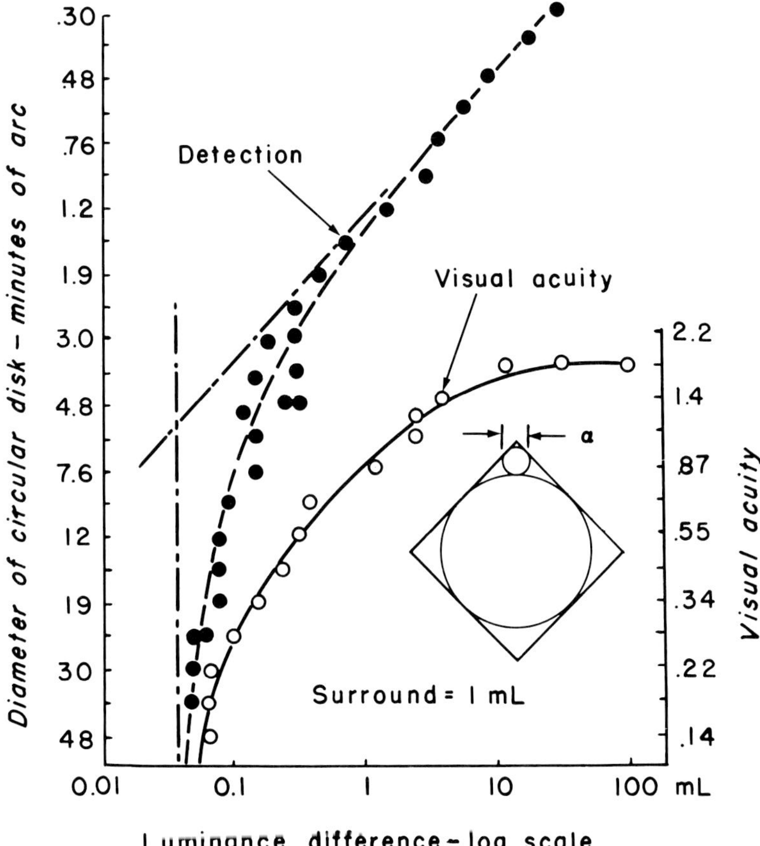

Figure 242. Data of Aulhorn (3) showing detection thresholds and form discrimination thresholds (visual acuity) for white circles and squares on a gray background.

visual acuity data, as usual, show the relationship between visual acuity (as Aulhorn defined it) and this luminance difference; these latter data are similar to those of Koenig and of Shlaer. The detection data bring out the well-known fact that, as the diameter of the circle is increased, the difference in luminance for detection approaches a constant value (46), and that for smaller diameters the threshold approaches a line described in Ricco's law. The critical angle (intersection of the two asymptotes) is about 5.1 minutes of arc. As would be expected, the luminance required for the discrimination of the form difference between the square and the circle of a certain area is much higher than the corresponding luminance required for detection of the circle or the square alone.

There appears to be every reason for believing that the relationship between visual acuity and illumination is extremely complex, that it varies with the type of target used, and that possibly no one physiologic mechanism can account for the relationship over the entire range of retinal illumination. We also recall that, when point light sources are used as test objects for resolution, the visual resolving power *decreases* with increasing contrast; i.e., for an adapting field of constant luminance, the resolving power decreases with increase in luminous intensity of the point sources.

It is pertinent to mention briefly several of the theories proposed to account for the phenomenon. It probably can be said that as of this date no single proposed theory is satisfactory. The problem is usually discussed in relation to test objects consisting of black details visible against an illuminated background.

1. One of the older theories assumes that there is a change in the visual response to the irradiation or illuminance spread from the image. The effective contour in the image moves closer to the image of the geometric edge as the illuminance heightens, because the contrast threshold increases. The separation of the spatial contours can then be decreased, which means increased acuity. Wilcox stated that "irradiation, or the apparent shift of contours, is the only cause of the variations of visual acuity with intensity" (72).

It has also been suggested that the scatter of light within the optical media of the eye, as well as that caused by aberrations of the eye, also reduces the contrast of the test detail. This degree of contrast change could not account for the variation in acuity over the wide range of luminances.

2. A theory of recruitment was proposed by Hecht (27), in which he assumed that the light thresholds varied greatly among the retinal receptors and that these thresholds were randomly distributed. As the retinal illuminance increases, more and more receptors become active, and with these changes the average separation between active receptors decreases. Correspondingly, there would be a decrease in the minimum angle of resolution, or an increase in visual acuity. At much higher illuminances all the receptors would become active; visual acuity would attain a maximum and remain at that level in spite of further increases in retinal illuminance. The random distribution of the light thresholds of the receptors was assumed to follow a Poisson distribution, and it appeared that two integrated distributions did in fact fit the data fairly well (Figure 241), one curve for the rod and the other for the cone system.

An objection to this theory was that it implied the existence of receptor elements known to be anatomically similar, especially at the fovea, but for which the sensitivities to light would have to vary over 7 log units of luminous intensity. Hecht's theory is still discussed in some texts as the correct explanation.

3. A third theory, discussed by Shlaer (64), is based on Hecht's photochemical stationary-state equation, namely

$$KI = x^n/(a - x)^m,$$

in which I is the retinal illumination, a the maximum concentration of the photochemical retinal pigment in the receptors when the eye is dark-adapted, and x is the concentration of the decomposed pigment at a given time due to the illumination I. K, m, and n are constants; $m = n = 2$. Shlaer found that, by assuming the visual acuity to be proportional to x^2 and by proper choice of the constants, he could obtain a curve that fitted closely the cone portion of the data (Figures 240 and 241). Similarly, with a change in constants he could fit the rod portion of the curve, though with less specificity in the choice of those constants. This result was taken as evidence that a photochemical process could account for the increase in acuity with illumination. However, Pirenne (54) has shown that, while this theory may account for the data in the higher levels of luminous intensity, it is inadequate at low intensities, where the change in pigment concentration for perception would be low.

4. Other theories are somewhat related to a common idea, namely that retinal receptors may apparently act in groups, the size of these sensorial groups increasing with decrease in retinal illuminance (25).

One theory postulates that this mechanism permits weak luminous excitations to be summated over a larger number of elements to activate a single ganglion sufficiently for the generation of a detectable nervous impulse.

Another interpretation of this apparent change in the area of the sensorial units with illuminance, suggested by Otero (cf. Aguilar & Yunta, 2), considers the transverse amacrine cells of the retina to play the principal role, since these cells may possibly intercept the impulses from the bipolar cells and hence effectively spread the area of response to particular ganglion cells. 'The amacrine cells are of various lengths; some connect near the bipolar cells while others reach out to more distant cells. According to the way one or the other is linked, we have sensorial units of smaller or larger sizes. This interpretation assumes that the amacrine cells are supersensitive and are only useful as a means for conducting the excitations for low retinal illuminances, and that they become less active as the illuminance increases. . . . This supersensitivity of the amacrines is assumed to increase with their length. The very large ones are active first, which means that only at low illuminances can widely separated receptors be united by connecting ganglions'* (2). As the illuminance increases, the number of ganglions whose excitations are summated decreases.

5. Pirenne (54) has suggested that detection of the gap in the Landolt ring (for example) results not from the light flux from the gap itself, but rather depends on small eye movements in which the black edges of the ring, if resolved, lead to perception through "off" neural stimuli. This is to say that, since the luminance of the gap and background is the same, it would be the movement of the images of the dark edges enclosing the gap over different retinal elements that leads to the perception of the gap through receptor "off" responses. "Thus the gap [in the ring] will be seen not because it is white, but because it is not black . . ." (54). This is a complex concept, and some ancillary information would be needed to account fully for the increase in acuity with retinal illuminance.

Experiments conducted within recent years indicate the existence in a receptor system of the retina of an area of inhibition surrounding the center of luminous excitation (58). Figure 243 illustrates a schematic excitation-inhibition response. In this and in similar discussions there is the suggestion that this phenomenon of spatial excitation-inhibition is also present in the fovea. The area, or spread, of the inhibition would expand with an increase in the strength of the excitation.

---

* Author's translation.

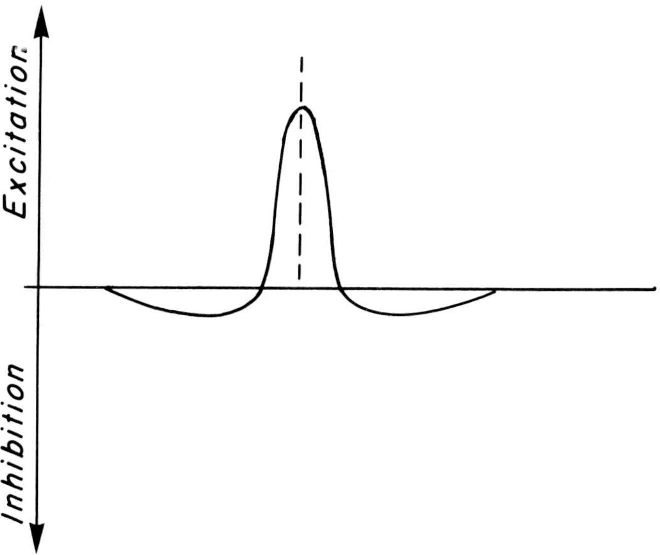

Figure 243. One of the possible schemes proposed to illustrate the excitation and inhibition effects surrounding a retinal light stimulus.

This increase in spatial inhibition would effectively reduce the area of the excitatory sensorial unit (neural units) (67), and a consequence would be an increase in visual resolution. In determining the detection threshold of small test areas, it has been shown that a neighboring light area has an additive interaction at low luminances, but this becomes inhibitory at higher luminances (6). The general concept was expressed by Pirenne (53): "... over a considerable part of the intensity-acuity range, the increase of acuity is due to the bringing into play of finer and finer retinal mosaics made up of smaller and smaller functional units, the *absolute* thresholds of the various units being reached successively as the retinal illumination increases." The role of the excitatory and inhibitory areas in the retina may also be affected by temporal factors.

Eye Movements and Visual Acuity

The fact that our visual acuity is so much finer than what we would expect from our knowledge of the size of the smallest optical blur disk on the retina and the size of the elements in the retinal mosaic has led many investigators to seek an explanation for this discrepancy in the well-known small involuntary physiologic nystagmoid eye movements. Pirenne's theory (53) has already been mentioned as an explanation of the mode of detection of the gap in the Landolt ring through these eye movements. There seems to be some clinical evidence that small voluntary scanning eye movements tend to improve slightly the visual identification of letters. There is also some evidence that the excursions of the involuntary saccadic eye movements increase as the stimulus details approach the threshold of discrimination (28).

When a subject attempts to fixate a point steadily, three different types of involuntary physiologic nystagmoid movements are identified: (*a*) small tremor-like movements with a frequency of about 50 cps (range 30 to 80), with an average amplitude of only about 15 seconds of arc (these rapid tremor movements would probably have little effect on acuity under any circumstances); (*b*) sudden flicks found at somewhat irregular intervals from 0.03 to 5 seconds, with amplitudes that vary but may be as much as 7 minutes of arc (flicks as large as 20 minutes have been recorded); and (*c*) drift movements occurring between the flicks, usually slow, but with amplitudes as large as 5 minutes of arc. Except for the minute rapid tremor movements, all of the horizontal physiologic nystagmoid movements are synchronous for the two eyes in binocular fixation.

Bryngdahl (9) has recently concluded from a purely theoretical treatment that the flick movements were of predominant importance in "supporting normal vision". Averill & Weymouth (4) found considerable decrease in visual acuity with decrease in exposure time of a test target, a finding they interpreted as resulting from a reduction of the effect of the involuntary nystagmoid eye movements. A systematic decrease of stereoscopic depth acuity was also found with decreasing exposure times of the test stimuli, from one second to about five milliseconds when the stereo-acuity leveled off at a minimum (51). Jones & Higgins (30) believed that results in their study of the detection of small rectangles visible against a luminous background supported the assumption that detection of change in "luminance in the visual field is dependent directly upon the temporal illuminance gradients to which the retinal receptors are subjected by virtue of the movement of the image with respect to the retinal mosaic." These physiologic nystagmoid movements were considered to provide an averaging mechanism

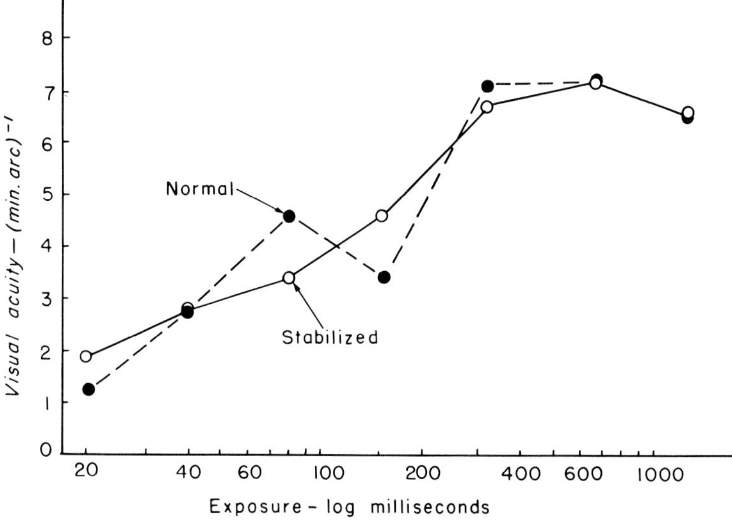

Figure 244. The data of Keesey (31) (replotted in terms of acuity), showing that visual acuity for a range of exposure times, as determined by the nonius (vernier) test, is the same with stabilized images and with normal vision.

which effectively rectified the blurred images on the retina; they provided the mechanism by which the variation in contrast on the receptor elements could be quickly changed from one illuminance level to another.

While measuring visual acuity with a grating test, however, Ratliff (57) also recorded the horizontal physiologic nystagmus; his preliminary results suggested that involuntary drifts during the exposure of the grating were detrimental to the monocular visual acuity. Even the small rapid tremor movements did not enhance the acuity for the grating.

In her most recent experiments, in which she used stabilized images (contact lenses in special instrumentation), Keesey (31) found almost no difference in visual acuity between stabilized and normal (unstabilized) vision, determined for a single vertical line, a nonius (vernier) alignment test, and a grating target for a range of exposure times from 20 milliseconds to 1.25 seconds (Figure 244). Similarly, data by Shortess & Krauskopf (65) showed no difference in stereoscopic acuity between vision with stabilized images and normal vision, for a wide range of exposure times of the test details.

These results, though not yet confirmed by other investigators, must be taken as strong evidence that physiologic nystagmus plays little, if any, role in enhancing visual acuity. However, they leave unexplained: (*a*) the basic problem of how, experimentally, the visual acuity can be so high when the retinal images are known to be so large; and (*b*) the decrease in visual acuity with a decrease in exposure time.

Visual Acuity and Pupil Size

Considerable importance is attached to the relationship between normal acuity and the size of the pupil. Optical theory would determine the size of the image on the retina for small pupils by diffraction and chromatic aberration of light alone, while the spherical aberration would play a dominant role for large pupils. This fact was brought out by Le Grand (33) in comparing visual resolution under normal conditions with that obtained by means of the interference fringes on the retina, with which retinal resolution is measured. He found that for *small* pupils the two resolutions were essentially the same, showing that normal resolution was more or less independent of the optical aberrations of the eye. For large pupils, however, while the *retinal* resolution was also the same as for small pupils, the normal acuity was greatly reduced, showing that the optical aberrations were playing a dominant role.

Figure 245 illustrates some results obtained by several investigators (8,16,17), showing clearly that the visual acuity remains nearly constant for pupil diameters larger than 2 mm. This constancy would imply in part that the decreasing effects of diffraction were offset by the increasing effect of the aberrations of the eye with increases in pupillary diameter greater than 2 mm.

For smaller pupils, the acuity rapidly decreases—an effect attributable to diffraction. The same trend is found when the luminance of the background is decreased in proportion to the increase of the pupil area, thus keeping the retinal illuminance essentially constant. Figure 245 shows two sets of data obtained by

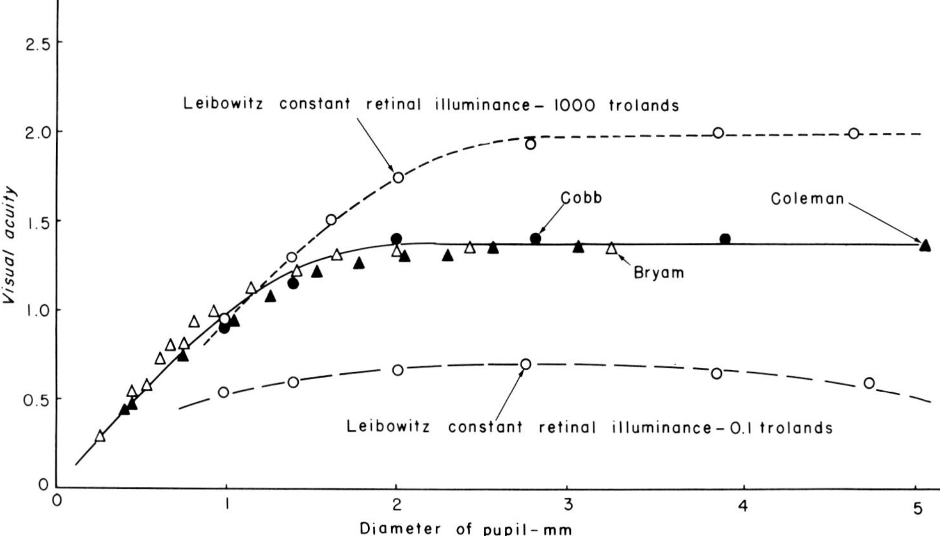

Figure 245. Data showing relationships between visual acuity and size of the pupil as determined in three studies by different investigators (8,16,17).

Leibowitz (36) with this constant retinal illuminance, one for a high luminance equivalent to 100 mL and the other for a low luminance of 0.01 mL. Both sets of data were obtained with a 2 mm artificial pupil, for retinal illuminances of 1000 and 0.1 trolands, respectively.

These data show that, to obtain a clinical estimate of visual acuity by the use of the "pinhole", the diameter of the hole should be no less than 2 mm if best acuity is to be found. Centering of the artificial pupil before the eyes may also be important, for studies on retinal acuity (14) from interference fringes show that visual acuity may decrease considerably when a vertical slit before the pupil is displaced laterally from the center of the natural pupil. This effect may be due to an aspect of the Stiles-Crawford phenomenon, namely that the light rays entering the eye near the pupil edge fall on the retinal receptors at an oblique angle, and are accordingly less effective.

It should be pointed out that pupil size does play a role in determining the cutoff spatial frequency for visual resolution of the grating test object (69). These results may also suggest that the grating type target is less useful for studies of visual acuity as it applies to our everyday surroundings.

Binocular versus Monocular Visual Acuity

Visual acuity is commonly found to be better with two eyes than with one eye when tested on a letter chart. It is a clinical impression that with two eyes the subject can identify the letters on the chart nearly one line lower than with one eye; this degree of increase in acuity would be about 30 per cent.

Little new information has been added to explain this phenomenon. In fact, some investigators doubt that a general rule in this regard can be made. If the vision in the two eyes of an emmetrope is 20/20 (6/6) or better, acuity with the two eyes is apparently not improved. A greater improvement is found with an ametropic or anisometropic subject whose two eyes have relatively low and different acuities (63).

The theories proposed to explain the superiority of binocular acuity over monocular acuity fall roughly into four types:

1. One theory pertains to the so-called peripheral factors, and assumes that in binocular vision accommodation is more accurate and the ability to fixate is subject to less variation.

2. A readily accepted theory, based on statistics (5), assumes that the visual acuity of each eye fluctuates from moment to moment around a statistical mean. The fluctuations in one eye are entirely independent of those in the other. According to the theory, therefore, at any particular moment, the mean binocular acuity would be better than the acuity of each eye by itself. This increase was estimated to be about 20 per cent. Bárány (5) found experimental evidence to verify this prediction.

3. A third theory assumes that by a cortical (psychologic, perhaps) process there is a type of "summing" of the visual acuity stimuli from the two eyes, i.e., that details within the image of one eye can be used to fill the "gaps" in the details within the image of the other eye.

4. Finally, a theory perhaps similar to the second one assumes that the responses from the two eyes are matched and summated, but in addition there are in the individual responses spurious signals (noise) that are random and uncorrelated between the two eyes. On a statistical basis, Campbell & Green (12) reasoned that "because the standard error of the sum of n independent measurements of a random or noisy process decreases as $\sqrt{n}$, an observer using two eyes can obtain two measurements which thus permit a $\sqrt{2}$ lower contrast to be detected." This would mean that the acuity should be 41 per cent better with two eyes than with one, and Campbell & Green presented data (using the sinusoidal grating) in which a 41 per cent improvement was indeed found.

It is rather doubtful that visual acuity in general will be enhanced to this degree, especially in emmetropia, with the usual acuity tests. As a matter of fact, other investigators have found a generally smaller improvement, often of only 6 to 10 per cent (61). Again, these results may vary greatly with the degree of uncorrected ametropia. One might even expect that, if a contour-inhibiting effect exists between the two eyes (21), some tests would show no improvement in acuity at all in binocular vision.

It is clear that more experimental work is needed on the question of binocular versus monocular visual acuity, using different types of test targets, control of illumination, and pupil size.

Visual Acuity in Amblyopia

Certain aspects of the visual acuity in amblyopic eyes are pertinent to this discussion. An eye is said to be amblyopic when there is no evidence of disease or pathologic anomalies but the visual acuity is subnormal and cannot be improved during the clinical examination with ophthalmic lenses or a pinhole. Amblyopia is variously classified: suppression or functional (hysterical), strabismic, and organic. In this brief discussion no distinction will be made among those.

It is factually difficult to explain this type of reduced visual acuity. Since there is evidence that the light sense of the amblyopic eye is essentially normal, the decreased acuity is assumed to be some anomaly of the form sense. One of the simplest explanations is that in the amblyopic eye there exists a functional scotoma at the fovea, and this eye fixates slightly extrafoveally, where the acuity is normally lower. In all studies of visual acuity of the amblyopic eye, one of the difficulties encountered by the examiner is locating the retinal point of fixation. Such a point may not always be the same.

Certain facts are fairly well substantiated. One pertains to the so-called crowding phenomenon or separation difficulty. The amblyopic eye is often able to discriminate or identify small symbols or letters when presented singly on a uniform background, but if the letters are presented in rows, much larger letters are necessary before it can recognize or identify them. The fact that contours in the vicinity of the Landolt ring tended to reduce the acuity (21) of normal individuals is consistent with the crowding phenomenon. It has also been shown that this crowding effect occurs in normal eyes to a certain extent, being greatly exaggerated in amblyopia (39,40). These results suggest that the effect might be due to an exaggerated spread of an inhibition (or a pronounced irradiation) around a stimulated element of the retina. In specifying the acuity of the amblyopic eye, one should indicate whether it is "Snellen acuity" (chart) or "single E acuity".

The influence of illumination on the visual acuity of the amblyopic eye has been inadequately studied. At low luminances and using optotypes, one study (68) showed that the acuity of amblyopic eyes was essentially the same as for normal eyes (Figure 246). As the luminance of the background was intensified, however, the acuity of the amblyopic eye increased rapidly at first, reaching a constant value and not improving much with further increases in luminance. For the normal eye the plateau of constant visual acuity was attained only for much higher luminances. It appeared from this study that for low illuminations the amblyopic eye was essentially normal. One could not infer from this, however, that the amblyopic eye acts, insofar as acuity is concerned, as though it had rod vision only.

Another study (60) suggests that, at least for children (ages 10 to 15 years), the visual acuity of the amblyopic eyes always remained less than that of the normal eyes, but increased with luminance (Figure 247). According to this curve, it is possible to obtain a given acuity, within limits, by merely changing the luminance. More data are needed on this problem, and with the advent of pleoptics it may be possible to ascertain where the amblyopic eye is fixating during the measurements.

Some types of amblyopia might be due to or associated with an abnormal Stiles-Crawford phenomenon (20). The experimental results are interpreted to indicate that the axes of the retinal elements (cones) at the fovea are aligned asymmetrically with respect to the visual axis of the eye. Apart from anatomic theories, the decreased visual acuity in amblyopic eyes has been assumed by

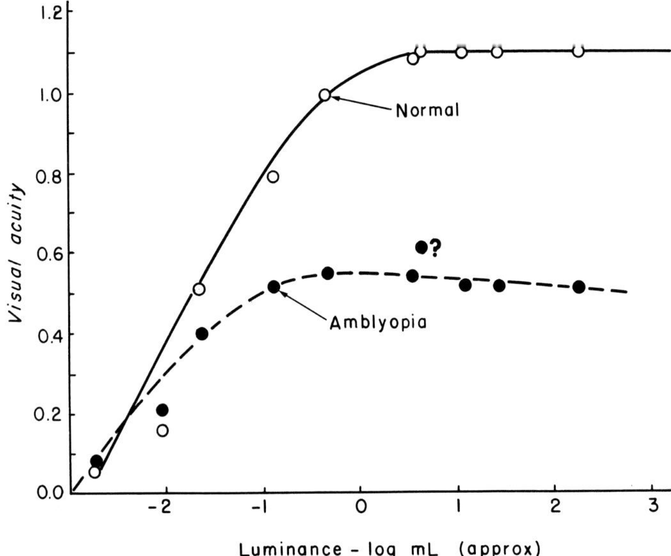

Figure 246. Data of Von Noorden & Burian (68) showing the change in visual acuity with change in luminance, in normals and amblyopes.

others to be (*a*) an active inhibition arising in the retinal structures, (*b*) "an active inhibition in the visual cortex" (10), (*c*) "a disturbance of the higher visual functions which results in an inability to integrate a sensed form into a meaningful percept" (10), or (*d*) evidence of an exaggerated "fixation difficulty." Burian and his associates (10) believed that amblyopia itself to be an exaggerated aspect of an already normally existing physiologic function. The fact that visual acuity in the amblyopic eye in many individuals can be increased greatly after the continued occlusion (patching) of the normal eye is certainly evidence of a normal underlying function.

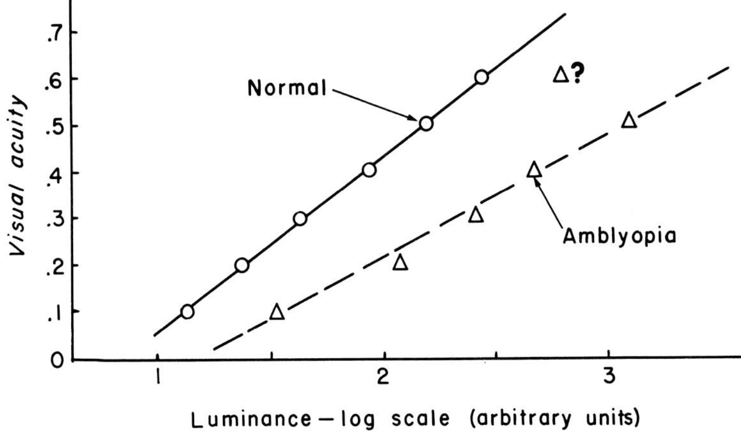

Figure 247. Data of Saiduzzafar & Ruben (60), for 25 amblyopic children, showing the change in visual acuity with illumination.

Kinetic or Dynamic Visual Acuity

Kinetic (or dynamic) visual acuity refers to the ability of a subject to discriminate (resolve) details on a rapidly moving target; the discrimination depends on pursuit movements of the eyes following the target. Using a mirror rotating on an axis at right angles to the plane of the movement of the target image, and a chart of Landolt rings, with a luminance of about 21 mL and angular velocities up to 170 arc degrees per second, Ludvigh and Miller (38,41) found that the visual acuity with movement in the horizontal meridian deteriorated greatly with angular velocity, although there were considerable individual differences. They also found that critical velocity varied between about 130 to 200 arc degrees per second. Figure 248 illustrates data obtained by Cutler & Ley (18) with the Landolt ring, showing the change in the minimum angle of resolution (reciprocal of visual acuity) with angular velocity of the moving test target. According to these results, acuity is better with binocular than with monocular vision; these investigators also found lower critical angular velocities.

The acuity does increase with intensification of the target luminance; in general, higher luminances were necessary for satisfactory acuity measurements. Pursuit movements in the vertical meridian were essentially similar to those in the horizontal meridian. The same results were obtained irrespective of whether it was the individual or the chart that was moved (rotated). One result was that little or no correlation was found between the static and the kinetic visual acuity.

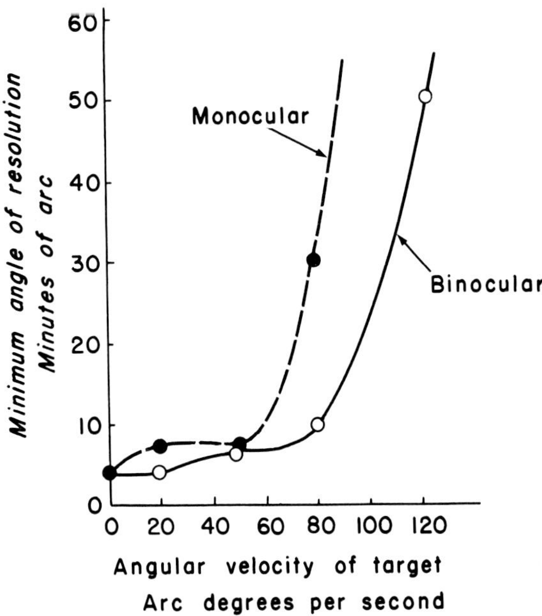

Figure 248. Data of Cutler & Ley (18), showing change in the minimum angle of resolution with angular velocity of a moving target.

It was concluded that kinetic visual acuity depended on the efficiency of the entire oculomotor pursuit mechanism and not on weakness or strength of individual muscles.

Emphasis has been placed by some writers on the value of kinetic (dynamic) visual acuity because it may represent the acuity with which we should be more concerned relative to such activities as automobile driving and flying.

SUMMARY

This paper presents a review of present knowledge of visual acuity. Following a treatment of the characteristics of the minimal blur disk on the retina, the critical problem of visual resolution is stated, namely how to account for the fineness of visual resolution when retinal images are so large. Fundamental considerations of visual resolution based upon the discrimination of point light sources lead to the important concepts of spatial excitation and inhibition areas of the retina, which enhance the physiological contrast at borders. Types of visual acuity targets, some well known, others less so, are then described. In each, the underlying physiological characteristics are stressed: point light sources, black dots and bars on light backgrounds, the grating, the checkerboard, the nonius (or vernier) lines, point alignment configuration, Landolt ring, Snellen hook, optotypes—letter charts. In the latter the important problems of design, gradation, acuity notations, and form discrimination are separately emphasized. The familiar relationship between visual acuity and illumination, though well documented, still defies an adequate physiological explanation. The use of stabilized images has suggested that some of our concepts regarding the effect of physiological nystagmoid movements upon visual acuity should be re-examined. Despite certain experimental results, there is still no satisfactory explanation of why binocular acuity is generally higher than monocular. Finally, kinetic (or dynamic) visual acuity is discussed in relation to pursuit eye movements.

REFERENCES

1. Adler, F. H., *Physiology of the Eye; Clinical Application* (4th ed.). Mosby, St. Louis, 1965.
2. Aguilar, M., and Yunta, J., Agrupación de receptores en la retina. *An. Real. Soc. Esp. Fis. Quím. Ser. A*, 1953, **49**: 281–290.
3. Aulhorn, E., Über die Beziehung zwischen Lichtsinn und Sehschärfe. *Graefe Arch. klin. exp. Ophthal.*, 1964, **167**: 4–74.
4. Averill, H. L., and Weymouth, F. W., Visual perception and the retinal mosaic. II. The influence of eye-movements on the displacement threshold. *J. Comp. Psychol.*, 1925, **5**: 147–176.
5. Bárány, E., A theory of binocular visual acuity and an analysis of the variability of visual acuity. *Acta Ophthal.* (Kobenhavn), 1946, **24**: 63–92.
6. Beitel, R. J., Jr., Spatial summation of subliminal stimuli in the retina of the human eye. *J. Gen. Psychol.*, 1934, **10**: 311–326.
7. Bennett, A. G., Ophthalmic test types; a review of previous work and discussions on some controversial questions. *Brit. J. Physiol. Opt.*, 1965, **22**: 238–271.

8. Bryam, G. M., The physical and photochemical basis of visual resolving power. II. Visual acuity and the photochemistry of the retina. *J. Opt. Soc. Amer.*, 1944, **34**: 718–738.

9. Bryngdahl, O., Effect of retinal image motion on visual acuity. *Opt. Acta* (London), 1961, **8**: 1–16.

10. Burian, H. M., Benton, A. L., and Lipsius, R. C., Visual cognitive functions in patients with strabismic amblyopia. *Arch. Ophthal.* (Chicago), 1962, **68**: 785–791.

11. Campbell, F. W., Visual acuity via linear analysis. In: *Proceedings of Symposium on Information Processing in Sight Sensory Systems.* California Institute of Technology, Pasadena, 1965: 177–193.

12. Campbell, F. W., and Green, D. G., Monocular versus binocular visual acuity. *Nature* (London), 1965, **208**: 191–192.

13. ———, Optical and retinal factors affecting visual resolution. *J. Physiol.* (London), 1965, **181**: 576–593.

14. Campbell, F. W., and Gregory, A. H., The spatial resolving power of the human retina with oblique incidence. *J. Opt. Soc. Amer.*, 1960, **50**: 831.

15. Cavonius, C. R., and Schumacher, A. W., Human visual acuity measured with colored test objects. *Science*, 1966, **152**: 1276–1277.

16. Cobb, P. W., The influence of pupillary diameter on visual acuity. *Am. J. Physiol.*, 1914, **36**: 335–346.

17. Coleman, H. S., Coleman, M. F., Fridge, D. L., and Harding, S. W., The coefficient of specific resolution of the human eye for Foucault test objects viewed through circular apertures. *J. Opt. Soc. Amer.*, 1949, **39**: 766–770.

18. Cutler, G. H., and Ley, A. H., Kinetic visual acuity. *Brit. J. Physiol. Opt.*, 1963, **20**: 119–127.

19. Dreyer, V., On the exactness of visual acuity determination charts with decimal, Snellen, and logarithmic notation. *Acta Ophthal.* (Kobenhavn), 1964, **42**: 295–306.

20. Enoch, J. M., Receptor amblyopia. *Am. J. Ophthal.*, 1959, **48**: 262–274.

21. Flom, M. C., Weymouth, F. W., and Kahneman, D., Visual resolution and contour interaction. *J. Opt. Soc. Amer.*, 1963, **53**: 1026–1032.

22. Foxell, C. A. P., and Stevens, W. R., Measurements of visual acuity. *Brit. J. Ophthal.*, 1955, **39**: 513–533.

23. Fry, G. A., Mechanisms subserving simultaneous brightness contrast. *Am. J. Optom.*, 1948, **25**: 162–178.

24. Fry, G. A., and Bartley, S. H., The effect of one border in the visual field upon the threshold of another. *Am. J. Physiol.*, 1935, **112**: 414–421.

25. Glezer, V. D., The receptive fields of the retina. *Vision Res.*, 1965, **5**: 497–525.

26. Goldmann, H., Objektive Sehschärfenbestimmung. *Ophthalmologica*, 1943, **105**: 240–252.

27. Hecht, S., A quantitative basis for the relation between visual acuity and illumination. *Proc. Nat. Acad. Sci. USA*, 1927, **13**: 569–574.

28. Higgins, G. C., and Stultz, K. F., Frequency and amplitude of ocular tremor. *J. Opt. Soc. Amer.*, 1953, **43**: 1136–1140.

29. *IES Lighting Handbook* (3rd ed.). Illuminating Engineering Society, New York, 1959.

30. Jones, L. A., and Higgins, G. C., Photographic granularity and graininess. IV. Visual acuity thresholds: dynamic *versus* static assumptions. *J. Opt. Soc. Amer.*, 1948, **38**: 398–405.

31. Keesey, U. T., Effects of involuntary eye movements on visual acuity. *J. Opt. Soc. Amer.*, 1960, **50**: 769–774.
32. Krauskopf, J., Light distribution in human retinal images. *J. Opt. Soc. Amer.*, 1962, **52**: 1046–1050.
33. Le Grand, Y., Sur la mesure de l'acuité visuelle au moyen de franges d'interférence. *C. R. Acad. Sci. D* (Paris), 1935, **200**: 490–491.
34. ———, L'espace visuel. In: *Optique Physiologique*, Vol. III. Editions de la Revue d'Optique, Paris, 1956: 79–120.
35. Lehmann, A., Versuch einer Erklärung des Einflusses des Gesichtswinkels auf die Auffassung von Licht und Farbe, bei direktem Sehen. *Pflüger Arch. ges. Physiol.*, 1885, **36**: 580–639.
36. Leibowitz, H., The effect of pupil size on visual acuity for photometrically equated test fields at various levels of luminance. *J. Opt. Soc. Amer.*, 1952, **42**: 416–422.
37. Ludvigh, E., Direction sense of the eye. *Am. J. Ophthal.*, 1953, **36**: 139–143.
38. Ludvigh, E., and Miller, J. W., Study of visual acuity during the ocular pursuit of moving test objects. I. Introduction. *J. Opt. Soc. Amer.*, 1958, **48**: 799–802.
39. Maraini, G., Pasino, L., and Peralta, S., L'acuité visuelle dans l'amblyopie. II. Difficulté de séparation. *Ophthalmologica*, 1963, **145**: 7–12.
40. ———, Separation difficulty in amblyopia. *Am. J. Ophthal.*, 1963, **56**: 922–925.
41. Miller, J. W., Study of visual acuity during the ocular pursuit of moving test objects. II. Effects of direction of movement, relative movement, and illumination. *J. Opt. Soc. Amer.*, 1958, **48**: 803–808.
42. Morris, A., Katz, M. S., and Bowen, J. D., Refinement of checkerboard targets for measurement of visual acuity limens. *J. Opt. Soc. Amer.*, 1955, **45**: 834–838.
43. Ogle, K. N., On the resolving power of the human eye. *J. Opt. Soc. Amer.*, 1951, **41**: 517–520.
44. ———, On the problem of an international nomenclature for designating visual acuity. *Am. J. Ophthal.*, 1953, **36**: 909–921.
45. ———, Blurring of the retinal image and contrast thresholds in the fovea. *J. Opt. Soc. Amer.*, 1960, **50**: 307–315.
46. ———, Foveal contrast thresholds with blurring of the retinal image and increasing size of test stimulus. *J. Opt. Soc. Amer.*, 1961, **51**: 862–869.
47. ———, Blurring of retinal image and foveal contrast thresholds of separated point light sources. *J. Opt. Soc. Amer.*, 1962, **52**: 1035–1039.
48. ———, The optical space sense. In: *The Eye, Vol. IV: Vision Optics and the Optical Space Sense* (H. Davson, Ed.). Academic Press, New York, 1962: 211–417.
49. ———, Visual resolution at the fovea for low contrasts. In: *Performance of the Eye at Low Luminances* (M. A. Bouman and J. J. Vos, Eds.). Excerpta Medica Foundation, Amsterdam, 1966: 71–82.
50. Ogle, K. N., and Schwartz, J. T., Depth of focus of the human eye. *J. Opt. Soc. Amer.*, 1959, **49**: 273–280.
51. Ogle, K. N., and Weil, M. P., Stereoscopic vision and the duration of the stimulus. *Arch. Ophthal.* (Chicago), 1958, **59**: 4–17.
52. Patel, A. S., Spatial resolution by the human visual system; the effect of mean retinal illuminance. *J. Opt. Soc. Amer.*, 1966, **56**: 689–694.
53. Pirenne, M. H., The absolute sensitivity of the eye and the variation of visual acuity with intensity. *Brit. Med. Bull.*, 1953, **9**: 61–67.
54. ———, Visual acuity. In: *The Eye, Vol. 2: The Visual Process* (H. Davson, Ed.). Academic Press, New York, 1962: 175–195.

55. PRINCE, J. H., Improvements in letter styles for sight-testing charts. *Texas Rep. Biol. Med.*, 1954, **12**: 370–382.
56. PRINCE, J. H., and FRY, G. A., The effects of spherical ametropia and astigmatism on visual acuity. *Brit. J. Physiol. Opt.*, 1957, **14**: 190–203.
57. RATLIFF, F., The role of physiological nystagmus in monocular acuity. *J. Exp. Psychol.*, 1952, **43**: 163–172.
58. ———, *Mach Bands: Quantitative Studies on Neural Networks in the Retina*. Holden-Day, San Francisco, 1965.
59. RIGGS, L. A., Visual acuity. In: *Vision and Visual Perception* (C. H. Graham, Ed.). Wiley, New York, 1965: 321–349.
60. SAIDUZZAFAR, H., and RUBEN, C. M., Visual acuity thresholds in amblyopes. *Brit. J. Ophthal.*, 1963, **47**: 153–163.
61. SAKIYAMA, A., Summation of visual acuity by binocular vision. *Ophthal. Lit.* (London), 1953, **7**: 398.
62. SCHWARTZ, J. T., and OGLE, K. N., The depth of focus of the eye. *Arch. Ophthal.* (Chicago), 1959, **61**: 578–588.
63. SÉDAN, J., JAYLE, G. E., and FARNARIER, G., De la supériorité de l'acuité visuelle binoculaire sur l'acuité visuelle monoculaire. *Ann. Oculist* (Paris), 1957, **190**: 385–400.
64. SHLAER, S., The relation between visual acuity and illumination. *J. Gen. Physiol.*, 1937, **21**: 165–188.
65. SHORTESS, G. K., and KRAUSKOPF, J., Role of involuntary eye movements in stereoscopic acuity. *J. Opt. Soc. Amer.*, 1961, **51**: 555–559.
66. SLOAN, L. L., Measurement of visual acuity; a critical review. *Arch. Ophthal.* (Chicago), 1951, **45**: 704–725.
67. VON BÉKÉSY, G., Neural inhibitory units of the eye and skin; quantitative description of contrast phenomena. *J. Opt. Soc. Amer.*, 1960, **50**: 1060–1070.
68. VON NOORDEN, G. K., and BURIAN, H. M., Visual acuity in normal and amblyopic patients under reduced illumination. II. The visual acuity at various levels of illumination. *Arch. Ophthal.* (Chicago), 1959, **62**: 396–399.
69. WESTHEIMER, G., Pupil size and visual resolution. *Vision Res.*, 1964, **4**: 39–45.
70. ———, Visual acuity. *Ann. Rev. Psychol.*, 1965, **16**: 359–380.
71. WESTHEIMER, G., and CAMPBELL, F. W., Light distribution in the image formed by the living human eye. *J. Opt. Soc. Amer.*, 1962, **52**: 1040–1045.
72. WILCOX, W. W., The basis of the dependence of visual acuity on illumination. *Proc. Nat. Acad. Sci. USA*, 1932, **18**: 47–56.
73. WILCOX, W. W., and PURDY, D. M., Visual acuity and its physiological basis. *Brit. J. Psychol.*, 1933, **23**: 233–261.

VISUAL FIELD DEFECTS IN RETINAL DISEASE

DAVID O. HARRINGTON
University of California School of Medicine
San Francisco, California

Retinal function, or vision, is measured clinically by the ability of the rods and cones to detect stimuli of varying size, degree of separation and luminance within the area of the visual field while the eye is steadily fixating a target placed in its visual axis.

Foveal vision, or central visual acuity, is generally measured by exposure to the retina of standard stimuli of varying size, such as Snellen letters or Landolt rings, at fixed distances under constant illumination. It is the function of the cones, which are concentrated in the macular area and whose threshold stimulus is high; they function most effectively under photopic conditions and their ability to discriminate between stimuli of minimal size and luminance is of a high order. Visual acuity in the macular or cone area is at its highest level in daylight.

Peripheral vision is measured by presenting stimuli of varying size and luminance in the field of vision of the steadily fixing eye. It is the function of the rods, which are diffusely spread throughout the retina except for the macular area, where they are totally absent. These photosensitive end organs are most effective under scotopic conditions, with low levels of illumination. Visual discrimination in the rod areas is low, partly because many rods are summated in a single bipolar cell and what they gain in sensitivity by such summation they lose in visual discrimination.

Cogan (8) has aptly differentiated the rods and cones by comparing them to the coarse and fine grains of photographic film: the coarse-grain film has greater sensitivity but lacks the qualities of detail of the fine-grain film.

Both central and peripheral vision depend upon the ability of the retina to change a minimal light stimulus into a photochemical reaction which in turn excites neuronal structures.

Visual acuity, whether in the rod or cone areas, varies with the illumination presented to the retina by the stimulus. This, in turn, depends on size and luminance of the test object (25), the contrast with its background, duration of stimulus exposure, size of the pupil, refractive state of the eye, clarity of the media through which the light from the stimulus must pass, and integrity of the photosensitive end organs, the rods and cones of the retina. The color of the stimuli and the degree of light or dark adaptation of the eye will also determine the size of the visual field and scotomatous areas within its boundaries. Finally, anatomical variations of the retina and its vasculature will affect the production of scotomata in case of disease. All these variables and their effects on the visual field, both normal and abnormal, are discussed in great detail in Dubois-Poulsen's elegant monograph (9), published by the French Ophthalmological Society in 1952.

Any disease process which damages the receptor organs of the retina will produce a relative or absolute loss of function in the portion of the visual field corresponding to the retinal area affected. Most of the diseases of the retina give rise to lesions that can be classified according to morphology, location and etiology, and are visible with the ophthalmoscope; because of dependence on this instrument for clinical diagnosis of retinal diseases, the study of their effect on function is often neglected. Functional loss may not, however, be proportionate to the apparent size and position of the ophthalmoscopically visible lesion. Sector defects in the visual field may change to island scotomata and vice versa. Analysis of the scotomata may therefore give much valuable information regarding the nature of the diseases which produced them, the total areas of retina affected, and the prognosis for improvement or decrease in function.

The variety of visual field defects produced by retinal disease is almost limitless, and there is probably no completely typical disturbance in function which is diagnostic of one lesion to the exclusion of all others. But careful analysis of a defect by a variety of perimetric techniques will usually give sufficient information regarding its density, position, sensitivity, progression, and actual size and shape as opposed to its visible characteristics, to guide the examiner in both diagnosis and prognosis. Such analysis may call for considerable flexibility in the examination and use of a variety of stimuli and instruments. For example, the central scotoma resulting from minimal and practically invisible macular edema may closely resemble that found with early retrobulbar neuritis when both are tested on a tangent screen. If monochromatic blue luminescent stimuli are exposed to ultraviolet light in the area of the scotoma, the defect resulting from retinal edema will be grossly exaggerated, whereas that from the neuritis will be unaffected. If the eye with the macular edema is subjected to a measured luminance stimulus (photostress), central visual acuity will be markedly depressed and the period of time required for recovery of the pre-exposure level of vision will be grossly prolonged (24); the eye with the optic neuritis will recover at an almost normal rate. Measurement of such a scotoma on the perimeter is almost useless because the short working distance (300 to 330 mm) of the instrument makes it virtually impossible to plot the defect, which may be so small as to lie entirely within the fixation target. At the same time, the retinal lesion which is barely visible at or near the ora serrata requires examination on the arc or hemisphere perimeter.

It becomes obvious that quantitative perimetric techniques are as important for the analysis of visual field defects due to retinal lesions as they are for diseases involving the rest of the visual pathway (17). Other examples will be discussed in the description of individual lesions to follow.

The retinal lesions that result in visual field defects, both peripheral and central, are probably best classified according to the pathology of the disease process, the portions or layers of the retina involved and, when possible, by the etiological agents causing the disease. This paper is concerned with the analysis of the various visual field defects produced by the following broad categories of retinal disease:

A. Vascular lesions affecting the arteries, veins, and capillaries of the retina and the choroid.

B. Inflammatory lesions of the retina and choroid.

C. Degenerative lesions of the various layers of the retina: hereditary, congenital, and acquired.

D. Toxic retinopathy and toxic lesions of the choroid secondarily affecting the retina.

E. Traumatic lesions of the retina and choroid.

F. Tumors of the retina and those of the choroid affecting retinal function.

G. Miscellaneous diseases affecting retinal function.

A. Vascular Lesions

Vascular affections of the retina are most important because they are both very common and, from the standpoint of retinal function, the most devastating. They consist of retinal arterial occlusion, both complete and partial, with resulting retinal ischemia and ischemic infarcts, capillary insufficiency, occlusion, and leakage; and venous occlusion, both partial and complete, with resulting hemorrhagic retinopathy and edema. In addition, there are the special retinal vascular manifestations of diabetes, the blood dyscrasias, arteriosclerotic changes without frank occlusion, vascular disease in the choroid with secondary circulatory insufficiency in the overlying retina (especially in the macular region), and damage to retinal function from circulatory insufficiency far removed from the retina itself.

1. Because the *central retinal artery* with its arborizations is an end artery, its occlusion causes complete ischemia of the retinal areas which it supplies, resulting in immediate and total blindness, usually permanent. If the eye is fortunate in having a cilioretinal artery arising from the choroid, the central area of the retina may be spared and a small island of central vision retained (Figure 249). On the other hand, occlusion of a cilioretinal artery produces a total centrocoecal scotoma within a normal peripheral field (5).

Obstructions of the retinal arterial system may be complete or may involve any part of the arterial tree from one half to a tiny twig near the macula or in the far periphery. These obstructions may be embolic, atherosclerotic, ischemic, or due to vasculitis.

Embolic obstruction of the inferior branch of the central retinal artery before it bifurcates into its nasal and temporal branches produces sudden loss of vision involving the entire superior field of vision (Figure 250A), with ischemia and cloudy swelling of the affected inferior retina. When the embolus (which may be a fragment of an atheromatous plaque from the internal carotid artery or possibly a rheumatic heart valve vegetation) lodges in an arteriole on the disk or in the

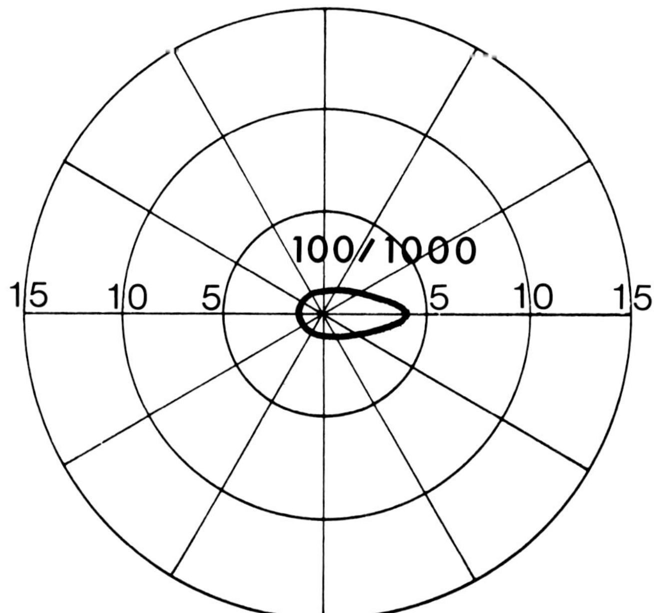

Figure 249. Total occlusion of the central retinal artery. The small central island of vision was preserved by a still patent cilioretinal artery.

anterior optic nerve, it may produce a typical nerve fiber bundle defect or Bjerrum scotoma (15) in the visual field (Figure 250B).

Occlusions of peripheral branches give rise to irregular sector defects, depending on the area of ischemic infarct in the retina. Although obstruction of minute arteriolar twigs near the macula, whether by emboli (common), atherosclerosis (rare), or vasospasm associated with hypertension, causes very small and almost invisible areas of infarction, the visual field defect may result in considerable loss of vision if it involves the macular area. Even if the scotoma is small and paracentral it may be very annoying to the patient because it is a positive scotoma and very dense. In time, many of these small scotomas become less noticeable, but some permanent defect in the visual field usually remains.

2. Embolus or atheromatous *obstruction of the choroidal vessels* supplying the foveal area of the retina causes marked and permanent loss of central vision with associated irregular central scotoma. These vary greatly in size, shape, and density, and the scotoma is often disproportionate in extent and density to what might be expected from the appearance of the macula.

There is good reason to believe that choroidal capillary insufficiency with secondary retinal ischemia is the primary cause of many macular holes. While it is sometimes difficult to ascertain whether these lesions are "cysts" or "holes", they always cause a progressive loss of central vision with a small, round, sharply outlined central scotoma. At first these defects are detectable only with small test objects, but later they may become so dense that no stimulus fitting within the boundaries of the scotoma is visible. It is also probable that this same capillary

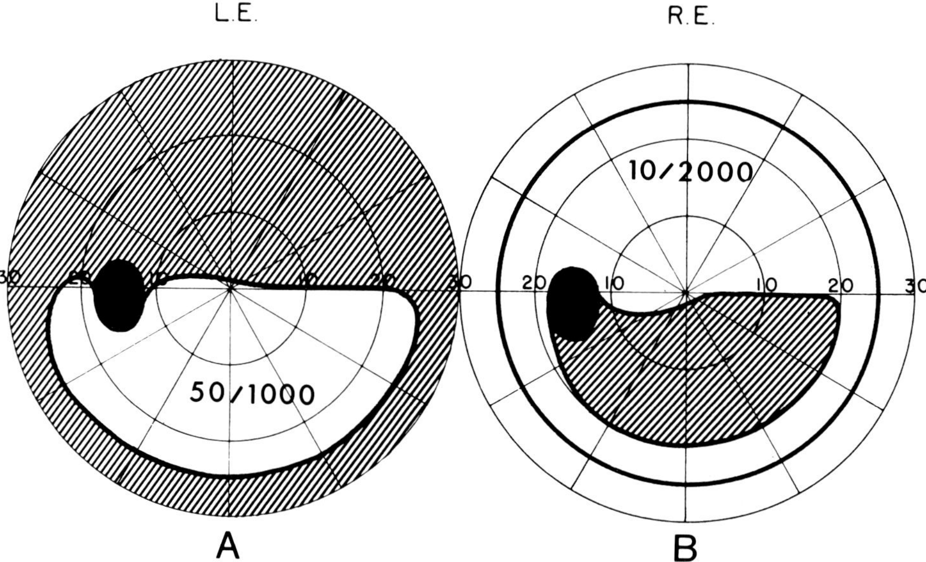

Figure 250. *A:* Altitudinal type hemianoptic defect produced by occlusion of the superior branch of the central retinal artery before it bifurcated into superior temporal and superior nasal branches. *B:* Bjerrum type scotoma resulting from an atheromatous plaque in the superior temporal artery at the disk margin; the occlusion followed an endarterectomy.

insufficiency is responsible to a large degree for the loss of retinal function in senile macular degeneration. It is not known whether this is due to pathological changes in the microvascular system supplying the macular region, or to deficient blood flow caused by faulty hemodynamics resulting in "blood sludging" and secondary to alteration in blood lipids. The work of Bloch (4) on the microvascular system is interesting in this regard.

The characteristic visual field defect in this condition is a "ragged", irregular central scotoma, often varying in density within its boundaries, slowly progressing in both size and density, usually unilateral in its onset but almost always eventually bilateral. The appearance of the macula frequently gives no real clue as to the extent of the scotoma; some of the worst-looking maculae have surprisingly good function. Whether this condition is, in fact, a true degenerative disease of the retina is still unsettled (8); I believe that it would be more reasonable to classify it as a disturbance secondary to vascular insufficiency, perhaps the result of arteriosclerotic or atherosclerotic changes in the choriocapillaries, but in any case due to decrease in blood flow to the very vulnerable fovea. This would explain the sometimes dramatic improvement in central vision and the scotoma when such cases are treated with rather small doses of heparin. Improvement in blood flow, probably due to lipid changes in the blood and not to the very transient anticoagulant effect of the heparin has, in my experience, often stopped or even reversed the progressive deterioration in visual acuity in early cases of senile macular degeneration. Intramuscular injection of only 200 mg (20,000 units) of aqueous sodium heparin twice weekly has improved retinal function in such a significant number of these patients that I believe it is a valid form of therapy. This supports the theory of capillary insufficiency in this disease. None of the cases thus treated showed a visible change in the appearance of the macula, but in many instances a discontinuance of the heparin resulted in an increase in the size and density of the scotoma and in a further progressive deterioration in visual acuity, which was again interrupted by resumption of treatment.

Evaluation of the effectiveness of such therapy is admittedly difficult, but in selected cases it has been most gratifying. Obviously, it is of no value in long-standing senile macular damage with irreversible destruction of the outer layers of the retina.

3. *Atheromatous obstruction of the retinal arteries* is probably rare. When it occurs it produces sector defects in the visual fields corresponding to its location in the retinal vascular tree. On the other hand, death of the ganglion cell layer of the retina from atheromatous occlusion of arteries relatively far removed from the retina may cause a variety of visual field defects. Thus, arterial obstruction in the ophthalmic artery and the arterioles supplying the optic nerve gives rise to segmental optic nerve atrophy and corresponding visual field defects; the most notable of these are typical and atypical nerve fiber bundle defects (15). These scotomata are rarely bilateral, and rarely multiple in a single eye. They may take the form of the typical Bjerrum scotoma and be indistinguishable from that seen in glaucoma (Figure 251); they may bisect fixation and break through into the peripheral field as a true altitudinal hemianopsia. In such cases, except that the defect is unilateral, the field loss may resemble that seen in the severe retinal ischemia associated with exsanguination (9,24) (Figure 252).

The same type of visual field defect, often preceded by increasingly frequent

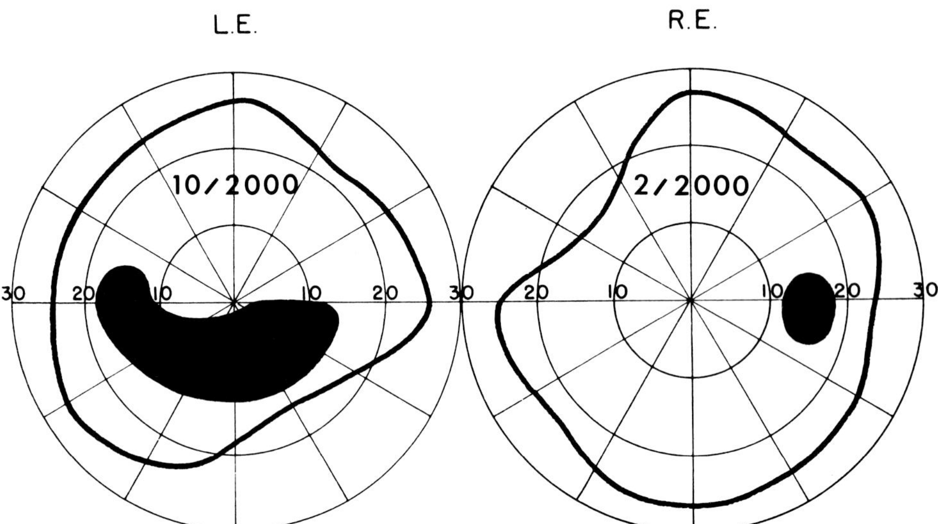

Figure 251. Nerve fiber bundle defect seen in a patient with stenosis and insufficiency of the left internal carotid artery. Intraocular pressure was normal, but retinal arterial blood pressure in the left eye was markedly lower than in the right.

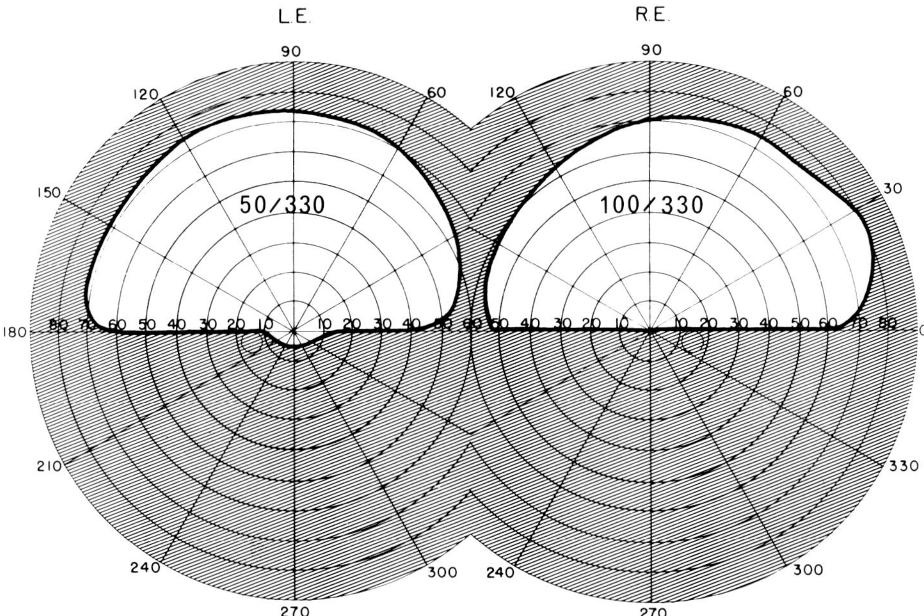

Figure 252. Bilateral inferior altitudinal hemianopsia following severe cerebral and retinal hypoxia from suffocation. An almost identical visual field defect was seen in a patient who was almost exsanguinated from massive hemorrhage from a peptic ulcer; similar bilateral altitudinal hemianopsia has been seen in two patients with long-standing pernicious anemia. Unilateral altitudinal field defects may be seen with superior retinal artery occlusion, whether due to atherosclerosis or to arteritis.

periodic transient "blackouts", usually of one eye, may result from gradual occlusion of the internal carotid artery (15). The visual loss, initially relatively infrequent and very transient partial or total in the eye on the same side as the occlusion, may increase in frequency and duration until suddenly there is prolonged obstruction with retinal ischemia, and either temporary or permanent visual field loss. The defect may obliterate the entire visual field, be altitudinal, with a narrow area of sparing of fixation, or involve only a part of the Bjerrum area. The scotoma may last for a few hours or it may be permanent. Frequently, there are other manifestations of neurological deficits such as hemiplegia or sensory loss contralateral to the occluded artery. In two such cases I have found a nerve fiber bundle defect in the visual field of the ipsilateral eye with a contralateral homonymous hemianopsia (14). Other signs of carotid artery occlusion may be present, such as a bruit over the affected artery, a lowered retinal arterial pressure on the same side as the occlusion when compared with the measurement of arterial pressure by ophthalmodynamometry in the opposite eye. Observations on the tonographic pulse wave as it is altered by carotid artery compression may also be useful in determining the side and even the site of the obstruction (2,11). This carotid-compression tonographic test should be carried out in cases of suspected carotid artery occlusion or in patients who have glaucoma-like nerve fiber bundle defects in the visual field without other evidence of glaucoma. I have used it in one such patient with "low tension glaucoma" and visual field defects to demonstrate the presence of ipsilateral carotid artery insufficiency.

Relief of the "blackouts" and, in some cases, reversal of the visual field defects associated with carotid and ophthalmic artery insufficiency has been accomplished with anticoagulant therapy. I have seen prompt and prolonged improvement in several patients treated with the low dosages of heparin described above; such improvement must be attributed to increased blood flow and was not related to the anticoagulant effect of the heparin nor to pressure changes in the retinal arteries as measured by ophthalmodynamometry.

4. *Arterial spasm* in the retina is generally associated with severe hypertension and is usually accompanied by varying degrees of hypertensive retinopathy. Whether it results in visual field defects is largely dependent on the location and severity of the spasm and on how much retinal ischemia or edema is produced by the arterial obstruction.

On occasion, one may see rather obvious localized narrowing of the larger retinal arteries near the disk with edema or perhaps cloudy swelling of the adjacent retina and disk margin. In such cases, careful tangent screen study of the area of visual field around the blind spot will reveal quite characteristic angioscotomatous-like defects (Figure 253). These may appear at first to be simple elongations of the blind spot, but careful analysis reveals that they are in fact due to broadening of an angioscotoma which can sometimes be followed well into the peripheral field.

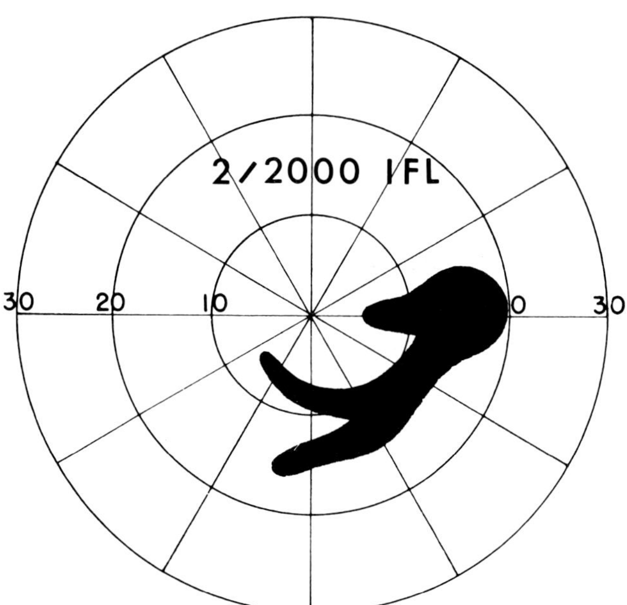

Figure 253. "Spasm" and severe localized narrowing of the superior temporal artery. The angioscotoma was easily demonstrated at two meters on the tangent screen with a 2 mm electroluminescent stimulus emitting 1 foot lambert of illumination (10).

When the angiospasm affects the smaller arterioles, especially those near the macula, the resulting retinal edema may cause a paracentral scotoma which in time spreads to the fixation area to affect central vision. These scotomata are generally not dense and their margins are sloping. When loss of vision is severe, a rather large defect may be expected to appear when tested with small targets, but with a denser central island of visual loss detectable with much larger stimuli.

Not uncommonly such eyes, in addition to the visible areas of retinal arterial spasm, will also show varying degrees of hypertensive retinopathy with deep and superfical retinal hemorrhages and exudates. Visual field studies are rarely done in such cases but examination, especially on the tangent screen at two meters, will reveal multiple small, irregular scotomata corresponding to the areas of deep retinal hemorrhage, occasionally also revealing sector-like defects probably due to unseen areas of infarction. It is obvious that the visual field defects found in hypertensive retinopathy are as variable as the degrees of retinal damage* from the disease.

5. The condition variously known as *central serous retinopathy*, *central serous detachment of the retina*, or *central angiospastic retinopathy*, is almost certainly vascular in origin. Whether it is an exudative retinopathy due to choroidal inflammation or angiospasm is a moot point. It is my belief that there may well be a variety of etiologic factors capable of producing this rather common and well described clinical entity. Cogan (8) has called it an exudative retinopathy and has listed it among the inflammatory affections of the retina, although he conceded that it may be an angioneurotic manifestation. Klien (21) calls the condition a serous chorioretinopathy and suggests that increased choroidal venous pressure may be its cause. I have felt (13) that the condition has been most frequently angiospastic in character, with the primary disturbance in the choriocapillaries and the clinical signs and symptoms being due to secondary retinal edema.

The typical ophthalmoscopic picture is one of central retinal elevation, sometimes as much as two diopters in height but more often of much lesser degree. The area of edema is surrounded by a bright ring reflex. The entire macular area may have a deeper and darker red coloration than normal. With minor differences, I have seen this ophthalmoscopic appearance in patients with macular edema from a variety of causes:

a. A minute area of macular choroiditis may give rise to overlying retinal edema sufficient to mask the inflammatory nature of the primary disease until the active inflammation and edema subside. At this time the pigmented choroidal scar becomes visible, and the true nature of the condition is evident. Considerable loss of central vision with dense steep-margined permanent central scotoma occurs.

b. The macular edema of commotic retina may, in its early stages, closely resemble this picture. The degree of edema, visual loss, and size and character of the central scotoma are naturally dependent on the severity of the contusion

---

* S. Severin, personal communication.

injury and the disruption of the outer retinal layers. In some cases, considerable degrees of edema may slowly regress, leaving relatively little functional loss.

c. Thermal burn of the retina may initially look like central serous retinopathy, but later stages reveal the minute foveal hole and ragged central scotoma to be described later.

d. The disturbance I prefer to call central angiospastic retinopathy is, I believe, a clinical entity distinct in many of its characteristics: it is usually unilateral but may be bilateral; it occurs in young persons, predominantly in males; it is usually fairly rapid in onset, and metamorphosia is a frequent and prominent presenting symptom, easily demonstrated on an Amsler grid. Visual loss may vary greatly, from 20/200 to 20/30. During the stage of maximum edema and visual loss there is a round, smoothly outlined central scotoma with density compatible with the degree of visual loss and with sloping margins; the scotoma is rarely very dense and can often be detected only by the most careful perimetry with small test objects, a working distance of two meters or more, and often only with reduced illumination of the stimuli.

One of the characteristics of the scotoma is its high degree of insensitivity to blue stimuli. Thus, if monochromatic blue test objects of luminescent phosphors are exposed to ultraviolet light, a small central scotoma, found only with difficulty with white targets, is greatly enlarged and intensified (Figure 254). In such circumstances, a 5 mm or even a 10 mm blue stimulus may reveal a larger scotoma

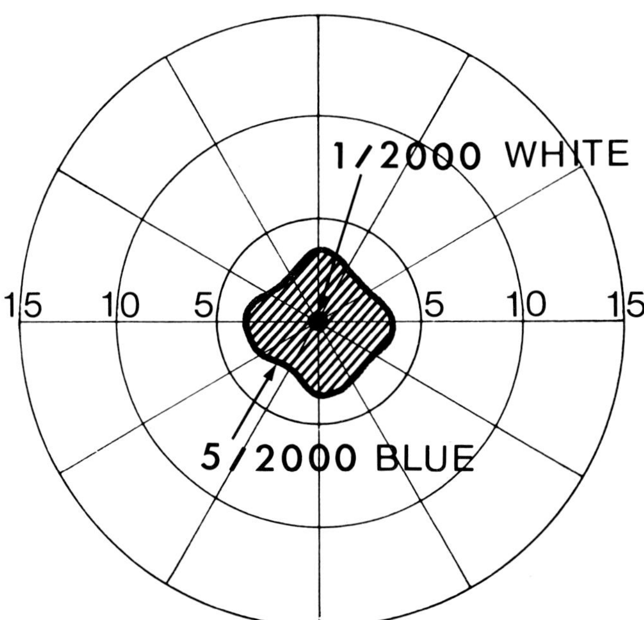

Figure 254. Angiospastic retinopathy with foveal edema (central serous detachment of the retina). The irregular, sloping margined central scotoma is best demonstrated on the tangent screen with monochromatic luminescent blue stimuli exposed to ultraviolet light. Positive photostress test (24).

than would a 1 mm target (18). As the edema subsides the scotoma regresses both in size and density. When such a macula is exposed to very bright light, as in the photostress test (24), the period of time required for vision to return to the pretest level is markedly prolonged (photofatigue), and the size and density of the scotoma are grossly exaggerated.

Many of these patients eventually recover completely. Vision returns to normal, the scotoma disappears and the only visible evidence of preexisting retinal disease is a faintly stippled or granular appearance in the macula. Permanent functional loss is rare and minimal in degree. In the other conditions listed above as giving rise to retinal edema, complete functional recovery is rare, and there is usually a permanent loss of central vision and a well-defined and permanent central scotoma.

Justification for considering this condition as angiospastic is found in its relatively transient character, the absence of any obvious pathological disturbance such as trauma, inflammation, or arterial occlusion, and its frequent and close association with autonomic nervous system imbalance (13).

6. *Hypertensive retinopathy* disturbs vision in a variety of ways, and the visual field defects associated with this condition usually reflect the picture seen with the ophthalmoscope. There may be isolated peripheral scotomata which result from hemorrhage into the outer retinal layers; superficial hemorrhage and exudates rarely give rise to scotomas. Ischemic infarcts of the retina may occur; their effect on vision and the visual field have already been described. Venous occlusion due to arterial compression at an arteriovenous crossing may cause severe retinal destruction and widespread visual field deficits (Figure 255); this will be discussed later.

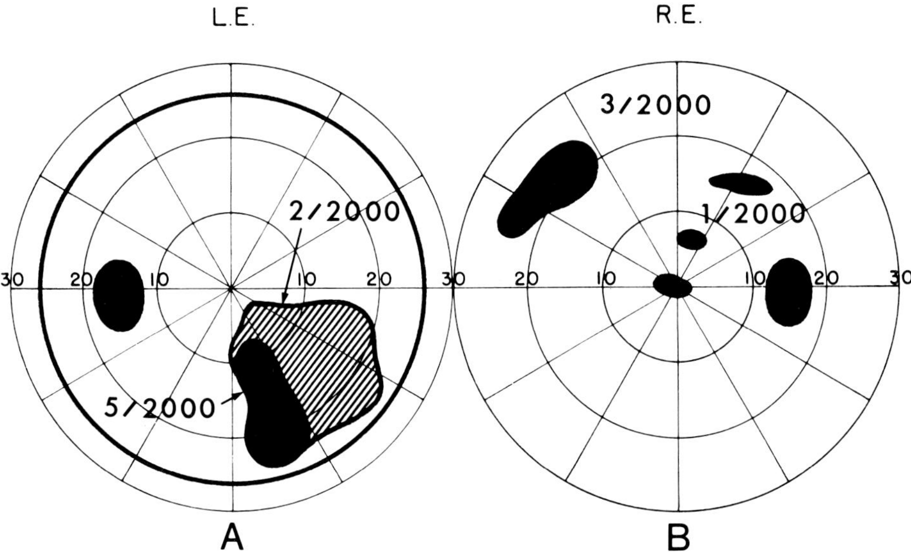

Figure 255. *A:* Occlusion of the superior temporal retinal vein with retinal hemorrhage. *B:* Hypertensive retinopathy with multiple deep and superficial retinal hemorrhages and isolated island-like scotomas.

7. *Papilledema* associated with hypertensive retinopathy may cause nerve fiber bundle defects in the visual field, possibly from arterial obstruction in the nervehead. Chronic papilledema with gliosis may also produce a Bjerrum scotoma (15). More commonly, edema of the disk, whether caused by increased intracranial pressure or as part of the picture of hypertensive retinopathy, produces generalized enlargement of the blind spots. In rapidly progressive edema, which may extend from the nervehead into the surrounding retina, the blind spot enlargement will take on the character of a centrocoecal scotoma with sloping edges and an apex pointing toward fixation. In chronic edema of the disk, the size of the blind spots may be enormous; the margins of the scotoma will be very steep (Figure 256). On occasion, the blind spot enlargement may be so gross that most of both temporal fields become involved, simulating a bitemporal hemianopsia.

8. *Vasculitis* or inflammatory involvement of the retinal vessels may take various forms. Most typical is the giant cell arteritis known as temporal arteritis, in which vision and the visual fields are frequently affected (6,26). This disease, characterized by general malaise, fever, leucocytosis, elevated sedimentation rate, and frequent pain and tenderness of the temporal arteries, may be widespread and involve the cerebral, ophthalmic, and retinal arteries, especially the central retinal artery in the optic nerve. Loss of vision is usually fairly sudden, total and permanent. The inflammatory occlusion of the ophthalmic and retinal arteries may not occur for several weeks after the onset of the disease. Both eyes may be affected, one after the other. I have seen one patient with a large central scotoma and the typical ophthalmoscopic picture of papillitis, in whom the diagnosis of giant cell arteritis was confirmed by temporal artery biopsy. Another case with widespread cerebral arteritis, confirmed at autopsy, had an altitudinal

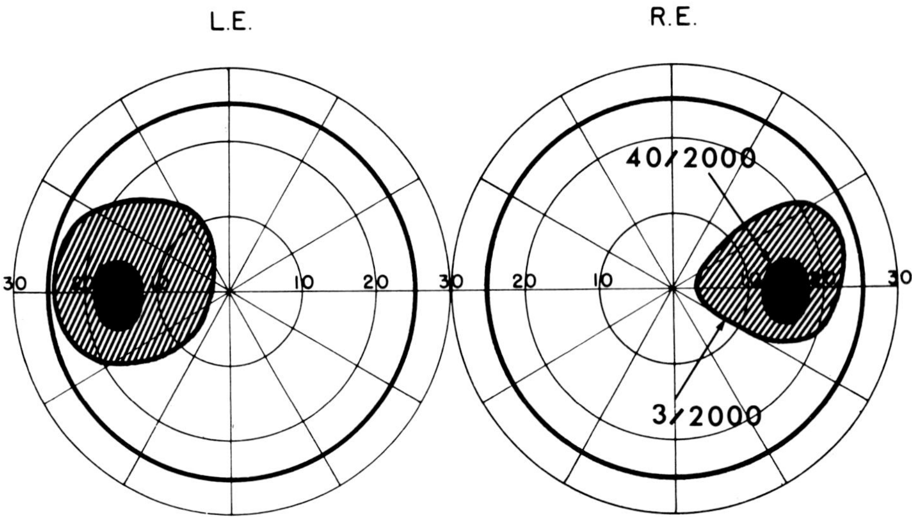

Figure 256. Gross enlargement of the blind spots in severe acute papilledema associated with increased intracranial pressure. The retinal edema extended almost to the fovea.

hemianopsia. A third patient with the typical clinical syndrome of temporal arteritis developed a double Bjerrum scotoma (15). Nasal and concentric contraction of the visual fields is common. Favorable response to steroid therapy may be expected and is often dramatic.

Cogan (8) has pointed out that many inflammatory processes may involve retinal arteries and veins, and that such conditions may therefore be classified as vasculitis. When the vessels in the optic nerve are involved, the condition may be indistinguishable from any papillitis. It is in fact quite likely that many cases of papillitis are due to vascular inflammation in the optic nerve which may then spread into the retinal vascular tree, producing arterial (or venous) sheathing and finally obstruction (23). In such cases, visual loss may be severe and the visual fields will show a dense central or centrocoecal scotoma or a marked contraction of the peripheral field depending probably on which vessels are involved. Visual loss may be greater than would be expected from the ophthalmoscopic appearance of the retinal vascular tree. Some of these cases appear to respond favorably to steroid therapy.

Occasional patients are seen with sheathing of a portion of the retinal vascular tree and with corresponding sector deficits in the visual field. It is not always possible to ascertain whether this condition is due to vasculitis.

Acute syphilitic vasculitis with ocular involvement, once very common, is now extremely rare. At one time it was responsible for many cases of blindness with a great variety of visual field defects.

9. *Diabetic retinopathy* is listed here because in it the main cause of visual loss is vascular in origin. In its early stages troublesome visual disturbance is rare (22). Even when there are large numbers of microaneurysms, numerous deep and superficial retinal hemorrhages, and some areas of retinal edema, complaints of visual loss are uncommon. Careful examination of the central area of the field on the tangent screen with small stimuli will sometimes reveal isolated and multiple scotomas corresponding to areas of hemorrhage and exudate (Figure 257). If the macula is involved there will be bothersome central scotoma and in some cases enlargement or irregularity of the blind spot will indicate optic nerve involvement.

Once the stage of proliferative retinopathy is reached there will be, of course, marked visual loss with extensive obliteration of large segments of the visual field. These defects are dense and steep-margined. Coincidental arteriosclerosis and hypertension are common with diabetes, and visual defects may be, in part, due to these conditions rather than to the diabetes.

10. *Retinal venous occlusion* occurring in the central retinal vein, usually at or just behind the lamina cribrosa, produces very severe hemorrhagic retinopathy with extensive deep and superficial retinal hemorrhages radiating out from the obscured optic disk in the so-called "firecracker fundus". Visual loss is sudden and marked but not total, and the prognosis for its reversal is very poor; in a relatively high percentage of cases, "hemorrhagic glaucoma" supervenes sooner or later, and many of these eyes are lost. There is no characteristic visual field defect in central vein occlusion but, when the field is examined on the arc or spherical perimeter with large stimuli, remnants of peripheral vision are usually

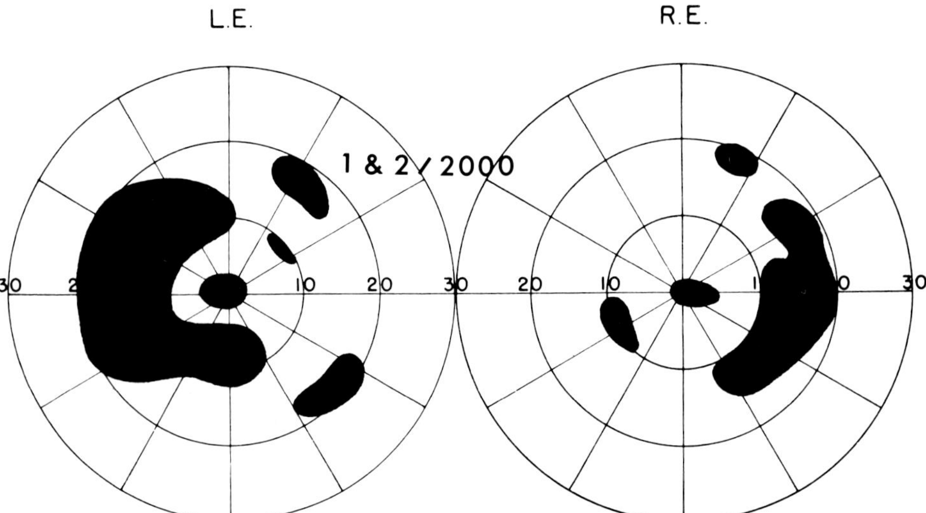

Figure 257. Multiple scotomas resulting from advanced diabetic retinopathy with hemorrhages, exudate and retinal edema.

found remaining around a large, dense, and ragged central scotoma. Even in severe cases of central retinal vein occlusion some vision is often detected in both central and peripheral fields if large enough stimuli are used in the examination.

Occlusion of branches of the central retinal vein occur mainly at arterial crossings of the vein, hence their usual association with arteriosclerosis. Both central vein and branch occlusion also occur rather commonly in diabetes, and may result from any systemic disease predisposing to increased blood viscosity and sludging, such as polycythemia, sickle-cell disease (12), and macroglobulinemia (1).

Visual loss and visual field defects depend on which branch is occluded, how close to the central trunk the occlusion occurs, and how severely the macular area is affected by hemorrhage and edema. For some reason, the superior tributaries seem to be more frequently affected than those in the lower retina. The result is an inferior altitudinal quadrant or sector defect (Figure 255A), often with severe macular involvement due to the exaggerated macular response to edema following obstruction (27). The field loss may or may not be proportionate to what might be expected from the appearance of the retina. Prognosis for return of considerable vision is good, and resolution of a good part of the visual field deficit may occur as hemorrhages and edema are absorbed. Intractable "hemorrhagic" glaucoma rarely occurs in branch occlusion of retinal veins, but primary glaucoma is not an uncommon coincident finding which has led to the feeling that there may be some connection between the two conditions.

Chronic retinal vein occlusion or insufficiency may produce little or no visual loss due to development of collateral circulation. There may be, however, considerable arborization and enlargement of angioscotomatous defects around the blind spot (9).

B. Inflammatory Lesions Affecting the Retina

These lesions, producing visual loss and visual field defects, have been mentioned in the discussion of vasculitis, but the majority of such defects are secondary to inflammatory lesions of the choroid with destruction of the overlying retinal cells.

1. *Harada's disease* may give rise to a peculiar exudative type of retinal detachment, usually bilaterally, affecting the lower peripheral retina and producing superior irregular quadrant or altitudinal defects in the visual fields.

2. *Toxoplasmosis* is a common cause of unilateral and bilateral chorioretinal damage with central scotoma and marked visual loss in children. The scotomata are irregular in size and outline, extremely dense and steep-margined. The area of field loss may also be peripheral and is dependent upon the area of toxoplasmic retinopathy.

3. *Choroiditis with associated retinitis* and severe visual loss may occur in diverse conditions and give rise to varying degrees of visual loss and a wide range of visual field defects, depending on the area of retina affected. Sympathetic ophthalmia may show both central scotoma and peripheral contraction.

4. The *disseminated choroiditis of syphilis* is responsible for profound visual loss when the macular area is involved. Peripheral island-like scotomata occur from widespread patchy chorioretinitis. The condition is relatively uncommon today.

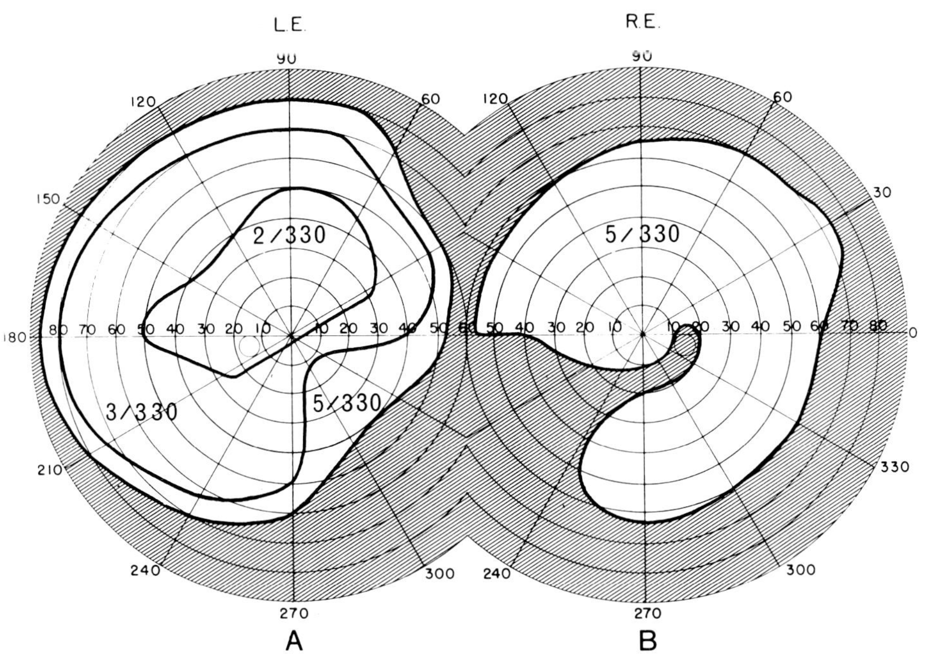

Figure 258. *A:* Visual field defect produced by malignant melanoma of the choroid with overlying retinal detachment. *B:* Nerve fiber bundle defect in the visual field resulting from acute choroiditis juxtapapillaris.

5. *Nonspecific choroiditis* always involves the overlying retina. In its acute stage visual loss may be severe, due in part to vitreous opacification but mostly to edema and cellular damage in the outer retinal elements. As there may be associated involvement of the optic nervehead, the condition is spoken of as neuroretinitis. In such cases the visual fields show scotomata with sloping edges in the areas of the field corresponding to the choroidal lesions. When the optic nerve is involved, there is almost always a fairly dense central scotoma. When a nerve fiber bundle is involved in a patch of choroiditis at the disk margin, the field defect which results may be a cuneate sector or wedge-shaped scotoma in the nasal field, or a typical arcuate or Bjerrum scotoma with nasal step and peripheral breakthrough (Figure 258B).

The occurrence of minimal foveal choroiditis with overlying macular edema has already been discussed in connection with angiospastic retinopathy. The central scotoma produced by this lesion is initially fairly large, but not dense, and has sloping edges. As healing takes place, the retinal edema subsides and the scotoma regresses until all that remains is a small, dense, steep-margined defect corresponding to the area of choroidal scar.

C. Degenerative Lesions of the Retinal Layers

Degenerative diseases involving the outer retinal layers may cause marked and progressive visual loss, both central and peripheral. Except for retinitis pigmentosa, the usual visual field defect is a progressively enlarging central scotoma.

1. Because *retinitis pigmentosa* initially and primarily involves the retinal rods, the earliest symptom is night blindness associated with a characteristic ring

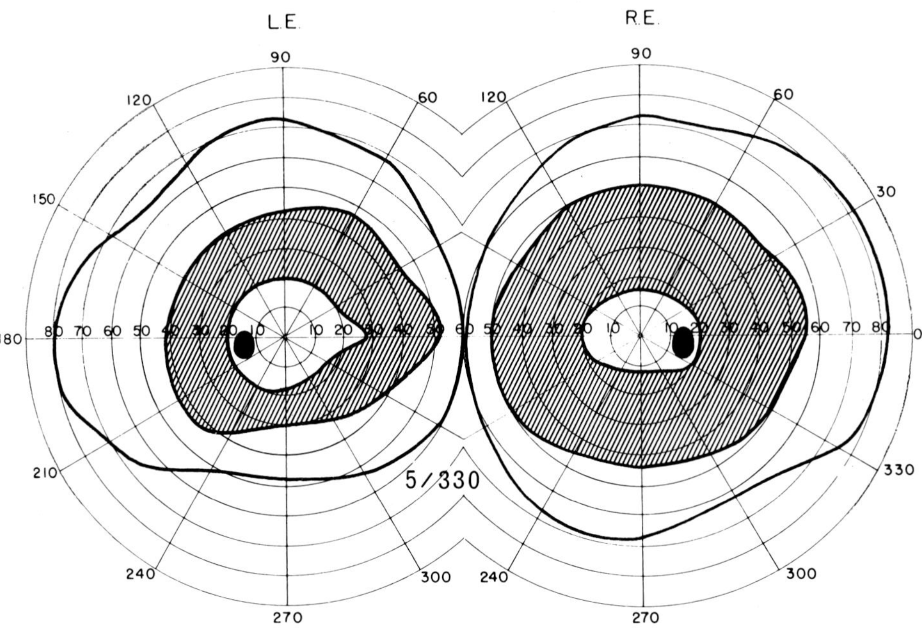

Figure 259. Typical equatorial ring scotoma in an early case of retinitis pigmentosa.

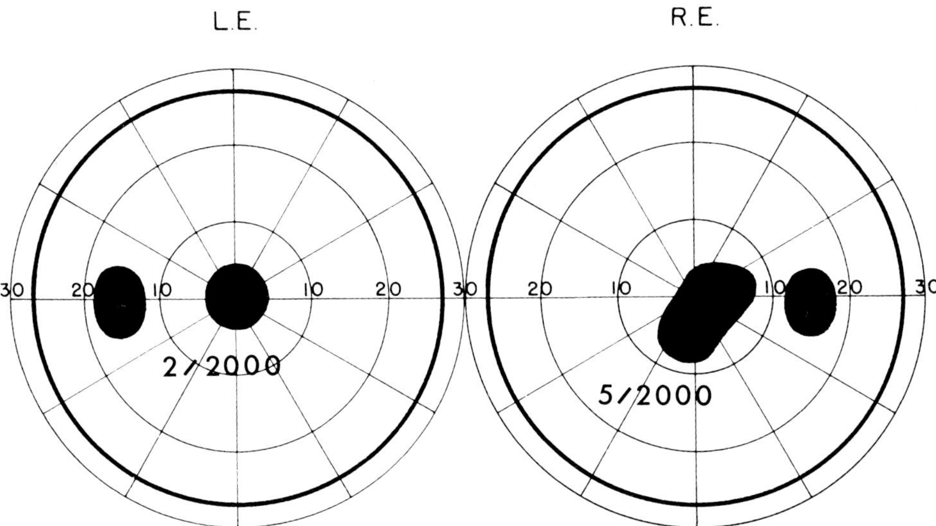

Figure 260. Bilateral central scotoma in a case of familial pigmentary degeneration of the macula. Two other siblings had identical macular disease and visual field defects. Only one generation of the family was affected.

scotoma occupying the midperiphery of the visual field. This scotoma usually starts as a group of isolated scotomata in the area 20 to 25 degrees from fixation (Figure 259). These defects gradually coalesce to form a partial and finally a complete ring. The outer edge of the ring expands peripherally at a fairly rapid pace, while the inner margin contracts towards fixation at a much slower rate. Long after the entire peripheral field is gone, there may remain a small oval remnant of intact central field, resembling the terminal field defect of glaucoma. There are numerous variants of typical retinitis pigmentosa, among them the Laurence-Moon-Biedl syndrome, in which condition there may be macular involvement with central scotoma in addition to widespread peripheral field loss; visual defects also tend to progress more rapidly.

2. *Familial or hereditary pigmentary degeneration of the maculae* is a fairly common condition that may affect several siblings. The condition is bilateral, with a gradual onset in the second decade of life. Central visual loss occurs early and progresses slowly. The visual field deficit is a round, sloping margined central scotoma (Figure 260). Occasionally, a minute area of vision is spared exactly at fixation, giving the scotoma the appearance of a doughnut. The condition may affect more than one generation of a family.

3. *Senile macular degeneration* has already been discussed in connection with vascular or capillary insufficiency in the macular area of the choroid. The degree of interruption of visual function may not parallel the appearance of the retina, but when retinal function is disturbed a central scotoma results. Aging maculae, whether they show visible degenerative changes or not, are more than usually vulnerable to photostress* and subject to severe photofatigue. Visual recovery

---

* S. Severin, personal communication.

after exposure to intense light is very prolonged; this is probably associated with the exaggerated macular response to retinal disease (27).

4. *Disciform degeneration* may occur at almost any age, although it is very much more common after the sixth decade of life. Senile macular degeneration may change gradually and almost imperceptibly to disciform degeneration. Until hemorrhage occurs around the disk-like yellowish white macular mass, visual acuity may be surprisingly good; eventually central visual acuity is reduced and an irregularly round central scotoma with sloping edges develops (Figure 261). The condition is always bilateral, although one eye may be involved long before the other. Visual loss and the scotoma are due to destruction of the outer retinal layers resulting from breaks in Bruch's membrane followed by hemorrhage from the choriocapillaris and proliferation of fibrous tissue from the pigment epithelium.

5. *Drusen*, invading the retinal pigment epithelium as excrescences from Bruch's membrane, cause relatively little visual disturbance and, unless they are very large and occur in great numbers, cause no visual field defect. Occasionally macular drusen produce small, rather vague scotomas in the fixation area. Drusen on or behind the optic disk, on the other hand, may give rise to irregularly contracted visual fields (17) or to typical Bjerrum scotomas (15).

D. Toxic Lesions of the Retina and Choroid

There are a few drugs and poisons which directly affect the retina and produce varying degrees of visual loss and characteristic visual field defects.

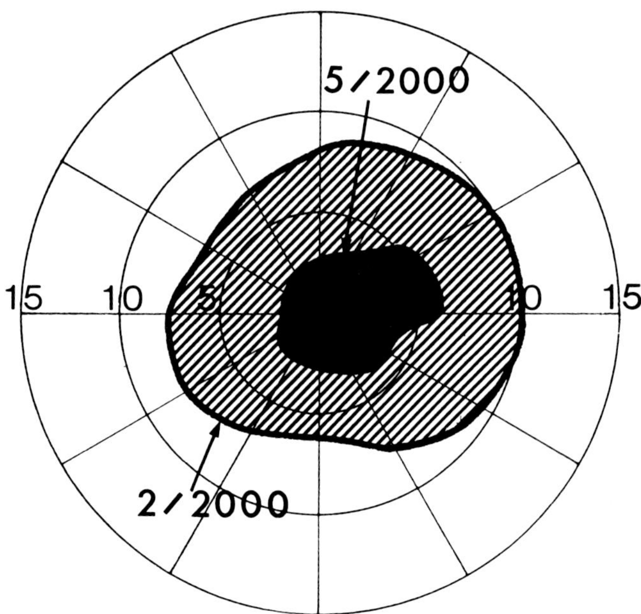

Figure 261. Large, irregular sloping margined central scotoma seen in a typical case of disciform degeneration of the macula. The other eye showed early senile degeneration of the macula with a very small and indefinite paracentral scotoma.

Quinine in large doses, such as those used in self-medication to induce abortion, produces marked attenuation of the retinal arterioles, probable secondary retinal hypoxia and death of the ganglion cells. The acute phase of poisoning results in blindness, followed later by partial restoration of vision but with markedly contracted visual fields.

Methyl alcohol poisoning, which causes severe optic atrophy and the development of large and very dense bilateral central scotomas, may affect the optic nerve primarily, or the ganglion cell layer of the retina, or both.

The amblyopia associated with severe nutritional deficiency is characterized by destruction of the ganglion cell layer of the retina and by the presence of bilateral central scotomas.

Pigmentary degeneration of the retina following prolonged and massive dosage of thoridiazine (Mellaril) may result in night blindness followed by loss of central vision and the development of bilateral central scotomata. The degree of disturbance is correlated with the dosage of the drug and the condition may be partially reversible when the drug is discontinued.

Much interest has recently centered on the effect on the retina of various quinoline drugs used in the treatment of rheumatoid arthritis and lupus erythematosus, of which the most widely used are chloroquine and hydroxychloroquine. When used in fairly large doses and for prolonged periods, chloroquine may produce a pigmentary degeneration of the retina which slightly resembles retinitis pigmentosa, but with macular involvement, and which is irreversible (19). Visual loss may be profound and the visual field defect is a characteristic ring-shaped scotoma with a minute area of macular sparing (Figure 262). The drug produces pigment migration from the pigment epithelium, arteriolar narrowing, and widespread destruction of rods and cones in the retina (3).

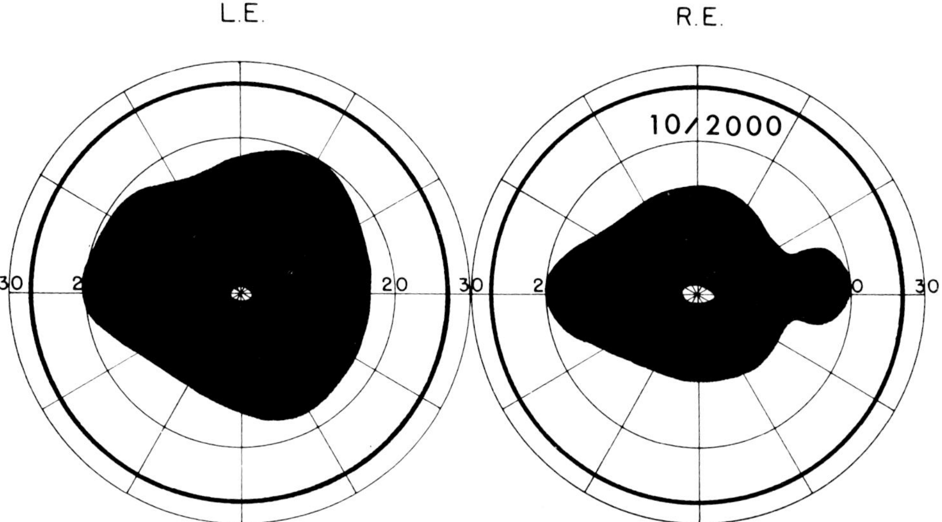

Figure 262. Large, dense central scotoma with a minute area of foveal sparing in a case of chloroquine retinopathy.

E. Traumatic Lesions of the Retina and Choroid

Lesions of the retina induced by trauma may be primary in the retina or secondary to choroidal injury.

1. *Contusion injury* of the globe without laceration, rupture, or intraocular hemorrhage may cause edema and subsequent temporary or permanent damage to the outer retinal layers, especially in the macular area. This "commotic retina" or "Berlin's edema" of the macula is probably due to the contra-coup effect of sudden and severe compression of the globe. Initial visual loss may be extensive. As the edema subsides somewhat, a fairly large central scotoma may be demonstrated (Figure 263). Finally, with complete absorption of the retinal edema, the macula may exhibit a granular pigmented appearance and, depending on the degree of destruction of the outer retinal layers, a permanent small central scotoma will result. The end result of a fairly severe commotio retina may resemble closely the final stages in angiospastic retinopathy.

2. *Traumatic choroidal rupture* which usually occurs (also by contusion of the globe) in the area between disk and macula, may be accompanied by severe retinal edema and resultant visual loss, especially in the central area of the field. At the same time, the damage to the outer retinal cells immediately over the rupture is usually profound. When the retinal edema and choroidal hemorrhage have subsided, the crescent-shaped, yellow choroidal tear (either single or

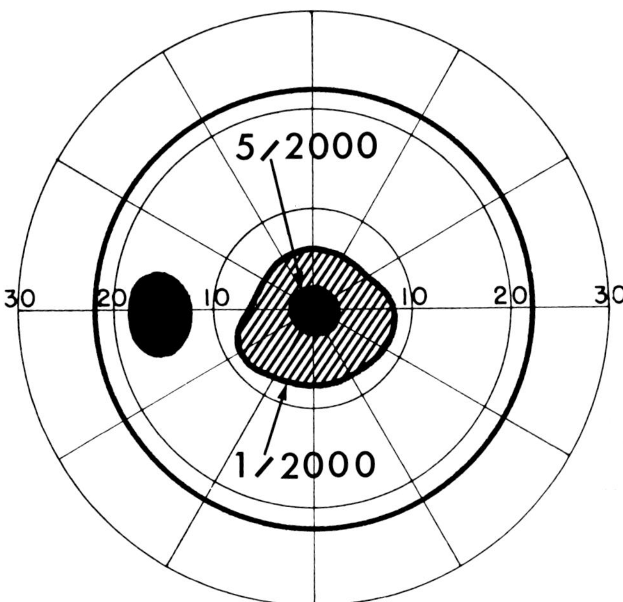

Figure 263. Sloping margined central scotoma due to commotio retina with macular edema following a contusion injury to the eye with a hard rubber handball. Visual acuity was restored to normal after subsidence of the macular edema.

multiple) may be seen; the visual field defect corresponds closely to the size and position of the rupture (Figure 264). The central scotoma frequently persists after all macular edema has disappeared.

3. *Thermal burns* of the retina are commonplace after every eclipse of the sun despite widespread publicity regarding the danger of watching solar eclipses through even the darkest filters. Similar burns of the retina have been reported after exposure to the light generated by atomic explosions (7). Minute irregular retinal "holes" or "cysts" occur in or immediately adjacent to the fovea in one or both eyes following exposure to direct sun rays, concentrated in the macular area by the condensing action of the lens. Immediately after exposure there is marked visual loss with intense "afterimage" blindness. This may subside fairly quickly, leaving a rather large diffuse central scotoma. In time, with the complete subsidence of edema, the characteristic foveal or parafoveal hole is seen, and the visual field defect (which is permanent) corresponds very accurately to the visible retinal lesion.

These scotomata are usually fractions of a degree in size and may be difficult to detect, but careful tangent screen examination using small stimuli and two-point discrimination at two, three or even four meters makes it possible to plot them very accurately (Figure 265). Another excellent method of mapping such small central or paracentral defects is the prism-displacement test of Irvine (20).

4. *Traumatic retinal tears* which allow the vitreous to seep into the subretinal space and produce retinal detachment will be considered separately.

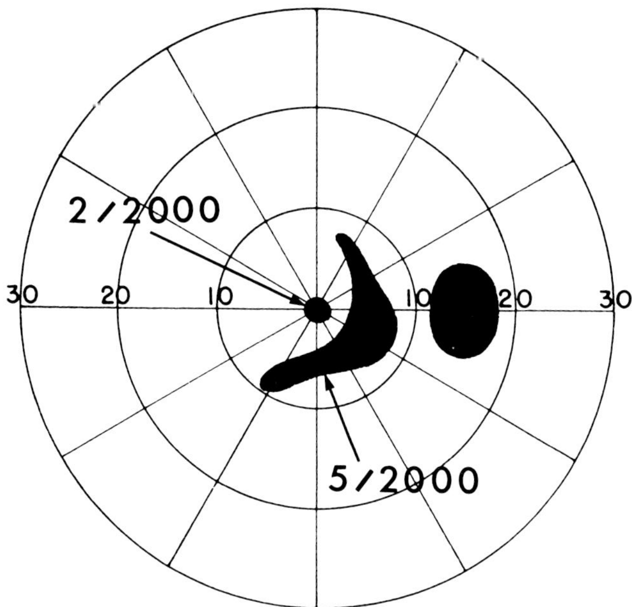

Figure 264. Crescent-shaped paracentral scotoma between fixation and the blind spot resulting from traumatic choroidal rupture. The macula was pigmented and showed a small, permanent central scotoma.

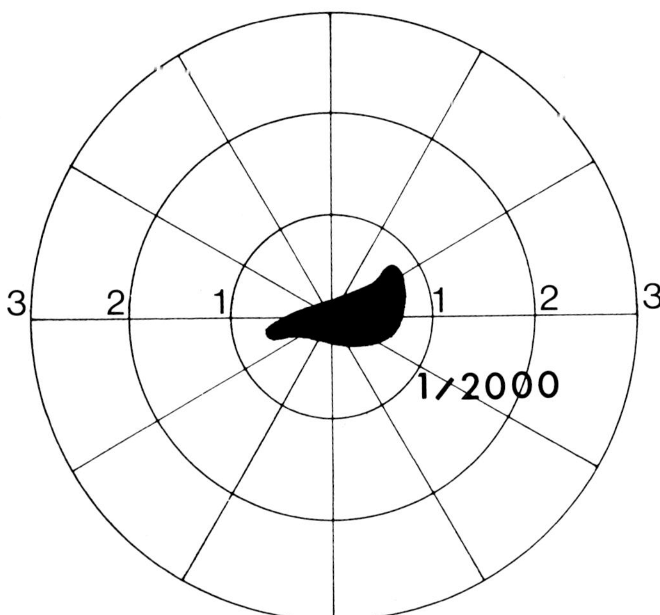

Figure 265. Minute, irregular central scotoma resulting from eclipse burn of the fovea; note that the defect is less than one degree in its widest diameter. Such defects are best elucidated on the tangent screen at distances of 2 or even 4 meters with very small test objects and fixation targets. They may also be accurately mapped out with the prism displacement test (20).

F. Retinal and Choroidal Tumors

Tumors involving the retina and the choroid produce visual loss and visual field defects entirely dependent on their size, location, duration, and degree of retinal separation overlying them.

1. A *malignant melanoma of the choroid* arising anterior to the equator with a minimal degree of "flat detachment" of the retina may show evidence of visual deficit in the field only when examined with small stimuli or with a low-luminance stimulus (17) (Figure 258A). A similar but perhaps considerably smaller tumor located at the disk margin and interrupting nerve fiber bundles in the retina or optic nerve may produce a much denser scotoma in the visual field, either corresponding to the shape and size of the tumor or arcuate in character (Figure 266).

2. *Retinoblastoma* is diagnosed with the ophthalmoscope. Because of the age of patients suffering this disease, visual field studies might have value but cannot in fact be done.

3. *Angiomatosis retinae* with or without cerebellar involvement causes severe visual loss and widespread damage to the visual fields, both central and peripheral (Figure 267). Both eyes are often affected. While the lesions are usually in the far periphery of the fundus and the corresponding visual field defects are also

peripheral, the central retinal area is frequently involved, probably due to "exaggerated macular response" (27), and central scotomas are common and disabling. Growth spread of the tumor and its vascular response eventually cause blindness.

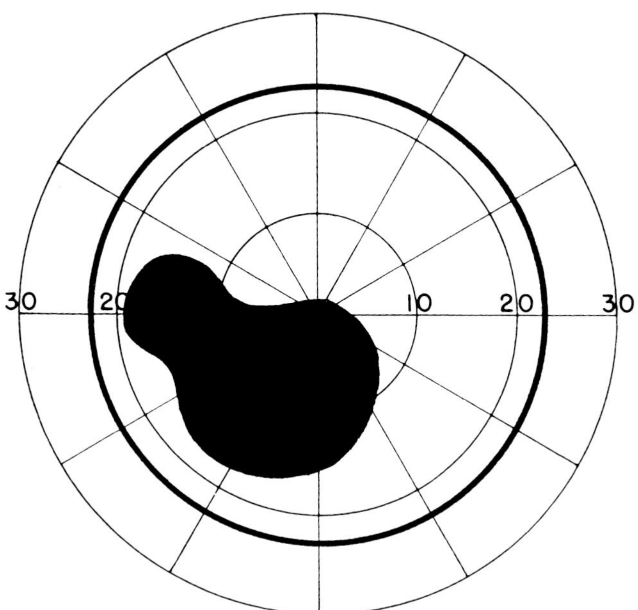

Figure 266. Malignant melanoma at the disk margin with overlying retinal edema and detachment.

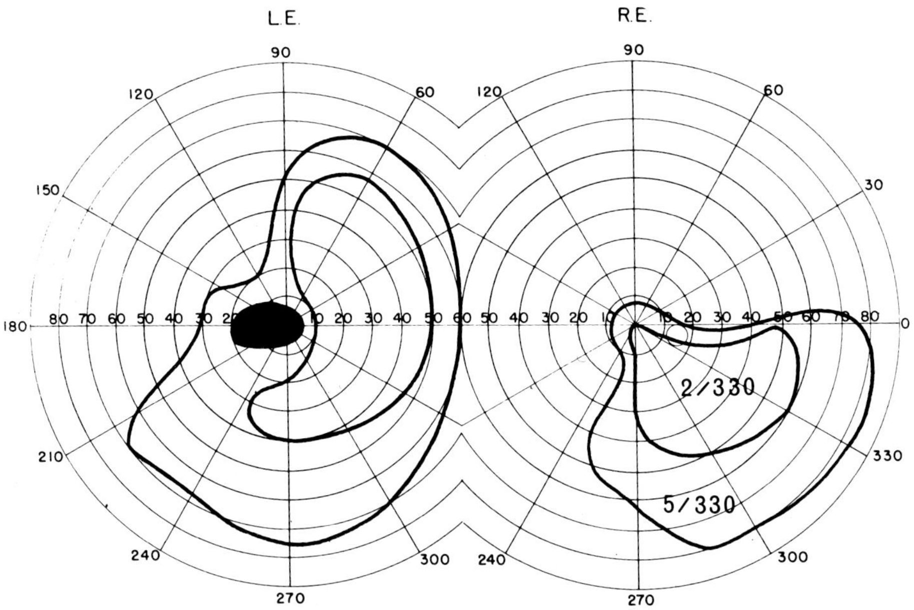

Figure 267. Visual field defects in a case of bilateral Von Hipple's angiomatosis retinae.

4. *Benign naevus of the choroid* producing a defect in the visual field should be viewed with great suspicion and subjected to frequent scrutiny. I have seen two such cases in which visual field studies with stimuli of low luminance revealed consistent deficits in the field corresponding to the area occupied by the naevus (16). These patients have been observed for several years without evidence of change in their visual fields or in the appearance of the lesion; I still feel, however, that they should be vigilantly watched.

G. Miscellaneous Diseases Affecting Retinal Function

Among these are carotid artery stenosis and insufficiency, anoxemia secondary to exsanguination and asphyxia, abnormal protein retinopathies (e.g., macroglobulinemia), the leukemias, retinal cysts, retinal schesis, myopia, posterior staphyloma and ectasia, and retinal detachment. A discussion of miscellaneous retinal diseases which may cause visual field defects must also consider a variety of congenital abnormalities such as coloboma of the choroid, retina and optic nerve, medullated nerve fibers, and optic nerve pits with ganglion cell atrophy.

1. For the most part, the *colobomas* cause extensive loss of the superior field of vision, usually involving fixation. Vision and fixation are usually so poor that accurate studies are almost impossible.

2. *Medullated nerve fibers* rarely cause visual loss, and field defects are uncommon. Occasionally, a patch of these medullated nerve fibers, isolated from the optic disk, will cause a defect in the visual field; differential diagnosis in such cases may be somewhat difficult.

3. *Optic nerve pits* which produce secondary retinal nerve fiber and ganglion cell layer atrophy may produce typical nerve fiber bundle defects in the field (15). These are dense and steep-margined, and are best detected on the tangent screen. They are often attributed to glaucoma even in the absence of elevated intraocular pressure.

4. High degrees of *myopia* with retinal stretching, atrophy and cell damage may cause a variety of visual field defects. Central scotoma is not uncommon; markedly enlarged blind spot secondary to abnormal "conus" about the optic nervehead is common and, on occasion, nerve fiber bundle interruption at the disk margin will produce a Bjerrum scotoma.

5. *Posterior staphyloma*, especially if it involves the macular area, will cause a relative central scotoma, in which case the difference in refraction between the disk and the macula may be several diopters. If the eye is corrected for its minimal myopia and the visual field is examined with small stimuli at one or two meters, an area of visual loss or depression will be found at fixation. Conversely, if correction is worn for the macular refraction, other areas of the retina will be over- or under-corrected and will show depression of the visual field. These areas have been called "refraction scotomas" (10) (Figure 268). The same type of scotoma may, of course, be demonstrated in the case of a macular tumor which has elevated the retina several diopters in a localized area. To some degree, even the visual field in retinal detachment in its earliest stage of development may be a "refraction scotoma".

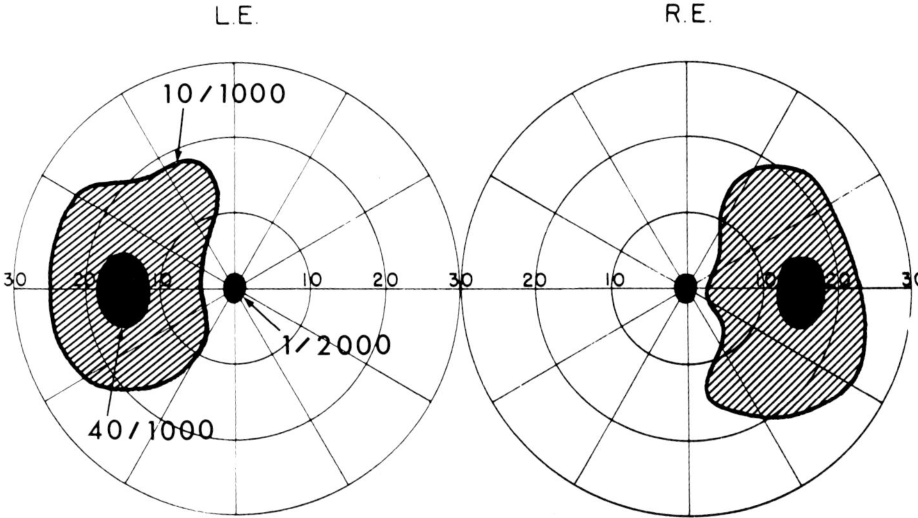

Figure 268. Extreme enlargement of the blind spots associated with posterior staphyloma or ectasia of the sclera around the optic nervehead. There was considerable choroidal and retinal atrophy. When the ectasia occupies the macular area the scotoma may be central. This "refraction scotoma" may represent a difference of five diopters between two portions of the retina.

6. The visual field defect of *retinoschisis* is characterized by its extreme density and steep margins, its bilaterality, and the fact that the nasal fields are almost always involved, more frequently above than below. The patient may be aware of the defect, and routine examination of the peripheral field will sometimes detect retinoschisis missed by ophthalmoscopy (Figure 269). Because of the density of the defect it is as readily detected with a 50 mm stimulus and as with one of 2 mm.

7. *Detachment of the retina*, or retinal separation from whatever cause, eventually destroys the outer retinal elements with resulting loss of vision in the area of separation. Traumatically induced retinal tears with subsequent retinal detachment have already been mentioned.

Visual field studies in retinal separation may be of considerable importance. The actual extent of the detachment may be more accurately judged by the field defect than with the ophthalmoscope, especially as detachments approach the macular area. When the visual field defect crosses fixation the prognosis is generally poorer than when fixation is spared. Occasionally, a very large and bulbous type of detachment of the superior retina will "hang down" over fixation, and yet the macular area may still have attached retina. In such cases it is worthwhile to have the patient lie flat for a period of time and then re-examine the field immediately and quickly after he resumes a sitting position; if the retina has "flattened out" during the reclining period but the visual field remains unchanged, the actual area of detachment may be outlined on the tangent screen.

Visual field defects in retinal detachment usually have sloping margins. They are exaggerated when the stimulus is presented under reduced illumination, and

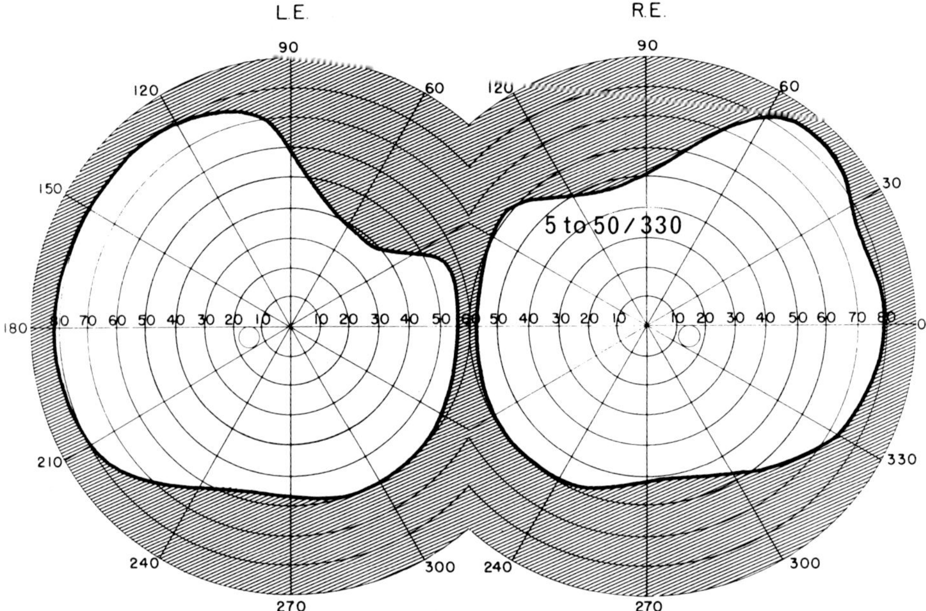

Figure 269. Dense, steep-margined peripheral nasal quadrant defects resulting from bilateral retinoschisis.

also with blue stimuli (Figure 270). Superior detachments usually have more extensive, denser, and steeper-margined defects than detachments involving the inferior retina and are also likelier to be noticed earlier and to be more disabling. An almost infinite variety of field defects may occur; in their early stages they are easier to detect with a perimeter than with a tangent screen. In addition to the more typical quadrantic or irregular hemianopic defects, many of them are altitudinal in type; there may be generalized contraction and, rarely, isolated scotomas.

Postoperative visual field studies for comparison with the preoperative field deficit are important for evaluating progress and prognosis and for medico-legal evidence.

8. No mention has been made of the visual field defects which may occur in association with the retinopathies of leukemia or of some of the retinopathies of unknown etiology, as they have no special characteristics. I have seen two patients, however, with long-standing pernicious anemia who have demonstrated dense bilateral inferior altitudinal hemianopsia (see Figure 252); in both cases the optic disks were partially atrophic and there was marked attenuation of the retinal arterial tree.

SUMMARY

The importance of visual field studies in retinal disease should be emphasized, for they frequently elicit information on the extent of the retinal lesion, its progress and its prognosis which is not obtainable by the ophthalmoscope or the measure-

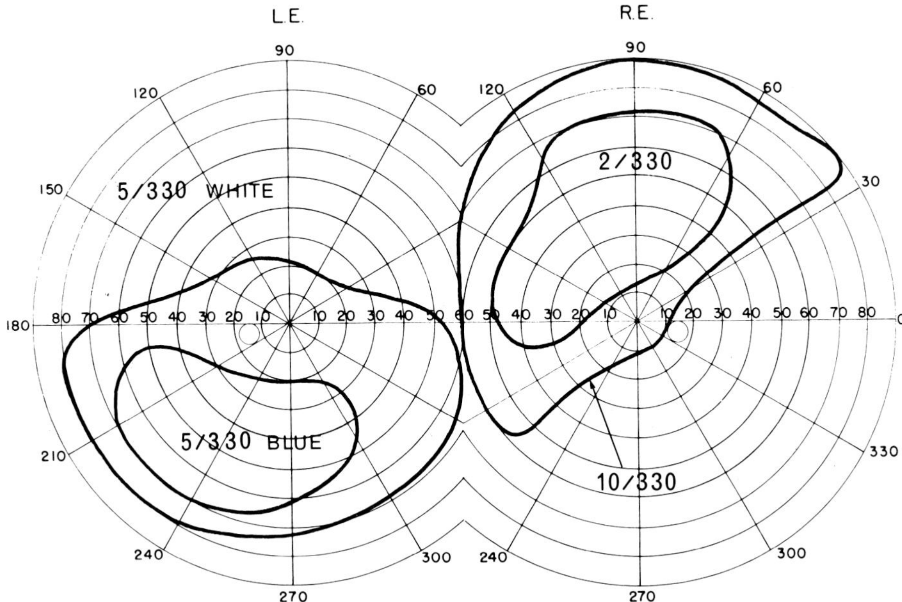

Figure 270. Two eyes with typical visual field defects resulting from retinal detachment. Note that the defects have very sloping margins and that the most marked deficit is demonstrated with blue stimuli.

ment of central visual acuity. A variety of perimetric techniques are necessary and should be utilized to obtain maximum information regarding the function of the retinal area affected by disease. Visual defects associated with several broad categories of retinal disease are discussed. Some of the visual field defects produced by retinal disease are illustrated.

REFERENCES

1. Ackerman, A. L., The ocular manifestations of Waldenström's macroglobulinemia and its treatment. *Arch. Ophthal.* (Chicago), 1962, **67**: 701–707.
2. Barrios, R. R., and Solís, C., Carotid-compression tonographic test; its application in the study of carotid-artery occlusions. *Am. J. Ophthal.*, 1966, **62**: 116–125.
3. Bernstein, H., Zvaifler, N., Rubin, M., and Mansour, A. M., The ocular deposition of chloroquine. *Invest. Ophthal.*, 1963, **2**: 384–392.
4. Bloch, E. H., Principles of the microvascular system. *Invest. Ophthal.*, 1966, **5**: 250–255.
5. Brosnan, D. W., Occlusion of a cilioretinal artery; with permanent central scotoma. *Am. J. Ophthal.*, 1962, **53**: 687–688.
6. Bruce, G. M., Temporal arteritis as a cause of blindness. Review of literature and report of a case. *Trans. Am. Ophthal. Soc.*, 1949, **47**: 300–316.
7. Byrnes, V. A., Brown, D. V. L., Rose, H. W., and Civis, P. A., Retinal burns—new hazard of the atomic bomb. *J. Am. Med. Ass.*, 1955, **157**: 21–22.
8. Cogan, D. G., *Neurology of the Visual System.* Thomas, Springfield, 1966.

9. Dubois-Poulsen, A., *Le Champ Visuel; Topographie Normale et Pathologique de ses Sensibilités*. Masson, Paris, 1952.
10. Enoksson, P. Perimetry in neuro-ophthalmological diagnosis. *Acta Ophthal.* (Kobenhavn), 1965, Supp. **82**.
11. Galen, M. A., and Harris, L., The ocular pulse in carotid-cavernous sinus fistula. *Am. J. Ophthal.*, 1966, **61**: 1472–1479.
12. Goodman, G., von Sallmann, L., and Holland, M. G., Ocular manifestations of sickle-cell disease. *Arch. Ophthal.* (Chicago), 1957, **58**: 655–682.
13. Harrington, D. O., The autonomic nervous system in ocular disease. *Am. J. Ophthal.*, 1946, **29**: 1405–1425.
14. ———, The pathogenesis of the glaucoma field; clinical evidence that circulatory insufficiency in the optic nerve is the primary cause of visual field loss in glaucoma. *Am. J. Ophthal.*, 1959, **47**: 177–185.
15. ———, The Bjerrum scotoma. *Trans. Am. Ophthal. Soc.*, 1964, **62**: 324–348.
16. ———, Tangent screen stimuli of variable luminance. *Arch. Ophthal.* (Chicago), 1964, **72**: 23–28.
17. ———, *The Visual Fields; A Textbook and Atlas of Clinical Perimetry* (2nd ed.). Mosby, St. Louis, 1964.
18. Harrington, D. O., and Hoyt, W. F., Ultraviolet radiation perimetry with monochromatic blue stimuli. *Arch. Ophthal.* (Chicago), 1955, **53**: 870–881.
19. Hobbs, H. E., Sorsby, A., and Freedman, A., Retinopathy following chloroquine therapy. *Lancet*, 1959, **2**: 478–480.
20. Irvine, S. R., Measuring scotomas with the prism-displacement test. *Am. J. Ophthal.*, 1966, **61**: 1177–1187.
21. Klien, B. A., Macular and extramacular serous chorioretinopathy; with remarks upon the role of an extrabulbar mechanism in its pathogenesis. *Am. J. Ophthal.*, 1961, **51**: 231–242.
22. Lee, P.-F., McMeel, J. W., Schepens, C. L., and Field, R. A., A new classification of diabetic retinopathy. *Am. J. Ophthal.*, 1966, **62**: 207–219.
23. Lyle, T. K., and Wybar, K., Retinal vasculitis. *Brit. J. Ophthal.*, 1961, **45**: 778–788.
24. Severin, S. L., Harper, J. Y., and Culver, J. F., Photostress test for the evaluation of macular function. *Arch. Ophthal.* (Chicago), 1963, **70**: 593–602.
25. Sloan, L. L., and Brown, D. J., Area and luminance of test object as variables in projection perimetry. *Vision Res.*, 1962, **2**: 527–541.
26. Wagener, H. P., and Hollenhorst, R. W., The ocular lesions of temporal arteritis. *Am. J. Ophthal.*, 1958, **45**: 617–630.
27. Wise, G. N., and Wangvivat, Y., The exaggerated macular response to retinal disease. *Am. J. Ophthal.*, 1966, **61**: 1359–1363.

CLINICAL ADAPTATION STUDIES OF THE HUMAN RETINA*

CHARLES J. CAMPBELL and M. CATHERINE RITTLER
Knapp Memorial Laboratory of Physiological Optics
Institute of Ophthalmology of Presbyterian Hospital
College of Physicians and Surgeons of Columbia University
New York, New York

This investigation is concerned primarily with adaptometric studies on patients with various retinal diseases. The report will include a description of the conditions and equipment employed and the normal values established for each of the specified testing conditions. A large number of retinal diseases, with a significant number of patients in most disease categories, were studied. The adaptometric findings will be related to the clinical diagnosis and to other functional attributes of the retina.

The perception of light is the most basic and elemental function of the retina and an essential aspect of the higher discriminatory visual functions. Adaptometry is closely related to light perception since it is concerned with the measurement of the threshold of the retina to light.

Due to the great sensitivity range of the retina, the various stimuli to which it responds, and the complexity of the information relayed to the central nervous system, the specification of retinal threshold values is extremely complex. Consequently, for threshold data to be meaningful, it is essential that standard conditions be selected and the mean and range of values for normal subjects be established. In this way, the emphasis in the clinical study can be directed toward altered threshold values in specific diseases.

The actual threshold value which may be obtained in any experimental situation depends on three different parameters. The first of these, *preadaptation*, refers to the exposure of the eye to a general illumination level before starting the period of dark adaptation, the rate of dark adaptation and the relative contributions of the rod and cone responses are influenced by the spectral composition, intensity, size, and duration of the preadapting exposure; preadaptation provides a common stimulus background for all subjects before starting threshold determinations. The second parameter which influences the threshold is the

---

* This research was supported in part by Grant-in-Aid #G-221 from The Fight for Sight-National Council to Combat Blindness, and by Grant NB-00879 from the National Institute of Neurological Diseases and Blindness, U.S. Public Health Service.

adaptation state of the eye after the preadapting exposure; this may be either photopic or scotopic. The third determinant of the threshold is the *nature of the testing stimulus* itself; as in preadaptation, the pertinent physical qualities in adaptation and in the stimulus are intensity, spectral composition, duration, and location and extent of the retina stimulated.

It is just as essential to specify the diagnostic criteria and the techniques employed in the clinical evaluation of each patient as it is to state the conditions for the threshold measurements. Normal subjects must be subjected to the same diagnostic evaluation as patients, and studied under the same adaptometric conditions. In this investigation the normal subjects and all patients had a complete clinical ocular examination in the Retina Clinic of Presbyterian Hospital, as well as an extensive series of retinal function studies. The clinical examination included a cycloplegic refraction and careful ophthalmoscopy.

The retinal function studies actually form a profile, and consist of perimetry, flicker perception, color vision testing, and electroretinography. In general, most patients were studied with three perimetric procedures. Peripheral visual fields were measured with a Goldmann or Airmark perimeter and central visual fields were mapped on a black tangent screen illuminated to 17 foot-candles; the patient was located either one or six meters from the black tangent screen, the latter distance constituting the macular visual field technique described previously (2). In flicker perimetry a gray tangent screen, illuminated to 6 foot-candles, was employed; the flickering stimulus was a neon stroboscopic lamp subtending an angle of 1.5 degrees; the flicker threshold (cff) was determined at the central fixation point and at selected points in eight meridians out to 25 degrees (1). Color vision was tested on all patients with the AO H-R-R Pseudoisochromatic Plates, the Tokyo Medical College Color Vision Test, and the Farnsworth Dichotomous Test. Selected individuals were studied further with the Nagel Anomaloscope, the Farnsworth-Munsell 100 Hue Test, and with color disk mixtures.

The electroretinographic data included in this study are only potentials of the scotopic type, and represent the response from a single flash. The patient was generally dark-adapted for seven minutes and subjected to a single flash at a frequency of 20 seconds. The stimulus was a xenon stroboscopic lamp used at full intensity and with neutral density filters. The data were recorded on a modified Grass electroencephalographic console.

Present Equipment, Technique, and Conditions

The adaptometer employed in this study has been described in detail in a previous publication (3). The instrument consists essentially of a modified Goldmann perimeter, the hemisphere of which is used for uniform adaptation and preadaptation. Any area of the retina may be investigated without requiring the subject to assume an eccentric direction of gaze. The intensity of the threshold stimulus may be varied continuously through a wide range. Finally, an effective device is provided for monitoring fixation under all levels of illumination.

The inside dome of the hemisphere is a white diffuser which can be illuminated by various combinations of six lamps mounted on its edge. This provides preadaptation and background illumination, which is highly uniform, and ranges from 0.001 to 500 millilamberts.

The head is positioned by a combination chin-forehead rest which has vertical and horizontal adjustments for centering either eye. Effective performance of this instrument depends on the conjugate relationship between points on the hemisphere and the retina. This can be assured only if the eye is properly in position and fixation is carefully controlled. A fixation point is provided with a small cystoscope lamp mounted centrally in the dome. By means of a potentiometer, the lamp is adjusted to present a barely detectable glowing filament to the subject.

An infrared viewing device was substituted for the optical telescope in the perimeter to monitor the patient's fixation. The source of the infrared illumination (a 12V automobile headlight combined with an infrared filter) is mounted behind the subject. The filter transmits radiation only above 8000 Å. This radiation is directed to the inside of the hemisphere so that the subject's eye is illuminated by reflection. A three-power telescope, incorporating an infrared converter, allows the examiner to have a clear, magnified view of the subject's eye for all conditions of adaptation, including darkness. It is thus possible to monitor fixation accurately at all times.

Near the top of the dome is a black housing for the tungsten stimulus lamp, which has a color temperature of 3010 degrees Kelvin. The light is relayed by an optical system mounted in the black casing and projected to the inside of the hemisphere. The stimulus subtends a visual angle of 1.5 degrees. The duration is controlled by a Compur shutter, located adjacent to the lamp housing and operated pneumatically permitting exposure times ranging from 1 to $\frac{1}{500}$ of a second. The location of the stimulus on the inside of the dome is controlled by a pantograph or lever system; one end of the pantograph is connected to the objective in the projector and the other end to a pointer which can be placed at any testing location on polar coordinate paper. The stimulus light is projected to any locus in the hemisphere simply by moving the pointer on the paper. As a consequence of the optical conjugacy between the retina and the hemisphere surface, on the one hand, and the mechanical relation between the stimulus optical system and pantograph, on the other, each retinal point has a unique locus on the polar coordinate paper.

Three controls on the back of the instrument regulate the intensity and spectral quality of the stimulus. These operate a neutral density wedge, neutral density filters, and color filters. They can be rotated into the light path either individually or in combination for an additive effect. The density of the wedge ranges from 0.15 to 1.30. The neutral density filters range from 1.0 to 5.0 density. It is also possible to interpose three color filters into the optical path, but in this study only two filters were used. One filter, a Wratten 89B, is deep red, the shortest wavelength it transmits being 6900 Å; it was employed when a predominantly cone response was desired. The second filter, a Corning 5113, is deep violet and transmits only wavelengths shorter than 4800 Å; it is useful in accentuating the rod component in the response, and its use results in a typical biphasic dark-adaptation curve.

In this clinical study the subject's eye was first preadapted to 500 millilamberts for three minutes. Since the entire hemisphere of the adaptometer was illuminated, virtually the entire retina was exposed to this level of luminance. After the preliminary light preadaptation, several testing procedures could be followed. In total darkness the thresholds with the blue or red filter could be measured at a point five degrees nasally from the fixation point to obtain a dark-adaptation curve. This might be followed by obtaining the scotopic thresholds in the horizontal meridian with the aid of the blue or red filter. If photopic thresholds were desired, these could be determined after only 10 minutes of dark adaptation or after the measurement of scotopic thresholds. The measurement of photopic thresholds requires that the patient be adapted to an illumination level of 0.015 millilamberts for three minutes before the photopic thresholds are determined. As a general rule, a predominantly cone response was obtained (*a*) under scotopic conditions with the 89B filter, and (*b*) under photopic conditions with the 5113 filter. For predominantly rod responses under scotopic conditions, a 5113 filter was employed.

The duration of the exposure time of the stimulus was fixed at one-fifth of a second. The stimulus was located only on points in the horizontal and vertical meridians.

Threshold values were specified as Log I Luminance, micro-micro-lamberts, and plotted as the ordinate. In the dark-adaptation curve the time in minutes in the dark was noted after preadaptation and plotted as the abscissa. When final thresholds were plotted across the horizontal meridian, the abscissa denoted the location of the stimulus in degrees from the fixation point.

Normal Subjects

The following data represent mean values as well as the total range of the normal series.

Figure 271 shows (below) a dark-adaptation curve for 12 subjects in which the stimulus was located five degrees in the nasal field from the fovea; the curve is biphasic and was obtained with the Corning 5113 filter. The cone threshold was reached at approximately seven minutes. Final rod threshold was achieved about five minutes later, and represented an increased sensitivity of 2.0 to 2.5 log units. The five-degree nasal field is an ideal site for these adaptation measurements because of the mixed receptor population in that location.

The upper curve in Figure 271 represents the data obtained on ten normal subjects with a Wratten 89B filter. This deep-red filter excludes most shorter wavelengths, and produces a response largely due to cone action. The curve was monophasic, and the threshold corresponded to that obtained at the seven-minute point with the Corning 5113 filter. The Wratten 89B filter is of value in determining the threshold primarily of the cone receptors.

Figure 272 illustrates the scotopic thresholds obtained at selected areas in the horizontal meridian from 17 normal subjects 30 minutes after adaptation in complete darkness. Thresholds were determined with two different filters, the Corning 5113 yielding primarily the rod response, and the Wratten 89B filter the

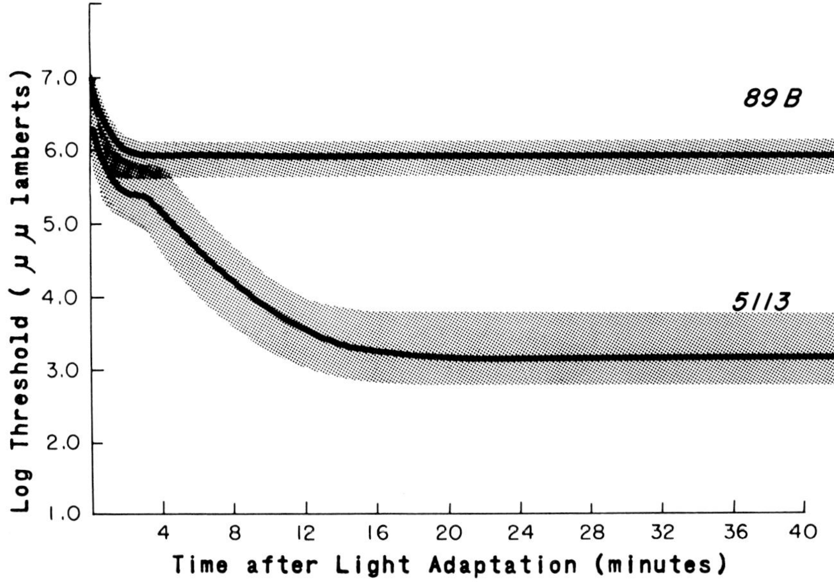

Figure 271. Dark-adaptation curves at 5° nasal field for normal observers (range and mean).

cone response. These two threshold values were separated by 2.5 to 3.0 log units except in the central area, where there was a decrease in rod sensitivity, corresponding to a reduction in the rod population in that area, and an increase in cone sensitivity.

Figure 273 illustrates the mean and range of normal values obtained during conditions of photopic adaptation. Threshold values were measured in five subjects

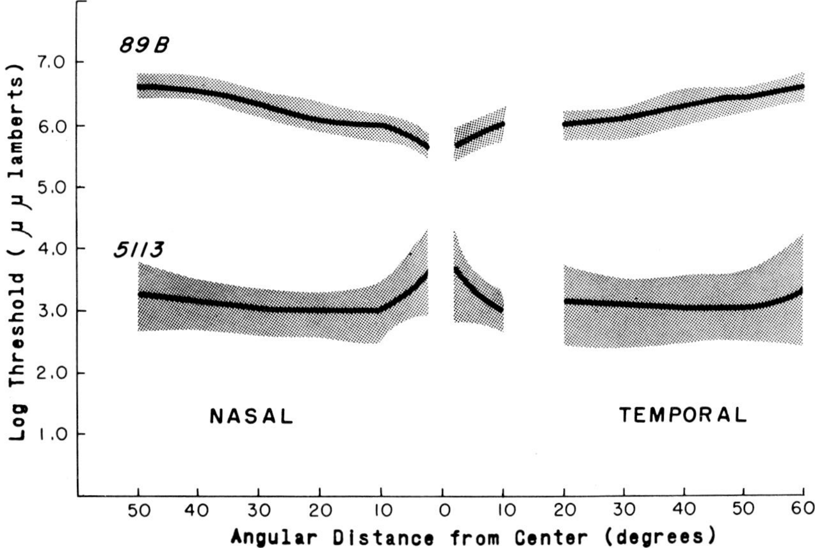

Figure 272. Scotopic thresholds for normal observers (range and mean).

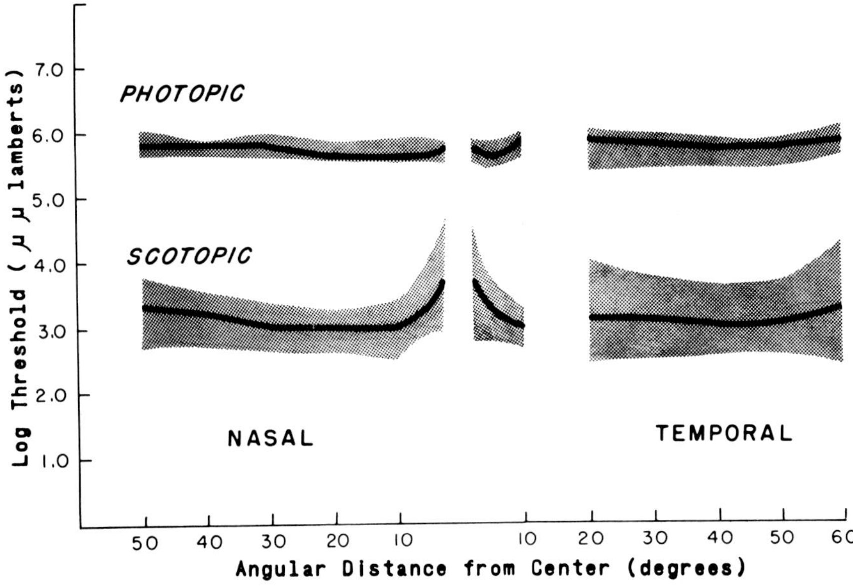

Figure 273. Comparison of photopic and scotopic thresholds with 5113 filter for normal observers (range and mean).

in the horizontal meridian, employing a Corning 5113 filter. Preadaptation was performed in the standard manner, the eye was dark-adapted for ten minutes, and then readapted to an illumination level of 0.015 millilamberts. Photopic adaptation was achieved after exposure of three minutes to this latter level of illumination. The photopic level of adaptation results in suppression of rod function, so that values were obtained which probably correspond approximately to cone threshold. For comparison purposes, the scotopic threshold values, obtained in the same condition of complete darkness as employed for the data illustrated in Figure 272, are included in Figure 273. The separation between the two groups of data is 2.0 to 2.5 log units, corresponding to the separation between threshold values obtained with a 5113 Corning filter and a Wratten 89B filter under scotopic conditions. Figure 273, then, illustrates a second technique of obtaining cone thresholds with the adaptometer.

Pathological Subjects

Previous publications (5,8) have dealt with adaptometric abnormalities in a limited number of patients. The total number (612) of patients included in this study provides significant numbers in most disease categories. Fifty-three normal subjects described previously are included. Table 30 itemizes the disease categories and the number of patients in each group. Each of the disease groups will be considered separately and the adaptometric findings reviewed in detail.

Macular Degenerations

The 237 patients with macular degeneration were divided into three groups according to age at onset of the disease. Generally, macular degenerations are

TABLE 30

Disease Categories	Number of Patients
Normal	53
Macular Degeneration	237
Primary Chorioretinal Degeneration	224
Uveitis	23
Retinal Vascular	24
Optic Atrophy	14
Congenital Anomalies	21
Toxic Agents	10
Undiagnosed	6
TOTAL	612

characterized by bilaterality, corrected visual acuity less than 20/25, and lesions in the macular regions detectable on clinical examination. Within each age group these degenerations were further divided into clinical subgroups based on the ophthalmoscopic appearance of the macular lesions. The terminology is sufficiently descriptive to identify each clinical group.

From the point of view of retinal function, all patients in these groups showed normal peripheral visual fields and normal flicker thresholds except in the central regions. The scotopic electroretinographic potentials were also normal with all stimulus intensities except for one group of senile macular degenerations which will be identified specifically. Color vision defects were present in most patients and were usually of a mixed variety, that is, both red-green and blue-yellow in type.

JUVENILE MACULAR DEGENERATION. This classification is defined as disease occurring in individuals less than 21 years of age. A total of 49 patients fell in this general category, itemized into clinical subgroups listed in Table 31.

The dark-adaptation curve and the scotopic thresholds obtained with the 5113 filter in the horizontal meridian were, with the exception of slight elevations of

TABLE 31

JUVENILE MACULAR DEGENERATION

Type	Number of Patients
Choroidal Atrophy	28
Colloid	10
Cyst	10
Vitelline	1
TOTAL	49

isolated areas, generally within the normal range. No adaptometric differences under any conditions of testing were apparent in comparing the results obtained from the various clinical subgroups in this general disease category.

In 63 per cent of the total group, scotopic thresholds were measured using the 89B filter in the horizontal meridian. Virtually all values obtained were slightly above the normal range. These elevations in threshold were especially marked centrally, and frequently covered a relatively large central zone.

A typical example of the scotopic thresholds with the red and blue filters is illustrated in Figure 274, showing a 10-year-old patient with central choroidal atrophy. Table 32 illustrates similar data obtained on a patient also with the clinical diagnosis of central choroidal atrophy but recorded at two different ages, 15 and 17 years. The values in the table represent departures of the thresholds in log units from the upper limit of the normal range. In the two-year interval between the threshold determinations, only slight further elevations in the threshold are demonstrated with the 89B and 5113 filters, the greatest elevations occurring in the central area with the red filter.

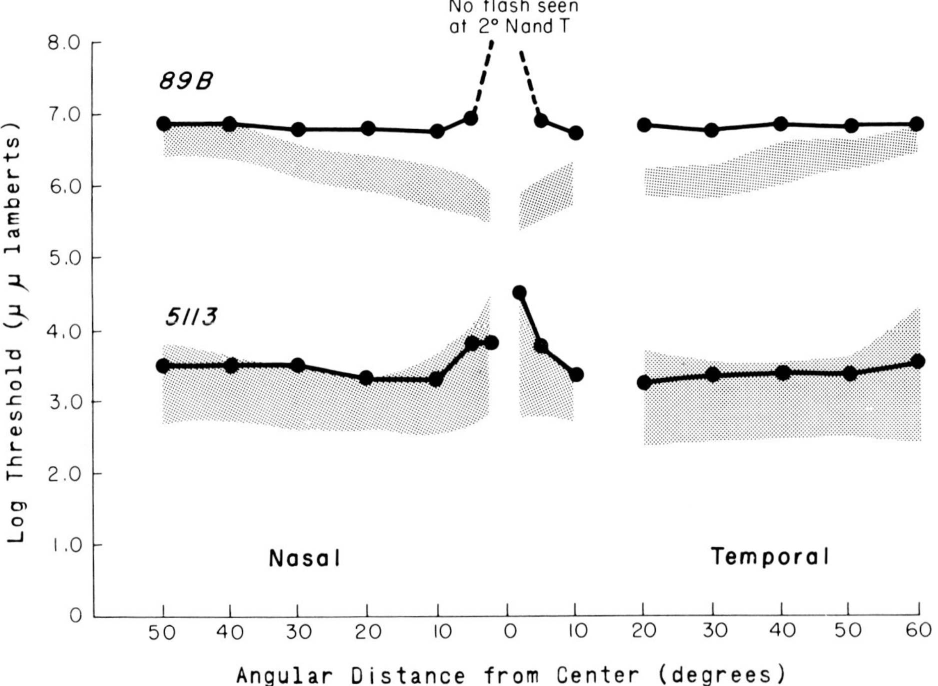

Figure 274. Scotopic thresholds with 5113 and 89B filters in juvenile macular degeneration.

Only three patients in this group were studied under photopic adaptation conditions with the 5113 filter. The threshold values were uniformly elevated in the horizontal meridian and did not manifest the relatively marked central elevation noted with the 89B filter under scotopic conditions. These findings are illustrated in Figure 275 for a 20-year-old patient with choroidal atrophy.

TABLE 32

Comparison of Elevations Above Normal Limit of Scotopic Thresholds in the Horizontal Meridian with 5113 and 89B Filters

Angular Distance (Degrees)	Elevation with 5113 Initial test	Elevation with 5113 2 years later	Elevation with 89B Initial test	Elevation with 89B 2 years later
Temporal				
60	N	N	N	0.1
50	N	LN	LN	0.2
40	N	LN	0.2	0.2
30	N	LN	0.5	0.5
20	N	LN	0.6	0.6
10	0.2	0.6	0.3	0.4
5	0.2	0.4	0.7	0.9
2	N	LN	1.1	>1.2
Nasal				
2	N	N	1.0	>1.1
5	N	LN	0.8	>0.9
10	LN	0.6	0.7	0.9
20	LN	0.5	0.4	0.5
30	LN	0.2	0.1	0.2
40	N	LN	N	N
50	N	LN	N	0.1

N: Average Normal; LN: borderline normal.

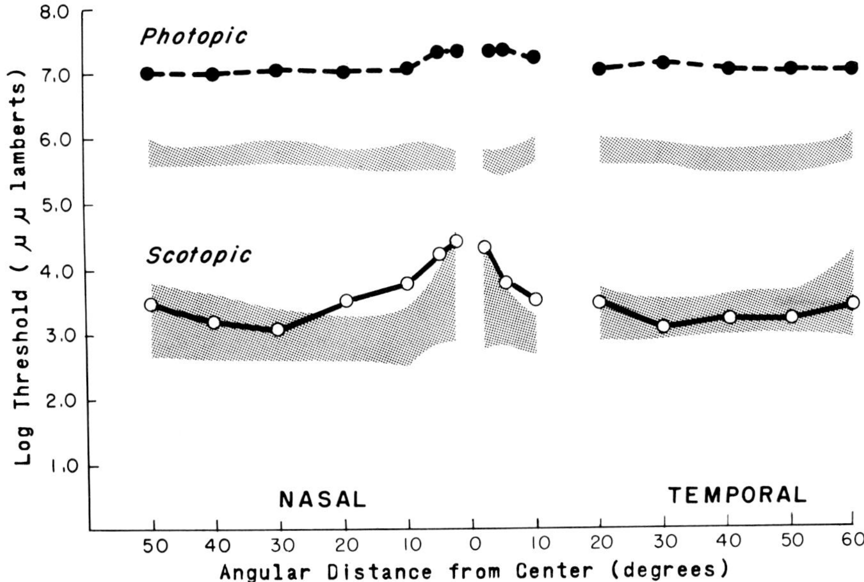

Figure 275. Comparison of photopic and scotopic thresholds with 5113 filter in juvenile macular degeneration.

These data indicate that juvenile macular degeneration is a disease involving elevations in the thresholds of the cone receptors in all areas of the retina most markedly in the central regions. Rod thresholds remain largely undisturbed.

Presenile Macular Degeneration. This group of macular degenerations was defined as occurring in individuals between the ages of 21 and 50. Sixty patients were studied and divided into clinical subgroups, itemized in Table 33. As in the

TABLE 33

Presenile Macular Degeneration

Type	Number of Patients
Choroidal Atrophy	32
Colloid	17
Cyst	4
Disciform	7
Total	60

juvenile macular degenerations, the adaptometric responses were similar regardless of the clinical classification of the degenerative process. The patients in this general disease category may be divided into two groups on the basis of the adaptometric findings.

The first group (two-thirds of the total number of patients) showed a response

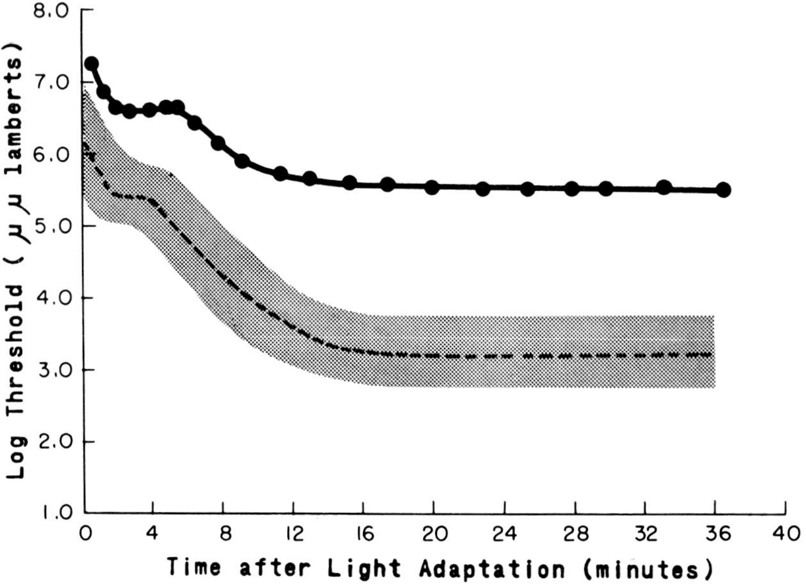

Figure 276. Dark-adaptation curve at 5° nasal field with 5113 filter in presenile macular degeneration.

generally similar to that noted for most of the individuals with juvenile macular degeneration. The dark-adaptation curve and the scotopic thresholds measured with the 5113 filter were either normal or slightly abnormal. The scotopic thresholds measured with the 89B filter showed a slight peripheral elevation associated with a somewhat more marked central elevation in thresholds.

The second group of patients (one-third of those with presenile macular degeneration) shows elevations not only in the dark-adaptation curve but in the scotopic thresholds measured with the 5113 filter. Figure 276 illustrates the elevation of the chromatic and achromatic thresholds of the biphasic dark-adaptation curve with the 5113 filter. Seven patients in this group had scotopic thresholds in the horizontal meridian, measured with both the red and blue filters. Three showed only mild elevations with the blue filter, but marked elevations with the red, particularly in the central regions. Figure 277 illustrates the results obtained from the other four patients; the scotopic thresholds with the 5113 filter were markedly elevated, while those with the 89B filter were so extremely elevated that no measurement could be obtained. This implies that in this second group of patients with presenile macular degeneration there is more generalized impairment in function than noted in the preceding group, and that the impairment involves both the rod and the cone receptors.

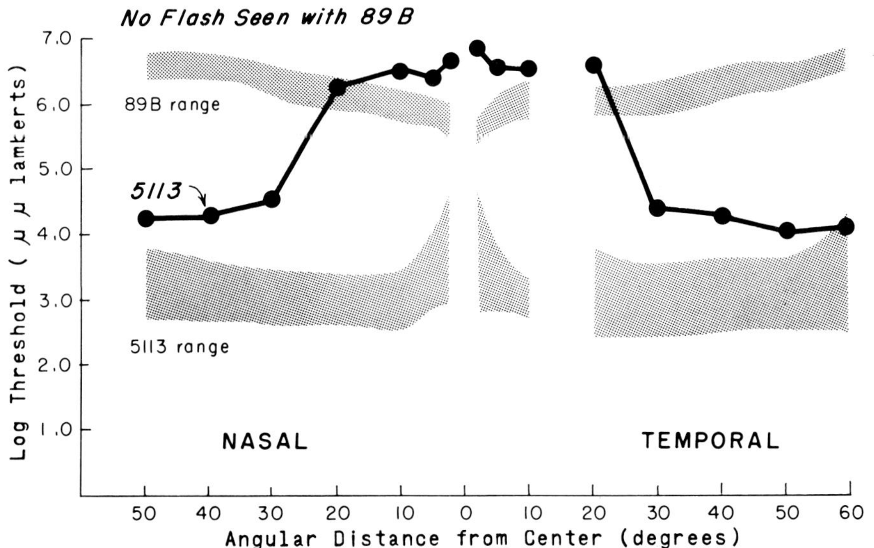

Figure 277. Scotopic thresholds with 5113 and 89B filters in presenile macular degeneration.

The two groups of patients with presenile macular degeneration show significant differences in the extent and degree of adaptometric impairment. Despite these rather marked differences, the peripheral visual fields in both groups of patients were normal and no significant electroretinographic abnormalities were detected.

Senile Macular Degenerations. There were 128 patients in this disease category, clinically classified in Table 34. From the adaptometric point of view, the patients with senile macular degeneration may be divided into three groups. The first, Group A, manifested adaptometric findings similar to those found in patients with juvenile macular degeneration. The dark-adaptation curve obtained with the 5113 filter and scotopic thresholds with this filter were both within normal limits or only slightly elevated. Scotopic thresholds obtained with the 89B filter were slightly elevated in the periphery and, as in the patients with juvenile macular degeneration, these elevations were more marked centrally. It is of interest to note that this group included approximately 30 per cent of the total number of cases with central atrophy, 30 per cent of those with a colloid type of degeneration, and 30 per cent of those with cystic macular degeneration. None of the patients with a clinical diagnosis of either disciform degeneration or circinate degeneration were found in Group A.

TABLE 34

Senile Macular Degeneration

Type	Number of Patients
Choroidal Atrophy	52
Colloid	45
Cyst	13
Disciform	12
Circinate	6
Total	128

The second group (B) of patients with senile macular degeneration was characterized by more marked adaptometric changes. In many cases the dark-adaptation curve plotted with the 5113 filter showed a slight elevation of the entire curve for both rod and cone components, as illustrated in Figure 276, but in 11 patients a multiphasic curve was obtained. (A multiphasic curve is characterized by more than two plateaus and will be illustrated in Figure 279 with a patient from Group C.) Group B was also characterized by slight elevations in the scotopic thresholds with both the 5113 and 89B filters. The 89B data are similar to those found in Group A. Group B included 30 per cent each of the patients with a clinical diagnosis of choroidal atrophy, colloid, and cyst. Also present, however, were 20 per cent of the patients with disciform degeneration and 33 per cent of those with circinate degeneration.

The third group of patients with senile macular degeneration, classified as Group C according to the adaptometric findings, is characterized by more profound changes in both rod and cone functions. The dark-adaptation curve obtained with the 5113 filter showed a more definite elevation of all values than in Group B for both the rod and cone components. This elevation was frequently about equal in magnitude for the two components. In the dark-adaptation curve these elevations varied somewhat from individual to individual. Figure 278 is an illustration of a patient with relatively marked colloid-type of macular degeneration, in whom the elevation in rod thresholds is significantly higher than that in cone thresholds.

In order to study further the defect in cone function, dark-adaptation curves with the red filter were obtained for seven patients. Marked elevations were seen in the final thresholds of all seven, and they were greater than those found with the blue filter.

Figure 279 is an example of a patient with a multiphasic dark-adaptation curve. There were approximately ten patients in Group C with curves of this type, from whom a final threshold was obtained only after prolonged dark adaptation. One patient was studied on two occasions separated by a two-year interval; he showed a biphasic curve with the final threshold at approximately the same elevated level, although the final threshold was reached in a shorter time at the second examination.

In the third adaptometric group (C) there were relatively marked elevations in the scotopic thresholds across the horizontal meridian measured with the 5113 filter; the scotopic thresholds with the 89B filter were so markedly elevated that in most individuals they were unmeasurable. Figure 280 illustrates a patient with colloid degeneration and a second patient with relatively advanced central choroidal atrophy. There were significant elevations in the rod thresholds, but cone function was so greatly depressed that the threshold could not be measured. Group C consisted of approximately 40 per cent of the patients with the clinical diagnosis of choroidal atrophy, colloidal degeneration, and cystic degeneration.

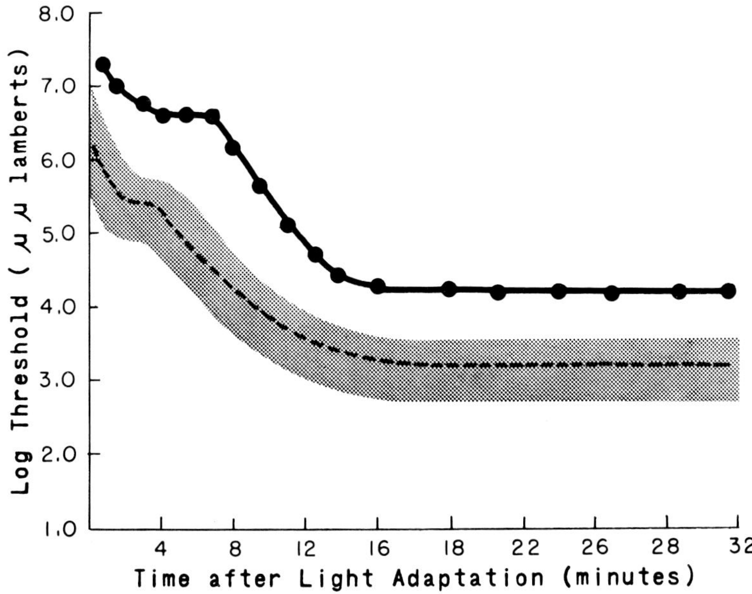

Figure 278. Dark-adaptation curve at 5° nasal field with 5113 filter in marked colloid-type senile macular degeneration.

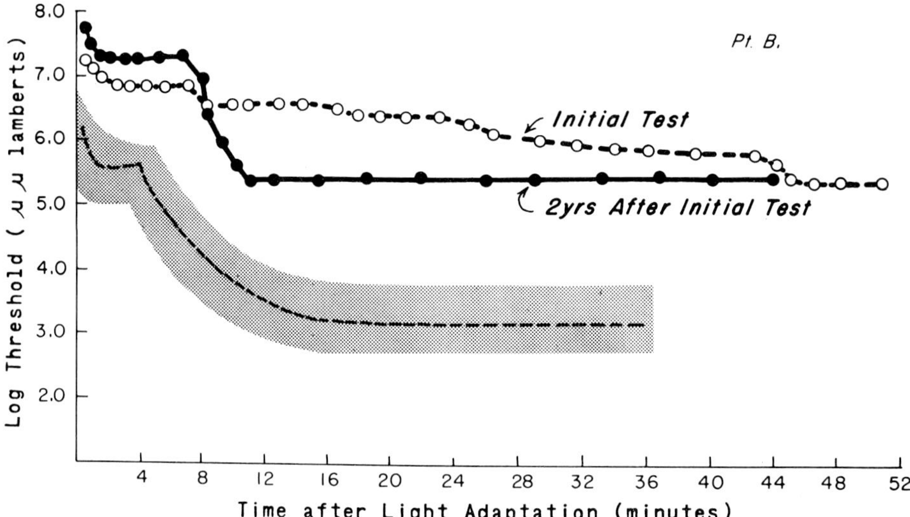

Figure 279. Multiphasic dark-adaptation curves at 5° nasal field with 5113 filter in senile macular degeneration.

Also included were 80 per cent of those with the disciform degenerations, and 67 per cent of the circinate degenerations.

The adaptometric classification of the senile macular degenerations resulted in their division into three groups based on increasing abnormalities. With greater defects there was evidence that not only the cone but also the rod receptors were involved, and that the abnormalities were not confined to the central regions, but were more extensive in nature. Furthermore, the clinical classification of the disease indicates that disciform and circinate degenerations are associated with

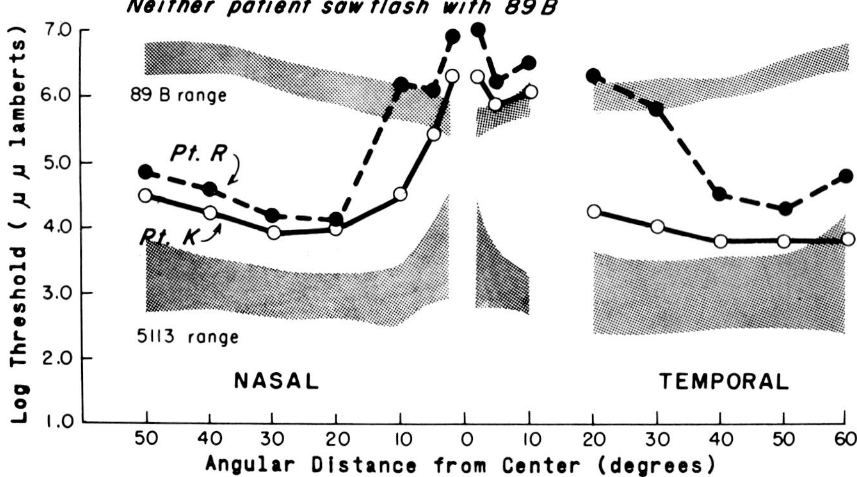

Figure 280. Scotopic thresholds with 89B and 5113 filters for two patients with senile macular degeneration.

more profound adaptometric changes than are the other clinical subdivisions. The other clinical subdivisions occurred with equal frequency in the three adaptometric classes.

It is also of interest to note the changes found in the retinal function profile. The patients in Groups B and C showed more marked color-vision defects than those in Group A. There was also a more significant impairment in visual acuity, and clinically the disease process was more marked. The electroretinographic responses, particularly when stimuli of reduced intensity were employed, were abnormally reduced in 50 per cent of the patients in adaptometric groups B and C. These electrical response abnormalities would confirm the adaptometric data that some patients with senile macular degeneration manifest more extensive generalized retinal involvement with the degenerative process.

Optic Atrophy

Fourteen patients with the clinical diagnosis of optic atrophy were studied. They had developed optic atrophy generally from central nervous system disease; diagnosis was established by ophthalmoscopic examination. From the adaptometric point of view they may be divided into two groups, based on the extent of the abnormality found.

The first group of patients (Group A) included 60 per cent of the cases, and represents the milder adaptometric changes. With the 5113 filter, both the dark-adaptation curves and the scotopic thresholds were within normal limits or slightly and irregularly elevated. With the 89B filter, however, moderate elevations were found in both the dark-adaptation curve and scotopic thresholds with more marked elevations centrally. Figure 281 (patient A) illustrates scotopic thresholds plotted with the 5113 filter for a patient in this classification.

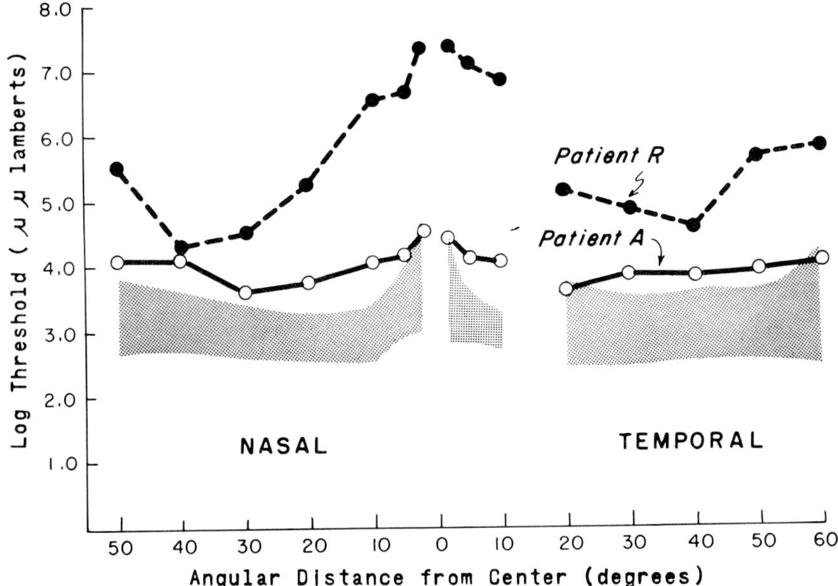

Figure 281. Scotopic thresholds with 5113 filter for two patients with optic atrophy.

The second adaptometric class (Group B) consisted of approximately 40 per cent of the optic atrophy patients. In this group the dark-adaptation curve and the scotopic thresholds measured with the 5113 filter were significantly elevated. Thresholds with the 89B filter were so markedly elevated that no measurement could be made. The elevated scotopic thresholds obtained with the 5113 filter are also illustrated in Figure 281 (patient R), thereby providing a comparison of representative patients from adaptometric classes A and B.

The patients in group B generally exhibited significantly greater visual impairment on clinical tests and manifested greater evidence of optic atrophy. In group A, color-vision defects were generally relatively mild but they were strong for the second group. The color vision defects were of the mixed variety, both blue-yellow and red-green in type. The electroretinographic potentials were normal in 90 per cent of the subjects of both groups. Minimal defects were present with reduced stimulus intensities in both groups and the electroretinographic abnormalities did not appear to be related to other functional findings.

Uveitis

Twenty three patients with the clinical diagnosis of uveitis were studied, itemized into clinical categories in Table 35.

All four patients with pars planitis showed mild to moderate elevations in all thresholds obtained with the 5113 filter. The functional profile studies are also of interest. The electroretinographic potentials were reduced to a moderate degree but were not of the extinguished variety. Slight constrictions in the peripheral field of vision were frequently found. There were color-vision abnormalities which were termed mild if the visual acuity was better than 20/30, and medium in extent if the visual acuity was less than 20/30. Figure 282 illustrates the data obtained in both eyes of a patient in whom the right eye corrected to 20/30 and the left eye to 20/60; the scotopic thresholds with the 5113 filter in the right eye are at the upper limit of normal, whereas in the left eye there is a generalized moderate elevation. The dark-adaptation curve of a second patient with pars planitis is illustrated in Figure 283; the visual acuity in this eye was 20/20; there was a moderate elevation in rod thresholds, and cone thresholds were also slightly elevated. The results obtained from other patients with active pars planitis were somewhat variable. They do indicate, however, that there is generalized retinal

TABLE 35

UVEITIS

Type	Number of Patients
Inactive Focal Chorioretinitis	13
Active Focal Chorioretinitis	6
Pars Planitis	4
TOTAL	23

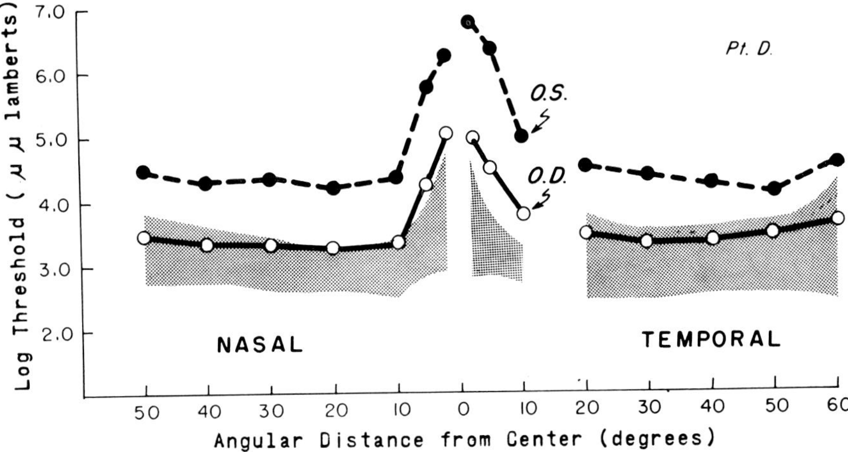

Figure 282. Comparison of scotopic thresholds with 5113 filter for both eyes of a patient with uveitis.

involvement in this inflammatory process and that there is impairment of both receptors.

There were six patients with the clinical diagnosis of active focal chorioretinitis. All patients in this group showed mild to moderate elevations in the dark-adaptation curves and in the scotopic thresholds obtained with the 5113 filter. The electroretinographic potentials were somewhat variable in this group, ranging from just below normal to moderate reductions. Occasionally, there were slight constrictions in the peripheral field of vision and mild color-vision defects

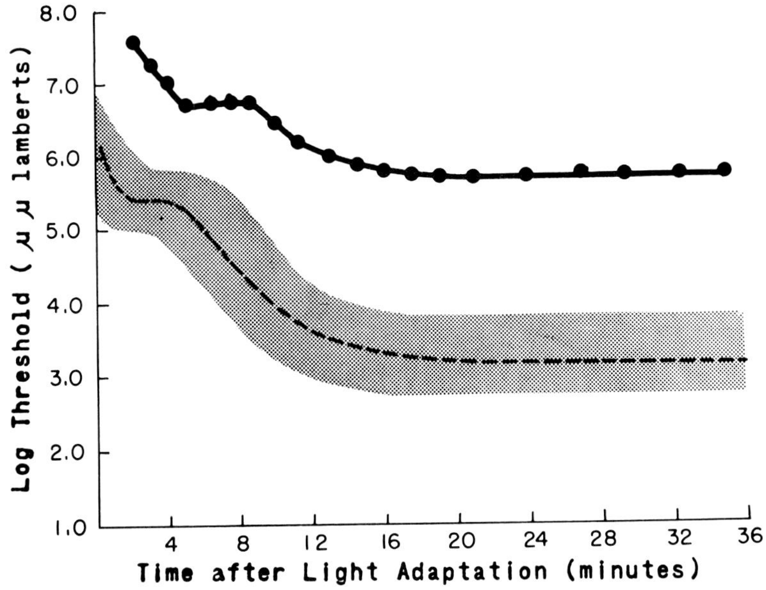

Figure 283. Dark-adaptation curve at 5° nasal field with 5113 filter in uveitis.

of a mixed variety. These findings are not dissimilar to those found in the pars planitis group. They emphasize that inflammatory disease, although confined clinically to one area, produces generalized impairment in retinal function.

Thirteen patients with inactive focal chorioretinitis were studied. From the adaptometric point of view, they may be divided into three groups. One-third manifested normal dark-adaptation curves and scotopic thresholds with the 5113 filter. Another third had slightly elevated dark-adaptation curves and scotopic thresholds with the blue filter, indicating some permanent impairment in function representing irreversible damage to the retina as a consequence of a remote lesion. The third adaptometric group, consisting also of about one-third of the patients, manifested marked elevations in both the dark-adaptation curve and the scotopic thresholds measured with the 5113 filter. Since the inflammatory process was inactive in this group, it further confirms that permanent irreversible damage does befall the retina as a consequence of a remote lesion. Clinically, the lesions in this group were generally more extensive than those in the second adaptometric group.

Retinal Vascular Diseases

Twenty-four patients with retinal vascular disease were studied; the subclassification of this group is indicated in Table 36. Most were diagnosed clinically as central serous retinopathy.

TABLE 36

RETINAL VASCULAR DISEASES

Type	Number of Patients
Central Serous Retinopathy	20
Periphlebitis	2
Retinal Vessel Occlusion	2
TOTAL	24

From the adaptometric point of view, central serous retinopathy may be divided into three groups depending on the extent of the functional impairment The first group (A) consisted of 40 per cent of the total number of patients, characterized by normal dark-adaptation curves and scotopic thresholds with the 5113 filter. There were slight elevations centrally with the 89B filter.

The second adaptometric group (B) which clinically showed evidence of more profound disease, consisted also of approximately 40 per cent of the total number of patients. The dark-adaptation curves measured with the blue filter showed a slight elevation, generally of the cone component, but occasionally of both rod and cone responses. The scotopic thresholds with the 5113 filter were slightly elevated centrally, and with the 89B filter more marked elevations were present centrally but only slight peripheral changes were found. In this group there was evidence of both central and peripheral functional impairment, which was more marked than in group A.

The remaining 20 per cent of the patients formed a third adaptometric group (C) in which more profound abnormalities were found. Both road and cone thresholds in the dark-adaptation curve with the blue filter were elevated. The scotopic thresholds with the 5113 filter were also substantially elevated, and the thresholds with the 89B filter were so elevated that they could not be measured. Clinically, the patients in this group showed more marked central changes on ophthalmoscopic examination and the reductions in visual acuity were greater.

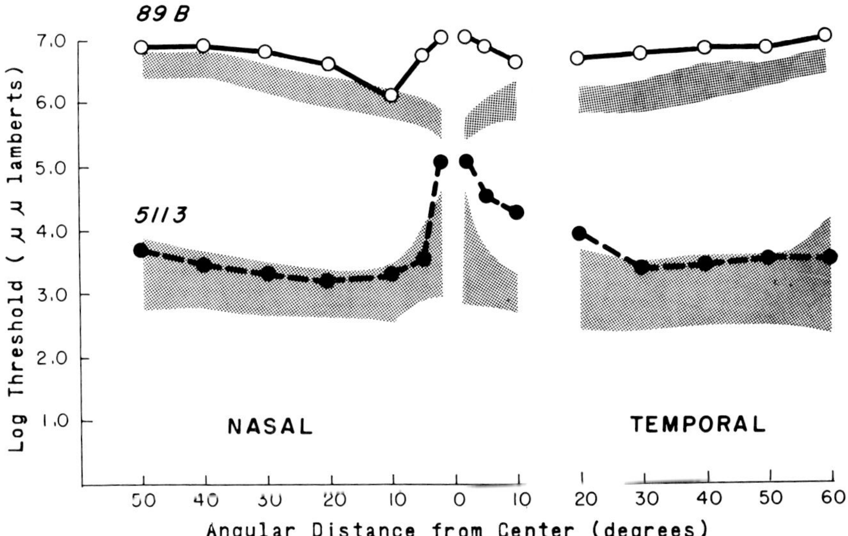

Figure 284. Scotopic thresholds with 89B and 5113 filters in central serous retinopathy.

Figure 284 illustrates data obtained from a patient in adaptometric Group B. The scotopic thresholds showed centrally mild to moderate elevations with both the red and blue filters. In the periphery, the thresholds were normal with the blue filter but slightly elevated with the red. In spite of the abnormal scotopic thresholds in the central regions, the corrected visual acuity in this patient was 20/15. Abnormalities were also detected with the Farnsworth-Munsell 100 Hue Test in some patients in this group even after the visual acuity had returned to normal.

The electroretinographic potentials were normal in patients with central serous retinopathy. Color-vision defects and macular visual field defects were more marked in adaptometric classes B and C than in class A. There were also abnormalities in flicker perception in adaptometric class C.

Toxic Agents

Table 37 itemizes the patients who presumably suffered retinal or optic nerve damage as a consequence of toxic agents. Retinal damage following chloroquine

TABLE 37

TOXIC AGENTS

Type	Number of Patients
Tobacco-Alcohol Amblyopia	1
Toxic Agent (Chloroquine)	8
Retrobulbar Neuritis	1
TOTAL	10

therapy has been reported in a number of publications (6,7,10). The largest group of patients, eight in number, had been treated for an extended period of time with this drug. Most individuals included in Table 38 had daily dosages in excess of 250 mg which in general were continued for longer than one year. The more severe impairments occurred in patients whose drug dosages were higher or else continued for substantially longer periods. The table indicates that significant widespread elevations in scotopic thresholds occur with this drug.

Some patients with chloroquine toxicity manifested typical perimacular pigment irregularities, and others showed no typical changes on ophthalmoscopic

TABLE 38

ELEVATION OF SCOTOPIC THRESHOLDS IN THE HORIZONTAL MERIDIAN ABOVE THE NORMAL LIMIT WITH 5113 FILTER

Angular Distance (Degrees)	E. H.	E. L.	J. D.		P. M.	M. B.	B. G.	M. D.	O.G.
			OD	OS					
Temporal									
60	0.6	0.6	0.3	LN	N	LN	2.0	LN	1.4
50	0.8	1.0	0.6	0.4	LN	0.4	2.7	0.5	2.3
40	0.3	0.8	0.3	0.2	0.4	0.6	2.3	0.5	2.3
30	0.4	0.7	0.5	0.4	0.4	1.2	2.1	0.7	2.2
20	0.4	0.9	0.2	0.2	0.3	1.4	1.8	0.8	LN
10	0.8	1.7	1.5	1.2	1.3	2.1	2.1	2.5	3.1
5	0.3	1.5	> 3.6	2.3	1.1	2.1	1.8	3.3	1.6
2	N	0.3	1.4	0.9	0.6	1.9	0.6	> 2.7	LN
Nasal									
2	N	LN	0.9	1.0	0.6	1.8	0.7	> 2.7	0.2
5	0.2	0.2	> 3.2	1.9	0.8	1.5	1.0	1.6	> 3.2
10	0.6	0.6	1.5	1.3	1.1	1.7	1.8	1.1	> 3.8
20	0.7	1.3	0.7	0.6	0.7	1.5	2.2	0.8	> 3.9
30	0.6	1.5	0.6	0.5	0.6	1.0	2.2	0.8	> 3.8
40	0.3	1.3	0.3	0.2	LN	0.6	2.3	0.5	> 3.6
50	0.3	1.2	0.3	0.2	LN	0.6	2.3	0.4	> 3.4
Age–Sex	56F	60F	49M		38F	35F	39F	43F	42F
V.A.	$20/15^{-3}$	$20/20^{-3}$	20/15	20/15	$20/25^{-3}$	$20/25^{-3}$	$20/25^{+2}$	$20/40^{+}$	$20/20^{+2}$

N: Average normal; LN: borderline normal.

examination. Visual field abnormalities were somewhat variable, and the electroretinographic potentials were generally within normal limits. There were only small changes in the visual acuity of most of the patients.

The adaptometric determinations were repeated on several patients with chloroquine toxicity at a relatively extended time after the initial examination. Although the drug was discontinued, there was no reversal of the elevated threshold, but no further deterioration occurred in any individual in this limited group.

These data suggest that adaptometric study is perhaps the most sensitive technique for detecting early chloroquine toxicity. Since the elevated thresholds may frequently be irreversible, it appears justifiable to suggest that patients receiving this drug for a sustained period of time should have periodic adaptometric evaluations. Carr, Gouras & Gunkel (4) also recommend adaptation as a sensitive test for early chloroquine retinopathy.

One patient was studied with the clinical diagnosis of retrobulbar neuritis resulting from an experimental drug; the data are summarized in Figure 285. The markedly elevated central thresholds are consistent with acute retrobulbar neuritis. The visual acuity in this patient was 20/400. Prompt total recovery did occur with cessation of the drug, and the thresholds returned to normal.

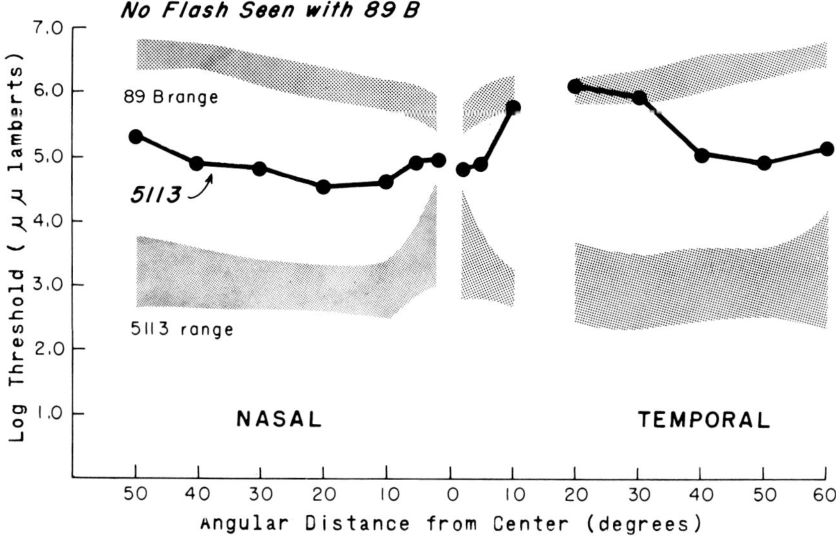

Figure 285. Scotopic thresholds with 5113 and 89B filters in retrobulbar neuritis.

Congenital Anomalies

Twenty-one patients with the clinical diagnosis of congenital anomaly were studied; the specific diagnoses are indicated in Table 39. All adaptometric findings were normal in these cases of albinism, dichromasy, anomalous trichromasy, and amblyopia ex anopsia.

TABLE 39

CONGENITAL ANOMALIES

Type	Number of Patients
Hereditary Night Blindness	3
Achromatopsia	5
Dichromasy	2
Anomalous Trichromasy	2
Albinism	2
Refractive Amblyopia	3
Amblyopia ex Anopsia	3
Coloboma of the Disk	1
TOTAL	21

The diagnosis of refractive amblyopia refers to those patients with a relatively high hypermetropic refractive error (generally greater than 6.00 diopters) in the eye with better visual acuity and without previous optical correction. This diagnosis was made in the eye with better visual acuity to reduce the possibility of confusion with amblyopia ex anopsia. With the blue filter there were mild elevations in both cone and rod thresholds in the dark-adaptation curve. Scotopic thresholds were slightly elevated centrally with the blue filter, but these elevations were more marked with the red filter. All functional studies were within normal limits, except for the reduced visual acuity and irregular defects found with the macular visual field technique.

On the basis of relatively limited numbers there does appear to be a significant adaptometric difference between patients with the clinical diagnosis of refractive amblyopia and amblyopia ex anopsia. The latter diagnosis is characterized by relatively normal retinal function except for the fovea itself, whereas there is more generalized impairment in central function in those patients with refractive amblyopia.

One patient with the clinical diagnosis of coloboma of the disk was studied. Marked elevations in scotopic thresholds measured with the blue filter were found only in the area corresponding to the scotoma plotted by conventional perimetry. All other areas of the retina manifested normal thresholds.

Two groups of patients in the congenital anomaly classification—those with hereditary night blindness and those with achromatopsia—are of particular interest. Three patients with hereditary night blindness were studied; the corrected visual acuities ranged from 20/20 to 20/30. Their visual field studies and flicker thresholds were all generally within normal limits. The scotopic electroretinographic potentials, however, were of the extinguished variety.

The dark-adaptation curve with the blue filter was monophasic in type, with the final threshold elevated to the level of the normal cone range or slightly above. Scotopic thresholds in the horizontal meridian with the blue filter were markedly elevated across the retina, approximately 2.0 to 2.5 log units. No flash was seen when a red stimulus was employed.

Two of the three patients with hereditary night blindness were studied under photopic conditions of adaptation with the blue filter. Their data were either normal or showed thresholds only slightly elevated above the normal range. Comparison of photopic and scotopic thresholds with the blue filter showed intermingling of the two curves similar to that found in the retinal degeneration shown in Figure 290. In these cases, however, the intermingling occurred generally within the photopic normal range.

Five patients with the clinical diagnosis of achromatopsia were studied and three of them manifested typical monophasic dark-adaptation curves with the blue filter. Their final thresholds were approximately within normal limits. One patient manifested a normal biphasic dark-adaptation curve, and one showed a biphasic curve with slight elevations in both rod and cone thresholds. However, those patients with biphasic curves identified the flash with blue stimulation as gray throughout the 30-minute period of dark adaptation. Scotopic thresholds in the horizontal meridian were normal with the blue filter. Scotopic thresholds were also plotted on two patients with a red stimulus; their thresholds were so greatly elevated in a central area subtending a half angle of 30 degrees that the stimulus could not be detected; peripheral to 30 degrees there were slight to moderate elevations in the thresholds.

Thresholds were also determined in two patients under photopic levels of adaptation. The thresholds were markedly elevated at two degrees and there were relatively mild elevations at five degrees. Peripheral to five degrees the thresholds were relatively normal.

The other functional studies in patients with achromatopsia are of interest. Their corrected visual acuities ranged from 20/50 to 20/400. Peripheral visual

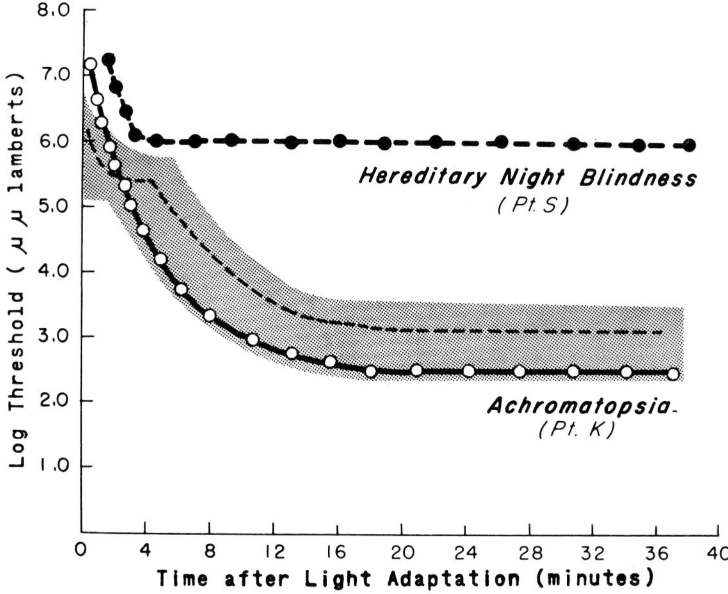

Figure 286. Comparison of dark-adaptation curves with 5113 filter in hereditary night blindness and in achromatopsia.

fields with a white test object were generally normal but the macular visual field technique disclosed relatively extensive central areas of impaired function. Flicker thresholds were so universally and substantially reduced that virtually all values were less than 20 per second. The scotopic electroretinographic potentials were normal.

The color vision of patients with achromatopsia was evaluated with all available testing procedures; marked color-vision defects, in fact, practically no evidence of color discrimination, were found. In the disk mixture study, three patients matched nine hues to gray; this matching occurred with colors at the five chroma level. The other two patients were uncertain that any exact matches to gray could be obtained. For each of the nine hues, either a trace of color was still present in the outer section or the inner gray section was seen as a complimentary color.

Adaptometric data obtained from a patient with achromatopsia are plotted in Figures 286 and 287 to be compared with threshold values from another patient with hereditary night blindness. Figure 286 shows typical dark-adaptation curves obtained with a blue stimulus, and Figure 287 gives plots of the scotopic thresholds obtained with a blue filter.

Primary Chorioretinal Degenerations

This retinal disease has been studied from the adaptometric point of view since 1941 (9,11,12), but most of the investigations have been concerned with the subgroup, pigmentary degenerations of the retina. A total of 224 patients in this general disease group category were studied by us, subclassified in Table 40.

CHOROIDAL DEGENERATIONS. Primary choroidal degenerations are characterized by retinal vessels of relatively normal caliber and no preretinal pigment deposits.

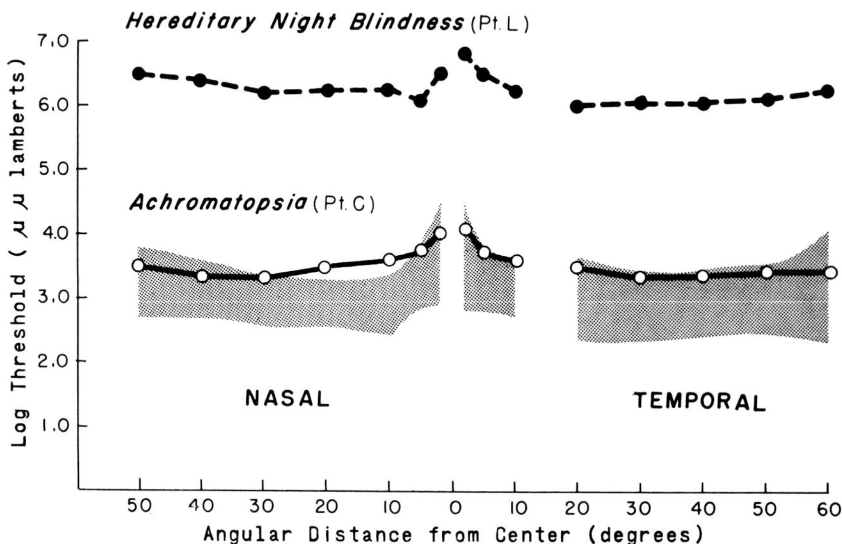

Figure 287. Comparison of scotopic thresholds with 5113 filter in hereditary night blindness and in achromatopsia.

TABLE 40

Primary Chorioretinal Degeneration

Type	Number of Patients
Choroidal Degeneration	62
Retinal Degeneration with Pigment	128
Retinal Degeneration without Pigment	17
Angioid Streaks	5
Myopic Degeneration	10
Choroideremia	1
Retinitis Punctata Albescens	1
Total	224

There are pigmentary disturbances but these appear to be deeper, approximately at the level of the pigment epithelium. They were often difficult to detect in our patients, and the changes were frequently extremely subtle.

Sixty-two cases with the clinical diagnosis of choroidal degeneration were divided into groups A (35 patients) and B (27 patients) relative to the magnitude of the defect shown adaptometrically under scotopic conditions. Figure 288 illustrates the difference between the two groups upon being tested under scotopic conditions across the horizontal meridian using the blue and red filters. The dark-adaptation curve at five degrees nasal field was sometimes normal for Group A, but the scotopic thresholds with both red and blue filters were elevated,

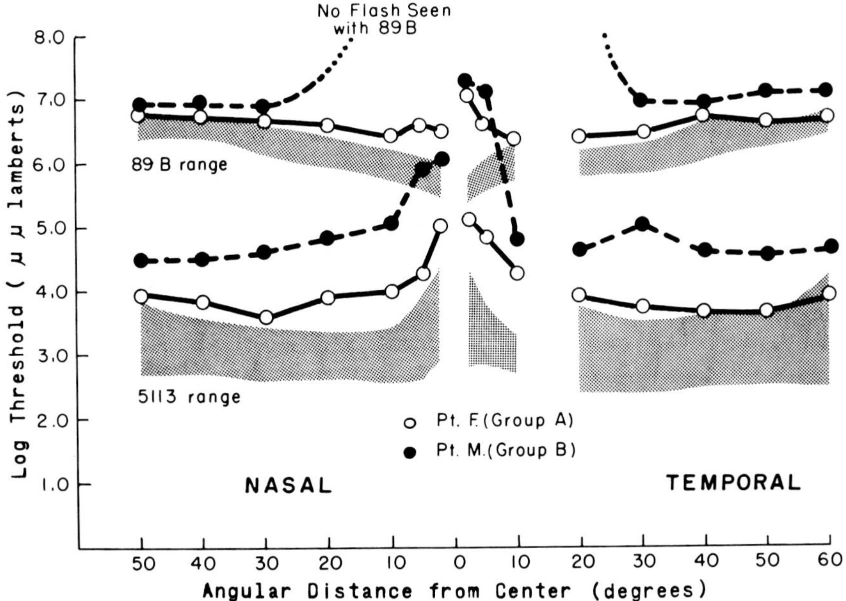

Figure 288. Scotopic thresholds with 5113 and 89B filters in choroidal degeneration.

particularly in the central area. While some cases in Group A showed peripheral abnormalities as well, all in Group B had definite central and peripheral elevations.

It is of interest to note the other retinal function studies in the patients with the diagnosis of primary choroidal degeneration. In Group A, 15 of the patients, or slightly less than half, showed relatively normal visual fields and normal electroretinograms. Sixteen manifested some reductions in the electroretinographic potentials and relatively mild perimetric defects. Only four patients of the total group of 35 showed significant visual field defects and marked abnormalities in the scotopic electroretinographic potentials. These ranged from very small potentials to the extinguished type.

In Group B of the primary choroidal degenerations, four patients showed normal scotopic electroretinographic potentials, but significant abnormalities were found in flicker perception and color vision; only mild abnormalities were present in the peripheral visual fields. Eleven patients showed definite but small abnormalities in the electroretinographic potentials, with similar findings in the other functional testing procedures. Twelve patients in the total group, or slightly less than half, had extinguished electroretinograms and evidence of relatively marked impairment in central visual function. The peripheral visual fields were only slightly abnormal.

Retinal Degenerations with Pigment. A second large group of 128 patients in the general category of primary chorioretinal degenerations had primary retinal degeneration associated with pigmentary changes. On ophthalmoscopic examination, these individuals were characterized by significantly narrowed retinal vessels and typical bone corpuscle superficial retinal pigmentation. The patients in this group may also be divided into two subgroups from the adaptometric point of view.

In the first subgroup (A) consisting of 34 patients, the dark-adaptation curve and the scotopic thresholds centrally with a blue filter were relatively normal, or there were only slightly elevated rod thresholds. The peripheral scotopic thresholds were abnormal, and in many patients were marked to the extent that little evidence of rod function could be demonstrated. The scotopic thresholds with the red filter were slightly elevated centrally and also showed marked peripheral elevations. The functional studies of the patients of this group showed evidence of impaired central and peripheral function. There were color-vision defects, and flicker perception in most individuals decreased markedly peripheral to 10 degrees The peripheral visual fields in general were also constricted to a moderate degree. The electroretinographic potentials were of the extinguished type in 54 per cent of the patients, were significantly reduced but not extinguished in 40 per cent, and 6 per cent showed normal potentials.

The second subgroup (B) of retinal degenerations associated with pigmentation, consisted of 94 patients. Their dark-adaptation curves with the blue filter showed moderate elevations of the cone thresholds and marked elevations of the rod thresholds. The rod thresholds were so elevated that in many individuals the curve was no longer biphasic in nature. The scotopic thresholds with the blue filter were markedly elevated, especially at five degrees, and so elevated with the red filter that the stimulus was frequently not visible.

Functional studies in this second group of patients with retinal degeneration were characterized by relatively marked generalized impairments. Flicker perception was decreased even centrally, and there were marked constrictions in the peripheral field of vision. The electroretinographic potentials were of the extinguished type in 97 per cent of the patients, and markedly abnormal in the remaining 3 per cent.

Several patients are of particular interest in the two subgroups. The first is illustrated in Figure 289 by two curves representing scotopic thresholds with the blue filter. One curve was obtained from the same individual five years previous to the second, which showed evidence of marked elevations in the thresholds throughout the entire field of vision. This individual would have been initially classified in subgroup A, but with the progression of the disease moved into subgroup B. At the time of the initial examination this patient was nine years old; there was slight narrowing of the retinal vessels but no retinal pigmentation; the peripheral visual fields were normal, but the electroretinographic potentials were extinguished. In the second examination, five years later, there was definite narrowing of the retinal vessels and some evidence of pigmentation; no visual field defects were found, but there was impaired flicker perception peripherally.

The second patient of particular interest serves as an example of the B subgroup of retinal degenerations (Figure 290). A blue stimulus was employed and the thresholds were plotted under both photopic and scotopic conditions. The photopic thresholds were slightly elevated centrally but, in general, there were only slight differences between the photopic and scotopic thresholds.

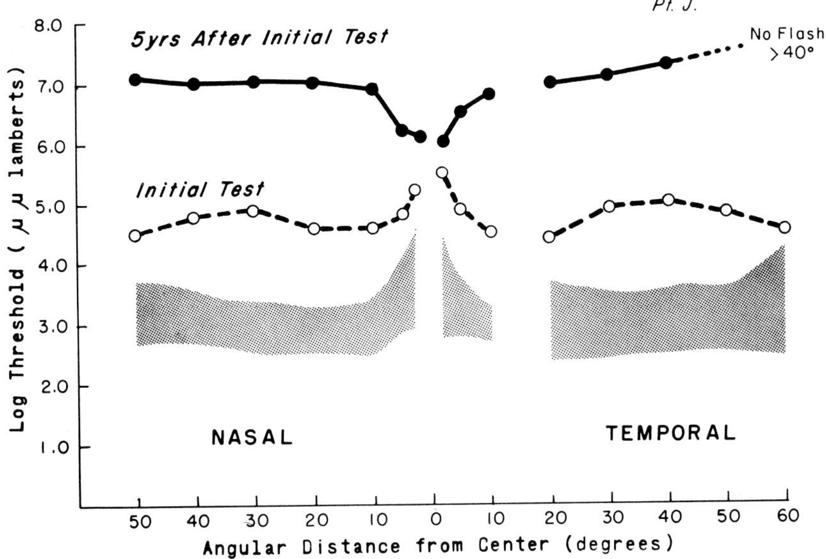

Figure 289. Scotopic thresholds with 5113 filter in retinal degeneration with pigmentation.

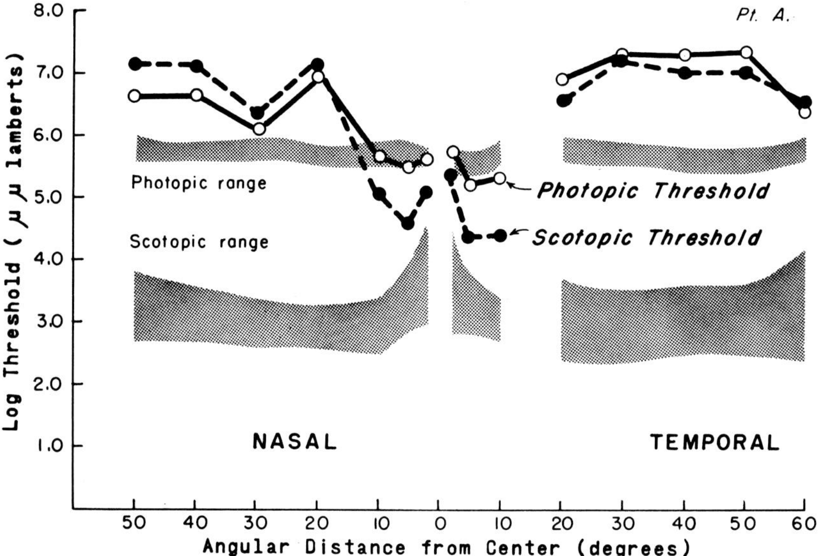

Figure 290. Comparison of photopic and scotopic thresholds with 5113 filter in retinal degeneration with pigmentation.

Figure 291 illustrates scotopic thresholds obtained with a blue filter in a patient with moderately advanced primary pigmentary degeneration in one eye, whose second eye appeared to be normal from the points of view of ophthalmoscopy, conventional visual fields, and even electroretinography. Significantly abnormal adaptometric thresholds were found, however, in both eyes at the time of the initial examination. Upon reexamination four years later, the "normal"

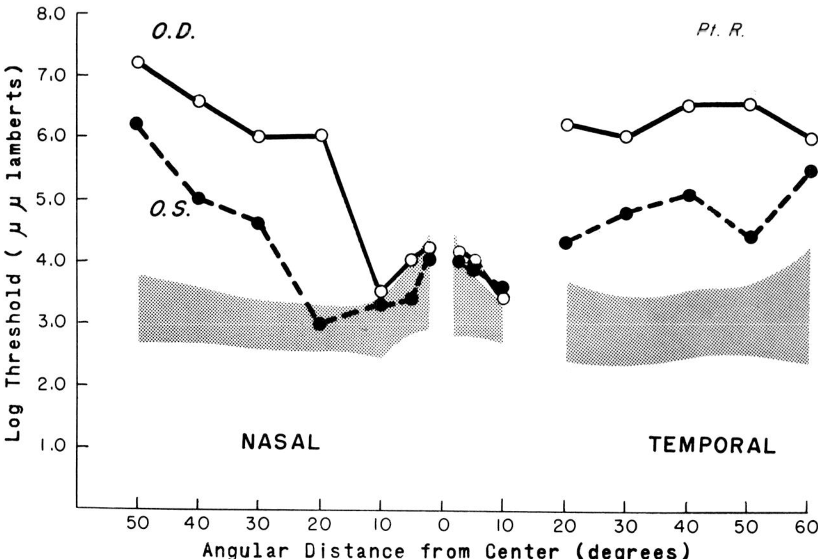

Figure 291. Comparison of scotopic thresholds with 5113 filter in pigmentary retinal degeneration.

second eye showed narrowing of the retinal vessels and peripheral deposits of pigment. The electroretinographic potentials had become extinguished in the second eye, and were virtually identical to the potentials in the first eye on the initial examination. The adaptometric studies in this individual are of particular value in the early detection of the disease process.

Retinal Degenerations without Pigment. Seventeen patients were classified clinically as primary retinal degeneration without pigment. This disease is characterized by narrowing of the retinal vessels with either no preretinal pigment deposits or very rare deposits.

From the adaptometric point of view, the patients in this disease class may be divided into two groups. The first group consisted of six patients, characterized by mild to moderate elevations in thresholds centrally and peripherally with red and blue filters. These abnormalities were found in the dark-adaptation curve and under scotopic conditions, and were somewhat more marked with the red stimulus. There were also moderate abnormalities in flicker perception and the peripheral visual fields varied from normal to moderate constrictions. The electroretinographic potentials were normal in one patient, extinguished in another, and abnormally reduced in four patients.

Eleven patients in the second group showed evidence of more profound abnormalities than those in the first group. There were marked elevations in the thresholds both centrally and peripherally, in the dark-adaptation curve, and in the measurements obtained under scotopic conditions with the blue filter. In general, the thresholds were so elevated that the red stimulus was not visible in any part of the field of vision. There were generally marked color-vision defects and abnormalities in flicker perception. The peripheral visual fields showed moderate to marked abnormalities. The electroretinographic potentials in ten patients were extinguished, and in one patient they were markedly abnormal.

Angioid Streaks. Five patients were studied with the clinical diagnosis of angioid streaks; the adaptometric findings in four were similar. They showed evidence of moderate to marked elevations centrally inside 10 degrees, and either normal thresholds or minimal abnormalities peripherally when the blue stimulus was employed under scotopic conditions. In general, the red stimulus was not visible under scotopic conditions.

The data in Figure 292 were obtained from a patient typical of this group of four patients, and illustrate the dark-adaptation curve obtained with a blue stimulus. The biphasic break in the curve, indicating rod-cone transition, was significantly delayed and, in this individual, occurred 17 minutes after the start of scotopic adaptation. The rod threshold was also significantly elevated, only slightly below the cone threshold.

Included in Figure 292 is a dark-adaptation curve of a typical individual from Group B with primary retinal degeneration without pigment. The cone threshold is reached in relatively normal time and the curve is monophasic, with a markedly elevated final threshold.

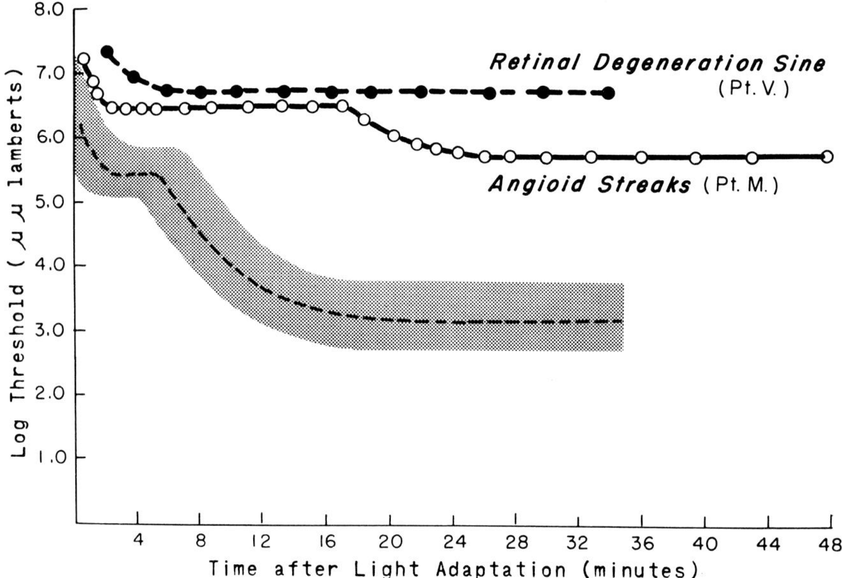

Figure 292. Comparison of dark-adaptation curves with 5113 filter in angioid streaks and retinal degeneration sine.

One of the five patients with angioid streaks was somewhat different adaptometrically, since the dark-adaptation curve and scotopic thresholds with the blue stimulus were normal.

Myopic Degeneration. We studied ten patients with the diagnosis of myopic degeneration, and in all of them the refractive error was greater than −20.00 diopters under a cycloplegic. All patients showed evidence of typical myopic degeneration on ophthalmoscopic examination.

Only one of the ten patients showed a completely normal dark-adaptation curve with the blue stimulus. There were slight elevations in the rod thresholds in three of the ten patients, and the remaining six individuals showed varying but significant elevations in both rod and cone thresholds.

Measurement of scotopic thresholds with the blue stimulus showed that six of the ten patients (Group A) had slightly elevated thresholds throughout. The remaining 40 per cent (Group B) showed more marked threshold elevations with irregular areas of rather greater elevations. Figure 293 shows the scotopic thresholds obtained with the blue stimulus for two patients, each representative of one of these groups. The irregular threshold elevations of patient C (Group B) present a characteristically spiked appearance resulting from local areas of depressed sensitivity; it was not possible to relate these areas of elevated threshold to pathology found on ophthalmoscopic examination.

All patients with myopic degeneration, when tested under scotopic conditions with the red stimulus, showed variability ranging from mild to marked elevations.

The results of the other retinal function studies in myopic degeneration were moderate abnormalities in flicker perception, in the peripheral field of vision,

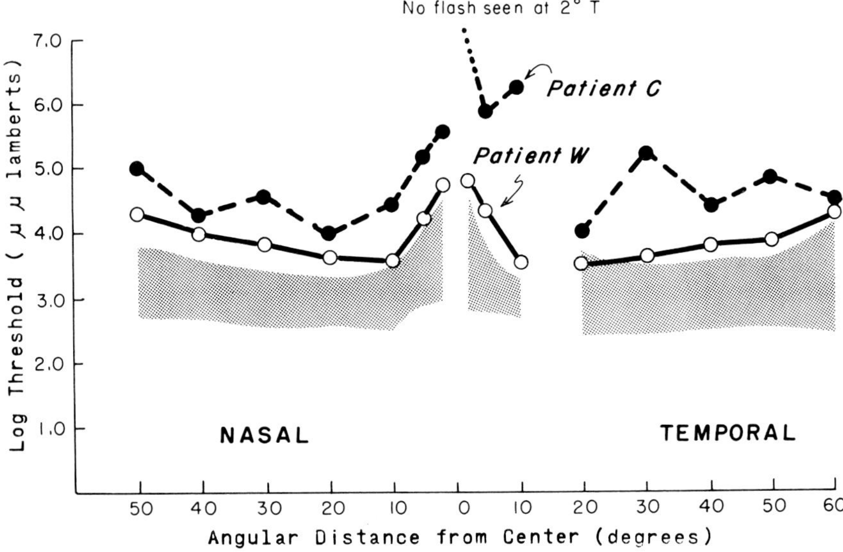

Figure 293. Scotopic thresholds with 5113 filter in myopic degeneration of the retina.

and in color vision. Approximately 50 per cent of the patients manifested normal electroretinographic potentials; the other 50 per cent showed only slight abnormalities.

Choroideremia. Only one patient with the diagnosis of choroideremia was studied. The dark-adaptation curve measured with the blue stimulus showed elevated cone thresholds and markedly elevated rod thresholds; in fact, there was no real evidence of rod function. The stimulus was not visible under scotopic conditions with the red filter, and with the blue filter the thresholds were markedly elevated. The visual fields were markedly constricted and there was a moderate impairment in visual acuity. The electroretinographic potentials were extinguished.

SUMMARY

A series of 612 patients with various eye diseases was studied from the adaptometric point of view, using equipment permitting the measurement of the threshold of any region of the retina. The adaptometer also provided means of varying the stimulus characteristics and adaptation level through relatively wide ranges. A description of the equipment, standard conditions, and techniques used in this investigation has been included.

Analysis of these data indicates that the testing procedure provides reproducible information that is both reliable and useful. The information permits a broader and more complete definition of the disease process, indicating that adaptometric studies are an essential part of any functional evaluation of the retina and contribute to the total picture of retinal function.

Alterations in adaptometric thresholds are extremely sensitive indicators of altered retinal physiology. As the adaptometric abnormalities are frequently among the earliest detectable changes, adaptometry is extremely valuable in the early diagnosis of some diseases. It also has proven to be useful in documenting the progression of the disease process by determining the changes that occur in retinal function with time. The characteristic adaptometric findings, which can be frequently related to one or the other receptor mechanism, are of differential diagnostic value in evaluating patients with impaired visual function.

The adaptometric studies have proven to be an essential adjunct to the clinical examination in the study of retinal pathology.

REFERENCES

1. Campbell, C. J., and Rittler, M. C., The diagnostic value of flicker perimetry in chronic simple glaucoma. *Trans. Am. Acad. Ophthal. Otolaryng.*, 1959, **63**: 89–98.
2. ———, Macular visual fields. *Arch. Ophthal.* (Chicago), 1959, **62**: 287–294.
3. Campbell, C. J., Rittler, M. C., and Kramer, W. G., A new projection adaptometer. *Arch. Ophthal.* (Chicago), 1963, **69**: 564–570.
4. Carr, R. E., Gouras, P., and Gunkel, R. D., Chloroquine retinopathy; early detection by retinal threshold test. *Arch. Ophthal.* (Chicago), 1966, **75**: 171–178.
5. Franceschetti, A., François, J., and Babel, J., *Les Hérédo-Degénérescences Chorio-Rétiniennes (Degénérescences Tapeto-Rétiniennes)*. Masson, Paris, 1963.
6. Henkind, P., Carr, R. E., and Siegel, I. M., Early chloroquine retinopathy: clinical and functional findings. *Arch. Ophthal.* (Chicago), 1964, **71**: 157–165.
7. Hobbs, H. E., Sorsby, A., and Freedman, A., Retinopathy following chloroquine therapy. *Lancet*, 1959, **2**: 478–480.
8. Jayle, G. E., Ourgaud, A. G., Baisinger, L. F., and Holmes, W. J., *Night Vision.* Thomas, Springfield, 1959.
9. Mandelbaum, J., Dark adaptation; some physiological and clinical considerations. *Arch. Ophthal.* (Chicago), 1941, **26**: 203–239.
10. Okun, E., Gouras, P., Bernstein, H., and von Sallmann, L., Chloroquine retinopathy; a report of eight cases with ERG and dark-adaptation findings. *Arch. Ophthal.* (Chicago), 1963, **69**: 59–71.
11. Sloan, L. L., Light sense in pigmentary degeneration of retina. *Arch. Ophthal.* (Chicago), 1942, **28**: 613–631.
12. Zeavin, B. H., and Wald, G., Rod and cone vision in retinitis pigmentosa. *Am. J. Ophthal.*, 1956, **42**(II): 253–269.

CLINICAL USEFULNESS OF ELECTROPHYSIOLOGICAL MEASUREMENTS*

ALBERT M. POTTS
University of Chicago
Chicago, Illinois

Our very cooperative 50-year-old patient sat before the light stimulus as electrodes were applied. We had explained very carefully that the machine was not going to send a current into her through the wires, but that the electricity from her eyes would make the machine operate. At the next visit, an ebullient patient was profuse in her thanks: "Doctor, I see so much better after that treatment you gave me!"

No one could fail to be impressed by the expensive hardware required to make electrophysiological measurements on the eye. The patient was convinced that such elaborate equipment must have been concocted only to treat her disease. Sometimes even the physician is carried away with the elegance of his methods and neglects to evaluate continuously the clinical worth of his activity. But the fact is that such clinical electrophysiological measurements have a sharply delimited set of applications. We thus take this opportunity to pause and evaluate our efforts, to show exactly where our techniques are useful and where they are not, and to look ahead a bit to possible future extensions of our methods which may gain us new capabilities.

In the glow inspired by space-age gadgetry, it should never be forgotten that the human visual system is the most elegant instrument of all; very many pieces of information on visual function are best obtained by asking the patient what he sees. Even in their somewhat simplified clinical form, the psychophysical measurements performed on a cooperative adult are usually the shortest route to the determination of visual function.

Thus, in considering clinical electrophysiological measurements we are only mildly interested in a catalog of all the disease situations where someone has reported a figure which departs from the normal. Such a catalog is of interest only because our highly significant situations will usually be contained in it and because improvements in technique may give significance to items now rated insignificant.

---

*The original work was supported in part by U.S. Public Health Service Research grants Nos. NB-02522 and NB-05505, from the National Institute of Neurological Diseases and Blindness; and by the National Council to Combat Blindness, Grant-in-Aid No. G-311.

Our main interest is centered on those measurements and disease situations where electrophysiology contributes something unique or a finding not easily obtainable by other methods. Measurements in children too young to cooperate with clinical tests are in this category, and this consideration extends to uncooperative adults, such as psychotic patients and malingerers. Our second area of interest depends on the capability of certain electrophysiological measurements to give information about involvement of a selected retinal layer or area in disease. Since psychophysical measurements require mediation of the entire visual system, there are only exceptional circumstances—as in nerve fiber bundle defects or central scotoma on visual field determination—where selective information is easily available. In certain electrophysiological measurements, information on involvement of specific retinal layers by disease is easily obtainable; the usefulness of such data in identification of retinal disease need not be belabored. Finally, there are the most important but rare situations where the electrophysiological measurement is uniquely valuable in detecting or diagnosing disease and no psychophysical measurement offers comparable information; the outstanding example of this circumstance is the extinction of the electroretinogram in certain heredoretinal degenerations as the earliest and most consistent finding.

What we want to know about visual function, particularly retinal function, is conditioned by several considerations. One of these is the duplex nature of the retina. If the sensitivity of the retina in the light is measured, and light sensitivity

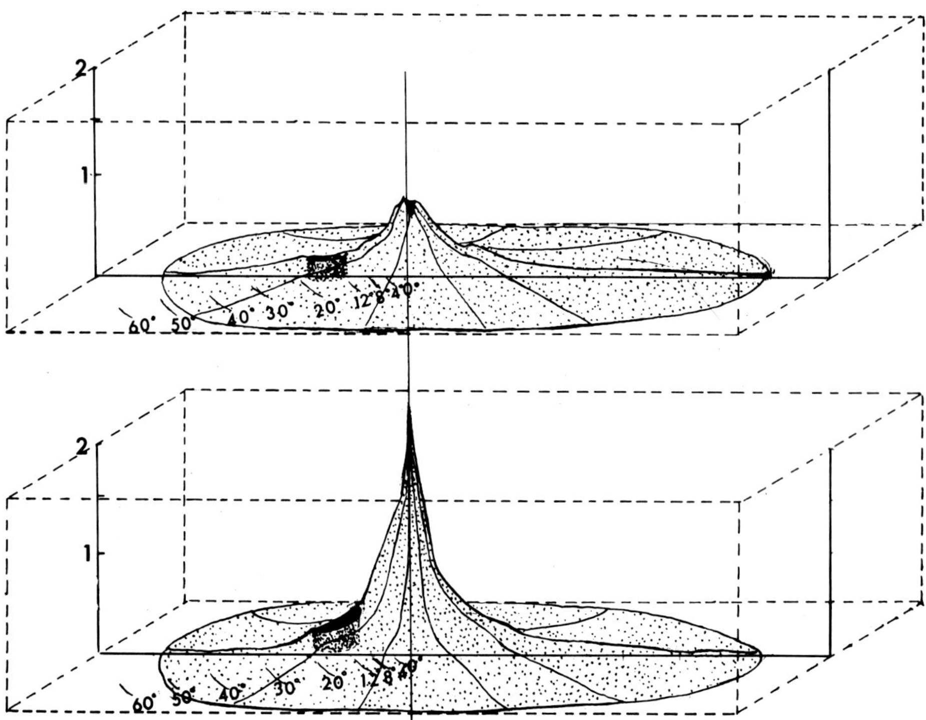

Figure 294. Visual acuity in the light-adapted (below) and dark-adapted (above) retina, expressed as a surface. (Data of Wertheim, 68.)

(minimum visibile) is plotted against position, the result is a rather complicated surface (Figure 294). If the same measurement is made in the dark, an equally complicated but markedly different surface is generated. If, instead of light sense, minimum separabile is measured, a similar but not identical set of surfaces is obtained (Figure 295). It is no secret, nor has it been since 1896 (66), that there is a marked correlation between the basic shapes of the surfaces just mentioned and those generated by the receptor cell population (Figure 296), the upper curve being similar to the rod population and the lower surface to the cone population. It is also evident that color sensitivity follows the lower surface. Perhaps the prime conditioning factor of all is embodied in the very peak of the "oriental hat" in the lower set of surfaces: receptor cell distribution and more central retinal organization determine that the half degree of axial fovea is the sole site of acute vision. Any test of maximum visual acuity must take cognizance of this fact. Other important data are: the contours of the surface itself, i.e., visual field; rate of shift from lower surface to upper surface, i.e., the rate of dark adaptation; and the spectral characteristics of the lower surface, i.e., color vision.

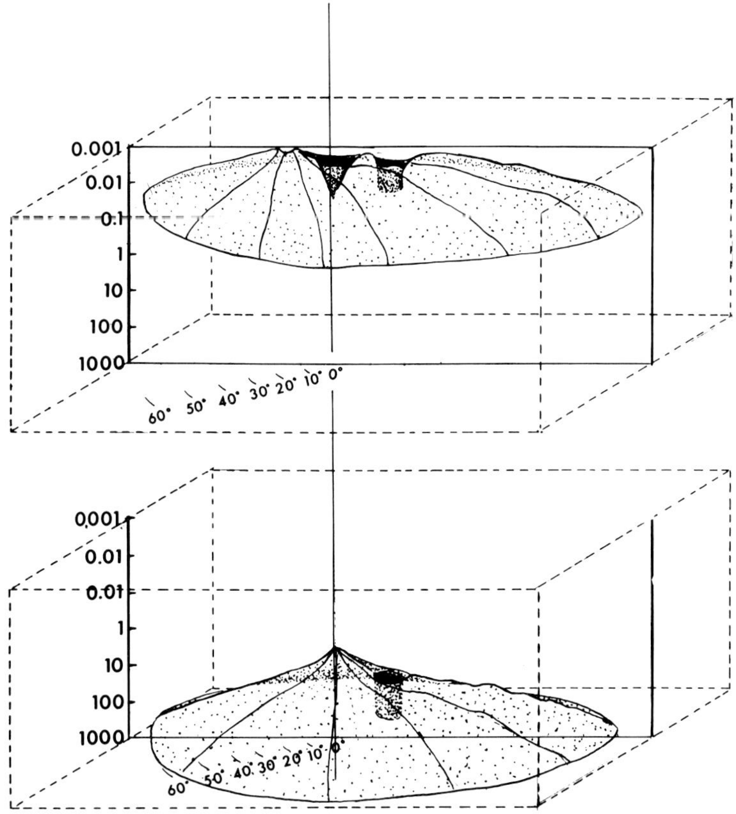

Figure 295. Light sensitivity (minimum visibile) in the light-adapted (below) and dark-adapted (above) retina, expressed as a surface. Note logarithmic ordinate scale. (After Aulhorn, 7.)

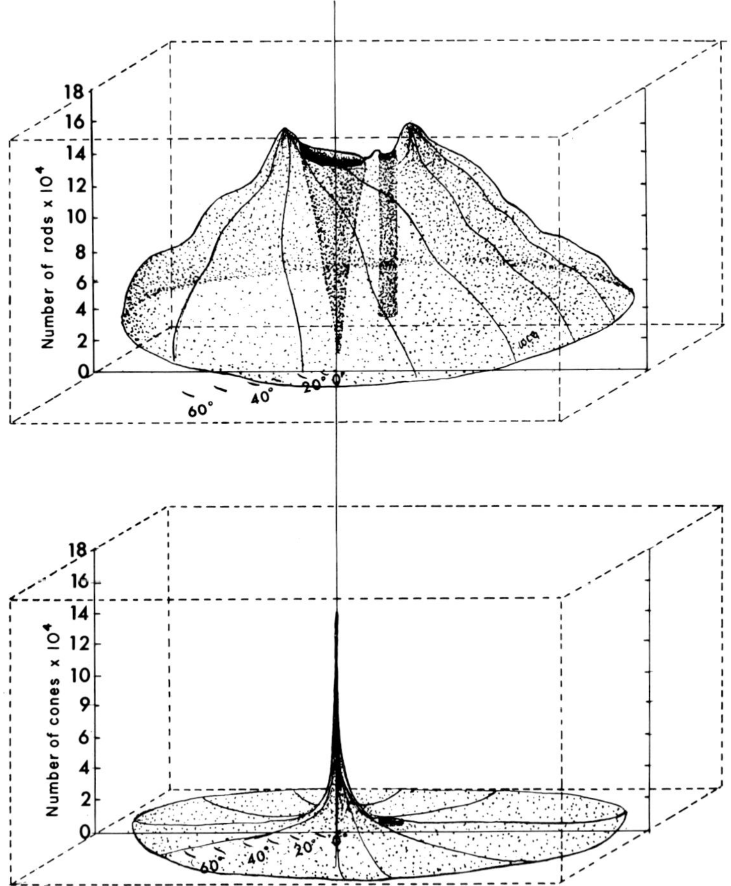

Figure 296. Population density of cones (below) and rods (above) in the human retina, expressed as a surface. (Data of Østerberg, 53.)

Electroretinography

The literature on electroretinography has grown apace; three books on clinical electroretinography are already in print (41,43,70). While there is no question about the usefulness of the electroretinogram (ERG) as an aid in ophthalmologic diagnosis, it is highly questionable whether either its special virtues or limitations are well understood. Since the nature of the electroretinogram has been discussed elsewhere in this symposium,* it should be sufficient to state that when electrodes are properly placed and a light stimulus properly applied an adequate amplifier and recorder will show a typical response.

Technique

It should be noted that, by almost universal agreement, the most convenient electrode for human electroretinography is some type of contact lens electrode—the dual contact type allowing for double-ended input being freest from extraneous

---

* See Dr. Brown's presentation, pp. 319–378.

electrical noise. The question of light stimulus will be treated under the section on standardization. There is no difference in amplifying and recording equipment between that used for animal work and that for human use. The state of the art in amplifiers has changed so rapidly that standards of performance and reliability vary almost from month to month. The A.C., coupled-battery-powered vacuum-tube amplifiers of the late 1940s are still adequate in many respects, but convenience, elegance, and certain aspects of performance favor the variously stabilized, line-operated, D.C.-solid state amplifiers of 20 years later. Recording data by photographing the cathode-ray oscilloscope screen on 35 mm film is well within the limits of accuracy required by electroretinography. However, new features such as the storage oscilloscope, polaroid photography, analog recording on magnetic tape, computer summation, and even on-line data reduction by computer add convenience and scope to electroretinography.

Standardization

Clinical electroretinography has shown least progress in the area of standardization of experimental conditions. In order to get a large measurable b-wave, it has been the usual clinical practice to dark-adapt the subject to various degrees and use an electronic flash tube to provide the light stimulus. The problem of adaptation is a real one. To obtain truly maximal response, dark adaptation of 20 to 30 minutes is required. After a stimulus is recorded, additional dark adaptation is necessary to reverse the light-adapting effect to the stimulus; otherwise the subject must be completely light-adapted and the dark-adaptation process repeated. Most laboratories have devised some empirical compromise that provides usable results, but because of differences in stimulus conditions it is impossible to compare one set of results with another. Consequently, the time sequence of questionably maximal flashes after *x* amount of dark adaptation to maintain equal responses is quoted as one second (41), two seconds (49), and four seconds (22) in three reports taken at random, none of which gives enough details to allow repetition of the experimental conditions that produced so precarious a maintenance of partial adaptation.

Most difficult of all is the matter of the light stimulus. The electronic flash is fired by condenser discharge, and until recently there was no practical equipment to measure its light output accurately. Recent phototransistor developments have allowed production of a calibrated device* which, with an oscilloscope, gives an accurate rendition of time-course and amplitude of light output over the millisecond or so that the flash lasts. The marked variation in output from the electronic strobe commonly in clinical use was described in (unpublished) discussion at the the Third Symposium (1964) of the International Society for Clinical Electroretinography (ISCERG). This, however, may seem a minute point in the face of much greater problems. Some clinical reports fail to give the distance from light source to subject and to indicate whether one or both eyes are illuminated through all or part of the visual field. The question of energy content of colored

---

* Lite Mike, Edgerton, Germeshausen & Grier, Inc.

stimuli, depending as it does on spectral energy content of the initial light source and band pass characteristics of each filter used, is beyond the scope of many clinical electroretinography laboratories.

The above still deals only with the amount of light delivered to the cornea; beyond this point the most important single factor is pupil size. It is now becoming general practice to dilate the pupil for electroretinography, but this still does not provide uniform pupil size by any means. One type of contact lens electrode designed for clinical use does provide an artificial pupil;* the usual contact lens electrodes have a plano surface, so that the problem of corneal curvature is eliminated. However, transmission of the ocular media, lens curvature, and axial diameter are variables not easily compensated for by any practical method.

As a consequence of these contingencies, the reporting of results in clinical electroretinography has been a qualitative rather than a quantitative matter. The rather fantastically detailed descriptions given by some authors—cf. Jayle, Boyer & Saracco (43: volume I, chapter 5)—are not justified by the techniques utilized. Nevertheless, each laboratory has an idea of the range of normal amplitudes of the b-wave and sometimes the a-wave under prevailing experimental conditions, and can therefore say whether b-wave amplitude is within the normal range, below it, or could not be elicited, i.e., is "extinguished" under conditions prevailing in that laboratory. Another qualitative configuration easily described is the "negative" electroretinogram. Under certain specific circumstances described below, the positive-going b-wave is selectively impaired, leaving the negative a-wave unopposed. The extreme instance of this is shown in the series of experimental electroretinograms of Figure 297; there is no vestige of b-wave in C, a small positive response at the base of the negative deflection appears in B, and in A the positive rise reaches the baseline but goes no farther. Any of these configurations is in the category which can properly be called "negative", implying partial or complete absence of the positive component—Granit's PII (36)—and leaving the negative component—Granit's PIII (36). This underlines the fact that the depth of the a-wave, as well as the height of the b-wave, is the algebraic sum of two opposing processes. One cannot tell by simple inspection what the extent of either would have been if the switch from negative to positive had occurred after the negative wave reached its full extent. An adequate quantitative measure of independent magnitude of a- and b-wave may require determination of amplitude and slope of each, or even rate of change of slope (i.e., the second derivative of the original curve). At all events, these considerations underline the irrationality of measuring the b-wave amplitude from the original baseline; it must be measured from the trough of the a-wave and even then with the reservations just discussed.

What is Being Measured

In evaluating the significance of the clinical electroretinogram, the next question to be answered is what processes we are measuring; for most of the answers

---

* Medical Workshop of Groningen, The Netherlands.

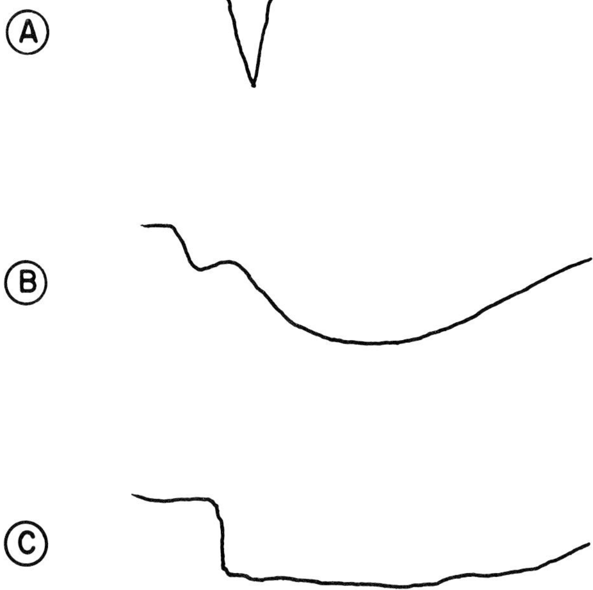

Figure 297. Forms of "negative" ERG encountered experimentally. *A:* Residual PII restores record only to baseline; *B:* tiny residue of PII seen in trough of a-wave; *C:* total absence of PII.

one must make use of the results of experimental electrophysiology. One major question pertains to the extent of retinal area being stimulated by a light stimulus of particular size—can a local area of retina be selectively stimulated? For a single flash the answer has been definitively negative (12,30). The scattered light plays such an important role in the dark-adapted eye that a stimulus entirely confined to the optic nervehead gave as large a response as the same stimulus falling on the posterior pole. Brindley (13) was able to obtain localization in the frog by illuminating the whole retina with light one log unit weaker than the stimulus, but until very recently this has not been clinically useful. With the use of summation techniques, Armington and coworkers (5) were able to demonstrate modest differences between retinal areas in the human subject, and by an extension of these techniques Brindley & Westheimer (16) have obtained electroretinograms which begin to differentiate retinal areas. It is too early to know what this refinement will add to clinical electroretinography. At present, standard clinical technique illuminates the whole retina with single flashes either by filling the pupil with a Maxwellian view using a focused source, or by using some approximation of ganzfeld stimulation.

The next question deals with the relationship of the configuration of the ERG to the retinal structures; the type of retinal abnormality signaled by a particular change in ERG is a highly desirable piece of information. We are far from being able to give a complete answer to this problem, but experiments, particularly of the last decade, have provided a partial answer. Perhaps the earliest and most definitive finding is that the retinal ganglion cell makes no great contribution to the ERG. The arguments on this point were originally indirect ones (36), but even when intracranial sectioning of the optic nerve was done—by Jacobson & Gestring (42), for example—there was no question of decrease of ERG, but only some uncertainty as to whether removal of centrifugal influences caused an increase in the amplitude of the normal pattern (15). Thus the ERG must be created entirely by structures distal to the ganglion cell.

An early notion that the a-wave was produced by cones and the b-wave by rods (65) was dispelled by experiments showing that ERGs from an all-rod retina such as the rat's (or, better, a night monkey's), or from an all-cone retina, such as the prairie dog's, both contain a- and b-waves (60). Later studies demonstrated closely overlapping components of the a-wave and similar overlapping components of the b-wave in the human ERG, attributable in a- as well as b-wave to rod and cone activity (4,6,38).

One definitive clue to the origins of the a- and b-waves came from a toxicological study done in my laboratory. Lucas & Newhouse (48) had found that administration of large amounts of sodium glutamate to newborn mice caused loss of vision and selective loss of the inner retinal layers with preservation of the outer layers. The electroretinogram of such animals showed loss of the b-wave and preservation of the a-wave (56). We therefore suggested that the a-wave was a function of receptor cell activity and the b-wave of bipolar cell activity—since, as mentioned above, the ganglion cells (also destroyed by glutamate) make no significant contribution to the ERG. Later experiments by Brown & Watanabe (18,19) on occlusion of the central retinal circulation in the monkey confirm this hypothesis from another direction.

We can summarize our scanty and hard-earned knowledge of the origin of the electroretinogram as follows:

a. The ganglion cell layer and optic nerve make little or no contribution to the ERG. If they do, it represents a very modest central inhibition of the ERG amplitude.

b. The receptor cells are responsible for the a-wave of the electroretinogram. Cone and rod contributions to the a-wave are identifiable as early and late subcomponents, respectively.

c. The b-wave originates from cells in the region of the bipolar cell layer. Cone and rod contributions to the b-wave are identifiable as early and late subcomponents, respectively.

Flicker

The use of a flickering stimulus is another modality which deserves mention because it has been increasingly introduced into clinical electroretinography in recent years. Over the course of experimentation with flicker it has been found that, under certain circumstances, discrete ERG responses may be obtained in human subjects at frequencies above the subjective fusion frequency. The optimal conditions necessary to obtain these results are: (*a*) use of square wave stimuli of equal on and off duration; (*b*) light adaptation; (*c*) the stimulation of large retinal areas; (*d*) the use of high-intensity stimuli. Under these conditions, it appears that the relatively rapid conduction times of the photopic retina allow the photopic b-wave and the positive-going portion of the off-effect to enhance one another, so that flicker ERG responses may be seen at 90 to 110 cps, while subjective flicker fusion has occurred at 60 to 68 cps. Such responses are a function of wide areas of retinal cone activity, and whereas they truly represent the photopic retina, they are in no sense a measure of foveal or even macular activity. Bornschein (10) has made a succinct review of this material. The clinical electroretinographer with his usual electronic flash stimulus is able to reproduce most of the conditions specified above, with the exception of the symmetrical square wave. Thus he does not reach the theoretical frequency limits mentioned, but he does have a tool good enough to give some independent measure of the activity of the cone system in the patient's eye. Here, again, computer summation is just beginning to be exploited and its potential contribution cannot yet be evaluated.

The ERG in Disease

The clinical electroretinographer has thus at his disposal tools which can indicate whether the ERG is normal, subnormal (dark-adapted b-wave), "negative", or "extinguished". He may also conclude that the flicker response is normal or below normal under his stimulus conditions. As suggested above, the "negative" electroretinogram signifies selective damage to the bipolar cell layer. The reduced or extinguished b-wave may be due to receptor damage alone or to nonselective damage in the outer retinal layer; indeed, loss of receptor function may be secondary to damage to the retinal pigment epithelium (see section on electro-oculogram, below). Selective damage to the cone system is signaled by subnormal response to flicker. In all these instances the electrical response is a function of the activity of large numbers of cells, and decrease in measured electrical response represents loss in function of a large number of cells. It is now of interest to consider specific disease entities in which study of the ERG makes a specific contribution to diagnosis.

THE HEREDORETINAL DEGENERATIONS. Many aspects of these conditions are still under study and no fully satisfactory classification has been proposed. Indeed, the appearance of the electroretinogram is part of the basis for classification. The order in which these diseases are discussed is largely arbitrary and follows in general the scheme of Franceschetti, François & Babel (28).

An important group of diseases known as "retinitis pigmentosa" may at least be subdivided into the classical, recessively inherited, pigmentary retinopathy, and the less usual dominant form. Karpe first reported that the classical recessive disease showed an "extinguished" electroretinogram (45), and that this could be found in affected infants before the appearance of physical signs and long before the age of possible subjective testing (9). The large majority of subsequent papers have confirmed these findings, but some reports have appeared which are ostensibly contradictory—a discussion which underlines the fact that "extinguished" is a relative term. Rubino & Ponte (63) and others (28) have discussed this topic. A small residual response may be elicited by an intense xenon flash when it is not seen with the incandescent bulb stimulus used at the Karolinska clinic. An even smaller residual response not detectable by even a strong flash may be made visible by summation techniques. Finally, a very small number of cases authentic in other respects appear to have normal electroretinograms. Franceschetti et al. (28) state that 10 per cent of cases show detectable but subnormal ERGs and less than one percent have normal responses.

Here is a prime example of the utility of clinical electroretinography. In the classic adult case with characteristic night blindness, defective dark adaptation, ring scotoma, retinal pigment deposits and recessive hereditary pattern, the absence or diminution of the electroretinogram is a moderately useful but by no means vital piece of corroborative information. In the case of the infant with hereditary predisposition and no other findings, it is the single focal fact which makes the diagnosis. Where the other findings are less clear-cut, the ERG plays a proportionately larger role. It should be mentioned that such patients may retain central field and normal or near-normal acuity for years despite the absent ERG.

The much more rare dominant form of pigmentary retinopathy (three to four per cent of total) appears to show a less profound and later effect on the electroretinogram (34). Nevertheless, the ERG is subnormal or not obtainable in a large number of these cases as well.

Congenital Amaurosis of Leber. This is another instance where the ERG is of primary value in making the diagnosis. When one is dealing with an infant

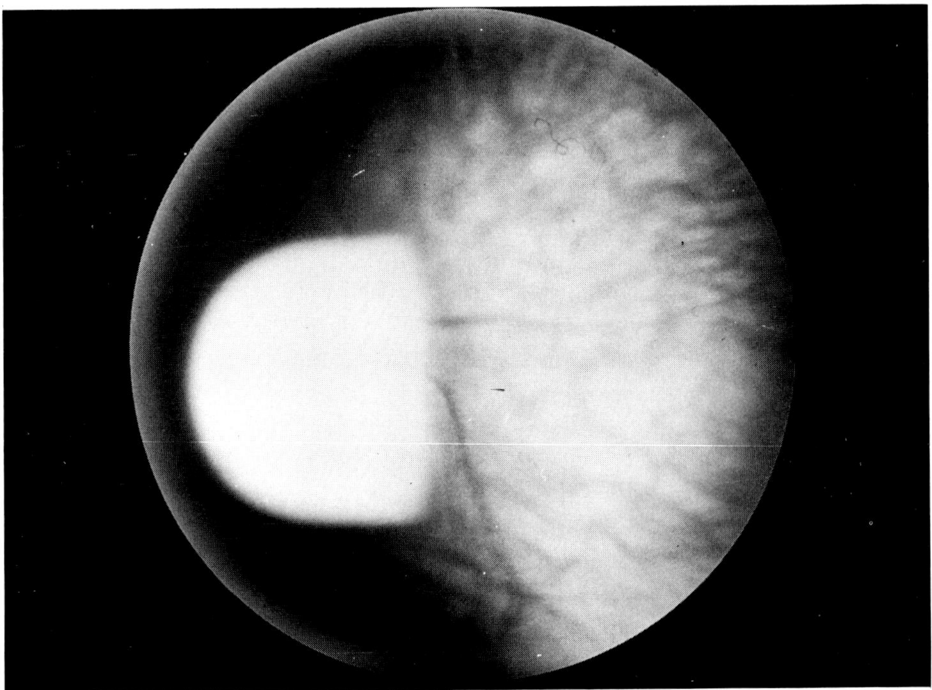

Figure 298. Fundus photograph of infant with congenital amaurosis of Leber. The ERG was "extinguished".

suspected of visual impairment, and ophthalmoscopy shows a pale disk and pepper-and-salt pigmentation of the retina, absence of the ERG renders the diagnosis certain. In the series of Alström & Olson (1), 92 per cent of the cases showed abolition of the ERG (Figure 298).

Flecked Retina Syndrome. The multiplicity of nomenclature in this set of abnormalities has been discussed by Krill & Klien (47). Current names for the three major subcategories are "fundus flavimaculatus", "fundus albipunctatus", and "drusen". Determination of the ERG responses in these categories may add confirmatory evidence to the diagnosis most easily made by ophthalmoscopy and determination of dark adaptation. The abnormalities have in common delayed dark adaptation, paralleled by a delay in the time required for the scotopic ERG to reach its normal height.

Toxic Retinopathies. In a number of instances of drug toxicity, the toxic effect appears to be exerted primarily on the pigment epithelium, and in severe enough cases there is extinction of the electroretinogram. Pigmentary retinopathy usually accompanies these effects, but it may require weeks or even months for its full development. Ordinarily, the history of administration of the drugs at toxic levels, coupled with the complaint of decreased visual acuity, is enough for a tentative diagnosis. In the early stages, before marked pigmentation is evident, absence of the ERG may be a useful additional clinical fact.

Some of the drugs under discussion, i.e., sodium iodate (8,52,62), the diaminodiphenoxyalkanes (51), and NP-207 (33), are no longer being administered to patients, and need concern us only as additional examples and as precautionary reminders. At least two drugs in the category, namely thioridazine and chloroquine, appear to be harmless at low dosages and important enough to warrant their continued availability. When toxic doses were still given, before the significance of dosage level was appreciated, extinction of the ERG was observed for both drugs (64,67).

Congenital Hemeralopias. In cases of dominantly inherited night blindness with no funduscopic findings, the significant electroretinographic finding is absence of the second component of the b-wave (11), but its unequivocal establishment is not within the capability of many clinical ERG laboratories. In nine cases of recessively inherited hemeralopia, Franceschetti and coworkers (28, Vol. II) found reduction of b-wave amplitude as well as loss of the late b-wave component. In the complete absence of other findings, the confirmatory electroretinogram might be a useful clinical adjunct in essential hemeralopias. Computer processing should make this routinely available in the future.

In the case of Oguchi's disease, the night blindness plus the characteristic funduscopic findings are unique, and the ERG without the late b-wave is only another confirmatory finding.

Retinal Detachment. The ERG in retinal detachment is an excellent example of how changes may be measurable without the measurement being fundamentally useful clinically. Rendahl (61) described the changes of the ERG in retinal detachment in considerable detail, and suggested that the diminution of the ERG is proportional to the percentage of retina detached and is an inverse measure of the prospects for operative success. This is not an unreasonable hypothesis—since the ERG reflects the results of a mass discharge of retinal receptors, diminution of the number of functional receptors, as in detachment, could well reduce the ERG amplitude proportionately. It is also reasonable that, all other factors being equal, the prospect of operative success is proportional to the amount of retina detached. However, a perfectly effective and much more accurate measure of the amount of retina detached is available in the subjective determination of visual field. Thus, the mere existence of an electrophysiological change does not automatically warrant its usefulness.

Retinal Destruction Visible Ophthalmoscopically. Complementing the foregoing categories, where the total extent of nonfunction is not visible ophthalmoscopically, there is a host of diseases in which the extent of retinal destruction is accurately shown by the ophthalmoscope, and where the disease is recognizable by funduscopic appearance. To mention a few, gyrate atrophy, choroideremia, chorioretinitis, and diabetes show diminution of the ERG in proportion to loss of retinal substance. The ERG contributes little to such cases.

Retinal Arterial Occlusion. In occlusion of the central retinal artery, the typical finding is a "negative" electroretinogram (39). In view of the fact that the b-wave is generated in the bipolar cell layer supplied by deep capillaries from the central retinal artery and the receptors are nourished by the choriocapillaris, it is easily understandable that the a-wave is accentuated and the b-wave diminished. Since the other characteristics of acute central artery occlusion are so typical, the ERG is of little use in diagnosing this condition. It is conceivable that in a new patient who is a poor historian and whose circulation has been re-established, the electroretinographic abnormality, if typical, could be of help in determining a diagnosis.

Siderosis. In siderosis bulbi the typical ERG is also negative (46), apparently due to selective action of the ferric ion on the bipolar cells. It is not likely that determination of the ERG could play a major role in diagnosis of siderosis, but it could conceivably be of some help in assessing ocular condition after delayed removal of a ferrous intraocular foreign body where cataract prevented psychophysical testing.

Discussion on ERG

The foregoing concrete examples have been cited to illustrate the three categories of usefulness of the electroretinogram. In the relatively rare entities of the retinitis pigmentosa group, in congenital achromatopsia and in Leber's amaurosis, the determination is of the highest importance and is the prime factor in establishing the diagnosis. In a second category of disease, exemplified by the flecked retina syndrome and the pigmented toxic retinopathies, the determination is useful as a confirmatory test. In a third category, exemplified by retinal detachment, there are measurable changes in the ERG, but other diagnostic procedures are more characteristic and there is no benefit to be gained by ERG determination. As one moves from the study of cooperative to uncooperative adults and on to young children, the relative importance of an objective test such as the ERG increases in relation to subjective tests, and the value of the ERG may move from a lower to a higher priority.

Furthermore, the technique of the ERG is today by no means at its ultimate state of perfection. Modifications of technique well within the capabilities of present-day technology may offer new diagnostic specificity not presently apparent. For one thing, the use of algebraic summation of repetitive responses, first done photographically by Heck & Rendahl (38) and more recently with special-purpose computers by Armington (4) and by Brindley & Westheimer (16), promises new information not yet utilizable. The subcomponents of the a-wave and b-wave are so close in amplitude to the electrical noise that one cannot measure them with confidence in a single-flash ERG. However, when many responses are summated, the background noise is averaged out and the subcomponents may be studied in detail. We already know that the early subcomponents are of cone origin and the late subcomponents come from rods, but we do not know the origin of the multiple b-wave subcomponents beyond this generalization. The ability to isolate these subcomponents, to identify their cells of origin, and possibly to attribute clinical significance to changes in them depends on the study of computer-summated records.

As such studies progress, the problem of data reduction looms increasingly larger. The amplitudes and latencies of each wavelet are of potential significance, requiring painstaking measurement. Automatic data reduction techniques applied to this material bring such calculations back to the realm of the possible. Indeed, other statistics on the waveforms, such as ratios, derivatives, integrals, may be obtained easily enough to be examined for significance.

The technology of D.C. amplifiers has advanced to the point where D.C.-coupled measurement of the ERG is readily possible. This will allow study of the neglected slow components such as the c-wave and—the necessary consequence of longer-duration stimuli—the off effect, which should have potential clinical usefulness.

Far from being a definitive statement about the clinical ERG as a non-modifiable method, the above is merely a progress report on what is very probably the kindergarten stage of the technique.

The Electro-Oculogram (EOG)

There have been a number of stages of interest in the standing (D.C.) potential across the axis of the globe. The c-wave of the electroretinogram, mentioned above, probably represents a slow change in this quantity. However, when the illumination level is held constant there is also a measurable axial potential difference, first described by DuBois-Reymond in 1849 (27).

Later studies have recognized that such a potential is the sum of a transcorneal (55), a lenticular (14), and a retinal (26) potential. Since the lenticular potentials across the anterior and posterior lens capsule tend to cancel each other, the corneal and retinal components are of the greatest significance. To isolate the retinal component and to facilitate measurement, it has been necessary to utilize not the potential itself but its change upon variation in illumination level. Since the potentials across transparent components will not be affected by visible light, the measurement of change in potential will sample the retinal component only. It has been found that electrodes on the skin adjacent to the eye are able to sample the corneo-retinal potential. If skin electrodes are placed just temporal and just nasal to the eye of interest, and the subject looks temporally, the two electrodes sample the corneo-retinal potential, with the temporal electrode being closest to the corneal end of the axis; when the subject looks nasally, the polarity is reversed and the nasal electrode is then closest to the corneal end of the axis. Employing nonpolarizable electrodes, the potential change obtained has been used as a measure of eye movement.

The term electro-oculogram (EOG) was introduced by Marg in a review of the early literature (50). The most practical adaptation of the EOG for purposes of measuring retinal function is that of Arden, Barrada & Kelsey (2), who utilized uniform-sized rhythmic oscillations of the subject's eyes elicited at command to generate an oscillatory potential with an easily measurable positive-to-negative peak height. The relation between the maximum light-adapted response and the minimum dark-adapted response can be expressed as a ratio; this at once eliminates the formidable problems inherent in measuring absolute values and abstracts the retinal component from the overall potential measurement. In our hands, the minimum response expected from a normal subject is a light-dark ratio of 2.

Microelectrode studies have located the retinal "standing potential" at the level of the pigment epithelium (21), and toxic agents which affect the pigment epithelium (cf., ERG section) abolish the standing potential (52). Thus, the clinical measurement of the EOG is primarily useful in those diseases which affect the pigment epithelium.

In the inherited pigmentary retinopathies in which the pigment epithelium is extensively involved, the EOG is abnormal (2,29). It markedly decreases in advanced cases of chloroquine toxicity (35), but there is considerable question as to whether the measurement is a useful tool for detecting early chloroquine damage, as was once claimed (3). In a severe case of thioridazine toxicity, the EOG response was abnormally low (L/D ratio = 1.2 O.D.; 1.4 O.S. versus minimum normal = 2.0) (54). One of two cases of inherited nyctalopia, which showed a dominant inheritance pattern, manifested decreased EOG response (23). Three out of three cases with recessive pedigree (35) and one recessive case (23) showed no abnormality.

In general, it appears that the value of EOG measurement is largely in the second category described above for the ERG, i.e., as a useful confirmatory test. It may conceivably become useful in differentiation of inherited nyctalopia, but more cases must be examined. The technique is too new in clinically usable form for its potential usefulness to be well defined, and much more work must be done before such definition can be made with confidence.

The Visual Evoked Response (VER)

Although it has been known for more than 30 years that an electrical response is detectable in the visual cortex after a flash of light is delivered to the eye (32), translation of a phenomenon recordable with intracortical electrodes into one reproducibly observed in the intact human subject has waited most of that time to be realized. The difficulty has been that the response to a single flash, when picked up with scalp electrodes, is of such low voltage (about 5 μV) that it is lost in the electronic and bioelectric "noise". Only with the advent of summating techniques have cortical evoked responses, among them the VER, been studied with some facility. The recent availability of small, relatively low-cost, special-purpose computers has brought the recording of the VER into the realm of the clinically possible. We are now in a period where numerous avenues for clinical exploitation are being investigated and conditions for standardization are being established.

The first attempt at clinical application of the VER was made by Copenhaver & Beinhocker (25), who were chiefly concerned with utilization of the technique for objective perimetry, and tailored their equipment to that purpose. Potts & Nagaya (57) later emphasized that the central retina plays a predominant part in the VER, and their studies have been directed toward exploiting that fact. It is evident that none of the electrophysiological methods discussed so far has been able to differentiate with ease between the narrow central spike representing foveal function in Figure 294 and the much larger area representing peripheral function. Since this small area is the only site of high visual acuity, it might be logical to hope that somewhere in the central nervous system its importance might require anatomical recognition compatible with its function. This is certainly not true in the retina, but it does appear to be true in the occipital cortex and visual association areas. As a result, stimulation of the fovea alone results in a respectable visual evoked response. Not only tiny stimuli, but even those that are small and dim, evoke a response if they are seen by the subject. In our work a 0.06 degree spot seen through an interference filter that peaks at 690 mμ gave excellent results. Indeed, there is a remarkable correlation between subjective foveal vision and the evoked response. It has not been mentioned before, but this is not true of the other electrophysiological measurements; the brightness threshold for the ERG, for example, is many times the psychophysical brightness threshold for a single flash—it may be possible, however, that summation technique will modify this in the future.

Despite all this, the VER is at best only as good as an acuity measurement done subjectively. Hence its utility is confined to special situations where subjective measurement is impractical, such as the testing of hysterical amblyopia. We have found (59) that hysterical amblyopes show no impairment of the visual evoked response, whereas in amblyopia (due to strabismus or to refractive error) there is marked impairment of the VER. This suggests, as does the work of Wiesel & Hubel (69), that amblyopia of disuse causes failure of large numbers of developing neurons to make connections at the geniculate or at the cortical level. Conversely, it suggests that in hysterical amblyopia the block lies cephalad to the calcarine cortex and the visual association areas.

The chief technical problem in recording the VER has to do with variability of response from trial to trial, even in the same subject. It was observed early that the factor of subject attention was important in this regard (31,37,40,44). Our efforts to standardize attention by using transilluminated alphanumeric characters of equal area as stimuli and requiring a response from the subject elicited intermittently by the characters have been described (58).

Additional applications of the VER include its use in malingering and in the study of children under two years of age who cannot give an adequate subjective acuity. In each of these situations it is imperative that the examiner control the placing of the stimulus ophthalmoscopically whether the patient is conscious or anesthetized. We have constructed such a stimulator, using the shell of a hand-held ophthalmoscope and a double coaxial fiber optics bundle. The larger outer portion is for general illumination and may be set at any desired level. The inner bundle transmits the central stimulus from an electronic flash synchronized with the computer. Results of these experiments will be described in the future.

Prospects

At their present state of the art, the electrophysiological measurements of the visual functions have varying utility, depending upon the specific circumstances. There are certain unusual instances where they are indispensable for diagnosis. In a second category of cases they are useful adjuncts and, together with other methods, help to establish the diagnosis. In a third category, although electrophysiological changes are observable, they make no significant contribution to diagnosis. In many instances the psychophysical methods developed in the 19th century are still the best and most accurate measure of visual function.

In my opinion, however, electrophysiological measurements have by no means reached their full potential. Study of the ERG by summation techniques, fuller exploitation of the VER (only possible with summation methods) and investigation of other parameters are for the immediate future. At least one of these parameters is the complex of responses known as the "early receptor potential" (ERP) (24). Although this phenomenon has been emphatically attributed to the receptors (20), there is evidence that at least a portion of it is due to the pigment epithelium and not to the receptor (17). ERP measurement in the human subject has not yet been reported, but it presents no inherent difficulty to prevent its being made. Regardless of whether the phenomenon originates in receptors or in retinal pigment epithelium, clinical applicability of the ERP will certainly follow.

A whole new level of achievement awaits the new order of data that will be made accessible by speed of automatic data reduction. It will be possible to do computations of complex parameters of individual and summated responses with such rapidity that numbers of such parameters may be explored and, if found significant, could even be computed in real time. The utilization of the presently perturbing influence of cerebration upon the VER promises information never before obtainable about processing of visual data anterior to the occipital cortex. The interaction of responses evoked by multiple sensory modalities will supply more information on the function of suprasensory cortex.

In brief, our present achievements in clinical electrophysiology of vision must be looked upon as accomplishments of very real but sharply limited utility. The very great possibilities for expansion of these accomplishments—many of them now within our grasp—must be realized by intensive application on the part of the present generation of researchers.

REFERENCES

1. Alström, C. H., and Olson, O., Heredo-retinopathia congenitalis. Monohybrida recessiva auto-somalis. *Hereditas*, 1957, **43**: 1–177.
2. Arden, G. B., Barrada, A., and Kelsey, J. H., New clinical test of retinal function based upon the standing potential of the eye. *Brit. J. Ophthal.*, 1962, **46**: 449–467.
3. Arden, G. B., Friedmann, A., and Kolb, H., Anticipation of chloroquine retinopathy. *Lancet*, 1962, **1**: 1164–1165.
4. Armington, J. C., A component of the human electroretinogram associated with red color vision. *J. Opt. Soc. Amer.*, 1952, **42**: 393–401.
5. Armington, J. C., Tepas, D. I., Kropfl, W. J., and Hengst, W. H., Summation of retinal potentials. *J. Opt. Soc. Amer.*, 1961, **51**: 877–886.
6. Auerbach, E., and Burian, H. M., Studies on the photopic-scotopic relationships in the human electroretinogram. *Am. J. Ophthal.*, 1955, **40**: 42–60.
7. Aulhorn, E., Über die Beziehung zwischen Lichtsinn und Sehschärfe. *Graefe Arch. klin. exp. Ophthal.*, 1964, **167**: 4–74.
8. Babel, J., and Ziv, B., Recherches sur les dégénérescences rétiniennes expérimentales. Étude histologique et électro-rétinographique. *Ophthalmologica*, 1956, **132**: 65–75.
9. Björk, A., and Karpe, G., The clinical electroretinogram. V. The electroretinogram in retinitis pigmentosa. *Acta Ophthal.* (Kobenhavn), 1951, **29**: 361–376.
10. Bornschein, H., Physiologische Aspekte des Flimmerelektroretinogramms: Komponenten und Frequenzcharakteristik. *Docum. Ophthal.*, 1964, **18**: 85–100.
11. Bornschein, H., and Vukovich, V., Das Electroretinogramm bei Mangelhemeralopie. *Graefe Arch. klin. exp. Ophthal.*, 1953, **153**: 484–487.
12. Boynton, R. M., and Riggs, L. A., The effect of stimulus area and intensity upon the human retinal response. *J. Exp. Psychol.*, 1951, **42**: 217–226.
13. Brindley, G. S., The effect on the frog's electroretinogram of varying the amount of retina illuminated. *J. Physiol.* (London), 1956, **134**: 353–359.
14. ———, Resting potential of the lens. *Brit. J. Ophthal.*, 1956, **40**: 385–391.
15. Brindley, G. S., and Hamasaki, D. I., Evidence that the cat's electroretinogram is not influenced by impulses passing to the eye along the optic nerve. *J. Physiol.* (London), 1962, **163**: 558–565.
16. Brindley, G. S., and Westheimer, G., The spatial properties of the human electroretinogram. *J. Physiol.* (London), 1965, **179**: 518–537.

17. Brown, K. T., and Gage, P. W., An earlier phase of the light-evoked electrical response from the pigment epithelium-choroid complex of the eye of the toad. *Nature* (London), 1966, **211**: 155–158.
18. Brown, K. T., and Watanabe, K., Isolation and identification of a receptor potential from the pure cone fovea of the monkey retina. *Nature* (London), 1962, **193**: 958–960.
19. ———, Rod receptor potential from the retina of the night monkey. *Nature* (London), 1962, **196**: 547–550.
20. Brown, K. T., Watanabe, K., and Murakami, M., The early and late receptor potentials of monkey cones and rods. *Sympos. Quant. Biol.*, 1965, **30**: 457–482.
21. Brown, K. T., and Wiesel, T., Intraretinal recording in the unopened cat eye. *Am. J. Ophthal.*, 1958, **46**(3/2): 91–98.
22. Burian, H. M., and Spivey, B. E., The effect of twin flashes and of repetitive light stimuli on the human electroretinogram. *Am. J. Ophthal.*, 1959, **48**: 274–286.
23. Carr, R. E., Ripps, H., Siegel, I. M., and Weale, R. A., Rhodopsin and the electrical activity of the retina in congenital night blindness. *Invest. Ophthal.*, 1966, **5**: 497–507.
24. Cone, R. A., Early receptor potential of the vertebrate retina. *Nature* (London), 1964, **204**: 736–739.
25. Copenhaver, R. M., and Beinhocker, G. D., Evoked occipital potentials recorded from scalp electrodes in response to focal visual illumination. *Invest. Ophthal.*, 1963, **2**: 393–406.
26. Dewar, J., and McKendrick, J. G., On the physiological action of light. *Trans. Roy. Soc. Edinburgh*, 1873, **27**: 141–166.
27. DuBois-Reymond, E., *Untersuchungen über thierische Elektricität.* Reimer, Berlin, 1849.
28. Franceschetti, A., François, J., and Babel, J., *Les Hérédo-Degénérescences Chorio-Rétiniennes (Degénérescences Tapeto-Rétiniennes).* Masson, Paris, 1963.
29. François, J., Verriest, G., and De Rouck, A., L'électro-oculographie en tant qu'examen fonctionnel de la rétine. *Progr. Ophtal.*, 1957, **7**: 1–67.
30. Fry, G. A., and Bartley, S. H., The relation of stray light in the eye to the retinal action potential. *Am. J. Physiol.*, 1935, **111**: 335–340.
31. García-Austt, E., Bogacz, J., and Vanzulli, A., Effects of attention and inattention upon visual evoked response. *EEG Clin. Neurophysiol.*, 1964, **17**: 136–143.
32. Gerard, R. W., Marshall, W. H., and Saul, L. J., Cerebral action potentials. *Proc. Soc. Exp. Biol. Med.*, 1933, **30**: 1123.
33. Goar, E. L., and Fletcher, M. C., Toxic chorioretinopathy following the use of NP 207. *Trans. Am. Ophthal. Soc.*, 1956, **54**: 129–139.
34. Goodman, G., and Gunkel, R. D., Familial electroretinographic and adaptometric studies in retinitis pigmentosa. *Am. J. Ophthal.*, 1958, **46**: 142–178.
35. Gouras, P., and Gunkel, R. D., The EOG in chloroquine and other retinopathies. *Arch. Ophthal.* (Chicago), 1963, **70**: 629–639.
36. Granit, R., *Sensory Mechanisms of the Retina.* Hafner, New York, 1947.
37. Haider, M., Spong, P., and Lindsley, D. B., Attention, vigilance, and cortical evoked-potentials in humans. *Science*, 1964, **145**: 180–182.
38. Heck, J., and Rendahl, I., Components of the human electroretinogram. An analysis in normal eyes and in colour blindness; preliminary report. *Acta Physiol. Scand.*, 1957, **39**: 167–175.

39. Henkes, H. E., Electroretinography in circulatory disturbances of the retina. II. The electroretinogram in cases of occlusion of the central retinal artery or of one of its branches. *Arch. Ophthal.* (Chicago), 1954, **51**: 42–53.
40. Hernández-Peón, R., and Donoso, M., Influence of attention and suggestion upon subcortical evoked electric activity in the human brain. In: *First International Congress of Neurological Sciences*, Vol. III (L. van Bogacrt and J. Radermecker, Eds.). Pergamon, London, 1959: 385–396.
41. Jacobson, J. H., *Clinical Electroretinography*. Thomas, Springfield, 1961.
42. Jacobson, J. H., and Gestring, G. F., Centrifugal influence upon the electroretinogram. *Arch. Ophthal.* (Chicago), 1958, **60**: 295–302.
43. Jayle, G.-E., Boyer, R.-L., and Saracco, J.-B., *L'Electrorétinographie, Bases Physiologiques et Données Cliniques*. Masson, Paris, 1965.
44. Jouvet, M., Schott, B., Courjon, J., and Allègre, G., Documents neurophysiologiques relatifs au mécanismes de l'attention chez l'homme. *Rev. Neurol.* (Paris), 1959, **100**: 437–450.
45. Karpe, G., The basis of clinical electroretinography. *Acta Ophthal.* (Kobenhavn), 1945, Supp. **24**.
46. ———, Early diagnosis of siderosis retinae by the use of electroretinography. *Docum. Ophthal.*, 1948, **2**: 277–296.
47. Krill, A. E., and Klien, B. A., Flecked retina syndrome. *Arch. Ophthal.* (Chicago), 1965, **74**: 496–508.
48. Lucas, D. R., and Newhouse, J. P., The toxic effect of sodium L-glutamate on the inner layers of the retina. *Arch. Ophthal.* (Chicago), 1957, **58**: 193–201.
49. Mahneke, A., Electroretinography with double flashes. *Acta Ophthal.* (Kobenhavn), 1957, **35**: 131–141.
50. Marg, E., Development of electro-oculography. *Arch. Ophthal.* (Chicago), 1951, **45**: 169–185.
51. Nakajima, A., The effect of amino-phenoxy-alkanes on rabbit ERG. *Ophthalmologica*, 1958, **136**: 332–344.
52. Noell, W. K., Experimentally induced toxic effects on structure and function of visual cells and pigment epithelium. *Am. J. Ophthal.*, 1953, **36**: 103–116.
53. Østerberg, G., Topography of the layer of rods and cones in the human retina. *Acta Ophthal.* (Kobenhavn), 1935, Supp. **6**.
54. Potts, A. M., Drug-induced macular disease. *Trans. Am. Acad. Ophthal. Otolaryng.*, 1966, **70**: 1054–1057.
55. Potts, A. M., and Modrell, R. W., The transcorneal potential. *Am. J. Ophthal.*, 1957, **44**: 284–290.
56. Potts, A. M., Modrell, R. W., and Kingsbury, C., Permanent fractionation of the electroretinogram by sodium glutamate. *Am. J. Ophthal.*, 1960, **50**: 900–905.
57. Potts, A. M., and Nagaya, T., Studies on the visual evoked response. I. The use of the 0.06 degree red target for evaluation of foveal function. *Invest. Ophthal.*, 1965, **4**: 303–309.
58. ———, Studies on the visual evoked response (VER). II. The effect of central influences. *Invest. Ophthal.*, 1966, **5**: 322.
59. ———, Studies on the visual evoked response. III. The VER in strabismus amblyopia and hysterical amblyopia. *Invest. Ophthal.*, in press.

60. Praglin, J., and Potts, A. M., The electroretinogram and spectral sensitivity of the eye of a pure cone mammal. *Fed. Proc.*, 1955, **14**: 116.

61. Rendahl, I., The clinical electroretinogram in detachment of the retina. *Acta Ophthal.* (Kobenhavn), 1961, Supp. **64.**

62. Roggenkämper, W., Akuter Pigmentzerfall der Netzhaut infolge Septojodintoxikation. *Klin. Mbl. Augenheilk.*, 1927, **79**: 827–828.

63. Rubino, A., and Ponte, F., The role of electroretinography in the diagnosis and prognosis of retinitis pigmentosa. *Acta Ophthal.* (Kobenhavn), 1962, Supp. **70**: 232–237.

64. Schmidt, B., and Müller-Limmroth, W., Electroretinographic examinations following the application of chloroquine. *Ibid.:* 245–251.

65. Svaetichin, G., Studies on the vertebrate ERG; on the relationship between the ERG and visual perception. *Acta Physiol. Scand.*, 1953, **29** Supp. 106: 601–610.

66. von Kries, J., Ueber die functionellen Verschiedenheiten des Netzhaut-Centrums und der Nachbartheile. *Graefe Arch. klin. exp. Ophthal.*, 1896, **42**(3): 95–133.

67. Weekley, R. D., Potts, A. M., Reboton, J., and May, R. H., Pigmentary retinopathy in patients receiving high doses of a new phenothiazine. *Arch. Ophthal.* (Chicago), 1960, **64**: 65–76.

68. Wertheim, T., Über die indirekte Sehschärfe. *Zschr. Psychol. Physiol. Sinnes*, 1894, **7**: 172–187.

69. Wiesel, T. N., and Hubel, D. H., Comparison of the effects of unilateral and bilateral eye closure on cortical unit responses in kittens. *J. Neurophysiol.*, 1965, **28**: 1029–1040.

70. Wirth, A., and Ponte, F., *Fisiopatologia e Clinica dell'Elettroretinogramma.* Industria Grafica Nazionale, Palermo, 1964.

CLINICAL ELECTRO-OCULOGRAPHY

PETER GOURAS
National Institute of Neurological Diseases and Blindness
Bethesda, Maryland

Clinical electro-oculography (EOG) depends upon a potential of several millivolts maintained across the eye, making the cornea more positive than the posterior pole. The existence of this potential and its alteration by light have been known for some time (23); although partly dependent upon the lens, cornea and ciliary body, its main source has always been considered to be in the retina. The responsible retinal structures were not clearly defined in the earlier literature, though the receptor-pigment epithelium complex was long considered to play an important role. This idea received support from the finding of a potential of opposite polarity in invertebrates, where the orientation of receptor cells to the pigment epithelium is reversed. The recent studies of Noell (32,33) and others (6,20,29) have demonstrated more clearly the importance of the pigment epithelium in maintaining the D.C. potential of the eye. This retinal potential is not determined solely by the pigment epithelium, however, since its alteration by light is controlled not only by the photoreceptors but also by more inner elements in the retinal neuropil (17,31).

Until recently the clinical application of this potential had been confined to the analysis of eye movements such as occur in nystagmus or during certain stages of sleep. The earliest accounts of its use as an actual retinal function test are those of François and his collaborators in 1955 (13), the Ten Doesschates in 1956 (35), and Heck & Papst in 1957 (20). The important demonstration of the extremely slow, oscillatory time-course of this potential in man following retinal illumination, made independently by Kris in 1958 (27) and Kolder in 1959 (25), provided the basis for a more quantitative retinal function test. Subsequently, Arden and his collaborators (1–5) succeeded in standardizing the EOG as a test of retinal function and in demonstrating its clinical value.

This presentation describes how the EOG can be recorded in man and how it behaves in a variety of retinal disorders. Both clinical and experimental changes in the EOG are compared with those in the ERG to demonstrate that these responses are testing different retinal mechanisms. When used in concert, these tests will be shown to provide considerably more information about retinal function than either one used alone, and make possible a type of differential diagnosis using only the electrical signals of the retina.

Recording Techniques

The EOG is a relatively easy test to perform, but requires 30 to 45 minutes for its satisfactory completion. Both eyes can be tested simultaneously by placing electrodes near the median and lateral canthus of each eye. In our studies, these electrodes are cupped silver disks, 9 mm in diameter, coated inside with electrode paste and fastened to the skin with adhesive tape. The subject sits erect, with his chin supported, and looks into a diffusing sphere (Figure 299) that provides a ganzfeld stimulus for either the EOG or the ERG. The ganzfeld enables the

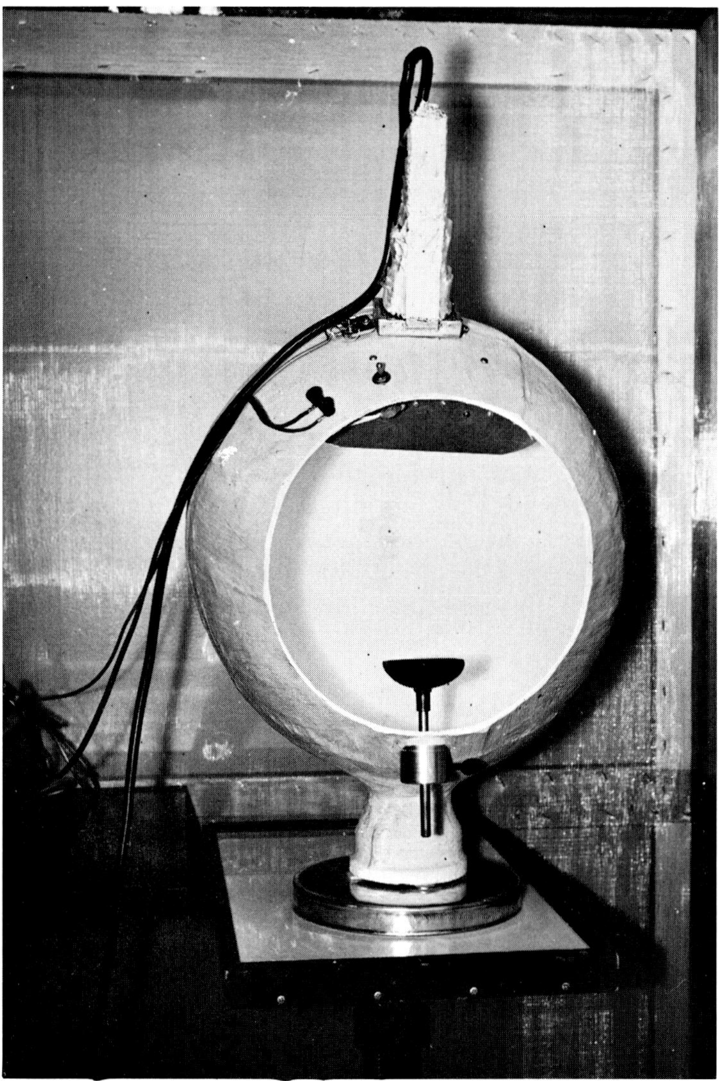

Figure 299. A diffusing sphere providing ganzfeld stimulation for either the EOG or the ERG. (Built in cooperation with Dr. R. D. Gunkel.)

effective stimulus to be expressed in units of retinal illumination without the troublesome problem of scattered light, and has the additional advantage of making psychophysical and electrical thresholds much more comparable.

The subject's eye level is adjusted to the horizontal equatorial plane of the sphere. On the oposite inner surface of the sphere are two quarter-degree, dim, red fixation lights, one central and the other 30 degrees to the right. The examiner alternately turns each light on and off every 10 seconds for short periods during each minute of the test. The subject is instructed to look at the light which is on while keeping his head still. His ocular movements generate a time-varying voltage directly related to the transocular potential of the eye (Figure 300) which can be amplified and recorded by a simple capacitance-coupled electrical system.

Measurements are made for 15 minutes after the room lights are off while the subject follows the dim red fixation light in the otherwise darkened sphere. Then the lights in the sphere are turned on, the brightness of the fixation lights simultaneously increased, and readings taken for an additional 15 minutes. The measurements for the entire test period are plotted and the line drawn through these points shows the overall time-course of the EOG response.

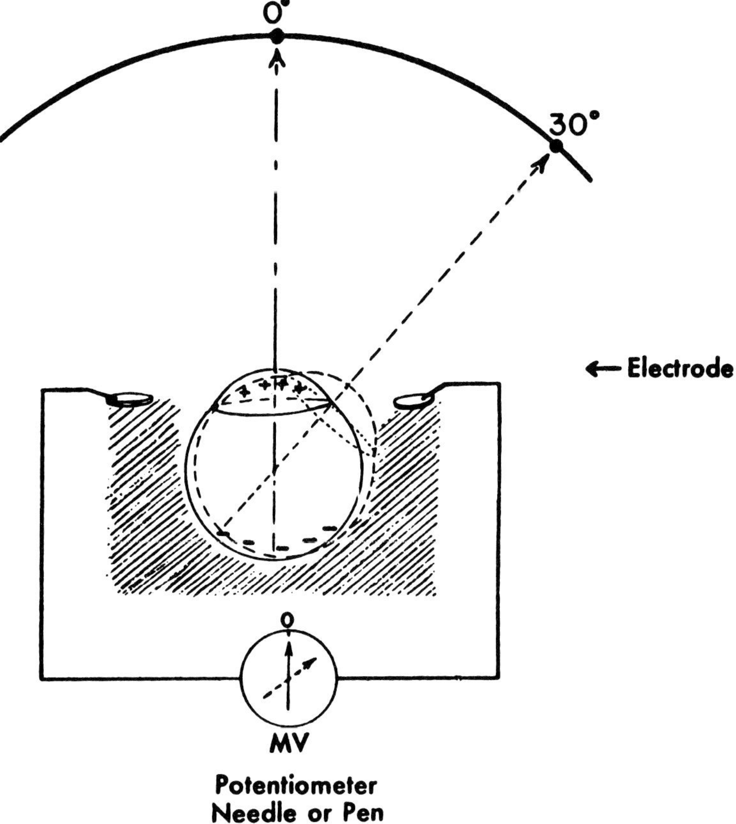

Figure 300. Schematic illustration of the method of measuring the transocular potential by means of eye movements. (From Kris, 28.)

The lights for the EOG stimulus are obtained from tungsten filament bulbs run from a 6 V lead sulfide battery. They are placed above and slightly behind the subject's forehead, thereby presenting him with a diffuse white field, homogeneous except for the fixation lights. The brightness in the sphere can be measured most easily with a Salford Electrical Instruments Exposure Photometer.

For recording the EOG in anesthetized subjects, a technique reported by Henkes & Verduin (21) is recommended, in which the eyes are moved to and fro by means of low-vacuum contact lenses attached to long shafts. For recording the EOG in an automatic way which obviates close participation by the examiner and provides an immediate record of the time-course of the entire response, the method proposed by Kolder & Scarpatetti (26) is recommended.

Normal EOG Responses

Figure 301 shows the slow, oscillatory time-course of normal EOG responses from the eye of a trained observer following changes in retinal illumination. The change from light to darkness or the reverse will alter the EOG potential for durations of an hour or longer. The latter change produces the larger potential and has been used most successfully as a standard clinical test. It must be understood that these large oscillations in the transocular potential are superimposed upon an already large steady potential. When there is no change in retinal illumination, the oscillations subside, and the transocular potential comes to an equilibrium level which is very similar in both light and darkness. When the changes in retinal illumination are considerable, the time needed to reach this equilibrium is accordingly long. Under all conditions the front of the eye always remains positive to the back.

Figure 302 shows the EOG response to stimuli of three different brightnesses

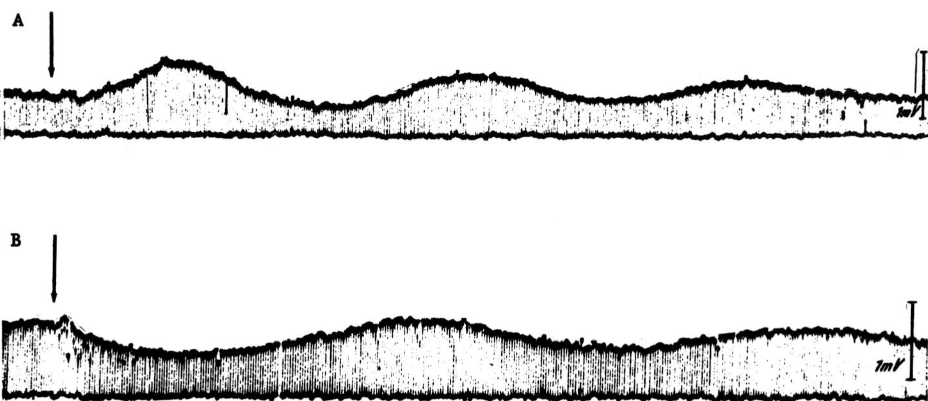

Figure 301. Records of the EOG response obtained by the automatic method of Kolder & Scarpatetti (26). *A:* The illumination is increased from darkness to 200 lm/m² at the arrow. *B:* The illumination has been decreased from 1000 lm/m² to darkness at the arrow. An upward deflection indicates increasing corneal positivity; the time markers are separated by 30 sec. (From Kolder, 25.)

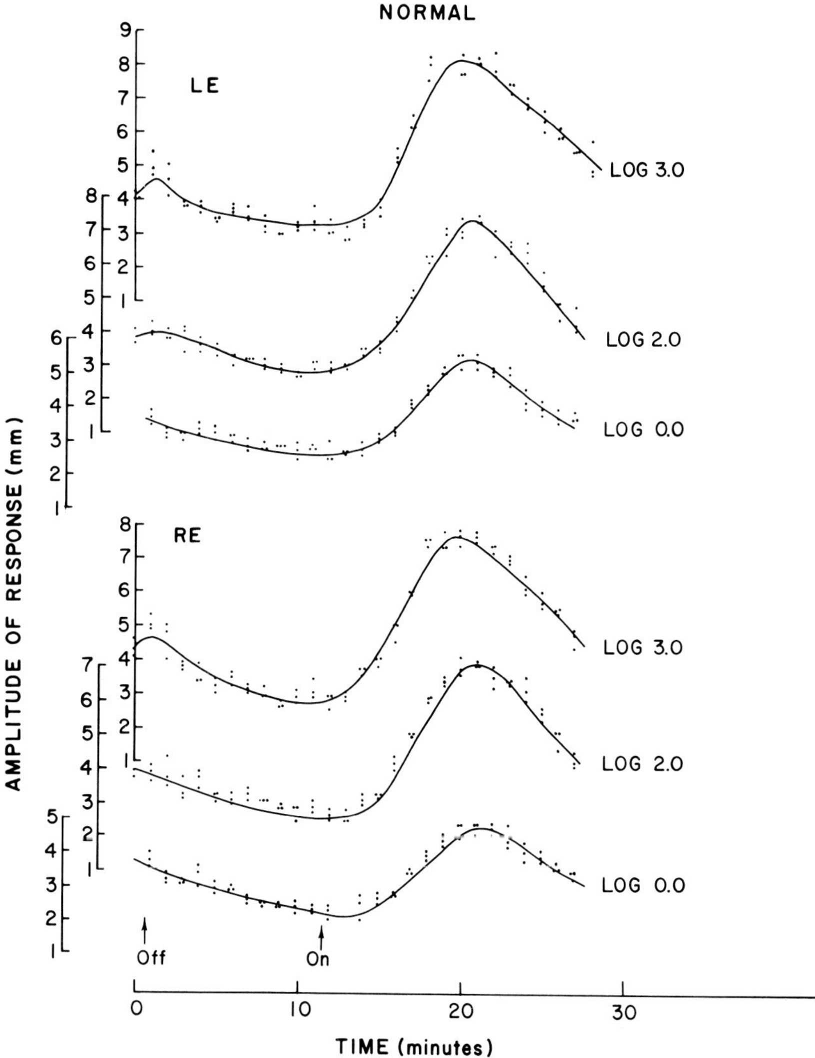

Figure 302. EOG responses from both eyes of a normal subject at three different luminance levels expressed in log foot-lamberts. Each unit on the ordinate scale equals approximately 100 mV/degree. (From Gouras & Gunkel, 19.)

obtained from both eyes of a normal subject during routine clinical tests made on separate days. The responses are usually similar in both eyes, but completely independent of each other. After the room lights are extinguished, the potential subsides to a low level called the "dark trough" (4) in 10 to 15 minutes. Upon reillumination, the potential rises to the peak of its first oscillation within 5 to 10 minutes, and then begins to subside more gradually. The amplitude of this light peak varies approximately linearly with the logarithm of retinal illumination (4,19,20,25). With stimuli brighter than about 10 ft. lamberts, the ratio of the potential at the light peak to that at the dark trough is normally greater than 1.8 (1). This ratio has been found to be more useful than the absolute value of the potentials. When the same routine is followed consistently, the absolute measurements are usually reproducible.

Figure 303 shows a frequency distribution of the actual potentials of normal subjects measured at the light peak and the dark trough under well-standardized conditions and with several test brightnesses. Even in the absolute measurements, a clear increase in the potential is apparent after light stimulation. The dark

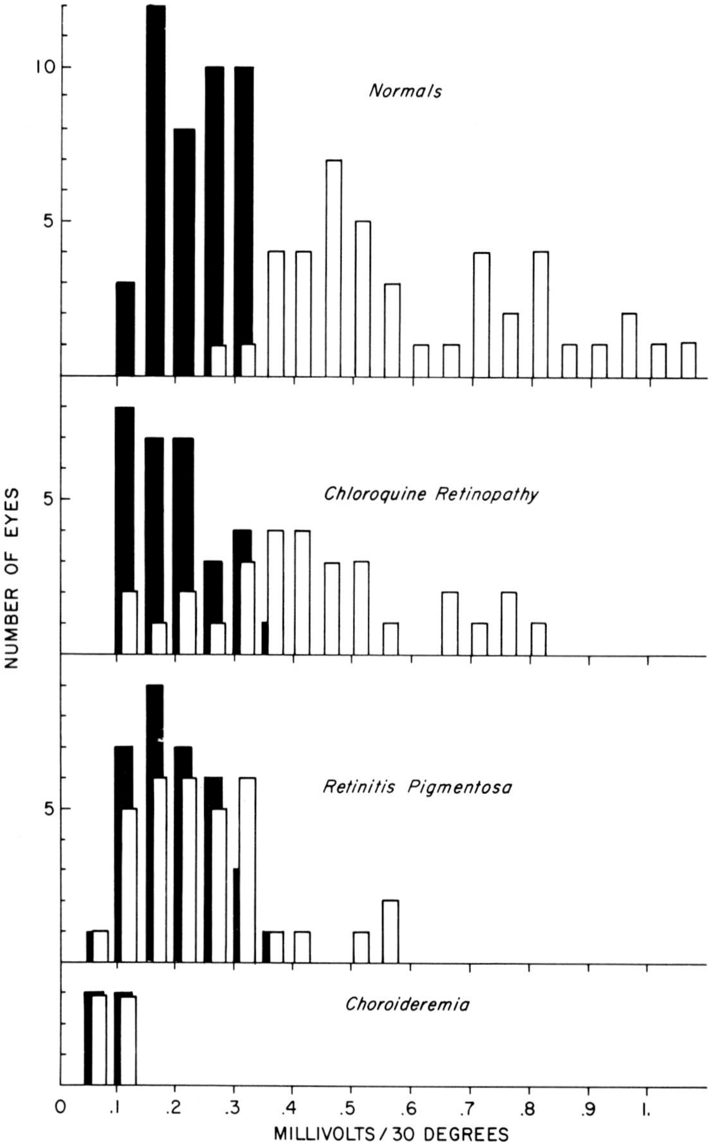

Figure 303. The frequency distribution of EOG potentials at the dark trough (black columns) and the light rise (white columns) from 9 normal subjects, 18 patients with retinitis pigmentation, 8 patients with chloroquine retinopathy (including 3 on chloroquine therapy), and 1 patient with choroidermia. Some subjects were repeatedly tested.

trough is more consistent, ranging from 100 to 350 μV/30 degrees. Changing the position of the electrodes will change these absolute values, but will not alter the ratio of the light peak/dark trough. Absolute measurements are necessary to evaluate the dark trough independently of the light peak.

Progressive Retinal Degenerations

Figure 303 also shows the EOG potentials at the light peak and the dark trough under the same conditions in patients with chloroquine retinopathy, retinitis pigmentosa and choroideremia. The former two disorders are represented by mild, moderate, and severe stages of degeneration. The results for choroideremia are from a 34-year-old patient with a moderately advanced disease, and illustrate what happens in a retinal degeneration which is assumed to damage the pigment epithelium layer early in its course.

In all three conditions, the light rise of the EOG is reduced, more so for retinitis pigmentosa and choroideremia than for chloroquine retinopathy, depending upon how widespread the disease has become. In some cases of chloroquine retinopathy the ratio of the light peak/dark trough was greater than 1.8; accordingly, these patients had much less of a visual deficit. The dark trough potential remains within the normal range for all cases of chloroquine retinopathy, and for all except the most advanced cases of retinitis pigmentosa. The patient with choroideremia showed a consistent reduction in both components of the EOG.

The ERG behaves similarly in these three types of retinal degeneration. In the advanced stages of the disease, the ERG is profoundly depressed, even though the dark-trough level of the EOG often remains within normal limits. In the earlier stages, some ERG responses are found; as in the case of the light rise of the EOG, this is more common in chloroquine retinopathy than in the other two degenerations. Again, this appears to be due to the fact that the damage from chloroquine is less widespread early in the course of the disease.

The ERG has long been considered to be a very sensitive index of early retinitis pigmentosa, being either undetectable or profoundly reduced in the relatively early stages of the disease. With the advent of the EOG, it was suggested that this test would be even more sensitive than the ERG for detecting retinitis pigmentosa; results indicating that the earliest abnormality in this disease occurs in the pigment epithelium of the retina (2) were offered as evidence. More recent studies have indicated that, on the contrary, the EOG can be within normal limits in this disease when the ERG is significantly depressed (16,31). In a group of especially selected subjects with early stages of retinitis pigmentosa, the rod component of the ERG was found to be abnormal, while the cone component and the EOG remained within normal limits (16). At present it does not appear that the EOG is any more sensitive than the ERG for detecting retinitis pigmentosa.

Early Detection of Chloroquine Retinopathy

Much of the impetus responsible for introducing the EOG into the clinic came from the report that it was a sensitive index of impending chloroquine retinopathy (3). Subsequent studies have not fully substantiated this claim (19,22,24).

Subjects on prolonged, high doses of chloroquine appear to have slightly lower than normal EOG responses (24). A complication surrounding this finding is that patients requiring chloroquine therapy for conditions such as rheumatoid arthritis and lupus erythematosus tend to have lower EOG potentials even when they are not receiving the drug (24). Patients who have widespread chloroquine retinopathy certainly do have abnormal EOGs, but many patients with clear-cut but mild retinal damage from chloroquine have EOG responses well within the normal range (19,22); these patients are usually no longer on chloroquine therapy. A question that remains unanswered is whether the EOG will herald the fact that a person being maintained on chloroquine is about to develop an irreversible retinal degeneration; this would be difficult to establish clinically.

What does appear clear at the present time is the considerable biological variation in the EOG, which makes one or a few of these examinations in a particular individual insufficient for detecting an incipient retinopathy. Careful baseline EOG levels should be established before therapy, followed by repeated testing, perhaps on a monthly basis, during the course of therapy, yet even this by itself may not insure the detection of an imminent retinopathy. A similar criticism can be made of the ERG, which is also affected either during long-term chloroquine treatment at high doses or in the more advanced stages of this retinal degeneration. In order to monitor carefully the retina for early damage from chloroquine, it appears even more important to include fundoscopy, perimetry, and certain special psychophysical examinations in the diagnostic armamentarium.

Stationary Retinal Abnormalities

Figure 304 compares the absolute levels of the EOG potential at the dark trough and light rise of normals with those of three types of stationary retinal disorders, rod achromatopsia (which involves a defect predominantly of the cone receptor system) recessive and dominant nyctalopias (defects and primarily of the rod receptor system).

The dark-trough potential is within the normal range in all cases. The light rise of the EOG tends to be reduced in the dominant or Nougaret form of night-blindness (8), but is normal in the recessive form as well as in rod achromatopsia. Normal EOG responses have been found recently in another class of recessive nyctalopia, Oguchi's disease (36).

The ERG, on the other hand, is quite abnormal in all these conditions. In stationary nyctalopia, the ERG is little influenced by the state of retinal adaptation, whereas in rod achromatopsia it is very strongly affected by adaptation. In Nougaret nyctalopia there are only small a- and b-waves in the ERG, whereas in the recessively inherited nyctalopias, including Oguchi's disease (7), the a-wave is much larger than the b-wave. In the latter conditions there is evidence that both the rods and cones are contributing to the a-wave of the ERG (14), while in the former all rod responses are absent.

Central Retinal Artery Occlusion

This condition is particularly interesting in regard to the EOG because the principal source of the transocular potential has been considered to be the pigment

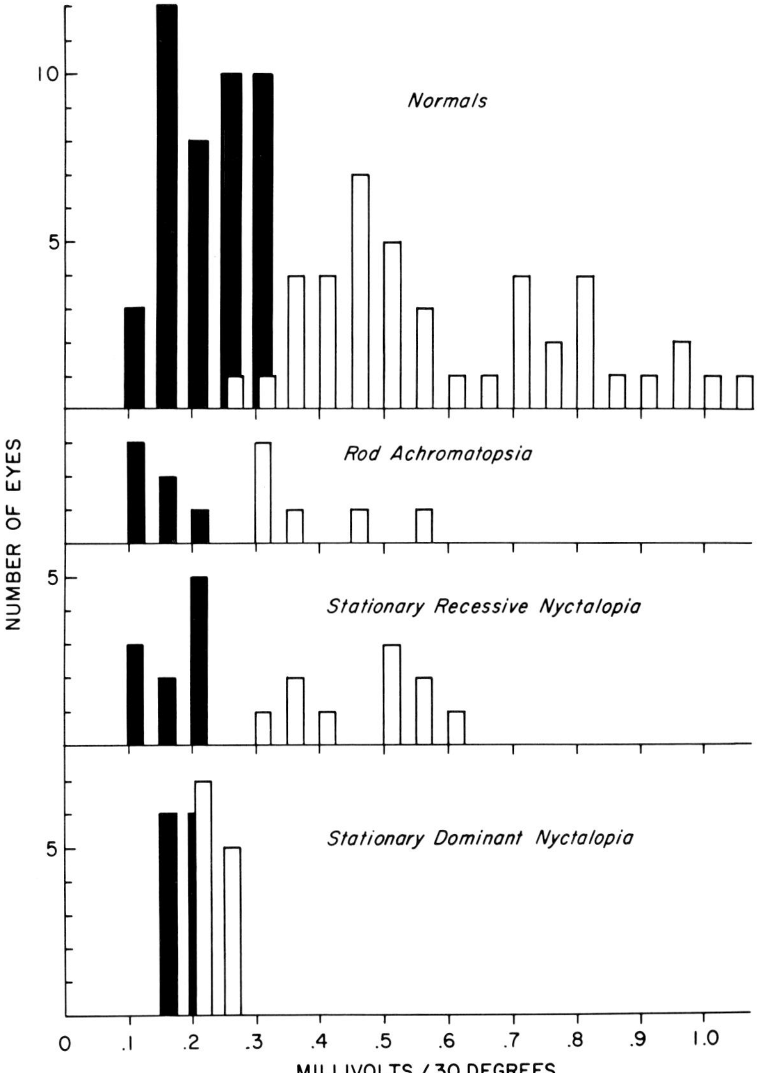

Figure 304. The frequency distribution of EOG potentials at the dark trough (black columns) and the light rise (white columns) from 9 normal subjects, 1 rod achromat, and 3 patients with stationary recessive nyctalopia. The dominant nyctalope has already been the subject of a previous and independent investigation (8). Some subjects were repeatedly tested.

epithelium under the influence of the photoreceptors. Central retinal artery occlusion provides an opportunity for testing this hypothesis, for both the receptors and the pigment epithelium tolerate the insult, whereas the more inner layers of the retina do not.

The transocular potential of monkey eyes has been examined before and months after central retinal artery interruption. Upon sectioning of the eyes, the histology showed severe degeneration of all the retinal layers inner to the external

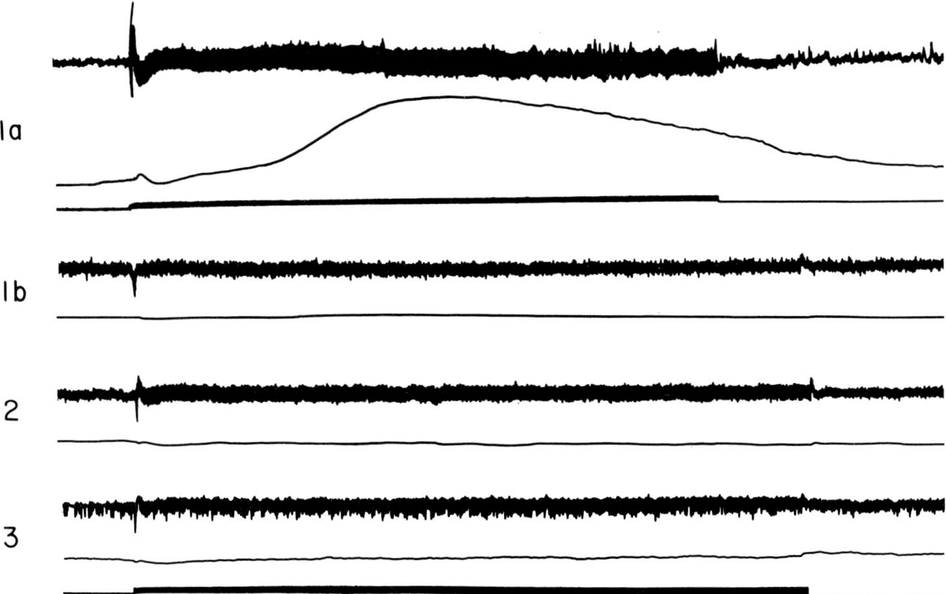

Figure 305. The ERG (upper trace) and transocular potential (middle trace) from the eyes of anesthetized Rhesus monkeys before and after central retinal artery interruption. The lowest trace in each set is the response of a photocell monitoring the light stimulus, a rectangular flicker of 4 cps with equal periods of light and darkness. *1a:* Normal responses; *1b:* the same animal 7 weeks postoperatively; *2* and *3:* other monkeys studied 5 and 13 weeks after operation, respectively. The vertical calibration signifies 0.14 mV for the upper and 1 mV for the middle traces of each set; the horizontal calibration represents 30 sec.; positivity is up. (From Gouras & Carr, 17.)

plexiform layer, while the photoreceptor and pigment epithelium layer remained intact. Nevertheless, the light rise of the EOG disappeared (Figure 305). The D.C. potential of the eye continued to respond normally to the intravenous administration of azide, indicating a functioning pigment epithelium layer. The b-wave of the ERG was extinguished, but the a-wave and a small negative potential maintained during light stimulation remained, indicating the presence of photoreceptor function (17).

Nagaya (31) has reported similar clinical results with the EOG and ERG following central retinal artery occlusion in man (Figure 306). Both the experimental and clinical results indicate that structures more proximal than the photoreceptor-pigment epithelium complex are responsible for the light rise of the EOG, whereas the dark-trough potential arises more distally in the retina, undoubtedly in the pigment epithelium.

Retinal Detachment

Clinical investigations have revealed that retinal detachment produces a reduction in the EOG potential and a loss of the light rise (5,20). The recent experimental work of Foulds & Ikeda (12) in the rabbit illustrates most completely the sequence of changes which occur in the EOG following a retinal

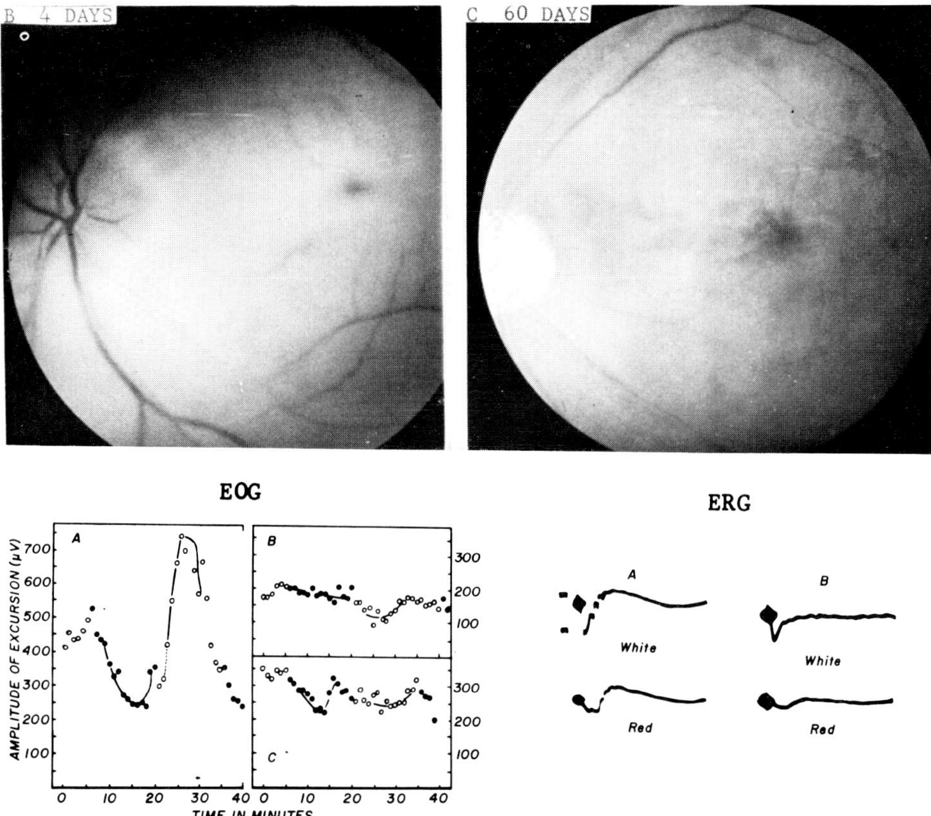

Figure 306. Fundus photographs and EOG and ERG responses of a patient, 4 and 60 days after occlusion of the central retinal artery. The light rise of the EOG was lost, whereas the dark-trough potential stayed within normal limits; only the a-wave of the ERG remained. (In part from Nagaya, 31.)

detachment. Immediately after detachment both the light rise of the EOG and the entire ERG are lost, results that would be expected if the photoreceptors were damaged. The level of the transocular potential is somewhat reduced, but a normal response to azide remains, indicating functioning pigment epithelium. Months later and concomitantly with a slow histological degeneration of the pigment epithelium, the residual EOG potential and the azide response disappear.

Sources of the EOG Potential

There appear to be at least two separate responses in the EOG. One is seen in the dark-trough potential, which seems to depend upon the pigment epithelium entirely and is extremely sensitive to azide. This component is resistant to many retinal disorders, being affected only in the late stages of abnormalities which eventually destroy the pigment epithelium layer.

The light-rise potential comprises a second component of the EOG, and depends upon the intactness of both the visual receptors as well as on structures in the more inner layers of the retina. This response is much more sensitive to most disorders than the dark trough of the EOG; it is always absent when the photoreceptors are damaged and sometimes even when receptor function is present. In this respect it resembles the b-wave of the ERG, but it is not produced by the same mechanism, since in certain forms of nyctalopia the b-wave is lost while the EOG remains normal.

There appears to be an additional component observable in the ERG which is revealed after loss of the light-rise potential following central retinal artery interruption. This is a small negative response maintained during illumination which appears as a continuation of the a-wave of the ERG. This potential is most likely produced by the photoreceptors, although the horizontal cells cannot be ruled out, since they also appear to tolerate central retinal artery interruption.* In the normal EOG, this small maintained negative response is obscured by the much larger light-rise potential.

The main barrier for current across the retina appears to be located at the pigment epithelium (37); electron microscopy also reveals that there are tight junctions between pigment epithelial cells (9),† where the dark trough or light-insensitive component of the EOG is presumably generated. The light rise or light-sensitive component of the EOG may also be determined by this same barrier, but it is clearly under the control of more inner layers of the neural retina. This control may depend upon the release of charged molecules or upon some inducer of pigment epithelium activity which is released after stimulation of the retina. On the other hand, the entire light response may be generated within the retinal neuropil.

The possibility that elements postsynaptic to the photoreceptors contribute to the slow, transient changes in the transocular potential must be given some consideration, since the retina isolated from the pigment epithelium is capable of generating extracellular potential changes as large as 10–15 mV (30). This occurs in the phenomenon of spreading depression and is accompanied by considerable changes in the impedance and transparency of the retina. Spreading depression involves an intense, abnormal sort of chain reaction of many retinal cells, and is presumably unrelated to the light rise of the EOG. On the other hand, some of the mechanisms involved in producing large, slow, transient D.C. changes within the retina in these two situations may be similar. It would be interesting to know whether changes in retinal impedance or refractive index accompany the light rise of the EOG.

Relationship to the ERG

The major components of the clinical ERG are the a- and b-waves, considered to be generated by the receptor cells and the bipolar cells of the retina, respectively. The dark-trough potential of the EOG thus provides information about pigment epithelium function, the a-wave about the receptors, and the b-wave and the light rise of the EOG about more inner structures of the neural retina, up to and including the bipolar cells.

An important difference between the EOG and the ERG is the manner in

---

* A. I. Cohen, personal communication.

† Also, A. Lasansky, personal communication.

which the rod and cone systems combine their signals in these responses. In the a- and b-waves of the ERG, these two receptor systems are completely independent (15), probably because there may be a separate set of bipolar and perhaps horizontal cells for both rods and cones, with little or no intercommunication between these two channels until after the b-wave of the ERG has been generated. The rod and cone receptor systems can therefore be studied independently in the ERG. Disorders which affect only rods alter the rod but not the cone a- and b-waves; the converse occurs in cone defects.

There has been no obvious separation into rod and cone components in the EOG, even though the cones contribute to this response (10,11,18). Defects which involve only the rods or only the cones and therefore produce totally different ERGs can produce, as in rod achromats and stationary recessive nyctalopes, the same type of EOG.

Clinical Application

Figure 307 illustrates diagrammatically where the various components of the EOG and ERG enter into the flow of information and material in the retina. A number of disorders are included, to demonstrate how they can be located within this system from the way they alter the electrical responses of the retina. The scheme is tentative and subject to change, presumably expansion, as new electrical manifestations of retinal function are uncovered.

The EOG, as the ERG, remains a test of more or less the entire retina—least useful for the study of localized disease and most useful for abnormalities which involve specific systems or mechanisms throughout the retina. The model proposed above for interpreting the significance of these responses is in large part academic in relation to the routine application of these procedures in clinical ophthalmology. While it usually is a question of whether or not there is widespread involvement of the external retinal layers by a disease process; if there is, either the EOG or ERG can be perfectly satisfactory, each having certain advantages over the other. By not requiring a contact-lens electrode, the EOG is less traumatic and can therefore be done relatively often and with little apprehension. The ERG is quick and can be done on patients who are either unconscious or unable to fixate properly.

Because these examinations test different retinal mechanisms, however, there are certain circumstances where their combined results can provide important new information on the underlying pathophysiology of a disease process. Some cases in point are already extant in the literature. Henkes & Verduin (21) were able to separate a true dysgenesis from an abiotrophy in cases of congenital retinal blindness with absent ERGs by means of the EOG. The dysgenesis leaves pigment epithelium intact and therefore exhibits some EOG response; the abiotrophe has neither pigment epithelium nor EOG. Three varieties of stationary nyctalopia have again been split into two separate functional categories based on the electrophysiology obtained from these two retinal tests (8). The functional damage after central retinal artery occlusion can be better interpreted with the use of both the EOG and the ERG than by using either alone (17,31).

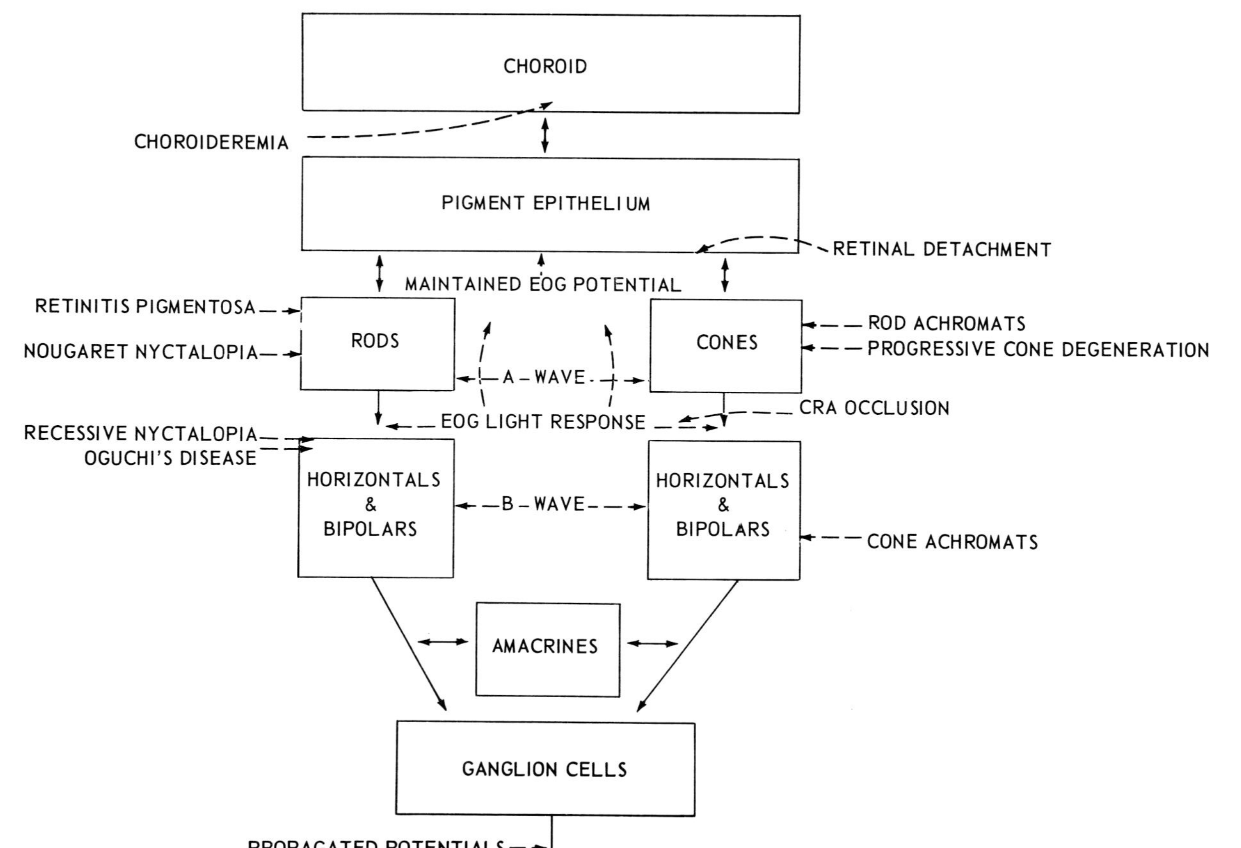

Figure 307. Diagram of location of sources of the various components of the EOG and ERG in the flow of events in the retina, derived from current knowledge of the physiology and microanatomy of the primate eye. The sites where a number of retinal disorders appear to be interrupting the system are also included. *CRA*: Central retinal artery.

Clinical electrophysiology has expanded its repertoire to provide new information about retinal function. The proper use of these objective diagnostic techniques provides a means of differentially diagnosing certain retinal mechanisms impossible with standard ophthalmological methods. Increasing awareness of the variety of hereditary defects involving specific biochemical abnormalities within the retina may eventually make this electrical approach even more valuable.

SUMMARY

This review deals with the present understanding of the physiology and the clinical applications of the electro-oculogram. The EOG is considered to have two major components: a maintained potential determined by the pigment epithelium and a slow response to light which depends upon the receptor and inner nuclear layers of the retina. The source of the latter potential is not clearly known. The maintained D.C. potential of the EOG can be measured without light stimulation, thus providing an index of pigment epithelium function which is not possible with the electroretinogram (ERG). The light-induced response of the EOG resembles the ERG in its dependence upon the neural retina. It is not produced by the same mechanisms which generate the ERG, however, as it is absent when the a-wave of the ERG is present and it is present when the b-wave of the ERG is not. A tentative scheme is proposed which associates the major components of the EOG and the ERG with specific cells comprising the rod and cone systems of the retina. The usefulness of this model for explaining a number of retinal abnormalities is demonstrated.

REFERENCES

1. Arden, G. B., Barrada, A., and Kelsey, J. H., New clinical test of retinal function based upon the standing potential of the eye. *Brit. J. Ophthal.*, 1962, **46**: 449–467.
2. Arden, G. B., and Fojas, M. R., Electrophysiological abnormalities in pigmentary degenerations of the retina. *Arch. Ophthal.* (Chicago), 1962, **68**: 369–389.
3. Arden, G. B., Friedmann, A., and Kolb, H., Anticipation of chloroquine retinopathy. *Lancet*, 1962 **1**: 1164–1165.
4. Arden, G. B., and Kelsey, J. H., Changes produced by light in the standing potential of the human eye. *J. Physiol.* (London), 1962, **161**: 189–204.
5. ———, Some observations on the relationship between the standing potential of the human eye and the bleaching regeneration of the visual purple. *Ibid.:* (London), 1962, **161**: 205–226.
6. Brown, K. T., and Wiesel, T. N., Localization of origins of electroretinogram components by intraretinal recording in the intact cat eye. *J. Physiol.* 257–280.
7. Carr, R. E., and Gouras, P., Oguchi's disease. *Arch. Ophthal.* (Chicago), 1965, **73**: 646–656.
8. Carr, R. E., Ripps, H., Siegel, I. M., and Weale, R. A., Rhodopsin and the electrical activity of the retina in congenital night blindness. *Invest. Ophthal.*, 1966, **5**: 497–507.

9. Cohen, A. I., A possible cytological basis for the 'R' membrane in the vertebrate eye. *Nature* (London), 1965, **205**: 1222–1223.
10. Elenius, V., and Lehtonen, J., Spectral sensitivity of the standing potential of the human eye. *Acta Ophthal.* (Kobenhavn), 1962, **40**: 559–566.
11. Enoch, J. M., Summary and discussion of: Elenius & Lehtonen (10). *Survey Ophthal.*, 1963, **8**: 544–547.
12. Foulds, W. S., and Ikeda, H., The effects of detachment of the retina on the induced and resting ocular potentials of the rabbit. *Invest. Ophthal.*, 1966, **5**: 93–108.
13. François, J., Verriest, G., and de Rouck, A., Modification of the amplitude of the human electro-oculogram by light and dark adaptation. *Brit. J. Ophthal.*, 1955, **39**: 398–408.
14. Goodman, G., and Bornschein, H., Comparative electroretinographic studies in congenital night blindness and total color blindness. *Arch. Ophthal.* (Chicago), 1957, **58**: 174–182.
15. Gouras, P., Rod and cone independence in the electroretinogram of the dark-adapted monkey's perifovea. *J. Physiol.* (London), 1966, **187**: 455–464.
16. Gouras, P., and Carr, R. E., Electrophysiological studies in early retinitis pigmentosa. *Arch. Ophthal.* (Chicago), 1964, **72**: 104–110.
17. ———, Light-induced DC responses of monkey retina before and after central retinal artery interruption. *Invest. Ophthal.*, 1965, **4**: 310–317.
18. ———, Cone activity in the light-induced DC response of monkey retina. *Ibid.*: 318–321.
19. Gouras, P., and Gunkel, R. D., The EOG in chloroquine and other retinopathies. *Arch. Ophthal.* (Chicago), 1963, **70**: 629–639.
20. Heck, J., and Papst, W., Über den Ursprung des corneo-retinalen Ruhepotentials. *Bibl. Ophthal.*, 1957, **48**: 96–107.
21. Henkes, H. E., and Verduin, P. C., Dysgenesis or abiotrophy? A differentiation with the help of the electro-retinogram (ERG) and electro-oculogram (EOG) in Leber's congenital amaurosis. *Ophthalmologica*, 1963, **145**: 144–160.
22. Henkind, P., Carr, R. E., and Siegel, I. M., Early chloroquine retinopathy: clinical and functional findings. *Arch. Ophthal.* (Chicago), 1964, **71**: 157–165.
23. Kohlrausch, A., Elektrische Erscheinungen am Auge. In: *Handbuch der normalen und pathologischen Physiologie*, Vol. 12/2 (A. Bethe, G. von Bergmann, G. Embden, and A. Ellinger, Eds.). Springer, Berlin, 1931: 1393–1496.
24. Kolb, H., Electro-oculogram findings in patients treated with antimalarial drugs. *Brit. J. Ophthal.*, 1965, **49**: 573–590.
25. Kolder, H., Spontane und experimentelle Änderungen des Bestandpotentials des menschlichen Auges. *Pflüger Arch. ges. Physiol.*, 1959, **268**: 258–272.
26. Kolder, H., and Scarpatetti, R., Registrierung von Änderungen des Bestandpotentials des menschlichen Auges. *Pflüger Arch. ges. Physiol.*, 1958, **267**: 295–298.
27. Kris, C., Corneo-fundal potential variations during light and dark adaptation. *Nature* (London), 1958, **182**: 1027–1028.
28. ———, Vision: electro-oculography. In: *Medical Physics*, Vol. III (O. Glasser, Ed.). Year Book Publishers, Chicago, 1960: 692–700.
29. Lasansky, A., and de Fisch, F. W., Potential, current, and ionic fluxes across the isolated retinal pigment epithelium and choroid. *J. Gen. Physiol.*, 1966, **49**: 913–924.

30. Martins-Ferreira, H., and de Oliveira Castro, G., Light-scattering changes accompanying spreading depression in isolated retina. *J. Neurophysiol.*, 1966, **29**: 715–726.
31. Nagaya, T., The standing potential of the eye in vascular and degenerative disease of the retina. *Bull. Yamaguchi Med. Sch.*, 1964, **11**: 187–201.
32. Noell, W. K., *Studies on the Electrophysiology and Metabolism of Vision.* USAF School of Aviation Medicine, Project 21–1201–004, 1953.
33. ———, Cellular physiology of the retina. *J. Opt. Soc. Amer.*, 1963, **53**: 36–48.
34. Schmidt, B., Müller-Limmroth, W., Heinmüller, G., Böke, W., and Bäumer, A., Veränderungen im Elecktroretinogramm des Menschen im Verlauf der Resochin-Langzeit-Therapie. *Klin. Wschr.*, 1961, **39**: 132–137.
35. Ten Doesschate, G., and Ten Doesschate, J., The influence of the state of adaptation on the resting potential of the human eye. *Ophthalmologica*, 1956, **132**: 308–320.
36. Ten Doesschate, J., Alpern, M., Lee, G. B., and Heyner, F., Some visual characteristics of Oguchi's disease. *Docum. Ophthal.*, 1966, **20**: 406–419.
37. Tomita, T., Murakami, M., and Hashimoto, Y., On the R membrane in the frog's eye: its localization, and relation to the retinal action potential. *J. Gen. Physiol.*, 1960, **43**(6): 81–94.

THE CLINICAL CHARACTERISTICS OF ACQUIRED COLOR-VISION DEFECTS

ARTHUR LINKSZ
New York University
New York, New York

This article will be concerned with the disturbances of color vision secondary to retinal disease and which are, in many instances, an integral part of clinical symptomatology. Discussion will be confined to general principles rather than to individual cases or details of individual disease entities; neither the normal characteristics of color vision nor those of the hereditary defects of color vision will be analyzed.

The symptomatology of the changes in color appreciation in diseases of the retina ("retina" is used here in a somewhat wider sense to include the optic nerve at least as far as the geniculate body) strongly supports the classification of these changes into two main groups. The defects of color vision caused by retinal pathology involve primarily either the red-to-green axis or the yellow-to-blue axis of the circle of appreciated colors. In this respect, they behave much like the ordinary hereditary defects. Red and green on the one side, yellow and blue on the other, are mutually exclusive color modalities, and that does not change with retinal pathology. Even a diseased eye never sees a reddish green or yellowish blue. But these are also inseparably associated. Even a diseased eye never becomes "red-blind" without becoming "green-blind" at the same time, and if it has become "blue-blind," its yellow vision is always involved. Be it inherited or disease-inflicted, a defect in color vision always manifests itself in terms of two opposing color modalities.

Still, there are certain peculiarities to these disease-induced "acquired" color vision disarrangements. According to the exposition of Jaeger & Grützner (9), the following features should be recognized:

a. Disturbances of color appreciation in the wake of retinal disease do not have the stability and immutability characteristic of hereditary defects. They represent *processes* rather than *conditions* as the latter do. They grow worse or better in a like manner as the disease process which causes them. Improvement on the one hand, deterioration on the other, blur the categories into which acquired color-vision defects can be classified. The disturbance may start with a state in which color vision is still trichromatic, suggesting a color anomaly; it may, for example, stimulate protanomaly. It might then progress toward a state of dichromacy, and finally culminate in total loss of color discrimination, a state reminiscent of one or the other form of achromatopsia. Therefore one cannot expect the characteristics of a certain red-and-green defect to be maintained throughout the course of, say, a degenerative process affecting the macular region.

b. A hereditary color-vision defect can be unilateral, though it seldom is; on the other hand, disease often affects only one eye, or one eye primarily. The other eye might be completely normal or show the defect to a much lesser degree. This will not, of course, apply to disturbances caused by toxic influences. Quinine, tobacco or wood alcohol will rarely affect only one eye; retrobulbar neuritis or central serous retinopathy can readily occur in only one eye. Moreover, one can have a color-vision defect involving the central area of the retina (as in central serous retinopathy) while other parts of the same retina remain more or less intact.

Judd (11) collected from the literature 37 more or less well-documented cases of unilateral color deficiency; ten were obviously acquired defects, five of which due to trauma to the head. It is certainly justified in the case of a unilateral color-vision defect to look for disease or trauma as its often not-so-apparent reason.* Genetic mosaicism or any other chromosomal disarrangement should be accepted only reluctantly as its ultimate cause.

c. One should also be aware of the fact that a diseased eye is a diseased eye and, therefore, other visual functions might also be affected. The central visual acuity might be poorer, the peripheral field might show defects, adaptation might be limited, or the electroretinogram might be abnormal. But signs or symptoms of ocular disease need not always accompany an acquired color defect. In certain stages of ocular disease color appreciation may be the only affected visual performance, with all the other visual functions seemingly still intact or already restored. Color vision might be the first visual function affected in pigment degeneration of the retina, or in juvenile macular degeneration; it is usually the last visual function to become normal during the remission period of a retrobulbar neuritis; it might be the only one permanently defective after a head trauma. Color vision in biological terms means the ability to discriminate the position of a visual stimulus in the visible spectrum. It is a late acquisition and therefore a vulnerable one. It follows the rule laid down for late phylogenetic acquisitions by the great Hughlings Jackson: it suffers early in any disease and is restored belatedly with remission or cure.

d. An interesting point noted by Jaeger & Grützner (9) should be especially emphasized: a person with a hereditary defect of color vision will generally call object colors by the same name used by normals. He will call a rose "red" and its leaves "green" even if he totally lacks these two color modalities. A person with acquired color-vision defect (assuming he had been color-normal before the onset of the disease) will usually state the color he actually sees. To one who is genuinely red-and-green blind both the rose and the leaves offer a certain familiar-

---

* Even the seemingly very well documented case of unilateral genetic deuteranopia which Graham and his associates (4) elaborately investigated might actually have been a unilateral acquired defect. (See Cox [2] on this topic.)

to-him modality of color—whatever that modality might be. (This problem will not be discussed here.) He is used to calling one of them "red", the other "green". The person with an acquired defect is aware of a change, of some strangeness in his vision, especially if the change occurred in only one eye. Many times have I had a patient with diabetes or general arterial hypertension report spontaneously that the color of familiar objects is different with each eye; this is for me sufficient justification for a thorough fundus study. There are, of course, some exceptions to this observation. As Jaeger & Grützner emphasized, if a person suffered a substantial loss of his visual functions, including much of the faculty of color discrimination, at an early age, he might have forgotten his childhood experiences of color and behave in this respect as a person with a hereditary defect would.

Two further details are worth mentioning, since they variegate the clinical picture and make the analysis so intriguing. First of all, since eight per cent of the male population is afflicted with some form of hereditary red-and-green defect, it would not be rare for a retinal disease process with a secondary disturbance in color vision to inflict itself upon an eye with a hereditary defect. This will naturally complicate the psycho-physiological data yielded by routine clinical color-vision tests.

There is another complicating element. Abnormalities, pathological changes within the eyeball, might act as a pre-receptorial, quasi-physical, obstacle for certain regions of the visible spectrum, and this too can affect color vision. For example, in central serous retinopathy a yellow-and-blue defect is typical; at the same time, especially in the earlier stages of the disease, the anomaloscope test reveals data reminiscent of protanomaly: the patient uses too much red light to set up a Rayleigh equation. This peculiarity can be explained by assuming that the retinal disease proper caused a defect in yellow-and-blue vision, while an intraretinal exudate acted as filter for the longer wavelengths of light.

In the normal aging person, increasing yellowness of the crystalline lens often causes an apparent decrease in sensitivity to the short wave end of the spectrum, thus mimicking a tritan defect. Vice versa, after removal of a cataractous lens, the retina becomes quasi-hypersensitive to the shorter wavelengths of light, even to light from the ultraviolet spectrum range (19).

This apparently decreased sensitivity of the elderly to light of shorter wavelength often manifests itself in the changing color values of aging painters. Citing two famed colorists—Turner and Monet—as examples in a paper on the intriguing subject, "The Influence of Eye Disease on Pictorial Art" (17), Trevor-Roper showed what such an apparently decreased sensitivity can do to a painter's palette. He also mentioned an interesting instance of the apparent hypersensitivity of the eye to the shorter wavelengths after cataract extraction as it manifests itself in a work of art by comparing two paintings of the same landscape, done by the same artist, in the same month, one before, the other a year after the removal of cataracts. The dominance of "colder" colors in the second painting was quite striking.

(It should probably be stressed again that these sensitivity changes are only apparent, due to a filtering effect or the lack of it and do not properly belong among those discussed in this paper.)

As previously mentioned, disease-induced defects of color vision present themselves mainly in two varieties—as deficiencies involving either the red-and-green axis of the color circle, or the yellow-and-blue axis. It was the German ophthalmologist, H. Köllner (12), who recognized the rather significant relationship between the site of the retinal affliction and the type of the associated color-vision defect. Köllner's name is still attached to the rule he established and, at least as a first order generalization, it can be stated that diseases of the optic nerve affect red-and-green vision, while diseases of the retina proper lead to a disturbance in the yellow-and-blue modalities. Thus, a red-and-green defect might be expected in a case of optic atrophy, retrobulbar neuritis, or head trauma, and a yellow-and-blue defect in a case of pigment degeneration.

One must, however, generalize with caution. There exists at least one type of optic nerve atrophy in which the color defect involves the yellow and blue modalities. Furthermore, color-vision defects caused by disease processes in the macular region do not seem to fit quite exactly into the narrow confines of Köllner's rule. This should not make us wonder unduly. The macular region of the retina has its anatomical special features and, as far as its nosology is concerned, it behaves differently from both the rest of the retina and the optic nerve. Most macular disease processes cause disturbance of yellow-and-blue vision, like disease processes of the rest of the retina, but at least one type of macular degeneration affects the two other opponent modalities.

In either case, color-vision defects associated with macular pathology feature some added clinical characteristics. (It is here where that first retinal fundamental shows itself primarily involved.) But the dichotomy always remains. Indeed, the structural *Aufbau* and *Abbau* of human color vision in terms of two sets of indivisible but opposing modalities is such a fundamental characteristic of our sensory physiology that even in pathology it allows for no exception.

Much new knowledge has accumulated since Köllner's time and at present, due primarily to the work of Jaeger & Grützner (9) and François & Verriest (3), it is known that neither the red-and-green defects nor the yellow-and-blue defects are entirely unitary in nature. The acquired red-and-green defects, and to a degree also the acquired yellow-and-blue defects, manifest themselves in two subgroups, just as the hereditary defects do. The relationship established by Köllner is still valid, but only with certain provisos. At least the first half of Köllner's rule should probably be restated as follows: If it is a red-and-green defect, then it is one particular type of red-and-green defect which is a clinical characteristic of diseases of the optic nerve.

According to the latest classification attempts by Verriest (18) and Jaeger & Grützner (9), the following main groups should be differentiated:

a. Acquired dyschromatopsia of the red-and-green axis with the normal spectral luminosity function retained (Type II of acquired red-and-green dyschromatopsia in the Verriest classification).

b. Acquired dyschromatopsia of the red-and-green axis with foreshortening of the effective spectrum of luminosity on its long-wave end (Verriest calls it Type I of acquired red-and-green dyschromatopsia).

c. Acquired dyschromatopsia involving the yellow-and-blue axis (according to Jaeger & Grützner, they should be further subdivided into two groups: one with normal luminosity functions, the other with the luminosity curve foreshortened at its long-wave end).

The characteristics of group *a* inevitably recall the class of hereditary defects labeled as "deutans". The similarities are indeed considerable. The rather normal distribution of the luminosity curve is common to both conditions. Their anomaloscope settings are also similar: by matching a yellow with a mixture of red and green both produce a mixture which the normal judges as greenish.

However, the reasons for the choice of similar proportions of red and green in the Rayleigh match are, to a degree at least, different in the two instances. As Rubin (15) pointed out, the deuteranomalous does not so much need *more* green, though this is the statement generally made, but rather *less* red because anomaloscope yellow contains, for him, only little red.* In contradistinction, the person with an acquired red-and-green defect of Verriest's Type II *does* need more green for an equation. For him the yellowish green area of the spectrum, already poorly saturated for the normal, is even further desaturated.†

I believe this to be a very important detail, deserving further discussion. It appears from the analysis of Jaeger & Grützner (9) that what most conspicuously differentiates the real deutan from these simulated deutans is the disposition of the most desaturated spectrum area. In ordinary hereditary red-and-green defects, in both deutans and protans, this area is to be found in the bluish green of the normal (1,20), at wavelengths less than 500 mμ, far from any of the three wavelengths (671 mμ for "red", 546 mμ for "green", and 589 mμ for "yellow") involved in the Rayleigh match. On the contrary, in the acquired red and green defects under discussion, the desaturation almost regularly involves the region of 546 mμ, the locus of anomaloscope green. It is quite likely that it is this desaturation which prompts those with this type of acquired defect to use more green in their attempts at a Rayleigh match.

The peculiarities of the maximally desaturated spectrum region in the two conditions offer still further evidence that, despite certain similarities, hereditary and acquired color-vision defects represent essentially different clinical entities. In hereditary red-and-green defects, in both deutans and protans, the maximally desaturated area always remains limited; in either variety it covers no more than a few spectrum wavelengths. This is true even in the case of complete red-and-green blindness, where maximum desaturation gives way to complete desaturation, to what is called a neutral area in the spectrum. One can, in fact, differentiate deuteranopia from protanopia by the very circumstance that the neutral point in

* According to Rubin's studies, the pure yellow of the color-normal is at 577 mμ, that of the deuteranomal at 583 mμ. Anomaloscope "yellow" is at 589 mμ—rather far toward orange for the normal, very close to pure yellow for the deuteranomal. Thus, the deuteranomal requires relatively less red to match it with a red and a green. Jaeger, Grützner & Oser (10) have also emphasized that the setting of the Rayleigh match by the deuteranomal is not caused by the isolated weakness of some green primary mechanism.

† Anomaloscope "green" is in reality a rather yellowish green and lies in this area of the spectrum, at 546 mμ. Hence the need for more of this ingredient in the making of a Rayleigh match.

the former is near 497 mμ, in the latter near 493 mμ, and that the two points never overlap. (Both the AO/H-R-R and the Farnsworth Panel D-15 tests are based on the fact that the axis of maximum desaturation in deutans and protans is acutely defined.*) The outline of the most desaturated spectrum area is sharp and definite because the yellow mechanism which covers the spectrum area *above* the maximally desaturated point and the blue mechanism which covers it *below* this point are and remain completely normal even in total red-and-green blindness. They both end quite sharply and abruptly at this point, leaving but the narrowest neutral "gap" between themselves.†

In dyschromatopsia caused by optic nerve pathology, the neutral area is never as well outlined, and selective involvement of the red and the green mechanism is only an initial feature. The very paleness of increasingly wider areas in the yellowish green suggests that the other color mechanisms do not long remain intact. One cannot, therefore, expect such clear-cut answers with either the AO/H-R-R or the Farnsworth tests as one usually obtains in the hereditary defects. (Sometimes there is no "axis" at all to the acquired dyschromatopsia, as *all* four color mechanisms appear more or less equally affected.)

Still, as long as the color-vision defect remains in a trichromatic or, at its worst, in a dichromatic stage, the Rayleigh equation retains a deutan character. The color-vision defect remains, at least predominantly, a red-and-green defect. Only quite late will the color defect turn into a more or less complete achromatopsia (indicating a manifest damage to the yellow-and-blue mechanism as well), while the luminosity function retains its normal photopic features. The defect in this stage is practically identical with that known as atypical total color blindness or "cone" monochromatism.

Since this form of acquired color deficiency occurs almost exclusively in diseases of the optic nerve, it is obvious—and Verriest (18) has especially emphasized this —that irregular light absorption by the refracting media of the eye or the retina proper cannot play any role in its causation. The disease process primarily damages the "color" transmitters in the optic nerve itself. Zanen (21) made the interesting observation that in afflictions of the optic nerve the so-called photochromatic interval becomes wider—an observation that further proves the differential effect of the disease process: it seems that only certain fibers (the ones transmitting a chromaticity message) are selectively damaged; other fibers (those that carry the message of luminosity) are not affected, or certainly not to a comparable degree. The separate nature of the luminosity function is, of course, one of the characteristic features of the Hering color-vision theory (8) and of Ladd-Franklin's phylogenetic hypothesis (13). The selective survival of the luminosity mechanism in diseases of the optic nerve speaks well for the separate existence of a photopic dominator.

This type of selective affection of the red-and-green sense is encountered in a number of disease conditions, for example in the retrobulbar neuritis of multiple

* For further details the reader is referred to the author's book, *An Essay on Color Vision and Clinical Color-Vision Tests* (14).

† Normally, this "gap" is filled by green. Trichromates have no neutral area in their spectrum.

sclerosis, the optic nerve atrophy in tertiary syphilis, the optic nerve involvement caused by tobacco, alcohol, and certain poisons. Of especial interest is hereditary optic nerve atrophy, usually known as Leber's disease.

The second group of acquired deficiencies in red-and-green color vision (the group called Type I in Verriest's classification) has foreshortening of the spectrum luminosity curve at its long-wave end as an added characteristic. Inevitably, this will suggest the hereditary "protan" defect, where the spectrum is also foreshortened at its long-wave end. Nor is this the only characteristic of this dyschromatopsia which parallels the protan condition: the relative maximum of the luminosity curve is displaced toward shorter wavelengths, as in protanopia. Moreover, at least in the earlier trichromatic stage of their color derangement, patients will require too much red to set up a Rayleigh equation, which is again reminiscent of protanomaly.

This picture might change considerably as the disease process progresses. The luminosity maximum usually becomes still further displaced toward shorter wavelengths and in the end might coincide with the scotopic-type luminosity curve of the typical total color blind. Also, as the disease progresses, the earlier trichromatic stage of the defect might turn into dichromacy, and the anomaloscope setting can be identical with that of the protanope. Finally, color vision can be totally lost. This acquired achromatopsia is more akin to the typical variety of total color blindness, not only in the form of the spectrum luminosity curve just discussed, but also in a very peculiar kind of anomaloscope match which both of them produce, and which is very different from that of either protanomaly or protanopia.

Mainly through the work of Grützner (5), it is known that this type of acquired red and green color vision defect does not seem to fit into Köllner's classification. It is primarily a red-and-green defect but not one patently associated with any optic nerve affection; even in this respect it is a type *sui generis*. It is a characteristic of certain hereditary degenerations of the macula proper; more precisely, of the juvenile type which in the German literature is often referred to as Stargardt's disease. Verriest (18) emphasizes that in these cases the affection of the color sense precedes any other manifestation of the degenerative process, and that it can be discovered while the visual acuity is still normal. Later on, the severity of the color-vision defect parallels the gradual loss of visual acuity. By the time visual acuity has dropped to 20/200 the color-vision defect becomes dichromatic in nature, and when the color-vision defect reaches the monochromatic stage visual acuity is generally less than 20/400. Besides, the disturbance of color vision manifests itself not only quite early, but also rather diffusely. One cannot actually say that in these cases the red-and-green sense is the only one affected. In this respect the defect stands quite apart from genuine protanomaly or protanopia. *All* retinal functions—all, including the photopic luminosity mechanism, the photopic dominator—suffer from some derangement, even if red-and-green vision is more prominently affected in the early stage of the disease. The eventual total loss of color vision and the final displacement of the luminosity curve into the scotopic range are only the consummation of a process which involves all photopic visual functions from the very beginning.

Stargardt's juvenile macular degeneration is indeed a unique clinical entity, especially with regard to the color-vision defect, which actually indicates that the ophthalmoscopically visible features of a retinal disease are only of a secondary nature. The defect could be secondary to either a degenerative process in the conducting retinal elements (in which case Köllner's rule would once more be upheld) or it could be secondary to an affection of the first of the three retinal pigments—the one sensitive to the longest wavelengths (in which case the protan character of the defect could be more easily explained). Other forms of macular degeneration do not share this characteristic. In senile macular degeneration, for instance, especially in the rather common Kuhnt-Junius type, the color-vision defect falls into the yellow-and-blue range, as in retinal diseases proper. This was described by Sloan as early as 1942 (16). In fact, the primary defect of color vision is in the yellow-and-blue in almost all other types of macular degeneration. Sometimes color vision is rather intact.

In macular degenerations the testing of color vision actually offers the most welcome means of differential diagnosis, and other juvenile macular degenerations can best be differentiated from Stargardt's disease by the very nature of their color-vision defect. They represent a different disease, probably with a different pathological, anatomical basis. More accurate scrutiny has in fact revealed that even their ophthalmoscopic appearance differs: they show disturbances in pigment distribution which do not occur in the real Stargardt's disease. Some macular degenerations with a yellow-and-blue defect are a quasi-macular subtype of those retino-choroideal or tapeto-retinal degenerations for which derangement of yellow-and-blue vision is, in fact, a clinical characteristic.

Color-vision studies have also helped in the differential diagnosis of the so-called hereditary optic nerve atrophies. It is now established that these are not a unitary disease condition. What might continue to be called Leber's disease is generally a sex-linked, recessive affliction manifesting itself in young male adults. This is the disease in which the disturbance of color vision is mainly, at least initially, along the red-and-green color axis. Another type of hereditary optic atrophy is transmitted as a dominant trend, becomes manifest at a much earlier age, and the color-vision defect associated with it is in the yellow-and-blue regions of the circle of colors. The type of color-vision defect itself suggests that what appears as a variant with a different transmission mechanism is, in reality, a different nosologic entity, most likely with different underlying pathology. Grützner (7) actually considers it primarily a retinal degeneration, with optic atrophy merely a secondary feature; thus, the exception from Köllner's rule would again be only an apparent one. The dominant variety has, in my experience a much better functional prognosis. Identifying it by any means is certainly a worthwhile endeavor.

In general, defects of the yellow-and-blue mechanism accompany affections of the retina proper, most of them peripheral, some mainly involving the macular area. In the latter eventualities there are usually some added disturbances to be expected. In cases where tapeto-retinal degeneration is primarily located in the macular region—a type of tapeto-retinal degeneration first described by Grützner

(6)—disturbances of the yellow-and-blue mechanism are combined with a displacement of the luminosity curve almost toward scotopic values. In the case of central serous retinopathy—a condition already mentioned—the anomaloscope reveals a kind of pseudo-protanomaly, most likely due to pre-receptorial absorption of the longest visible wavelengths by intraretinal exudate.

In case of peripheral retinal involvement, especially of the deeper retinal layers, the retinal rods will also necessarily be affected. In pigmentary or tapeto-retinal degenerations, hemeralopia is certainly one of the most distressing symptoms.

Verriest, in his outstanding monograph on acquired color-vision defects (18), discusses at length a number of conditions in which the yellow-and-blue mechanism is affected, some of which have already been briefly mentioned. The following are the more important or most interesting ones: pigment degeneration of the retina, choroideremia, senile macular degeneration, malignant myopia, central serous retinopathy, retinal detachment, hypertensive and diabetic retinopathy, vascular occlusion, papilledema, glaucoma. Since many of these are conditions encountered in daily practice, many cases of affected color vision are probably being missed. Admittedly, the study of color vision will hardly add to differential diagnosis or influence the management of most of these diseases, and only some special interest will prompt a clinician to investigate color vision in most of these conditions. There are, of course, cases where the study of color vision can be of significance: it might help in the differential diagnosis of papilledema and papillitis and serve to admonish that not all is well in cases of diabetes, glaucoma or hypertension. Since it comes early in the course of a disease, it is an aid in counseling families with hereditary eye defects such as pigment retinopathy or macular degeneration. It may help to prove that a person who allegedly suffered a head injury is not malingering for compensation benefits. And in a case undergoing prolonged chloroquine or isoniazid therapy, a warning voice can be rasied before other signs and symptoms of toxicity become manifest. Such examples seem to warrant the occasional use of an Ishihara chart or the smaller Farnsworth test despite the many demands on an ophthalmologist's office time.

REFERENCES

1. Chapanis, A., Spectral saturation and its relation to color-vision defects. *J. Exp. Psychol.*, 1944, **34**: 24–44.
2. Cox, J., Unilateral color deficiency, congenital and acquired. *J. Opt. Soc. Amer.*, 1961, **51**: 992–999.
3. François, J., and Verriest, G., Les dyschromatopsies acquises. *Ann. Oculist.* (Paris), 1957, **190**: 713–746; 812–859; 903–943.
4. Graham, C. H., Sperling, H. G., Hsiz, Y., and Coulson, A., The determination of some visual functions of a unilaterally color-blind subject: methods and results. *J. Psychol.* (London), 1961, **51**: 3–32.
5. Grützner, P., Typische erworbene Farbensinnstörungen bei heredodegenerativen Maculaleiden. *Graefe Arch. klin. exp. Ophthal.*, 1961, **163**: 99–116.
6. ———, Maculäre Form der diffusen tapeto-retinalen Degeneration. *Graefe Arch. klin. exp. Ophthal.*, 1962, **165**: 227–245.

7. Grützner, P., Über Diagnose und Funktionsstörungen bei der infantilen, dominant vererbten Opticus-Atrophie. *Ber. Deutsch. Ophth. Ges. Heidelberg*, 1963, **65**: 268–273.
8. Hering, E., *Outlines of a Theory of the Light Sense* (L. M. Hurvich and D. Jameson, Transl.). Harvard Univ. Press, Cambridge, 1964
9. Jaeger, W., and Grützner, P., Erworbene Farbensinnstörungen. In: *Entwicklung und Fortschritt in der Augenheilkunde* (H. Sautter, Ed.). Enke, Stuttgart, 1963: 591–614.
10. Jaeger, W., Grützner, P., and Oser, W., Wie erklärt sich der Unterschied der Einstellungen von Protanomalen und Deuteranomalen am Anomaloskop? *Graefe Arch. klin. exp. Ophthal.*, 1961, **164**: 63–71.
11. Judd, D. B., Color perceptions of deuteranopic and protanopic observers. *J. Res. Nat. Bur. Stand.*, 1948, **41**: 247–271.
12. Köllner, H., *Die Störungen des Farbensinnes, ihre klinische Bedeutung und ihre Diagnose.* Karger, Berlin, 1912.
13. Ladd-Franklin, C., Evolutional theory of color sensation. In: *The American Encyclopedia and Dictionary of Ophthalmology*, Vol. VI (C. A. Wood, Ed.). Cleveland Press, Chicago, 1915: 4559–4562.
14. Linksz, A., *An Essay on Color Vision and Clinical Color-Vision Tests.* Grune & Stratton, New York, 1964.
15. Rubin, M. L., Spectral hue loci of normal and anomalous trichromates. *Am. J. Ophthal.*, 1961, **52**: 166–172.
16. Sloan, L. L., The use of pseudo-isochromatic charts in detecting central scotomas due to lesions in the conducting pathways. *Am. J. Ophthal.*, 1942, **25**: 1352–1356.
17. Trevor-Roper, P. D., The influence of eye disease on pictorial art. *Proc. Roy. Soc. Med.*, 1959, **52**: 721–744.
18. Verriest, G., Les déficiences acquises de la discrimination chromatique. *Mém. Acad. Roy. Med. Belg.*, 1964, **4**: 35–327.
19. Wald, G., Human vision and the spectrum. *Science*, 1945, **101**: 653–658.
20. Walls, G. L., and Heath, G. G., Neutral points in 138 protanopes and deuteranopes. *J. Opt. Soc. Amer.*, 1956, **46**: 640–649.
21. Zanen, J., L'intervalle photochromatique en pathologie oculaire. *Bull. Soc. Franç. Ophtal.*, 1959, **72**: 498–527.

NAME INDEX

SUBJECT INDEX

D

E

M

N

Q

R

T